Delmar's
English
Pocket

for Health
Professionals

Rochelle K. Kelz, Ph.D.
Dean of Liberal Arts and Sciences
Mott Community College

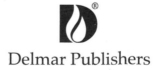

Delmar Publishers

an International Thomson Publishing company I(T)P®

Albany • Bonn • Boston • Cincinnati • Detroit • London • Madrid
Melbourne • Mexico City • New York • Pacific Grove • Paris • San Francisco

Cover Design: Charles Cummings Advertising/Art, Inc.

Delmar Staff

Acquisitions Editor: Marion Waldman
Developmental Editor: Jill Rembetski
Project Editor: Coreen Filson
Production Coordinator: Cathleen Berry

Art and Design Coordinator: Richard Killar
Editorial Assistant: Sarah Holle
Marketing Manager: Dawn Gerrain

For more information, contact Delmar, 3 Columbia Circle, PO Box 15015, Albany, NY 12212-0515 or find us on the World Wide Web at http://www.delmar.com

International Division List

Japan:
Thomson Learning
Palaceside Building 5F
1-1-1 Hitotsubashi, Chiyoda-ku
Tokyo 100 0003 Japan
Tel: 813 5218 6544
Fax: 813 5218 6551

Australia/New Zealand
Nelson/Thomson Learning
102 Dodds Street
South Melbourne, Victoria 3205
Australia
Tel: 61 39 685 4111
Fax: 61 39 685 4199

UK/Europe/Middle East:
Thomson Learning
Berkshire House
168-173 High Holborn
London
WC1V 7AA United Kingdom
Tel: 44 171 497 1422
Fax: 44 171 497 1426

Latin America:
Thomson Learning
Seneca, 53
Colonia Polanco
11560 Mexico D.F. Mexico
Tel: 525-281-2906
Fax: 525-281-2656

Canada:
Nelson/Thomson Learning
1120 Birchmount Road
Scarborough, Ontario
Canada M1K 5G4
Tel: 416-752-9100
Fax: 416-752-8102

Asia:
Thomson Learning
60 Albert Street, #15-0
Albert Complex
Singapore 189969
Tel: 65 336 6411
Fax: 65 336 7411

Library of Congress Cataloging-in-Publication Data
Kelz, Rochelle K.
    English/Spanish pocket dictionary for health professionals /
Rochelle K. Kelz.
        p. cm.
    ISBN 0-8273-6171-8 (alk. paper)
    1. Medicine—Dictionaries—Spanish. 2. Spanish language—Dictionaries—English.
3. Medicine—Dictionaries—English. 4. English language—Dictionaries—Spanish. I. Title.
R121.K323 1996
610'.3—dc20   96-17894
                                                  CIP

To the sources of my strengths and inspiration
—past, present, and future
Florence & Samuel, Arnold, Max & Melissa

A las fuentes de mis fuerzas e inspiraciones
Florence y Samuel, Arnold, Max y Melissa

Acknowledgments

From the start of this endeavor I have had the advantage of being able to draw on the wealth of knowledge of countless health care professionals, patients, and students of mine from so many different Spanish-speaking countries. I am indebted for their contributions of information and answers to my many queries. I am grateful to María Paz Díaz de Martínez for her counsel and patient reading of parts of this manuscript.

I wish to thank all of the reviewers, for their input and constructive suggestion:

Adie DeLaGuardia
Coordinator, Medical
Assisting
Center for Health Science
Education
Broward Community College
Davie, Florida

Ines Bello Paris, MS, RN
President, Health Systems
Consultants, Inc.
Bronx, New York

Alcira B. Park, RN
El Paso Community College
El Paso, Texas

Josie Reese, LPN, PNT
HHA Instructor/Supervisor
Visiting Nurse Association
Denver, Colorado

Carol Lee Sendell
Medical Spanish Instructor
Apson Adult Education
Aptos, California

Elda N. Vasquez, C.M.A., B.S.
Medical Assisting Adjunct
Instructor and Lab Technician
San Antonio College
San Antonio, Texas

Special thanks to Jill Rembetski and Cori Rogers, my editors, whose perceptions I value, and whose commentary and suggestions helped. Sincere appreciation to the production and art departments of Delmar Publishers, whose care and expert workmanship turn out beautiful and well-made books.

If I have failed to mention anyone who should have been listed, it is an unintended oversight. To all, my thanks.

And, finally, to Arnold Abrams, for support, encouragement, assistance, and doing the dishes, special and profound thanks!

Preface

After many years of teaching and translating, the author realized that communication between health care workers and their patients, especially when one group speaks English and the other Spanish, can still be improved. Consequently, out of this need she created a comprehensive English–Spanish/Spanish–English medical–dental dictionary, which will help facilitate such communication. This dictionary is the result of countless hours and many years of patient and delicate work. The author knows, nevertheless, that, in spite of her care, omissions, errata, and errors are absolutely inevitable. Therefore, she would like users to send her any comments, suggestions, or observations to improve the dictionary. These will be utilized to improve future editions.

Let us concede that a dictionary is nothing more than a catalog of words placed alphabetically in which the meaning or specific grammatical or idiomatic aspect is given. This particular medical–dental dictionary, therefore, is one that offers a compilation of equivalents in English and in Spanish of terms used in the health care field. Each symptom, sign, syndrome, disease and illness, and procedure, etc., is expressed with a term that makes possible knowledge and communication between physicians, dentists, health care workers, their patients, and others. To these words are added the technical terms, the regional expressions, the paramedical vocabulary, the vocabulary of the related and helping sciences, and the most frequent synonyms.

Although in spoken language we can express ourselves freely with quite a bit of latitude, for health care purposes we have to use the word or words that most closely fit the very specific meaning or thought. Even for native speakers of Spanish (or of English) one word or expression may mean one thing to the speaker and quite something else to the listener. Also, because of the delicacy of the problems, the goal always remains the same—to be able to communicate. Therefore, it is necessary to ask questions, to think, to allow one's memory or inspiration to bring to mind the sought-after word. If possible, it is much easier to consult a medical–dental dictionary. The dictionary's purpose is to inform, document, teach, and, without lengthy explanations or rhetoric, provide knowledge to someone who requires it. Nevertheless, it would not be possible to include the totality of all definitions nor is there any intention to present an encyclopedia of scientific knowledge.

The main purpose is to gather expressions and words with a pragmatic criteria. The important thing is not to omit anything that may be fundamental for medical interpretation. And this is the premise that guided this author: introduce words of general acceptance in the health care field. Definitions are only given when there is no equivalent or occasionally for a term that is somewhat unfamiliar. It is not surprising that exact equivalents are sometimes hard to find. Many words used in the health care field have other meanings. It is always a judgment call as to how to handle them. Some words that are generally useful have been included. Those that are unrelated to health care in general have usually been omitted. In listing phrases, the author has tried to avoid "padding" the book with obvious combinations of verb and noun or adjective and noun.

This dictionary contains tens of thousands of words and phrases that are used by Spanish-speaking people throughout the world as well as an equal number used by English-speaking health care workers. Today medical/dental terminology reflects both the new technology and the new "folk medicine" of the media, especially television and radio. The dictionary contains technical terminology, common everyday terminology, colloquialisms, slang, vulgarisms, and newly coined words.

Spanish slang is an extremely complicated subject and not one which can possibly be addressed in a work such as this. Every country and every region where Spanish is spoken has different slang. Many terms that are used colloquially in one region of a country are never heard in another region of the same country. The slang that this work includes is clearly a partial listing. It represents "standard" slang that can be heard on the streets, on TV and radio shows, records, etc., or that is widely read in newspapers and (comic) books. There is one type of slang that should specifically be noted: caló. It derives from the language of the Spanish gypsies and generally now refers to the underground language from the poor barrios. It can be likened to the British Cockney slang and is always changing.

Spanish is spoken in the southwestern part of the United States (in Arizona, California, Colorado, New Mexico, and Texas) by millions of Mexican–Americans or *Chicanos*. It is also spoken by Mexicans who live on the U.S. side of the border. When the language of either the Mexicans or the Mexican–Americans is influenced by English, the language is often referred to as "Spanglish" or *fronterazos* or *el español chicano*. "Spanglish" is considered to be a degenerative form of Spanish by the Royal Spanish Academy. One example might be a Spanish word like *colegio* which technically means "secondary school" but which starts being used to mean "college" because of imitation of American usage. English words are also "Spanglishized," as in *tonsils* or *huacha* meaning "watch." Such language has little value for travelers but is highly useful for health care personnel who must interact with these individuals.

After a great deal of discussion and deliberation the author decided to include many words that are considered vulgar and even obscene because these words are commonly heard. Health care workers should be aware that they should not use such language at work in either language. However, the inclusion of this vocabulary is meant to help since it is useful to know what is meant by words that one hears—and to know what words to avoid repeating. One must also remember that words, especially slang, change meanings in different countries. What may be perceived as a serious insult in one country may be common and relatively tame in another, and possibly even a compliment in still another country.

The rapidly increasing Spanish-speaking population has always challenged health care workers attempting to serve them. In the United States, immigration and increased life expectancy, along with the high birth rate and low infant mortality of the Spanish-speaking population, add to the number of Spanish speakers now living in the United States. Spanish speakers from all parts of the Hispanic world currently live in the United States, although the majority seem to come from Mexico, Puerto Rico, Cuba, Central America, and the Dominican Republic. Consequently, vocabulary and idioms have been selected which are best understood by people of these areas. However, this dictionary contains many regional or local variations within Spanish. Terms unique to a specific country or area are so labeled. Regional dialect differences have always affected health care communication. If there are health care terms that have regional meanings other than those given, the author feels their omissions are not serious.

The work also contains scientific words which, because of the same classical Greek or Latin origin, are cognates in both Spanish and English. However, because lay people frequently are unfamiliar with the scientific terminology, whether in Spanish or in English, their translation does not always assist communication. Health care workers and lay people, especially Spanish speaking lay people, do not always use the same basic premises of scientific medicine. Therefore, simple translations are not enough because ideas are not shared. Consequently, lay terms serve a more useful purpose than the scientific ones.

Communication problems also occur between health care worker and patient when there are different ideas about pathology and physiology of illness and well-being. Many Spanish speakers, therefore, are unable to communicate about the folk diseases from which they suffer. Also affected are the herbal treatments for these diseases and the administering curers (*curanderos*). These are "ethnological" problems of communication. This dictionary attempts to provide information to the health professional that will aid in this, and all other problems of communication.

That is why I feel so honored to present the most complete and compact dictionary of its type. Undoubtedly, a more extensive dictionary would be more complete. Nevertheless, considering its inconvenience, difficulty of management, and even complexity, a more extensive work would be too cumbersome to be readily useable. Readers will understand the inescapable need to accommodate a manageable format, in spite of the difficulty in finding the exact meaning. In order to achieve this I have selected words from everyday language which, in this way, imperceptively further one's interest so that it might be easily used, extremely practical for all who use it. My intention is to make this task easier.

This type of dictionary is irreplaceable as an aid to the physician, dentist, social worker, pharmacist, patient, and translator/interpreter. I hope that the good use and application of the present dictionary will produce abundant fruits of enrichment and that it may facilitate the desire to serve as much as possible all those who may use it. May it serve as a valuable reference work for everyday activity!

General Remarks

Spanish is pronounced the way it is written. Spanish letters are treated as feminine nouns, and each has one sound except for *C*, *D*, *E*, *G*, *N*, *O*, *S*, *X*, and *Y*, which have at least two sounds. The letters *K* and *W* appear only in foreign words. Excluding prefixes and suffixes, *C*, *R*, and *L* are the only three consonants that may be doubled in Spanish.

The Spanish alphabet is divided into vowels (**vocales**) and consonants (**consonantes**). The vowels *A*, *E*, *I*, *O*, and *U* are the same as in English. *Y* is a vowel when it is the last letter in a word and a consonant when it begins a word or a syllable. Thus, *Y* serves two functions. An example of *Y*'s use as a vowel is **hoy** (today); as a consonant, **inyección** (injection).

All vowels in Spanish are short, pure sounds. *A*, *I*, and *U* each have one sound, although there will be slight variations according to placement within the phrase or word.

The Spanish Alphabet

The Spanish alphabet has thirty letters. They are:

Letter	Name
A	a
B	be
C	ce
(CH)*	che/ce hache
D	de
E	e
F	efe
G	ge
H	hache
I	i
J	jota
K	ka
L	ele
(LL)*	elle/doble ele
M	eme
N	ene
Ñ	eñe
O	o
P	pe
Q	cu
R	ere
RR	erre
S	ese
T	te
U	u
V	ve/uve
W	doble ve
	doble u
	ve doble
X	equis
Y	i griega
Z	zeta

•Prior to 1994, the Spanish alphabet had thirty letters. With the exception of the **rr**, which never occurs at the beginning of a word, each letter was a separate entity in the Spanish alphabet and was listed in their proper order in a dictionary. In 1994, however, the Royal Academy of the Spanish Language eliminated two letters from the alphabet, the **ch** and the **ll**, in order to bring the Spanish alphabetical order more in line with those used in other languages. (The **k** and **w** are usually used with words of foreign origin.) This change allowed Spanish speakers to better adapt to the computer age. Consequently, dictionaries written and published after 1994 may not include the **ch** and **ll** as separate entries found after all **c** and **l** entries respectively.

Because the Royal Academy of the Spanish Language made these alphabetical order changes so recently, it is common to hear or use both **che** or ce hache and **elle** or **doble ele**. Native speakers use and understand all.

About the Author

Rochelle (Shelle) K. Kelz, PhD., is Dean of Liberal Arts & Sciences at C.S. Mott Community College in Flint, Michigan. Prior to that she was Director of Extension Programs and Evening College for North Park College & Theological Seminary, and later Director of Extension Programs at Roosevelt University, both in Chicago, Illinois. She held the academic title of Professor of Spanish, English as a Second Language, and French at North Park and was Professor of Languages and Education at Roosevelt. In addition, she served as Visiting Assistant Professor of Medical Spanish at the University of Illinois at Chicago Campus as well as at the University of Illinois at Chicago Medical Center for over eight years. In 1987 she was selected "Outstanding University Professor of Spanish in the United States" by the American Association of Teachers of Spanish and Portuguese.

She is also a sought-after medical–legal translator of Spanish and English, serving most of the medical and dental professional organizations. She also serves as a consultant to establish Medical Spanish Programs in hospitals, professional training institutions, and colleges and universities. She has published *Conversational Spanish for Medical Personnel*. Using her talents as a language educator and translator as well as her tremendous resources, she has compiled this very useful Spanish–English/English–Spanish health care dictionary.

List of Abbreviations Used in this Dictionary

Lista de Abreviaturas Empleadas en este Diccionario

The gender of Spanish nouns is indicated only when they do not end in the masculine -o or the feminine -a. Adjectives ending in -o and -a are only given in the masculine form.

El género de los sustantivos españoles se indica solamente cuando no terminan o en la forma masculina de -o o en la forma femenina de -a. Los adjetivos que terminan o en -o o en -a se dan solamente en la forma masculina.

adjective	*adj*	adjetivo
adverb	*adv*	adverbio
anatomy, anatomical	*Anat*	anatomía, anatómico
auxiliary	*aux*	auxiliar
biology	*Biol*	biología
cardiology	*Card*	cardiología
chemistry	*Chem*	química
dentistry/odontology	*Dent*	odontología
electricity	*Elect*	electricidad
ethnic	*ethn*	étnico
euphemism	*euph*	eufemismo
familiar, colloquial [given because term may be used by patient; not suitable for health worker to use]	*fam*	familiar, coloquial
feminine noun	*f*	sustantivo femenino
formal	*form*	formal
interjection	*inter*	interjección
invariable	*inv*	invariable
juvenile	*juv*	juvenil
masculine noun	*m*	sustantivo masculino
masculine or feminine noun according to the individual's sex or masculine and feminine noun	*m/f*	sustantivo masculino o femenino según el sexo sustantivo masculino y femenino
medicine	*Med*	medicina

noun	*n*	nombre/sustantivo
obstetrics	*Obst*	obstetricia
oneself	*o.s.*	a sí mismo
orthopedics	*Ortho*	ortopedia
past participle	*pp*	participio pasado
pediatrics	*Ped*	pediatría
pharmacy, pharmaceutical	*Pharm*	farmacia, farmacéutico
phrase	*phr*	locución
plural	*pl*	plural
preposition	*prep*	preposición
pronoun	*pron*	pronombre
psychology	*Psyc*	psicología
singular	*sg*	singular
slang	*slang*	argot
someone	*s.o.*	alguien
something	*sth.*	algo
surgical	*Surg*	cirugía
used more as feminine	*Ú.m.c.f.*	úsase más como femenino
used more as masculine	*Ú.m.c.m.*	úsase más como masculino
used more in plural	*Ú.m.e.p.*	úsase más en plural
variation	*var*	variación
veterinary science	*Vet*	veterinaria
vulgar	*vulg*	vulgar, grosero

Unless specified, words ending with **-a** are feminine, words ending with **-o** are masculine.

Since Spanish is normally a phonetic language and is pronounced as it is written, this dictionary does not provide phonetic pronunciation for its nearly 20,000 entries.

A causa del hecho de que normalmente el español es una lengua fonética y se pronuncia como se escribe, no se ofrecen en este diccionario las pronunciaciones fonéticas de los casi 20,000 artículos.

Special words used to indicate regional occurrences

Palabras especiales usadas para indicación regional

Argentina	*Arg*	la Argentina
Bolivia	*Bol*	Bolivia
Central America [Guatemala, El Salvador, Honduras Costa Rica, Nicaragua]	*CA*	Centroamérica [Guatemala, El Salvador, Honduras, Costa Rica, Nicaragua]
Caribbean [Cuba, Puerto Rico, Dominican Republic]	*Carib*	Caribe [Cuba, Puerto Rico, la República Dominicana]
Chicano [southwestern U.S.]	*Chicano*	Chicano
Chile	*Chi*	Chile
Colombia	*Col*	Colombia
Costa Rica	*CR*	Costa Rica
Cuba	*Cu*	Cuba
Dominican Republic	*DR*	la República Dominicana
Ecuador	*Ec*	el Ecuador
El Salvador	*El Sal*	El Salvador
Guatemala	*Guat*	Guatemala
Honduras	*Hond*	Honduras
Mexico	*Mex*	Méjico
Nicaragua	*Nic*	Nicaragua
Panama	*Pan*	Panamá
Paraguay	*Para*	Paraguay
Peru	*Perú*	el Perú
Puerto Rico	*PR*	Puerto Rico
Río de la Plata Region [Eastern Argentina, Uruguay]	*Ríopl*	Río de la Plata [la Argentina oriental, el Uruguay]
Santo Domingo	*S.D.*	Santo Domingo
Spanish America/South America	*SpAm*	América del Sur/ Sudamérica
Spain	*Spain*	España
United States of America	*EEUU*	Estados Unidos de América
Uruguay	*Ur*	Uruguay
Venezuela	*Ven*	Venezuela

Reconocimiento

Desde el principio de este esfuerzo he jugado con ventaja de poder aprovecharme del gran conocimiento de innumerables profesionales en el cuidado de la salud, de pacientes, y de estudiantes míos de casi todos los países de habla español. Agradezco su ayuda y sus contribuciones de información y respuestas a mis muchas interrogantes. Estoy en deuda con María Paz Díaz de Martínez por su consejo y su lectura cuidadosa de partes del manuscrito.

Quisiera dar mis gracias a todos los críticos, por sus sugerencias valiosas:

Adie DeLaGuardia
Coordinator, Medical Assisting
Center for Health Science
Education
Broward Community College
Davie, Florida

Ines Bello Paris, MS, RN
President, Health Systems
Consultants, Inc.
Bronx, New York

Alcira B. Park, RN
El Paso Community College
El Paso, Texas

Josie Reese, LPN, PNT
HHA Instructor/Supervisor
Visiting Nurse Association
Denver, Colorado

Carol Lee Sendell
Medical Spanish Instructor
Apson Adult Education
Aptos, California

Elda N. Vasquez, C.M.A., B.S.
Medical Assisting Adjunct Instructor and Lab Technician
San Antonio College
San Antonio, Texas

Les estoy agradecida a Jill Rembetski y a Cori Rogers, las redactores de mi obra, cuya sensibilidad estimo mucho, y cuyos comentarios y sugerencias me han ayudado. Aprecio el esmero y artesanía experta de los departamentos de fabricación y arte de Delmar Publishers que producen libros tan bellos y bien hechos.

Si no mencioné a alguien que merecía mención, fue por descuido no intencionado. A todos, mis gracias.

Y finalmente, a Arnold Abrams, por su apoyo, su ánimo, su ayuda, y por lavar los platos durante estos años, ¡unas gracias especiales y profundas!

Prólogo

Después de muchos años de enseñar y trabajar como traductora e intérprete médica–dental la autora no sólo ha podido familiarizarse con toda suerte de comunicación medica–dental, ha tenido numerosas oportunidades para constantes observaciones de las deficiencias incurridas por los profesionales del cuidado de la salud y sus pacientes, especialmente respecto a exactitud y claridad de expresión, factores considerados de evidente importancia tanto en la medicina como en la odontología cuando un grupo habla inglés y el otro español. Dichas observaciones y las dificultades que la autora ha tenido que vencer tanto para interpretar y traducir como para contestar de una manera satisfactoria tan varia conversación así como el "stock" de experiencia práctica que hoy reúne, se hallan entre las razones suyas para responder a esa urgente necesidad, que tanto se hace sentir en las relaciones médicas–dentales cada día más crecientes entre los países de habla española e inglesa para crear este diccionario y que ofrece como seguro "instrumento de trabajo" a las personas de habla española o inglesa que tienen suficiente conocimiento de ambos idiomas para desempeñar el puesto de traductor/comunicante. Este diccionario es resultado de muchísimas horas y muchos años de paciente y delicado trabajo. La autora sabe, sin embargo, que, a pesar de su cuidado, son absolutamente inevitables las omisiones, erratas y errores. Por eso, agradecerá a los lectores toda la información que puedan facilitarla sobre omisiones, erratas y errores. Que sepan que serán tenidas en cuenta para mejorar este diccionario en ediciones futuras.

Digamos que un diccionario no es otra cosa que un catálogo de palabras puestas alfabéticamente en el que se especifica el significado o ciertos aspectos gramaticales o idiomáticos. Este diccionario médico–dental, por lo tanto, es aquel que nos ofrece ordenadamente grupos de palabras de igual significado tanto en inglés como en español. Cada síntoma, signo, síndrome, enfermedad, y acto médico, etc., se expresa con un término que posibilita el conocimiento y la comunicación entre los médicos, dentistas, trabajadores en el cuidado de la salud, sus pacientes, y otros. A ello se suman los tecnicismos, los modismos regionales, los vocablos paramédicos, los de las ciencias afines y auxiliares y los sinónimos más frecuentes.

Aunque en la lengua hablada podamos expresarnos con más libertad o menos precisión, para metas médicas hemos de adoptar la palabra que más se ajusta al significado propio y específico de la idea o del pensamiento. Aun en cuanto a las personas de habla española (o inglesa) una palabra o un modismo puede significar una cosa al hablante y otra para el oyente. También, a causa de la delicadez de los problemas, la meta siempre queda igual—poder comunicar. Por consiguiente, es necesario preguntar, pensar, dejar que el recuerdo o la inspiración nos traiga a la mente la palabra buscada. Mucho más fácil es consultar un diccionario médico–dental. El diccionario informa, documenta, enseña y, sin largas explicaciones ni retórica, aporta el saber a quien lo requiere. Sin embargo, no sería posible incluir la totalidad de las definiciones, ni es intención presentar una enciclopedia del conocimiento científico.

Lo esencial es reunir expresiones y vocablos con un criterio pragmático. Lo importante es no omitir nada que sea fundamental para la interpretación de la medicina. Y ésta es la premisa que guió a la autora de la presente obra: introducir los términos de aceptación generalizada en el cuidado de la salud. Hay definiciones solamente cuando no hay equivalentes o a veces porque un término queda poco corriente. No es sorprendente que a veces es difícil encontrar equivalentes precisos. Muchas palabras que se usan en la medicina y la odontología tienen otros sentidos. Depende de la opinión cómo tratarlas. Se han incluido algunas palabras de uso general. Aquellas palabras que no se relacionan nada al cuidado de la salud por lo común no se incluyen. Al presentar las expresiones y frases, la autora ha hecho un esfuerzo de resistir incluir combinaciones obvias de verbo y sustantivo o de adjetivo y sustantivo.

Este diccionario contiene miles de palabras y expresiones que son usadas por personas de habla española por todo el mundo así como igual número usadas por profesionales del cuidado de la salud de habla inglesa. Hoy día la terminología médica–dental refleja tanto la nueva tecnología como los nuevos "remedios caseros" de los medios de información, especialmente la televisión y la radio. El diccionario contiene terminología técnica, terminología de uso cotidiano, expresiones familiares, argot, vulgarismos, y palabras recientemente creadas.

El argot español es bien complicado y no merece explicación aquí. Es diferente por todas partes del mundo de habla española. Nunca se oyen palabras y expresiones en una región de un país que se usan familiarmente todos los días en otra región del mismo país. Este diccionario presenta solamente una lista parcial del argot. Representa lo que se oye por las calles, en los programas de televisión y radio, en los discos y cintas, etc., o lo que se lee en los periódicos y tebeos e historietas. Existe un tipo de argot especial que merece mención—caló. Proviene del idioma de los gitanos españoles y ahora generalmente se considera una lengua clandestina de los barrios pobres. Se compara un poquito con el lenguaje característico de los barrios bajos de Londres y siempre cambia.

El español es hablado en el sudoeste de los Estados Unidos (en Arizona, California, Colorado, New Mexico, y Texas) por millones de mejicano–americanos o *chicanos*. También es hablado por los mejicanos que viven en la frontera dentro de los Estados Unidos. Cuando hay influencia del inglés, se refiere al idioma muchas veces como "Spanglish" o *fronterazos* o *el español chicano*. La Academia Real Española considera el "Spanglish" como una forma degenerativa de español. Hay muchos ejemplos de esto. Aunque tal lenguaje tiene poco valor para los viajeros, sirve mucho para el personal médico que tienen que comunicar con estos individuos.

Después de pasar mucho tiempo tratando de decidir si debiera incluir muchas palabras vulgares y groseras o no, la autora decidió incluirlas porque se oyen estas palabras con frecuencia. Los profesionales deben darse cuenta de que no deben usarlas ni en español ni en inglés cuando trabajan. Se incluyen porque ayuda saber lo que significan las palabras que se oyen y para saber qué palabras no se debe repetir. También, es importante recordar que ciertas palabras, especialmente el argot, tienen un sentido diferente según el país. Lo que se considera un insulto grave en un país puede ser común y aún soso en otro, y posiblemente un cumplido en todavía otro país.

A causa del aumento rápido de la población de habla española, los profesionales en el cuidado de la salud han tenido que buscar otras maneras de servirla. La inmigración y la esperanza de vida creciente, así como la alta natalidad y la baja mortalidad infantil de la población de habla española añaden al número de personas de habla española que habitan los Estados Unidos. Allí vienen de todas partes del mundo hispano, aunque la mayoría parece venir de Méjico, Puerto Rico, Cuba, la América Central, y la República Dominicana. Por lo tanto, se han escogido el vocabulario y los modismos que mejor se comprenden personas de estas áreas. Sin embargo, este diccionario contiene todos los términos, de uso y aplicación médicos y dentales, por los cuales se designan en Hispanoamérica con diferentes nombres las voces correspondientes castellanas. Se llaman regionalismos del español. Se indica claramente si el vocabulario pertenece específicamente a ciertos países o áreas. Estas diferencias de dialectos regionales siempre han tenido un papel en la comunicación para atención médica–dental. Si existen otros sentidos para las palabras y expresiones del cuidado de la salud, opina la autora que sus omisiones no son graves.

El diccionario también contiene palabras científicas que palabras afines tanto en español como en inglés a causa de la misma raíz griega o latina. Sin embargo, porque la mayoría de personas no conoce ni sabe la terminología científica, ni en español ni en inglés, su traducción directa no siempre resulta en comunicación. Los que trabajan en la medicina en comparación con la gente común, especialmente las personas legas de habla española, no se sirven de la misma premisa básica de la medicina científica. Por eso, traducciones sencillas muchas veces no son suficientes porque las ideas no se comparten. Por lo tanto, mejor usar palabras legas que las científicas.

Problemas de comunicación también ocurren cuando hay diferentes ideas por parte de los médicos y los pacientes en cuanto a la patología y la fisiología de enfermedad y salud. En consecuencia, muchas personas de habla española no pueden discutir las enfermedades caseras de las cuales sufren. Esto también afecta los remedios caseros herbarios y los curanderos. Estos son problemas etnológicos de comunicación. Este diccionario trata de proveer información al profesional de salud que ayudará en este tipo de comunicación así como en otros problemas de comunicación.

Por ello me siento honrada en presentar un diccionario tan completo y tan chiquito en su género. No hay duda de que un diccionario sumamente extenso ha de ser más completo. Sin embargo, si se piensa en su incomodidad, su difícil manejo y hasta en su complejidad, comprenderán los lectores en la ineludible necesidad de acomodarse a un formato manual, pese a la dificultad de acertar en el punto exacto. Para lograrlo he escogido las palabras del lenguaje básico que, de este modo, se acrecentarán insensiblemente, que fuera de fácil manejo, sumamente práctico para cuantos se usan. Hacer más fácil esta tarea es mi propósito.

Este tipo de diccionario es insustituible como auxiliar del médico, del dentista, del trabajador social, del farmacéutico, del paciente, y del traductor/intérprete. Espero que el buen uso y el empleo del presente diccionario produzca abundantes frutos de enriquecimiento y facilite el deseo de servir lo mejor posible cuantos lo manejen. ¡Que sirva de obra de consulta y de referencia valiosa para la actividad diaria!

Observaciones Generales

A diferencia del español, con mucha frecuencia el inglés no se pronuncia como se escribe. En efecto, algunas de las veintiséis letras inglesas representan más de un sonido. Además, la pronunciación varía mucho según las regiones y los países de habla inglesa.

El alfabeto inglés se divide en vocales (**vowels**) y consonantes (**consonants**). Las vocales son como en español: **A**, **E**, **I**, **O**, **U** y a veces **Y**. En los Estados Unidos existe la nasalización de las vocales antes y después de las consonantes nasales.

Puesto que este diccionario es un trabajo norteamericano, conviene advertir que existen muchas diferencias entre el inglés hablado en los Estados Unidos de América, el Canadá, Australia y Nueva Zelanda, Sudáfrica, etc., y el de Inglaterra y el de las regiones del Reino Unido. Conviene advertir que aun dentro del inglés norteamericano hay notables diferencias regionales. Hay el inglés de Nueva Inglaterra, el del Sur, el del Mediooeste, el de California, etc.

Acentuación

Las palabras que tienen dos sílabas o más después del acento principal llevan un acento secundario en el inglés de los Estados Unidos. A diferencia del español, no existen reglas sencillas y claras para dividir una palabra en sílabas.

El Alfabeto Inglés

El alfabeto inglés tiene veintiséis letras. Son:

Letra	Nombre
a	ei
b	bi
c	si
d	di
e	i
f	ef
g	dzi
h	eich
i	ai
j	dzei
k	que
l	el
m	em
n	en
o	o
p	pi
q	kju
r	ar
s	es
t	ti
u	yu
v	vi
w	dabelyu
x	eks
y	wai
z	si

Antes de 1994 el alfabeto español contuvo treinta letras. Con la excepción de la **rr**, que nunca ocurre al principio de una palabra, cada letra constituía una entidad propia y separada en un diccionario. Sin embargo, en 1994 la Real Academia Española eliminó dos letras del alfabeto, la **ch** y la **ll**, para alinear el orden alfabético español más con el orden usado por otros idiomas. (Por lo común, la **k** y la **w** se hallan solamente en palabras de origen extranjero.) Este cambio permitía que los de habla española se adaptasen a la edad informática. Por consiguiente, los diccionarios españoles y bilingües escritos y publicados después de 1994 no se incluirán la **ch** y la **ll** como entidades propias que siguen su ordern correspondiente después de la **c** y la **l** respectivamente.

A causa de que la Real Academia Española hizo estos cambios tan recientemente, todavía se oye y se usa tanto la **che** como la **ce hache** y la **elle** or la **doble ele**. Los hispanohablantes indígenas comprenden y usan todas.

Acerca de la Autora

Rochelle (Shelle) K. Kelz, PhD., es la Decana de Bellas Artes y Ciencias a C.S. Mott Community College en Flint, Michigan. Antes de eso fue la Directora de Programas de Extensión y la Universidad Nocturnal a North Park College & Theological Seminary, y más tarde, la Directora de Programas de Extensión a Roosevelt University, ambas en Chicago, Illinois. Tuvo el título lectivo de Profesora de español, inglés como segundo idioma, y francés a North Park y Profesora de idiomas y de educación a Roosevelt. Además, sirvió de Profesora Asistente Venida de Fuera de español médico a la Universidad de Illinois a Chicago así como al Centro Médico de la Universidad de Illinois a Chicago por más de ocho años. En 1987 fue nombrada "Profesora universitaria de español más sobresaliente de todos los Estados Unidos" por la Asociación Americana de Profesores de Español y Portugués.

Además es una solicitada traductora médica–legal de español e inglés, sirviendo la mayoria de las organizaciones profesionales médicas y dentales. También sirve de consultante para establecer Programas de Español Médica en hospitales, facultades de medicina y de odontología, y universidades. Publicó *Conversational Spanish for Medical Personnel*. Sirviendo de sus talentos como educadora de idiomas y traductora así como de sus recursos tremendos, compiló este diccionario médico-dental español/inglés, inglés/español.

A.A., Alcohólicos Anónimos

abandon, to, abandonar

abandoned (*person*), guacho *adj*, *Chi, Perú, Ríopl*

abatement, decaimiento; extenuación *f*; reducción *f*; remisión *f*

abbreviation, (*shortened form*) abreviatura; (*initials*) sigla; table of **~s** cuadro de abreviaturas

abdomen, abdomen *m*, *form*; barriga *fam*; estómago *fam*; panza *fam*; vientre *m*; **acute ~** abdomen agudo

abdominal, abdominal *adj*; **~ binder** vendaje abdominal *m*; **~ cramps** calambres abdominales *m*; cólico

able, to be, poder (ue)

able-bodied, apto *adj*; fornido *adj*; robusto *adj*; sano *adj*

able-minded, inteligente *adj*; listo *adj*

abnormal, anormal *adj*; **~ cellular division** división anormal de células *f*

abort, to, abortar; hacer abortar (una fiebre)

abortion, aborto; engendro; malparto; **induced ~** aborto inducido; aborto provocado; **spontaneous ~** aborto espontáneo; **therapeutic ~** aborto terapéutico; **threatened ~** aborto inminente; amenaza de aborto; **tubal ~** aborto tubárico

abrade, to, raer *Med*

abrasion, razpón *m*; lascadura *Mex*; **~** (*graze, sore*) desolladura; **~** (*scrape, scraping*) raspado; **~** (*scratching*) raspadura; **~** (*scratch, graze*) raspón *m*; **~** (*scratch*) rozadura; raedura *Med*

abruptio placentae, desprendimiento de la placenta

abscess, absceso; apostema (*var. de postema*); flemón *m*; furúnculos *fam*; grano *fam*; hinchazón *f*, *fam*; nacidos *fam*; postema; totuma *Chi*; **dental ~** postemilla; **milk ~** absceso en la mama; **to form an ~** apostemar

abscessed, apostemado *adj*

abscess, to, (*become full of pus*) apostemarse

absence, ausencia

absent-minded, despistado *adj*; distraído *adj*; olvidadizo *adj*; ido *adj*, *SpAm*; **to be ~** eslembarse *PR*; esparlotear(se) *PR*

absentmindedness, enajenación *f*

absorb, to, absorber; abstraerse; preocupar

absorbency, absorbencia

absorbent, absorbente *adj*; pasoso *adj*, *Col, Chi, Guat, Perú, Ven*; **~ cotton** algodón absorbente *m*; algodón hidrófilo *m*

abstain, to, abstenerse; **~ from sexual relations** abstenerse de las relaciones sexuales

abstention, abstención *f*

abundant, abundante *adj*

abuse, abuso; maltrato; seducción *f*; violación *f*; **child ~** abuso infantil

abuse, to, abusar de; dañar; injuriar; maltratar

abuttal, puente de apoyo dental *m*

Acapulco gold (*marijuana*), colombiana; grifa; grifo; Juana; Juanita; lucas; mariguana[1]; monte; mota; sinsemilla; yerba; yesca; zacate

acceleration, aceleración *f*

accept, to, aceptar

access, acceso; **wheelchair ~** acceso para sillas de ruedas

accident, accidente *m*; **airplane ~** accidente de aviación; **car ~** accidente de coche; **highway** ~ accidente de carretera; **industrial** ~ accidente de trabajo; ~ **insurance** seguro contra accidentes; ~ **rate** tasa de accidentes; **to meet with an** ~ sufrir un accidente; **traffic** ~ accidente de circulación

account, cuenta; **current** ~ cuenta corriente; **on** ~ a cuenta; **to settle an** ~ liquidar una cuenta

accountable, responsable *adj*

accumulation, acumulación *f*

accurate, exacto *adj*

accurately, con exactitud

acetaminophen, acetaminofén *m*

ache, dolencia; dolor de (+ *part of the body*) *m*; pena

ache, to, doler (ue); tener dolor de (+ *part of the body*)

aching, dolorido *adj*; doloroso *adj*; doliente *adj, Med*; ~ **all over** *fig.* molido *adj, fam*

acid, ácido; ~ (*LSD*) aceite *m*, *slang*; ácido; azúcar *m*; LSD; **acetic** ~ ácido acético (puro); **acetylsalicylic** ~ ácido acetilsalicílico; **amino** ~ aminoácido; **arsenic** ~ ácido arsénico; **ascorbic** ~ ácido ascórbico; **boric** ~ ácido bórico; **carbolic** ~ ácido carbólico; **cyanhydric** ~ ácido cianhídrico; ácido prúsico; **deoxyribonucleic** ~/**DNA** ácido desoxirribonucleico/ADN; **fatty** ~ ácido graso; **folic** ~ ácido fólico; **gastric** ~ ácido gástrico; **inosinic** ~ ácido inosínico; **lactic** ~ ácido láctico; **oxalic** ~ ácido oxálico; **p-aminosalicylic** ~/**PAS** ácido paramino salicílico; **phosphoric** ~ ácido fosfórico; ~**-proof** a prueba de ácidos; **ribonucleic** ~/**RNA** ácido ribonucleico/ARN; **salicylic** ~ ácido salicílico; **strong** ~ ácido fuerte; **sulfuric** ~ ácido sulfúrico; **uric** ~ ácido úrico

acidifiers, urine, acidificantes de la orina *f*

acidity, acidez *f*; **blood** ~ acidez de la sangre

acknowledgment, reconocimiento

acne, acné *f, form*; barros *fam*; cácara *Chicano*; espinillas *f, fam*; ~ **rosacea** acné rosácea *f*

acrylic, acrílico *adj*

Act of God, caso de fuerza mayor

act with restraint, to, templarse

acting-out, acto impulsivo; transformación de impulsos en acción directa *f*

action, acción *f*; movimiento; **to put into** ~ poner en movimiento; poner en práctica; **reflex** ~ acto reflejo

activate, to, activar

activated charcoal, carbón activado *m*

active, activo *adj*; **to be very** ~ cabrear *fam*

activity, actividad *f*; **field of** ~ esfera de actividad; **strenuous** ~ actividad fuerte

actual, ~ (*current*) actual *adj*; existente *adj*; ~ (*legitimate*) real *adj*

acuity, agudeza; **visual** ~ agudeza visual

acupuncture, acupuntura

acute, agudo *adj*; ~ **abdomen** abdomen agudo; ~ **care** primeros auxilios; ~ (*critical*) grave *adj*; **to become more** ~ agudizarse

acyclovir, aciclovir *m*

Adam's apple, bocado de Adán *m*; cogote *m, fam*; manzana *Mex*; nuez de Adán *f*; nuez de la garganta *f, fam*

add, to, agregar; añadir

added, adicional *adj*

addict (**drug**), adicto; adicto a droga(s); adicto a las drogas narcóticas; drogadicto; farmacodependiente *form*; morfinómano[2]; tecato[2]; toxicómano[2]; yeso[2]; ~ **in search of a fix** buscatoques[2] *sg, m/f*

addicted, adicto *adj*

addiction (**drug**), adicción *f*; dro-

gadicción *f*; farmacodependencia; hábito; toxicomanía
addictive, adictivo *m*, *adj*
adenoid, adenoide *f*; vegetación adenoide *f*; adenoideo *adj*
adenoidal expression, wearing, eslembao *adj*, *PR*
adenoidectomy, adenoidectomía
adenoma, adenoma *m*
adequate, adecuado *adj*; suficiente *adj*
adhesion, adherencia
adhesive, adhesivo *adj*; pegajoso *adj*; ~ **plaster** emplasto adhesivo; tafetán inglés *m*; ~ **strip** cinta adhesiva; esparadrapo; ~ **tape** cinta adhesiva; esparadrapo; tela adhesiva
adipose, adiposo *adj*
adjoining, adyacente *adj*; contiguo *adj*
adjust, to, adaptarse
adjustable, adaptable *adj*; ajustable *adj*
adjustment, ajuste *m*; corrección *f*; modificación *f*
administer, to, administrar; ~ **a purgative to** purgar *Med*; ~ **marijuana to someone** amarihuanar[2]; engrifar[2]; enmarihuanar[2]; marihuanar[2]
administrative, administrativo *adj*; ~ **counsel** junta administrativa
admission (*to the hospital*), admisión *f*; ingreso
admit, to (*to the hospital*), ingresar (en); internar (en)
admittance, no, prohibida la entrada; se prohibe la entrada
admitted, to be (*to the hospital*), ingresarse; internarse; ser internado *adj*
admitting, admisión *f*; ingresos *m*, *pl*
adolescence, adolescencia
adolescent, adolescente *m/f*, *adj*; púber *m/f*, *adj*
adopt, to, adoptar
adoption, adopción *f*

adoptive, adoptivo *adj*
adrenal, suprarrenal *adj*
adrenalin(e), adrenalina
adult, adulto
advance, avance *m*
advanced, avanzado *adj*; adelantado *adj*; ~ **in years** entrado en años *adj*; ~ **stage of pregnancy** estado avanzado de gestación
advancement, adelanto
advancing, progresivo *adj*
advantage, ventaja
adverse, adverso *adj*
advice, aviso; consejo; consulta; dictamen *m*; parecer *m*
advise, to, aconsejar
aerobics, aeróbicos *m*, *pl*
aerophagia, aerofagia
aerosol, aerosol *m*
affect, to, afectar; ~ **the health of** desmejorar *Med*
affection, afecto; cariño; afección *Med*, *f*; dolencia; enfermedad *f*
affectionate, afectuoso *adj*; cariñoso *adj*
afflict, to, afligir
afflicted with, to be, estar aquejado de; sufrir de
affliction, ~ (*of old age*) achaque *m*; aflicción *Med*, *f*; enfermedad *f*; mal *m*; ~ (*suffering*) sufrimiento
afflictive, doloroso *adj*
afraid, atemorizado *adj*; medroso *adj*; miedoso *adj*; **to be** ~ temer; tener miedo (de); juyir(se) *PR*
after-effects, consecuencias; efectos tardíos; secuelas; reliquias *f*, *pl*, *Med*
afterbirth, alumbramiento; expulsión de las secundinas *f*; placenta *form*; secundinas *pl*, *Mex*; segundo parto *Chicano*; sobreparto
aftercare, convalecencia; postcura; tratamiento postoperatorio
afterpains, dolores del alumbramiento *m*, *pl*; entuertos *pl*

aftertaste, gustillo; mal sabor de boca *m*; regusto

age, edad *f*; **awkward ~** edad del pavo; edad del chivateo *Chicano*; **middle ~** edad madura; **old ~** vejez *f*; **to be of ~** ser mayor de edad; **to be under~** ser menor de edad; ser demasiado joven; **to look one's ~** representar la edad que se tiene

age, to, envejecer

aged, envejecido *adj*; anciano *adj*

aging, envejecimiento

ageless, siempre joven *adj*

agent, agente *m*; ~ (*causal*) portador *m*

aggravation (*from an illness*), retroceso *Med*

aggravate, to, agravar; ~ **a problem** espetar la uña *fam, PR*

aggression, agresión *f*

aggressive, agresivo *adj*

agitate, to, agitar; **agitated**, agitado *adj*; **to become ~** agitarse

agonize, to, agonizar; angustiarse; penar

agony, agonía; angustia; dolor *m*

agree, to, acordar (ue); ~ **with one** caer bien; ~ (**with**) estar de acuerdo (con)

aid, auxilio; ayuda; **hearing ~** aparato para sordos; **medical ~** asistencia médica; **to go to the ~ of** ir en auxilio de

aid, to, ayudar

aide, asistente *m/f*; auxiliar *m/f*; ayudante *m/f*; **nurse's ~** asistente de enfermera

AIDS/Acquired Immune Deficiency Syndrome, SIDA / Síndrome de inmuno[logía] deficiencia adquirida *m*

ailing, achacoso *adj*; enfermizo *adj*

ailment, dolencia; enfermedad benigna *f*; indisposición *f*; malestar *m*; padecimiento

air, aire *m*; "**bad**" ~ mal aire; ~ **chamber** cámara de aire; ~ **conditioner** acondicionador de aire *m*; ~ **con-**ditioning aire acondicionado *m*; ~ **duct** tubo de ventilación; ~ **dressing** método de tratamiento de las heridas; **foul ~** aire viciado; **fresh ~** aire fresco; ~ **hammer** martillo neumático; ~ **hunger** falta de aire; ~ **intake** toma de aire; ~ **passages** vías aéreas; ~ **pollution** contaminación del aire *f*; ~ **pressure** presión atmosférica *f*; ~ **sack** alvéolo pulmonar; ~**sick** mareado *adj*; atacado de mal de altura *adj*; ~ **sickness** mal de los aviadores *m*; mareo (en viaje aéreo); ~ **vent** orificio de aeración; respiradero; **to put on ~s** dar(se) patas

air, to, ~ (*to expose to the air*) airear; ventilar; ~ (*to hang out to dry*) orear

airborne, llevado por el aire *adj*

air-condition, to, instalar aire acondicionado en

airtight, hermético *adj*; herméticamente cerrado *adj*

airway, conducto de ventilación; vía respiratoria

alarm, alarma

alarmed (*frightened*), **to become**, alarmarse

alarming, alarmante *adj*

alarmist, alarmista *m/f*

albino, albino *m, adj*

albumen, albumen *m*; albúmina

alcohol, alcohol *m*; bebidas alcohólicas; ~ **abuse** abuso del alcohol; ~ **consumption** consumo del alcohol; **denatured ~** alcohol desnaturalizado; **ethyl ~** alcohol etílico; **methyl ~** alcohol metílico; **rubbing ~** alcohol para fricciones; **wood ~** alcohol de madera; **to give up ~** estar en el dique *PR*

alcoholic, alcohólico *m, adj*; **chronic ~** atómico *fam*; botellero *fam*; **straight shot of an ~ drink** juanetazo *fam, PR*; palo *fam*

Alcoholics Anonymous, Alcohólicos Anónimos

alcoholism, alcoholismo
alert, alerta *adj*; enérgico *adj*; vivaracho *adj*; vivaz *adj*; **not to be ~** estar como un paslote *PR;* estar en nada *fam*
alertness, viveza
alert, to, alertar
algae, algas[3] *pl*
align, to, alinear(se)
alignment, alineamiento
aliment, alimento
alimentary, alimenticio *adj*; **~ canal** tubo digestivo
alive, vivo *adj*
alkali, álcali *m*
alkaline, alcalino *adj*
alkalize, to, alcalizar
allay, to, aliviar; calmar
allergen, alergeno
allergic, alérgico *adj*; **~ reaction** reacción alérgica *f*; trastorno alérgico
allergist, alergista *m/f*; alergólogo
allergy, alergia
alleviate, to, aliviar; calmar; mitigar; paliar
allow, to, dar lugar a; permitir; **~ for** tener en cuenta
alloy, aleación *f*
almond-eyed, de ojos rasgados *adj*
aloe, áloe *m*
alone, solo *adj*
aloud, en voz alta
A.L.S., E.L.A. (*See amyotrophic lateral sclerosis.*)
alteration, alteración *f*; alternancia
alternate, alterno *adj*; **on ~ days** cada dos días; en días alternos
alternate, to, alternar
alternative, alternativa
alveolar, alveolar *adj*; **~ bone** hueso alveolar; **~ ridge** proceso alveolar
alveolus, (*pl, alveoli*) alvéolo; alveolo
amalgam, amalgama
amblyopia, ambliopia
ambulance, ambulancia; **~ box** botiquín *m*; **~ service** servicio de ambulancias

ambulatory, ambulatorio *adj*; **~ patient** paciente ambulatorio
amenorrhea, amenorrea
amino acids, aminoácidos
aminoglycoside, aminoglucósido
ammonia, amoníaco; amoniaco
amnesia, amnesia
amnesic, amnésico *m, adj*
amniocentesis, amniocentesis *f*; prueba del saco amniótico
amnion, amnios
amniotic, amniótico *adj*; **~ fluid** agua[3] del amnios; **~ sac** bolsa amniótica; bolsa de aguas *fam*; saco amniótico
amoeba, ameba; amiba
amoebic dysentery, disentería amibiana
amoxacillin, amoxacilina
amphetamine, anfetamina; a; ácido *sg*; bombido[2]; bombita[2]; estimulante *m*; naranjas[2]; pepas *slang*
ampicillin, ampicilina
amplification, amplificación *f*
amplified, amplificado *adj*
amplify, to, amplificar
ampoule/ampule, ampolleta; ámpula; pomo (*término de las drogas*); tubo de jeringuilla
amputate, to, amputar; cortar; desmembrar; resecar *Med*
amputated, broco *adj, PR*
amputation, amputación *f*
amputee, ñoco *fam, PR*; simiñoco *fam, PR*; tuco *fam*
amuse oneself, to/have a good time, divertirse (ie)
amyotrophic lateral sclerosis/ALS, esclerosis lateral amiotrófica /ELA *f*
anabolic, anabólico *adj*
anal, anal *adj*
analgesia, analgésico; medicina para dolor; **continuous caudal ~** analgesia caudal continua; **infiltration ~** analgesia por infiltración; **surface ~** analgesia de superficie
analgesic, analgésico *adj*

analysis, análisis *m*; to do an ~ hacer un análisis
analyst, psicoanalista *m/f*
analyze, to, analizar
anaphylactic, anafiláctico *adj*
anaphylaxis, anafilaxia
anatomic, anatómico *adj*
anatomical, anatómico *adj*
anatomy, anatomía
ancestor, antepasado
anemia, anemia; sangre clara *f*, *fam*; sangre débil *f*, *fam*; sangre pobre *f*, *fam*; poca sangre *f*, *fam*; (atrophic) aplastic ~ anemia (atrófica) aplástica; (acute) febrile ~ anemia (aguda) febril; (acute) hemolytic ~ anemia hemolítica (aguda); iron deficiency ~ anemia ferropriva *form*; anemia por deficiencia de hierro; pernicious ~ anemia perniciosa; sickle cell ~ anemia de células falciformes; anemia drepanocítica; drepanocitemia; thalassemia ~ talasemia
anemic, anémico *adj*; papujo *adj*, *Mex*
anesthesia, anestesia; balanced ~ anestesia equilibrada; block ~ anestesia de bloque; caudal ~ anestesia caudal; compression ~ anestesia por compresión; epidural ~ anestesia epidural; general ~ anestesia general; anestesia total; inhalation ~ anestesia por inhalación; local ~ anestesia local; regional ~ anestesia regional; saddle block ~ anestesia en silla de montar; spinal ~ anestesia espinal; anestesia raquídea; twilight sleep ~ sueño crepuscular
anesthesiologist, anestesiólogo
anesthesiology, anestesiología
anesthetic, anestésico *m*, *adj*; insensibilizador *m*, *adj*, *Med*
anesthetize, to, anestesiar *Med*; insensibilizar *Med*
aneurysm, aneurisma *m*; abdominal ~ aneurisma abdominal; aortic ~ aneurisma aórtico; arteriovenous ~ aneurisma arteriovenoso; branching ~ aneurisma ramificado; cardiac ~ aneurisma cardíaco; cirsoid ~ aneurisma cirsoideo; dissecting ~ aneurisma disecante; embolic ~ aneurisma embólico; false ~ aneurisma falso; aneurisma espurio; fusiform ~ aneurisma fusiforme; mycotic ~ aneurisma micótico; sacculated ~ aneurisma saculado; silent ~ aneurisma silencioso; true ~ aneurisma verdadero; ventricular ~ aneurisma ventricular
aneurysmogram, aneurismograma *m*
angel dust/PCP, cucuy; fenciclidina; líquido; PCP; polvo *slang*
anger, cólera; coraje *m*; rabia *fam*; rencor *m*; fit of ~ viaraza *Col*, *Guat*, *Ríopl*
anger, to, encolerizar; enfadar; enojar; irritar; entripar *Arg*, *Col*, *Ec*
angina, angina; ~ abdominis angina abdominal; acute ~ angina aguda; follicular ~ angina folicular; ~ pectoris angina del pecho; angina péctoris; unstable ~ angina inestable; Vincent's ~ angina de Vicente
angiocardiography, angiocardiografía
angiocardiopathy, angiocardiopatía
angiogram, angiografía; angiograma *m*
angioplasty, angioplastia; percutaneous transluminal ~ angioplastia transluminal; coronary ~ percutánea coronaria
angiomate (red dots on skin), cabecita de vena *Chicano*
angle, ángulo; ~ of aperture ángulo de abertura; carrying ~ ángulo de porte; ~ of convergence ángulo de convergencia; coro-

nary ~ ángulo coronal; **costal** ~ ángulo costal; ~ **of deviation** ángulo de desviación; **elevation** ~ ángulo de elevación; ~ **of incidence** ángulo de incidencia; ~ **of the jaw** ángulo de la mandíbula; ángulo mandibular; **optic** ~ ángulo óptico; ~ **of polarization** ángulo de polarización; ~ **of reflection** ángulo de reflexión; **visual** ~ ángulo visual

angry, corajudo *adj, fam*; enfadado *adj*; enfogonado; enojado *adj*; china *adj, CA, Cu*; ~ (*a bit more than irritation*) enfadao *adj, PR*; inflamado *adj, Med*; **to be** ~ estar chino *adj, CA, Cu*; tener un chino *Arg, CA, Cu*; **to get** ~ (*See mad, to get.*) tener el moño parao *fam*; tener los grifos parao *fam*; encachorrarse *Col*; engranarse *Arg*; renegar (ie) *Mex, Perú, Ríopl*

anguish, ~ (*mental*) angustia; ~ (*physical*) congoja

animal, animal *m*; ~ **fats** grasas de animal

animated, to become, animar

ankle, maléolo; tobillo; guayaba *Ec*; ~ **fracture** fractura maleolar; ~ **support** tobillera; ~ **bone** astrágalo; taba *Anat*

anoint, to, ungir *Med*

annoyance, ~ (*state*) irritación *f*; ~ (*thing*) molestia; **to demonstrate** ~ hacer buche *fam*

annoy, to, chimar *Mex, Nic*; chingar *Mex, El Sal*

annoyed, pujilateao *adj, PR*

annoying, fastidioso *adj*; molesto *adj*; chocante *adj, SpAm*

annual, anual *adj*

anomaly, anomalía; **developmental** ~ anomalía congénita

anorexia, anorexia; ~ **nervosa** anorexia nerviosa; anorexia mental

ant, hormiga

antacid, antiácido *m, adj*

antagonist, antagonista *f, adj*

anthrax, ántrax *m*

antibiotic, antibiótico *m, adj*; **broad-spectrum** ~ antibiótico de alcance amplio; antibiótico de espectro amplio; **limited-spectrum** ~ antibiótico de alcance reducido; antibiótico de espectro reducido; ~ **supplements** suplementos de antibióticos

antibody, anticuerpo; **anaphylactic** ~ anticuerpo anafiláctico; **blocking** ~ anticuerpo bloqueador; **(in)complete** ~ anticuerpo (in)completo; **inhibiting** ~ anticuerpo inhibidor; **neutralizing** ~ anticuerpo neutralizante; **sensitizing** ~ anticuerpo sensibilizante

anticholinergic, anticolinérgico *m, adj*

anticoagulant, anticoagulante *m, adj*

anticonvulsant, anticonvulsivo *m, adj*

antidepressant, antidepresivo *m, adj*

antidote, antídoto; antifármaco; contraveneno; **chemical** ~ antídoto químico; **mechanical** ~ antídoto mecánico; **physiological** ~ antídoto fisiológico; **universal** ~ antídoto universal

antiemetic, antiemético *m, adj*

antifreeze, anticongelante *m*

antigen, antígeno

antigenic, antigénico *adj*

antihemorrhagic, antihemorrágico *adj*

antihistamine, antihistamínico *m, adj*; droga antihistamínica

antihistaminic, antihistamínico *adj*

antihypertensive, antihipertensivo *m, adj*

antiinflammatory, antiinflamatorio *adj*

antimalarial, antipalúdico *adj*

antiphlogistic, antiflogístico *m, adj*

antipyretic, antipirético *m, adj*; febrífugo *m, adj*

antipyrine, antipirina

antiseptic, antiséptico *m, adj*
antispasmodic, antiespasmódico *m, adj*; antiespástico *m, adj*
antitetanic/anti-tetanus, antitetántico *adj*
antitoxic, antitóxico *adj*
antitoxin, antitoxina; contraveneno
anuria, anuria
anus, agujero *vulg, Chicano*; ano *form*; culo *vulg*; fundillo *Mex*; istantino *fam*; ojete *m, slang*; recto *fam* (*used incorrectly as rectum*) trasero
anxiety, angustia *fam*; ansias *f, pl, fam*; ansiedad *f*; desesperación *f*; nervios *fam*; inquietud *f*; subsidio *Col, Ec*; ~ **attack** crisis nerviosa *f*
anxious, ansioso *adj*; nervioso *adj*; intranquilo *adj*; **to be** ~ desgonzarse *fam*; estar alterado *fam*; estar desesperado *fam*; estar nervioso; intranquilizarse; tener angustia *fam*; tener ansias *fam*
aorta, aorta
aortic, aórtico *adj*; ~ **insufficiency** insuficiencia aórtica; ~ **murmur** murmullo aórtico; ~ **sounds** ruidos aórticos; ~ **stenosis** estenosis aórtica *f*
apathetic, apático *adj*; indiferente *adj*; esguabinao *adj, PR*; **to be** ~ **toward** no mostrar (ue) interés alguno en; ser indiferente a
apathy, apatía
apex, ápice *m*
Apgar score, escala de Apgar
aphasia, afasia
aphonia (*hoarseness*), afonia; ronquera
apnea, apnea; **sleep** ~ apnea del sueño
apoplexy (*stroke*), apoplejía
apparatus, aparato; instrumento; **prosthetic** ~ aparato prótesis; **urinary** ~ aparato urinario; **urogenital** ~ aparato urogenital
apparition, aparición *f*
appearance, ~ (*outward*) apariencia; ~ (*looks*) aspecto

appendicitis, abdomen agudo *m, slang*; apendis *m, fam*; apendicitis *f*; mal del apendis *m, fam*; panza peligrosa *slang*
appendix, apéndice *m*; apendis *m, fam*; apendix *f*; tripita *fam*
appetite, apetito; ganas de comer *f*; ~ **change** cambio de apetito
apple, manzana
appliance, aparato
applicator, aplicador *m*
application, aplicación *f*; solicitud *f*
apply to (oneself), to, aplicar(se)
apply for admission, to, solicitar admisión a
appointment, cita; turno; **to make an** ~ hacer turno/cita; **to make an** ~ **with** coger hora para *fam*
appreciate, to, apreciar
approach, to, acercar(se) a
appropriate, apropiado *adj*
approximately, aproximadamente *adv*
apricot, albaricoque *m*
apron, delantal *m*
aqueous humor, humor acuoso *m*
ARC/AIDS related complex, CRS/complejo relacionado al SIDA
arc, arco; ~ **of the aorta** cayado de la aorta; **deep femoral** ~ arco crural profundo
arch, arco; ~ **of the foot** arco del pie; ~ **support** soporte para el arco del pie *m*
A.R.D.S./adult respiratory distress syndrome, S.I.R.A./síndrome de insuficiencia respiratoria del adulto *m*
area, área[3] *f*; campo
arm, brazo; **bend of the** ~ flexura del brazo; ~ **sling** cabestrillo
armpit, arca[3] *Mex*; axila *form*; hueco axilar; sobaco *fam*
arouse, to, ~ (*to awaken*) despertar (ie); ~ (*sexually*) excitar
arrange, to, arreglar
arrangement, arreglo; preparativo
arrears, in, atrasos; atrasado *adj*

arrest, paro; detención *f*; **cardiac ~** paro cardíaco; **respiratory ~** paro respiratorio

arrhythmia, cardiac, arritmia cardíaca

arse, (*anus*) *slang* ojete *m*

arsenic, arsénico

arterial, arterial *adj*

arteriosclerosis, arterio(e)sclerosis *f*

arteriosclerotic, arterio(e)sclerótico *adj*

arteriovenous, arteriovenoso *adj*

artery, arteria; vaso arterial; (*See page 499.*); **ascending aorta ~** arteria aorta ascendente; **brachial ~** arteria humeral; **(common) (external) carotid ~** arteria carótida (primitiva) (externa); **coronary ~** arteria coronaria; **deep auricular ~** arteria auricular profunda; **descending (thoracic) aorta ~** arteria aorta (torácica) descendente; **external (internal) mammary ~** arteria mamaria externa (interna); **femoral ~** arteria femoral; **interventricular ~** arteria interventricular; **posterior ulnar recurrent ~** arteria recurrente cubital posterior; **pulmonary ~** arteria pulmonar; **radial ~** arteria radial; **subclavian ~** arteria subclavia; **superior intercostal ~** arteria intercostal superior; **temporal ~** arteria temporal; **transverse facial ~** arteria facial (transversa)

arthritis, artritis *f*; reuma *m, fam*; **rheumatoid ~** artritis reumatoidea *f*

arthrogram, artrograma *m*

arthroscopy, artroscopia

articulation, articulación *f*; coyuntura; (*See joint.*)

artificial, artificial *adj*; plástico *adj*; postizo *adj*; **~ limb** miembro artificial; **~ respiration** respiración artificial *f*

artillery, (*drug term*) equipo hipo-

dérmico; estuche *m*; herramienta; herre *f*; R *f*

arthrosis, artrosis

articular, articular *adj*

asbestos, asbesto

ascend, ascender (ie)

ascending, ascendente *adj*

ASD/atrial septal defect, CIA/comunicación interauricular *f*

asexual, asexual *adj*

ashamed, to be ~ avergonzarse; tener vergüenza; **to feel ~** espicharse *Mex*

ashtray, cenicero

Asiatic flu, influenza asiática

ask, to, ~ (**for**) (*to order, request*) pedir (i); **~** (**for**) (*to request*) solicitar; **~** (*questions*) hacer preguntas; preguntar

asleep, adormido *adj*

asparagus, espárrago

aspect, aspecto

asphyxia, asfixia

asphyxiate, to, asfixiar(se); sofocar

aspirate, to, aspirar

aspiration, aspiración *f*; **needle ~** aspiración con aguja

aspirator, aspirador *m*

aspirin, aspirina; Mejoral *m, Mex*; **children's ~** aspirina para niños; Mejoralito, *Mex*

ass, culo *vulg*; roto *vulg, PR*

assault, asalto; golpiza; retratao *PR*; **~ and battery** asalto con lesión

assault, to, asaltar

assigned, asignado *adj*

assistance, asistencia; ayuda; concurso; socorro

assistant, asistente *m/f*; ayudante *m/f*; **nurse ~** enfermera auxiliar; **~/assisting surgeon** cirujano auxiliar

associated, asociado *adj*

association, asociación *f*

assume, to, asumir

assure, to, asegurar

asthenia, astenia

astigmatism, astigmatismo

asthma, ahoguío *fam, Mex*; asma[3]

form; mal del pecho *m*; fatiga *slang*; **bronchial ~** asma³ bronquial

asthmatic, asmático *m*, *adj*; **~ attack** ataque asmático *m*; **~ wheeze** resuello asmático

astigmatism, astigmatismo

astringent, astringente *m*, *adj*

asylum, asilo; **insane ~** manicomio

asymptomatic, asintomático *adj*

athlete, atleta *m/f*; **~'s foot** infección de serpigo *f*; hongos del pie; pie de atleta *m*

athletic supporter, suspensorio

atmosphere, atmósfera

atrial, auricular *adj*; **~ fibrillation** fibrilación auricular *f*

atrioventricular/A.V., auriculoventricular/A.V.

atrophy, atrofia

atrophy, to, atrofiarse

atropine, atropina

attach, to, adherir (ie); ligar; unir

attack, acceso (*fit*); ataque *m*; **heart ~** ataque cardíaco; ataque al corazón; **renewed ~** retroceso *Med*; **TIA/transient ischemic ~** isquemia cerebral transitoria/ICT

attend, to, asistir (a)

attendant, asistente *m*; asistenta

attending, asistente *m/f*, *adj*; **~ physician** médico a cargo; médico de atendencia; médico de cabecera

attentive, atento *adj*

attenuated, atenuado *adj*

attitude, actitud *f*

attribute, to, atribuir

atypical, atípico *adj*

audiogram, audiograma *m*

audiologist, audiólogo

audiology, audiología

audiometer, audiómetro

audiometry, audiometría

auditory, auditivo *adj*; **~ tube** conducto auditivo

augment, to, aumentar

auricular fibrillation, fibrilación auricular *f*

authorization, autorización *f*; permiso

authorize, to, autorizar

autism, autismo

autistic, autístico *adj*; autista *m/f*

autoclave, autoclave *m*

autoimmune, autoinmune *adj*

autoimmunity, autoinmunidad *f*

autopsy, autopsia

A.V./atrioventricular, A.V./atrioventricular

available, disponible *adj*; listo *adj*, *fam*; presto *adj*, *fam*; utilizable *adj*, *fam*

avascular, avascular *adj*

average, promedio *m*, *adj*; **~ deviation** promedio de desviación; **~ height** altura promedio

aversion, aversión *f*; piquiña *PR*; repugnancia

avoid, to, evitar

awake, despierto *adj*

awaken (s.o.), to, despertar (ie); **to ~ oneself** despertarse (ie)

awareness, conciencia; conocimiento; noción *f*

awkward, incrúspido *adj*, *Col, Mex, Nic*

---

¹ I have followed the spelling given in the *Diccionario de la lengua española*, RAE, 21st edition, 1990. Spanish does recognize variations using *j* and *h*.

² This is new vocabulary, not necessarily listed nor yet recognized by the Royal Academy of Spanish Grammar. It is understood that this vocabulary is primarily slang. Unless otherwise indicated, the gender of nouns is assumed to be obvious.

³ For pronunciation purposes, the masculine definite and indefinite articles, *el* and *un*, not *la* or *una*, are used when the article immediately precedes the feminine singular noun which begins with stressed *a* or any other that begins with stressed *ha*.

B

babble, ~ (*of a baby*) balbuceo; ~ (*confused speech*) farfullo

babble, to, balbucear; ~ (*to utter incoherently*) farfullar

Babinski's law, reflex, sign, syndrome, ley *f*, reflejo, signo, síndrome de Babinski *m*

baby, (**infant**) baby *m*, *Chicano*; bebé *m*; chipe *m/f*, *CA*, *Col*, *Mex*; criatura; guagua *m/f*, *Chi*, *Ec*, *Perú*, *Bol*, *Arg*, *Ur*; lactante *m/f*; nena; nene *m*; recién nacido; semilla *Chi*; tierno *CA*; **blue** ~ lactante azul *m/f*; **newborn** ~ **girl** chancleta *PR*; infantil *adj*; ~ **rash** eritema de los pañales *m*; ~ **teeth** dientes de leche *m*

babyish, ~ (*infantile*) de niño *adj*; infantil *adj*; ~ (*childish*) pueril *adj*

bachelor, jamón *m*, *PR*; soltero

bacillus, (*pl*, **bacilli**) bacilo; **Calmette-Guérin** ~/**BCG** bacilo de Calmette-Guérin/BCG

bacitracin, bacitracina

back, ~ (*of hand*) dorso; ~ (*of a person*) espalda; ~ (*spine, backbone*) espinazo *fam*; ~ (*of an animal*) lomo *fam*; **lower** ~ parte baja de la espalda *f*; **the** ~ **of** la parte de atrás de; ~ **of knee** corva; **on one's** ~ boca arriba; ~ **reflex** reflejo lumbosacro; ~ **strain** esguince vertebral *m*; **to be on one's** ~ (*See be on one's back.*); **to stand with one's** ~ **to** dar la espalda a; **to walk** ~ volver (ue) andando

backache, dolor de espalda *m*

backbone, columna *fam*; columna vertebral; espina dorsal; espinazo; raquis *m*

backdate, to, antedatar

backflow, flujo retrógrado; **pyelo-venous** ~ flujo retrógrado pielovenoso

backhand, ~ (*sports*) dado con el revés de la mano *adj*; ~ (*handwriting*) letra inclinada hacia la izquierda

backing, respaldo *Dent*; refuerzo; sostén *m*; **alloy** ~ de aleación *Dent*

backside, posaderas, *f*, *pl*, *Anat*; posas *f*, *pl*

backward, atrasado *adj*; lerdo *adj*; tardo *adj*

backwardness, atraso mental

backup, respaldo

backyard, traspatio

bacon, tocino

bacteremia, bacteriemia (*presencia de bacterias patógenas en la sangre*)

bacteria, (*sg*, **bacterium**) bacterias; ~ **count** recuento de gérmenes

bacterial, bacteriano *adj*; bactérico *adj*

bacteriologist, bacteriólogo

bacteriology, bacteriología; **hygienic** ~ bacteriología higiénica; **pathological** ~ bacteriología patológica; **sanitary** ~ bacteriología sanitaria; **systematic** ~ bacteriología sistemática

bacterioscopy, bacterioscopia (*estudio microscópico de las bacterias*)

bacterium, (*pl*, **bacteria**) bacteria; **acid-fast** ~ bacteria acidorresistente; (*higher*) (*lower*) ~ bacteria (superior) (inferior); **infectious** ~ bacteria infecciosa; **parasitic** ~ bacteria parásita; **pathogenic** ~ bacteria patógena; **toxic** ~ bacteria tóxica; **virulent** ~ bacteria virulenta

bad, malo *adj*; nocivo *adj*; ~ (*harmful*) dañoso *adj*; ~

(*rotten*) podrido *adj*; ~ **cold** resfriado fuerte; ~ **for one's health** malo para la salud; nocivo para la salud; ~ **judgment** mal juicio; **in a** ~ **mood** de mal humor; ~-**tempered** (*permanent*) de mal genio; ~-**tempered** (*occasionally*) de mal humor *adj*; malhumorado *adj*; ~ **trip** experiencia mala en el uso de drogas; mal viaje *m*

badly, mal *adv*

baffled, confundido *adj*; confuso *adj*

bag, bolsa; paquete *m*; saco; **doctor's** ~ maletín (médico) *m*; **hot-water** ~ bolsa de agua caliente; ~ **of bones** costa de huesos *m*, *fam*; ~ **of marijuana** funda² *PR*; ~ **of waters** aguas *f*, *pl*; bolsa de las aguas; bolsa membrosa; fuente *f*, *fam*; **paper** ~ bolsa de papel; **shopping** ~ bolsa para la compra; **large shopping** ~ funda; ~ **under the eye** bolsa (debajo de los ojos)

bake, to, ~ (*in an oven*) cocer en el horno; ~ (*to dry*) secar

baked, (cocido) al horno *adj*; horneado *adj*; ~ **tongue** lengua tostada

baking powder, levadura (en polvo)

baking soda, bicarbonato de sosa; bicarbonato (sódico)

balance, ~ (*scientific*) balance *m*; **acid-base** ~ balance acidobásico; **energy** ~ balance energético; **enzyme** ~ balance de enzimas; **fluid** ~ balance líquido; **neutron** ~ balance de neutrones; balance neutrónico; ~ (*scales*) balanza; ~ (*physical, mental, etc.*) equilibrio

balance, to, equilibrar

balanced, balanceado *adj*; equilibrado *adj*; ~ **diet** alimentación equilibrada *f*; **mechanically** ~ **occlusion** oclusión balanceada mecánicamente *f*

balancing contacts, contactos de balance *Dent*

balancing occlusal surfaces, superficies oclusales de balance *f*

bald, calvo *adj*; cocopelao *adj*, *PR*; lauco *adj*, *Chi*; ~ **head** pelada *Chi*, *Ríopl*; ~ **patch** calva; ~ **spot** (*on the head*) luquete *m*, *Chi*; ~ **tongue** lengua depapilada

baldness, calvicie *f*; lauca *Chi*; laucadura *Chi*

ball, bola; corpúsculo esferoidal; esfera; ~ **and socket joint** articulación de rótula *f*; ~ **of eye** globo ocular; ~ **of finger/fingertip** pulpejo; punta del dedo; yema del dedo; ~ **of the foot** antepié *m*, *fam*; eminencia metatarsiana; ~ **of thumb** eminencia tenar

ballistic, balístico *adj*

ballistics, balísticas; **wound** ~ balísticas de las heridas

balloon, ~ (*of a Foley catheter, etc.*) balón *m*; ~ (*of heroin*) cimbomba² *slang*; globo²

balloon, to, abombar; distender una cavidad con aire para facilitar su examen o limpiarla; (*See angioplasty.*); ~ (*to swell out*) hincharse

balls, (*See testicles.*) bolas *vulg*; bolones *m*, *pl*, *vulg*; cojones *m*, *pl*, *vulg*; güebos *pl*, *vulg*; huevos *pl*, *vulg*, *common*; lerenes *m*, *pl*, *vulg*; testículos

balm, bálsamo; melisa; ungüento; **lip** ~ ungüento para los labios

balsam, bálsamo; ungüento

bamboo, bambú *m*

banana, banana; guineo *PR*; plátano

band, cincha; cinta; faja; venda; **absorption** ~ banda de absorción; **amniotic** ~ brida amniótica; **arm** ~ brazalete *m*; **elastic** ~ goma

band, to, vendar

bandage, vendaje *m*; envoltura *fam*; ~ (*for the eyes*) tapaojo

SpAm; **abdominal** ~ vendaje abdominal; **circular** ~ vendaje circular; **compression** ~ vendaje compresivo; **immobilizing** ~ vendaje inmóvil; **plaster** ~ vendaje enyesado; **pressure** ~ vendaje a presión; **protective** ~ vendaje protectivo; ~ **scissors** tijeras de vendaje; **T** ~ vendaje en T; ~ (*dressing*) apósito (ligado con vendas); cura; **adhesive absorbent** ~ apósito absorbente adhesivo; ~ (*the material*) venda; **Ace** ~ venda Ace; **adhesive** ~ venda adhesiva; **elastic** ~ venda elástica; vendaje elástico; **gauze** ~ venda de gasa; **swathing** ~ faja abdominal

bandage, to, fajar; vendar

Bandaid, (*trademark*) bandita *PR*; Curita (una marca); parchecito; venda

bands, (*braces, Dent*) frenos; frenillos; ganchos

bandy-legged, con las piernas arqueadas *prep phr*; patizambo *adj*

bang, to, (*drugs*) clavarse[2] *fam*; componerse[2] *fam*; curarse[2] *fam*; filerearse[2]; jincarse[2]; picarse[2]; rayarse[2]; shootear[2]

bank, banco; **arteries, bone, eye, skin** ~ banco de arterias, huesos, ojos, piel; **blood** ~ banco de sangre

bankrupt, quebrado *adj*; **to go** ~ declararse en quiebra

bar, barra, obstáculo; **arch** ~ barra en arco *Dent*; ~ **clasp arm** brazo de barra de gancho

barbed wire, alambre de púas *m*

barbital, barbital *m*; **sodium** ~ barbital sódico; **soluble** ~ barbital soluble

barbiturate, barbiturato; barbitúrico; cacahuate *m, slang*; colorada *slang*; globo *slang*

bare, desnudo *adj*; viringo *adj, Col, Ec*; ~**foot** descalzo *adj/adv*; sin zapatos; ~ **from the waist down** desnudo de cintura para abajo *adj*; ~ **from the waist up** desnudo de cintura para arriba *adj*; ~**headed** con la cabeza descubierta *adj/adv*

barf, to, *vulg* (*to vomit*) arrojar; deponer *Mex*; devolver (ue); tener vasca; vomitar; (*See vomit, to.*)

barium, bario; ~ **arsenate** arseniato de bario; ~ **chloride** cloruro de bario; ~ **sulfate** sulfato de bario

bark, corteza

barking, ladrido; ~ **cough** tos perruna *f*

barley, cebada; **pearl** ~ cebada perlada

barrel, ~ (*of a syringe*) barril *m*; ~ **chest** tórax en tonel *m*; tórax globoso *m*; ~ **of the ear** caja del tímpano; (**green**) ~**s**/(**the**) **beast** aceite[2] *m*; ácido[2]; azúcar[2] *m*; LSD

barren, estéril *adj*; infecundo *adj*

barrier, barrera; **blood-brain** ~ barrera hematocefálica; **placental** ~ barrera placentaria

basal, basal *adj*; ~ **body temperature** temperatura corporal basal; ~ **ganglia** ganglios basales; ~ **metabolic rate/B.M.R.** valuación del metabolismo basal *f*/V.M.B.*f*; ~ **seat** (*outline*) (diseño del) asiento basal *Dent*

base, base *Chem, Pharm, etc. f*; ~ **of the cranium** base del cráneo *f*; ~~**line** línea de referencia; punto de referencia; punto de partida; ~~**line** (*lab value*) nivel habitual *m*; ~~**line** (*physical/behavioral exam of patient*) estado habitual; **oil** ~ a base de aceite; **water** ~ a base de agua; ~ **material** material de base *m, Dent*

baseplate, placa base *Dent*; base de estudio

based, to be, basarse

baseline, (*See base-line.*)

basement, sótano

bashful, ruboroso *adj*; tímido *adj*

basic, básico *adj*
basin, bacinete *m*; bandeja; cubeta; ~ (*for washing up*) barreño; ~ (*washbowl*) jofaina; palangana; tazón *m*; vasija; **emesis** ~ escupidera; riñón *m*; riñonera
basket, cesta
bassinet, moisés *m*, *fam*
bat, murciélago
bath, baño; **acid** ~ baño ácido; **air** ~ baño de aire; **warm air** ~ baño de aire caliente; **alcohol** ~ baño de alcohol; **bran** ~ baño de salvado; **chemical** ~ baño químico; **cold** ~ baño frío; **cool** ~ baño fresco; **emollient** ~ baño emoliente; **foot** ~ baño de pies; **half** ~ baño medio (*de las caderas y las piernas*); **herb** ~ baño aromático; **hot** ~ baño caliente; ~ **mat** alfombra de baño; **medicated** ~ baño medicinal; baño medicamentoso; **milk** ~ baño de leche; **mustard** ~ baño de mostaza; **oatmeal** ~ baño de harina de avena; **oil** ~ baño de aceite; **potassium permanganate** ~ baño de permanganato de potasio; **saline** ~ baño salino; **shower** ~ baño de regadera *Chicano*; ducha; **sitz** ~ baño de asiento; semicupio; **sodium** ~ baño de sodio; **sponge** ~ baño de esponja; baño de toalla *Chicano*; **starch** ~ baño de almidón; **steam** ~ baño de vapor; **sulfur** ~ baño de azufre; baño sulfuroso; **sweat** ~ baño de sudor; **tar** ~ baño de brea; **tepid** ~ baño tibio; ~ **towel** toalla de baño; **vapor** ~ baño de vapor; **water** ~ baño de agua; **whirlpool** ~ baño de torbellino
bathe, to, bañar; higienizarse *Arg*; ~ **oneself/to take a bath**, bañarse; ~ (*a wound*) lavar
bathing, no, prohibido bañarse
bathrobe, albornoz *m*; bata de baño

bathroom, cuarto de baño; temascal *m*, *CA*, *Mex*; **to go to the** ~ ir al baño
bathtub, bañera; bañadera *Cu*; tina
battered child syndrome, síndrome del niño golpeado *m*
battery, batería (eléctrica); **storage** ~ acumulador eléctrico *m*
battle casualty, baja de batalla
b.b.a./born before arrival, nacido antes de la llegada *adj*
B.B.B./Blood-brain barrier, barrera hematoencefálica; barrera sanguíneo-cerebral
BBT/basal body temperature, temperatura basal
be, to, estar; ser; ir *Med*; (*How are we today?*) (¿Cómo vamos de salud hoy?); ~ (**non)habit forming** (no) crear vicio; ~ ___ **years old** tener ____ años; ~ **afraid** tener miedo; ~ **ashamed** tener vergüenza *f*; ~ **accustomed to** soler (ue); ~ **blue** tener murria; ~ **called** (*to be named*) llamarse; ~ **careful** tener cuidado; ~ **carrying narcotic drugs** andar carga[2]; andar cargado; cargar[2]; traer carga[2]; ~ **characterized** caracterizarse; ~ **cold** tener frío; ~ **gowned** vestirse (i) de bata de hospital; ~ **guaranteed** ser garantizado; ~ **guilty/~ at fault** tener la culpa; ~ **high** andar (+ *adj*) (*See high.*); ponerse (+ *adj*) (*See high.*); ~ **hungry** tener hambre *f*; ~ **in a hurry** tener prisa; ~ **in the habit of** soler (ue); ~ **late** tener retraso; ~ **on one's back** (*literally*) estar acostado boca arriba *adj*; ~ **on one's back** (*to be ill*) estar encamado *adj*; ~ **on the nod** (*to be under the influence of heroin*) cotorear[2]; ~ **on the road to recovery** estar recuperándose; ~ **quiet** callarse; ~ **right** tener razón *f*; ~ **sleepy** tener sueño; ~ **successful** tener éxito; ~ **thirsty**

tener sed *f*; ~ **under the weather** estar pachucho, *Spain*; ~ **up and about after an illness** andar andando; ~ **warm** tener calor *m*; ~ **wrong** no tener razón *f*

bead, abalorio; cuenta; **rachitic ~** abalorio raquítico (rosario); **~ing of the ribs**, rosario raquítico

beam, (*x-ray, etc.*) rayo

bean, haba

bear, to, ~ (*a child*) dar a luz; parir *esp. Carib, fam*; ~ (*to endure*) aguantar; sostener; tolerar; ~ **down** hacer bajar por fuerza; pujar

beard, barba; piocha

bearded, barbudo *adj*

bearing, porte *m*; ~ **down** contracciones expulsivas *f*; pesadez pélvica *f*; ~ **down pain** dolor expulsivo *m*

beat, ~ (*blow*) golpe *m*; ~ (*heart, pulse*) latido; ~ (*heart*) palpitación *f*; **ectopic ~** latido ectópico; **premature ~** latido prematuro

beat, to, (*heart*) latir; palpitar; pulsar; ~ (*physically*) golpear; pegar; **to be badly ~en** coger pela *fam*

beating, golpiza; paliza; retratao *PR*; ~ (*of the pulse*) pulsación *f*, *Anat*

beauty mark, lunar *m*

become, to, ~ (*something*) hacerse (+ *noun of profession*); ~ (*turn*) (+ *adj*) ponerse (+ *adj of emotional/mental state*) ; ~ *acute again* reagudizarse *Med*; ~ **bloated** abotagar; ~ **cancerous** cancerarse *Med*; ~ **detached** desprenderse; ~ **infected** infectarse; ~ **lost in thought** ensimismarse; ~ **transformed** transformarse

bed, cama; ~ (*fig. deathbed, etc.*) lecho; **air ~** cama neumática; **capillary ~** lecho capilar; **nail ~** lecho de la uña; **water ~** cama de agua; **to go to ~** acostarse (ue); aniarse *PR*; **to go to ~/to**

hit the sack ir al sobre *PR*; **to put to ~** acostar (ue); **to stay in ~** guardar cama; quedarse en cama

bedbug, chinche *f*

bedclothes, ropa de cama

bedpan, bacín *m*; bacinilla; chata; cómodo *Mex*; cuña; loro *Chi*; paleta; pato *slang*; orinal *m*; silleta; vasín de cama *m*

bedrail, barandal *m*; baranda

bedridden, (confinado) en cama; encamado *adj*; postrado en cama *adj*

bedroom, alcoba; cuarto de dormir; habitación *f*; recámara *SpAm*

bedsore, llaga de cama; úlcera por decúbito

bed-wetting, enuresis *f, form*; (el) orinarse en la cama

bee, abeja

beef, carne de res *f*

beeper, busca *m*; bíper *m, Chicano*

beer, cerveza

beet, acelga

beg, to, rogar (ue)

begin, to, comenzar (ie); empezar (ie)

beginning, comienzo; principio

behave, to, comportarse; portarse

behavior, comportamiento; conducta; **automatic ~** conducta automática; **(in)variable ~** conducta (in)variable; ~ **modification** modificación de la conducta *f*

belch, eructo

belch, to, eructar; erutar; regoldar; regurgitar; repetir (i); tener eructos

belching, eructación *f*

belief, creencia

believe, to, creer; pensar (ie)

bell, timbre *m*

Bell's palsy, parálisis facial *f*

belladonna, belladona

belly, *fam*, abdomen *m*; barriga; guata *Arg, Chi, Perú*; panza *fam*;

~ **band** fajita; ~ **binder** faja abdominal; fajero; fajita; ombliguero; (*See binder.*); **big** ~ prominente; **big-bellied** barrigón *adj*; ~ **button** ombligo

bellyache, cólico; dolor de barriga *m*; dolor de tripa *m*; dolor de vientre *m*

belt, cinturón *m*; faja; **seat ~/safety** ~ cinturón de seguridad *m*

bend, ángulo; curva; doblez *m*; ~ **of the arm** flexura del brazo; ~ **of the elbow** fosa cubital; sangradura; ~ **of the knee** corva; flexura de la pierna

bend, to, doblar; ~ **back** inclinarse hacia atrás; ~ **down** doblarse; inclinarse; ~ **over** agacharse; doblarse; empinarse; ~ **one's head down** agachar la cabeza; bajar la cabeza

bends, enfermedad de los buzos *f, sg*; enfermedad por descompresión *f*; trancazo *fam*

beneficial, beneficioso *adj*; **to be** ~ hacer provecho

benefit, beneficio; bien *m*; **for your** ~ por su bien

benign, benigno *adj*

bent, chueco *adj, CA, Mex, Ven*; ~ **inward** varo *adj, Med*

benzedrine, bencedrina; **bennies/benz/benzies** (*amphetamines*) blancas[2]; anfetaminas; bencedrinas

benzene, benceno

benzoin, benjuí *m*; benzoína

benzoyl peroxide, peróxido de benzoílo

beriberi, beriberi *m*

berserk, to go, andar volando

beset with anxiety, transido de angustia *adj*

beta, beta; ~ **blocker** beta bloqueador *m*; ~**hemolytic** beta-hemolítico *adj*

better, mejor *adj*; **to get** ~ mejorarse; refrescar *Mex, Med*

bewildered, atontado *adj*

bewitch, to, echar al bote

bewitchment, hechicería

bib, babero

bicarbonate, bicarbonato; **blood** ~ bicarbonato sanguíneo; ~ **of soda** bicarbonato de soda; salarete *m*

biceps, biceps *m, Chicano*; conejo *slang, Chicano*; mollero *fam*

bichloride of mercury, cloruro mercúrico

bicuspid, bicúspide *m, adj*; diente premolar *m*

b.i.d./bis in die/twice a day, dos veces al día

bidet, bidé *m*

biennial, bianual *adj*

bifocals, bifocales *m, pl*

bifurcate, bifurcado *adj*

bifurcation, bifurcación *f*

big, grande *adj*; ~ **C** (*cocaine*) carga[2]; coca; cocaína; nieve[2] *f*; perico[2] *Cu*; talco[2] *Texas, Cu*; ~**-bellied** barrigón *adj, fam*; ~**-boned** huesudo *adj, fam*; ~ **bosomed** pechugón *adj, Arg, Mex, PR*; ~ **breasted** tetuda *adj, fam*; ~**-eared** orejudo *adj*; ~ **toe** dedo gordo; dedo grueso

bigger, to get, ponerse más grande

bilateral, bilateral *adj*

bile, hiel *f*; biliar *adj*; ~ **acids** ácidos biliares; ~ **duct(s)** conducto(s) biliar(es); ~ **pigments** pigmentos biliares; ~ **salt** sal biliar *f*

biliary, biliar *adj*; biliario *adj*; de la bilis *prep phr*; ~ **stones** piedras en el vesículo

bilingual, bilingüe *adj*

bilious, bilioso *adj*; ~ **attack** trastorno bilioso

bilirubin, bilirrubina

bill, (*charges*) cobro; cuenta

bind, to, ~ (*clothes, etc.*) apretar (ie); ~ (**up**) (*to bandage*) vendar; ~ (*to constipate*) estreñir; ~ (*to tie up*) amarrar; atar; ~ (*to unite*) unir; vincular

binder, cintura; faja; vendaje abdominal *m*; **obstetric** ~ faja obstétrica

bindle, (*quantity of marijuana or narcotics*) bolsita²; paquete² *m*

binge, borrachera

biochemical, bioquímico *adj*

biochemistry, bioquímica

biodegradable, biodegradable *adj*

biofeedback, biorretroalimentación *f*

biological, biológico *adj*

biologist, biólogo

biology, biología

biophysics, biofísica

biopsy, biopsia; **aspiration** ~ biopsia por aspiración; **needle** ~ biopsia con aguja; **punch** ~ biopsia de sacabocado

biorhythm, ritmo biológico

biostatistics, bioestadística

bipara, bípara *f, adj*

bipolar, bipolar *adj*

bird, pájaro; ~**-arm** brazo de pájaro; ~**-face** cara de pájaro; ~**-leg** pierna de pájaro

birth, (*childbirth*) alumbramiento; nacimiento; parto; ~ **at term** ~ a término; ~ **canal** canal del parto *m*; ~ **certificate** acta³ de nacimiento; certificado de nacimiento; partida de nacimiento; ~ **control** anticoncepcionismo; control de la natalidad *m*; limitación de la natalidad *f*; regulación de nacimientos *f*; ~ **control methods** métodos anticonceptivos para no tener niños; **Billing's method** método de Billing; **cervical cap** gorro cervical; **coil** coil *m, Chicano*; **coitus interruptus** interrupción de coito *f*; retirarse *m*; salirse *m, slang*; **condom** condón *m*; forro *vulg, Arg*; goma *slang*; hule *m, slang*; preservativo *slang*; profiláctico; **diaphragm** diafragma (anticonceptivo) *m*; **IUD** aparatito *Chicano*; aparato intrauterino; dispositivo in-

trauterino; DIU *m*; **loop** alambrito; asa; lupo; ~ **control pill** pastilla (anticonceptiva); píldora (anticonceptiva); píldora de anticoncepción; **rhythm** método de ritmo; ritmo; **rubber** *slang* forro *Arg, vulg*; goma *slang*; hule *m, slang*; **sterilization** esterilización *f*; **tubal ligation** ligadura de tubos; ligadura de trompas; **vaginal cream** crema vaginal; **vaginal foam** espuma vaginal; **vaginal jelly** jalea vaginal; **vasectomy** vasectomía; **multiple** ~ nacimiento múltiple; **natural** ~ parto natural; ~**place** lugar de nacimiento *m*; **postterm** ~ nacimiento tardío; **premature** ~ nacimiento prematuro; **to be about to give** ~ estar para desembarcarse *fam*; **to give** ~ aliviarse *Mex, fam*; alumbrar; dar a luz; desocuparse *Arg, Chi, Ven*; parir; salir de su cuidado *Chicano*; sanar *euph*

birthday, cumpleaños *m, inv*

birthmark, estigma *m, slang*; lunar *m*; marca de nacimiento

birthrate, natalidad *f*

birthweight, peso al nacer; peso de nacimiento

bisexual, bi² *m/f*; bisexual *adj*

bite, (*wound*) mordedura; **human** ~ mordedura humana; **scorpion** ~ mordedura de escorpión; **snake** ~ mordedura de serpiente; ~ (*animal*) mordida; **cat** ~ mordida de gato; **dog** ~ mordida de perro; mordisco dentellado *Dent*; **closed** ~ dentellada cerrada *Dent*; **open** ~ dentellada abierta *Dent*; **over** ~ sobre dentellada *Dent*; ~/**sting** (*insect*) picada; picadura; piquete *m*; picotada; picotazo; **spider** ~ picadura de araña; ~ (*snack*) bocado

bite, to, ~ (*ice, frost*) quemar; ~ (*cold, wind*) cortar; ~ (*ani-*

mals) morder (ue); morder (ue) a dentelladas *Dent*; ~/**to sting** (*fish*, *insect*, *snake*) picar; ~ **one's lips/nails/tongue** morderse (ue) los labios/las uñas/la lengua; ~ **down** apretar (ie) los dientes *Dent*; ~ **something** dar dentelladas a *algo*

bitter, amargo *adj*; ~ (*cold*) penetrante *adj*; ~ (*disappointment*) agudo *adj*; ~ (*enemy*) implacable *adj*; ~ (*person*) resentido *adj*; ~ (*sour*) agrio *adj*

bitters, amargo *m*; **Angostura ~** amargo de Angostura

black, ~ (*color*) negro *adj*; ~ (*person*) moreno; negro; ~ **and blue** amoratado *adj*; lleno de moretones; moreteado *adj*; ~ **eye** esquimosis de los párpados *f*, *form*; hematoma periorbitario *m*; ojo amoratado; ojo morado; **lamp ~** negro de humo; ~ **widow spider** araña capulina; viuda negra

black out, to, desmayarse; perder (ie) el conocimiento

blackhead, comedón *m*; espinilla

blackout, ~ (*fainting*) desmayo; ~ (*lapse of memory*) laguna mental

bladder, vejiga (de la orina); vesícula; **gall ~** vesícula biliar; vejiga de la bilis; "**heat in**" ~[4] calor en la vejiga[4] **urinary ~** vejiga urinaria; ~ **worm** cisticerco

blade, ~ (*knife*) cuchilla; hoja; **razor ~** cuchilla de afeitar; ~ (*tongue*) depresor *m*; **shoulder ~** escápula; espaldilla; omóplato; paletilla

blame, (*responsibility*) culpa

bland, (*food*) no picante *adj*; sin sabor fuerte *prep phr*

blanket, cobija *CA*, *Mex*, *Ven*, *Col*; frazada; fresada; friza *PR*, *DR*; manta

blasted, to be, andar botando[2]; andar elevado a-mil[2]; andar hasta las manitas[2]; andar hasta las manos[2]; andar hypo[2]; andar lo-

co[2]; andar locote[2]; andar pasado[2]; andar prendido[2]; andar servido[2]; andar subido a-mil[2]

blastoderm, blastodermo

bleach, blanqueador *m*; blanqueo; cloro

bleach, to, blanquear(se)

bleb, ampolla; vejiga

bleed, to, sangrar; sangrear; ~ **excessively** desangrar; ~ **to death** desangrarse; morir (ue) de desangramiento

bleeder, hemofílico; sangrador *m*

bleeding, *n* flujo de sangre; hemorragia; pérdida de sangre de poca intensidad; sangrado; sangría; **breakthrough ~** flujo de sangre por la vagina inesperadamente; hemorragia inesperada; **functional ~** hemorragia funcional; **internal ~** hemorragia interna; **occult ~** hemorragia oculta; ~ **tendencies** tendencias a sangrar *f*; ~ **time** tiempo de sangrar; tiempo de hemorragia; ~ **to excess** desangramiento; sangrante *adj*; sangriento *adj*; sanguíneo *adj*; ~ **ulcer** úlcera sangrante

blemish, lunar *m*; mancha

blepharitis, blefaritis *f* (*inflamación de los párpados*)

blind, ciego *adj*; ~ **in one eye** tuerto *adj*; a ciegas *adv*

blindness, ceguedad *f*; ceguera; **color ~** acromatopsia *form*; ceguera para los colores *fam*; daltonismo *form*; dificultad en diferenciar ciertos colores *f*; **day ~** ceguera diurna; hemeralopia *form*; **functional ~** ceguera funcional; **night ~** (*nyctalopia*) ceguera nocturna *fam*; nictalopía *form*; **river ~** (*onchocerciasis*) ceguera del río; oncocercosis *f*, *form*

blink, parpadeo

blink, to, parpadear

blister, flictena; pupa *Med*; vejiga; vesícula; ~ (*on the skin*) ampolla; bulla; **fever ~** ampolla en los labios; fuego *fam*; vesícula febril; ~ **on sole of foot** sietecueros *m, inv, fam*; ~ (**on a surface**) burbuja

blister, to, ampollar(se); levantar ampollas en; cubrirse de ampollas; formarse ampollas; producir ampollas en

blistering, vesicación *f*

bloat, to, entumecerse; hinchar(se)

bloated, abotagado *adj*; aventado *adj*; hinchado *adj*; inflado (del estómago) *adj*

block, ~ (**large piece**) bloque *m*; ~ (**obstruction**) obstrucción *f*; bloqueo *Pharm*; **bundle branch** ~ bloqueo de rama; **cardiac/ heart** ~ bloqueo cardíaco; **nerve** ~ bloqueo nervioso; **residual neuromuscular** ~ bloqueo neuromuscular residual

block, to, bloquear *Pharm*; obstruir *Anat, Surg*; tapar *fam*; ~ **the nerve** obstruir el nervio

blockage, obstrucción *f*; **to have an internal** ~ atascarse *Med, SpAm*

blocked intestine, tripa ida *slang*

blocker, bloqueador *m*; **adrenergic** ~ bloqueador adrenérgico; **beta** ~ betabloqueador *m*; bloqueador(es) beta *m*; **calcium channel** ~ bloqueador de los canales de calcio; **neuronic** ~ bloqueador neuronal

blocking, bloqueo

blond, rubio *adj*; güero *adj, Mex*

blood, sangre *f, form*; chicha *Ríopl*; colorada *slang, Chicano*; sanguíneo *adj*; ~ **analysis** análisis de sangre *m*; **arterial** ~ **gas** gasometría; gases arteriales *m, pl*; ~ **bank** banco de sangre; ~ **borne** transmitido a través de la sangre *adj*; ~ **brother** hermano carnal; ~ **cell** glóbulo; ~ **chemistry** análisis de (la) sangre *m*; ~ **circulation** circulación sanguínea *f*; ~ **clot** coágulo de sangre; coágulo san-

guíneo; cuajarón *m*; cuajarón de sangre *m*; cuajo; ~ **clot reaction time** tiempo de retracción del coágulo; ~ **coagulation time** tiempo de coagulación; ~ **component** componente de sangre *m*; componente sanguíneo *m*; **cord** ~ sangre umbilical *f*; ~ **corpuscles** corpúsculos de la sangre; ~ **count** biometría hemática; hematimetría; recuento hemático; recuento sanguíneo *fam*; **differential** ~ **count** hematimetría que indica la proporción de cada tipo de leucocitos en porcentaje; **white** ~ **cell count** recuento de glóbulos blancos; ~ **culture** hemocultivo; ~ **disease** enfermedad sanguínea *f*; ~ **donor** donante de sangre *m/f*; **excessive flow of** ~ sangría suelta *Med*; **film of** ~ extensión de sangre *f*; ~ **flow** circulación sanguínea *f*; flujo sanguíneo *form*; ~ **group** grupo sanguíneo; **universal donor** ~ **group** donante universal *m/f*; **universal recipient** ~ **group** receptor universal *m/f*; ~ **in the sputum** esputo sangriento; ~ **in the urine** sangre en el orín *f*; ~ **lavage** lavado de la sangre *fam*; **occult** ~ sangre oculta *f*; **oxalated** ~ sangre oxalatada *f*; ~ **oxygen analyzer** analizador del oxígeno de la sangre *m*; ~ **plasma** plasma sanguíneo *m*; ~ **platelet** plaquetas; ~ **poisoning** envenenamiento de la sangre *fam*; intoxicación de la sangre *f, fam*; sepsis *f*; septicemia; toxemia; ~ **pressure** presión arterial *f, form*; presión sanguínea *f*; tensión arterial *f*; ~ **pressure cuff** aparato para medir la presión *fam*; baumanómetro; esfigmomanómetro; manguito de presión sanguínea; tensiómetro; **high** ~ **pressure** hipertensión arterial *f*;

presión arterial alta *fam*; presión arterial elevada *fam*; **low ~ pressure** hipotensión arterial *f*; presión arterial baja *fam*; **~ relative** carnal *m/f*; **~ sample** muestra de sangre; **~ screening** prueba selecta de (la) sangre; **~ serum** suero sanguíneo; suero de sangre; **~ smear** extensión de sangre *f*; frotis sanguíneo *m*; **~ studies** exámenes hematológicos *m*; **~ sugar** azúcar sanguíneo *m*; glicemia *form*; glucemia *form*; **~ test** análisis de (la) sangre *m*; examen de (la) sangre *m*; **tinged with ~** sanguinolento *adj*; **(mismatched) ~ transfusion** transfusión de sangre (incompatible) *f*; transfusión sanguínea (incompatible) *f*; **~ type** grupo sanguíneo *form*; **~ typing** determinación del grupo sanguíneo *f*; **~ urea** uremia; **~ vessel** vaso sanguíneo; vena; **whole ~** sangre entera *f*; sangre pura *f*; **to lose a lot of ~** desangrarse

bloodshot, (*eyes*) sanguinolento *adj*; **~ eye** ojo inyectado de sangre; **to have ~ eyes** tener los ojos a millón *fam*; tener los ojos de pescao de nevera *fam*; tener los ojos de un gato que lambe aceite *PR, fam*

bloodstain, mancha de sangre

bloodstained, manchado de sangre *adj*; sanguinolento *adj*

bloodstock, depósito de sangre

bloodstream, corriente sanguínea *f*; torrente circulatorio *m*; torrente de sangre *m*; torrente sanguíneo *m*

bloody, cruento *adj*; sangriento *adj*; sanguinolento *adj*; **~ nose** sangrado por la nariz; hemorragia nasal; **~ show** mucosidad teñida de sangre *f*; muestra de sangre; sangrado vaginal; secreción mucosa mezclada con sangre *f*; tapón de moco *m, Mex*; **~**

sputum esputo sanguinolento; **~ stool** heces sanguinolentas *f*

blotches, **skin**, manchas oscuras en la piel

blotchy, (*skin*) pinto *adj*

blow, (*hit*) bimbazo; golpe *m*; ~ (*to a person's body, car*) cantazo *fam*; ~ (*specifically to head*) cocotazo; ~ (*with the fist*) guantón *m, SpAm*; jinquetaza *PR*; ~ (*with a club, etc.*) leñazo; ~ (*by policeman's nightstick*) macanazo; ~ (*of air*) soplo; ~ (*wound*) tarrajazo *Guat*; **~ to the stomach/belly** panzazo *Arg, Para, Perú*

blow, to, sonar (ue); ~ (*to breathe out air forcefully*) soplar; **~ a child's nose** sonar (ue) las (narices) a un niño; **~ one's nose** sonarse (ue) la nariz; soplarse la nariz *Carib*; **~ snow** *slang* aspirar cocaína

blue, **~** (*color*) azul *adj*; **~ angels, blue devils, blue dolls, blue heavens, blues** (*amobarbital sodium*) *slang* amital *m*; cápsulas azules[2]; **~ star** (*morning glory seeds*) dompedro[2]; semillas de dondiego de día[2]; **~** (*sad*) triste *adj*

blunt, obtuso *adj*; romo *adj*

blur, to, (*vision*) borrarse (la vista); empañarse

blurred, borroso *adj*; empañado *adj*; **~ vision** vista nublada *fam*

blurry, borroso *adj*; empañado *adj*

blush, to, ababacharse *PR*; achongar(se) *PR*; enrojecerse; ponerse rojo *adj*; ruborizarse

B.M./bowel movement, defecación *f, form*; (*See bowel.*)

B.M.R./basal metabolic rate, intensidad del metabolismo basal *f*

board, junta

body, cuerpo; **acetone bodies** cuerpos acetónicos; **cancer bodies** cuerpos de cáncer; **ciliary ~** cuerpo ciliar; **~ heat** calor corporal *m*; **~ hygiene** higiene

corporal *f*; ~ **odor** mal olor corporal *m*; ~ **part** parte del cuerpo *f*; ~ **position** posición del cuerpo *f*; **spongy** ~ cuerpo esponjoso; **vitreous** ~ cuerpo vítreo; ~ **weight** peso corporal
bodybuilder, fisicoculturista *m/f*
boil, absceso (de la piel); carbunclo; chichón *m*; chupo *SpAm, Med*; chupón *m, Col*; divieso; flemón *m*; forúnculo *var*; furúnculo *form*; grano enterrado; nacido *Carib, fam*; postema *Med, Mex*; sisote *m*; tacotillo *Chicano*
boil, to, ~ (*food*) cocer; ~ (*water*) hacer hervir; hervir (ie); ~ **the bottles** hervir (ie) las botellas
boiled, hervido *adj*
boiling, hirviendo *adj*; hirviente *adj*
bond, enlace *m*; ligadura; unión *f*; vínculo; **high energy phosphate** ~ unión de alta energía *f*; **hydrogen** ~ unión de hidrógeno *f*; **peptid** ~ unión peptídica
bond, to, formar un enlace con
bonding, enlazamiento *form*
bone, ~ (*of body*) hueso; óseo *adj*; **accessory** ~ hueso supernumerario; **ankle** ~ astrágalo; **breast** ~ esternón *m*; **brittle** ~**s** osteogénesis imperfecta *f*; **calf** ~ peroné *m*; **cheek** ~ hueso malar; **collar** ~ clavícula; ~ **disease** enfermedad de los huesos *f*; ~ **fragments** fragmentos óseos; **hip** ~ hueso coxal; hueso ilíaco; **(lower) (upper) jaw** ~ maxilar (inferior) (superior); ~ **marrow** médula (ósea); médula del hueso; tuétano; **metatarsal** ~**s** huesos metatarsianos; **rounded** ~ chueca *Anat*; ~ **splinter** astilla ósea; esquirla; **tarsal** ~**s** huesos del tarso; **thigh** ~ fémur *m*; ~ (*of a fish*) espina
bonesetter, sobador *Col, Mex*; sobandero *Col, Ven*
bony, óseo *adj*
booklet, folleto
bookworm, estofón *m, PR*

booster shot, búster *m, Chicano*; inyección de refuerzo *f*; inyección secundaria *f*; reactivación *f*; revacunación *f*
boot, bota
booze, *vulg* bebida alcohólica
borax, bórax *m*
border, borde *m*
borderline case, caso límite
bore, to, taladrar
boric acid, ácido bórico
boring, terebrante *adj*; ~ **pain** dolor terebrante *m*
born, to be, nacer
bosom, senos *m, pl*
botany, botánica; **medical** ~ botánica médica
bother, to, molestar; chimar *Mex, Nic*
bothersome, incómodo *adj*
bottle, botella; envase *m*; ~ (*for pills*) frasco; pomo; **baby** ~ biberón *m*; bote *m, slang, Chicano*; botella; mamadera *SpAm*; pacha *Chicano, CA*; pepe *m, Guat, Hond*; pezonera *Arg*; tele *f, Chicano*; ~ **cap** chapa *PR*; ~ **feeding** lactancia artificial; **hot water** ~ bolsa de agua caliente
bottle up, to, (*feelings*) reprimir
bottom, (*buttocks*) nalgas *fam*; sentaderas *fam*
botulism, botulismo
bouillon, caldo
bounce back, to, recuperarse
bound, ligado *adj*; unido *adj*
bouquet, ramillete *m*
bout, ataque *m*
bow-leg, pierna en paréntesis; pierna chueca *SpAm*
bow-legged, cambado *adj, Arg, Col, Ven*; cascorvo *adj*; con (las) piernas arqueadas; corvo *adj*; ñangado *adj, Cu*; perniabierto *adj*; zambo *adj, fam*
bowel, intestino inferior; tripa *fam* (*often pl*); **large** ~ intestino grueso; **small** ~ intestino delgado; ~ **movement** aguas mayores

f, pl, euph; caca *fam* (*best understood by children*); cagada *vulg*; cámara *f, slang*; defecación *f, form*; deposiciones *f, SpAm, slang*; evacuación del vientre *f*; excremento; heces fecales *f, pl*; materia fecal; miércoles *m, sg, euph*; mierda *vulg*; pase del cuerpo *m*; **to have a ~ movement** dar del cuerpo *Carib, fam*; defecar *form*; evacuar; excretar; exonerar el vientre; hacer caca *slang* (*best understood by children*); hacer del baño *Mex, fam*; hacer popó *slang, Ped*; hacer pupú *slang, Ped*; obrar *Mex, CA, fam*; **~ obstruction** abdomen agudo *m, slang*; obstrucción de la tripa *f*; panza peligrosa *slang*; **~s** entrañas; tripa *fam*

box, caja

boy, ~ (*child*) (*See child.*); **large young ~** potranco *PR*; **~** (*heroin*) azúcar[2] *m, Arizona, Texas*; caballo[2]; carga[2]; chiva[2]; cohete[2] *m*; heroína

B.P./**blood pressure**, presión sanguínea *f*

b.p./**boiling point**, punto de ebullición

brace, corsé *m, fam*; **~** (*truss*) braguero

braces, aparato ortodóntico *Dent*; frenillos; frenos; aparatos ortopédicos *Ortho*

bradycardia, bradicardia

braid, to, trenzar

Braille, Braille *m*

brain, cabeza *fam*; cerebro; coco *fam*; sesos *fam*; **~ cancer** cáncer del cerebro *m*; cáncer cerebral *m*; **~ fever** encefalitis *f*; **~ matter** materia cerebral; **~ stroke** derrame cerebral *m*; hemorragia cerebral; **~ tissue** tejido cerebral; **~ tumor** tumor cerebral *m*; **~ wave** onda cerebral; **~ wave test** electroencefalograma *m*

braincase, caja del cráneo; caja encefálica

brainstem, bulbo raquídeo; tallo cerebral; tronco cerebral

bran, afrecho; salvado

branch, rama; ramificación *f*; **~ of medicine** rama de medicina

branched, ramificado *adj*

brassiere, brasiere *m*; ajustador *m, Cu*; corpiño *SpAm*; sostén *m*

brassy cough, tos bronca *f*; tos metálica *f*

brawl, escarceo *PR*

bread, American, pan especial *m*

break, fractura *Ortho*; quebradura *Ortho*; rotura *Ortho*; **~** (*chromosome*) rompimiento *Ortho*

break, to, quebrantarse; resentirse (ie); **~** (*to damage*) escrachar(se) *PR*; *Ortho* fracturar(se); quebrar(se); partir(se) *Cu*; romper(se) *Carib*; **~ down** descomponer; **~ out** brotar; salirle barros; salirle granos

breakthrough bleeding, hemorragia de disrupción *fam*

breakable, quebradizo *adj*; rompible *adj*

breakbone fever, dengue *m*

breakdown, colapso; **nervous ~** colapso nervioso; crisis nerviosa *f*; depresión nerviosa *f*

breakfast, desayuno; **to have ~** desayunar(se)

breast, agarraderas *f, Chicano*; busto; chichas *CR*; chiche *f*; chichi *f, Mex*; mama; pecho; pechos *m, fam*; seno; tele *f, Chicano*; teta *slang*; **~** (*of a wet nurse*) chiche *m, Mex, Guat*; **big ~s** petacas *Mex, Anat*; **caked ~** mastitis por estasis *f*; pezón enlechado *m*; **~ cancer** cáncer del seno *m*; **to ~ feed** amamantar *form*; criar con pecho *Chicano*; dar chiche; dar de mamar; dar de pecho; dar el pecho; mamar; **~ feeding** (el) dar pecho; lactancia maternal;

lactancia natural; **gathered ~** absceso de mama; mastitis flemonosa *f*; **heaviness in ~s** pechos pesados; senos pesados; **painful ~** seno doloroso; **~ pump** bomba de ordeñar; mamadera; sacaleche *m*; tiraleche *m*; **~ self-examination** auto exploración de las mamas *f*; autoexamen mensual de los senos *m*

breastbone, esternón *m*; hueso del pecho

breath, aliento; **bad ~** mal aliento; **bad ~ from alcohol** tufo *PR*; **~ holding** espasmos respiratorios; pausas apneicas; **short of ~** corto de resuello; **shortness of ~** ahogos; corto de respiración; falta del aire; sensación de ahogo *f*; **to be short of ~** faltarle el aire; faltarle la respiración; **to draw one's last ~** exhalar el último suspiro; **to get one's ~ back** recobrar la respiración; **to get out of ~** quedarse sin aliento; **to hold one's ~** aguantar la respiración; detener la respiración; **to take a deep ~** hacer una respiración profunda; respirar profundo

breathalyser, alcohómetro; alcoholímetro

breathe, to, resollar (ue); **~** (*through mouth*) respirar (*por la boca*) *fam*; **~ hard** resoplar; **~ heavily** dar resoplidos; **~ in** inhalar; inspirar *form*; respirar *fam*; tomar aire *fam*; **~ out** botar aire *Carib, SpAm, fam*; expulsar aire *form*; sacar aire *fam, Mex, CA*

breathing, respiración *f*; resuello; **difficulty in ~** respiración dificultosa; **~ exercise** ejercicio respiratorio; **noisy ~** resoplido; **~ tube** tubo de respiración

breathless, jadeante *adj*

breathlessness, desaliento; disnea *form*

breech, (*buttocks*) nalgas *f*, *pl*; trasero; **~ birth** (*frank birth*) presentación de nalgas *f*; presentación trasera *f*; **~ delivery** parto de nalgas; **~ presentation** presentación pélvica *f*, *form*

brewer's yeast, levadura de cerveza

brick, (*slang, usually a kilo of marijuana or narcotics*) ladrillo[2]

bridge, puente *m*, *Dent, Mex, Carib, Ríopl*; **fixed ~** puente fijo; **removable ~** puente movible; **~ of the nose** dorso de la nariz; caballete *m*

bridgework, prótesis dental *f*; puente dental *m*

brief, breve *adj*

bright, brillante *adj*; claro *adj*

bring, to, traer; **~ a patient through** operar con éxito a un paciente; **~ on** causar; provocar

brittle, frágil *adj*; quebradizo *adj*; deleznable *adj*; **~ bones** osteogénesis imperfecta *f*; **~ diabetes** diabetes lábil *f*

broach, escariador *m*, *Dent*

broad-spectrum, amplio espectro; (*See antibiotic.*)

broiled, asado *adj*

broken, quebrado *adj*; roto *adj*; **~** (*health*) arruinado *adj*; deshecho *adj*, *Med*; estragado *adj*; quebrantado *adj*; **~** (*language*) chapurreado; **~ down** hundido *adj*; colapsado *adj*

bromide, bromuro

bromine, bromo

bromocriptine, bromocriptina

bronchial, bronquial *adj*

bronchiole, bronquíolo; **alveolar ~** bronquíolo alveolar; **respiratory ~** bronquíolo respiratorio; **terminal ~** bronquíolo terminal

bronchitis, bronquitis *f*; inflamación de los pulmones *f*; pechuguera *Bol, Col, Mex*; **acute ~** bronquitis aguda; **chronic ~** bronquitis crónica; **croupous ~**

bronquitis crupal; **exudative ~** bronquitis exudativa; **productive ~** bronquitis productiva; **secondary ~** bronquitis secundaria

bronchodilator, bronquiodilatador *m*

bronchology, broncología

bronchopneumonia, bronconeumonía

bronchoscope, broncoscopio

bronchoscopy, broncoscopía; broncoscopia

bronchospasm, broncoespasmo; broncospasmo

bronchospirometer, broncospirómetro (*aparato usado para medir la capacidad respiratoria de cada pulmón*)

bronchospirometry, broncospirometría

bronchus, (*pl*, **bronchi**) bronquio

bronze-skinned, trigueño *adj*

broom, escoba

broth, caldo

brother, hermano; **~-in-law** (*pl*, **brothers-in-law**) cuñado

brow, **~** (*eye*) ceja; **~** (*forehead*) frente *f*

brown, pardo *adj*

bruise, contusión *f*, *form*; lastimadura; magullamiento; morete *m*, *Mex*, *Hond*; patacón *m*, *Chi*; ramalazo; raspón *m*, *SpAm*; totuma *Chi*; verdón *m*, *Arg*; **~** (*contusion*) magulladura; moretón *m*; **~** (*on the body*) cardenal *m*

bruise, to, causar moretones; hacerse moretones

bruised, contusionado *adj*; magullado *adj*; **~** (*all over*) moreteado *adj*, *Chicano*; **~** (*in one area*) amoratado *adj*; que tiene moretón

bruit, ruido; soplo; **aneurysmal ~** soplo aneurismático; **~ placentaire** soplo placentario; **systolic ~** soplo sistólico

brunette, moreno *m*, *adj*; trigueño *m*, *adj*

brush, cepillo

brush, to, **~ one's hair** cepillarse el pelo; **~ one's teeth** cepillarse los dientes

brushing, cepillado

bubble, burbuja

bubblegum, goma

bubbling rale, estertor de burbujas *m*

bubo, (*pl*, **buboes**) búa; bubón *m*; ganglio; incordio; seca *fam*

bubonic plague, peste bubónica *f*

buccal, bucal *adj*; **~ surface** superficie bucal *Dent*, *f*

buccolingual, bucolingual *Dent*, *adj*; **~ relationship** relación bucolingual *f* (*la posición de un diente en relación a la lengua y el carrillo*)

buck tooth, diente salido *m*; diente saliente *m*; diente saltón *m*

bucket, balde *m*; cubo

buckle, hebilla

buckle, to, abrochar(se); **~** (*knees*) doblarse; **~ up** ceñirse el cinturón de seguridad

bud, yema; **end ~** yema terminal; **taste ~** botón gustativo; bulbo gustativo

buffer, amortiguador *m*; tampón *m*

buffered, amortiguado *adj*

buffering, amortiguamiento

bug, **~** (*slang*, *germ*) microbio; **~** (*insect*) bicho; insecto

build, físico; **~ up** acumulación *f*; depósito

build up, to, acumularse; **~** (*one's strength*, *etc.*) fortalecer; **~** (*one's resistance*) aumentar

bulb, bulbo; **auditory ~** bulbo auditivo; **gustatory ~** bulbo gustatorio; **olfactory ~** bulbo olfatorio; **syringe ~** pera; perilla; **tooth ~** bulbo dental; **~** *Elect* bombilla; **~** (*of thermometer*) ampolleta

bulging, abombado *adj*; protuberante *adj*; **~** (*eyes*) saltón *adj*; **~ eyes** ojos capotudos *Chicano*; ojos saltones

bulimia, bulimia
bulimic, bulímico *adj*
bullet, bala; ~ **wound** balazo; plomazo *CA, Mex*
bump, bola; bolita; camote *m, CA, Chi*; chibola *CA*; chibolo *Col, Ec, Hond, Perú*; pecota *Chi, Anat*; pelota; poporo *Col, Ven*; porcino *Med*; protuberancia *form*; totuma *Chi*; tolondro *Med*; ~ (*due to trauma, esp. head*) chichón *m*; ~ **on the back** totuma *Chi*; totumo *Chi*; ~ **on the head** testarada *fam*; testarazo *fam*; totumo *Chi*
bump one's head, to, darse una testarada
bunch, (*of hair*) mechón *m*
bundle, fascículo; ~ **branch** rama fascicular; ~ **branch block** bloqueo de rama; **muscle** ~ fascículo muscular
buns, (*buttocks*) cachas, *slang, pl, PR*
bunion, juanete *m*
bur, astilla (de metal)*Dent*; fresa
burdened with pain, agobiado de dolor *adj*
burn, quemadada; quemadura; quemazón *m*; **acid** ~ quemadura por ácido; **alkali** ~ quemadura por álcali; ~ **center** centro para víctimas de quemaduras; **chemical** ~ quemadura química; **dry heat** ~ quemadura por calor seco; **flame** ~ quemadura por llama; **flash** ~ quemadura por explosión; **friction** ~ quemadura por fricción; quemadura por frotamiento; **radiation** ~ quemadura causada por radiaciones calóricas, rayos x, cuerpos radiactivos, etc.; ~ (*scald*) escaldadura; **sun** ~ eritema solar *m*; quemazón *m*; solanera
burn (oneself), to, quemar(se); ~ (*to sting*) arder; ~ **out** consumir(se)
burning, ardiente *adj*; quemante *adj*; urente *adj, Med*; ~ **sensation** ardor *m*; ~ **on urination** ardor al orinar *m*
burp, eructo; regüeldo
burp, to, eructar; erutar; repetir (i) *fam*; urutar *Chicano*; ~ (*a baby*) hacer eructar; sacar (el) aire *Chicano*
burping, (*sour*) eructo acedo
burr, (*See bur.*)
bursa, bolsa
bursitis, bursitis *f*; **Achilles** ~ bursitis aquiliana *f*
burst, to, reventar(se) (ie)
bus, guagua *PR*; autobús *m*
bust, busto *slang*
busted, to be, ser arrestado; ser torcido
busy, en la movida *PR*; ocupado *adj*; ~ (*place*) de mucho movimiento
Butazolidin, Butazolidina
butt, *vulg* nalgas; (*See buttocks.*)
butt, to, topar *Dent*
butter, mantequilla
butterfingers, to have, tener un sapo en la mano *PR*
buttock, anca; aparato *Chicano*; bombo *Ur*; (*buns*) cachas *pl, PR*; común *m, Mex*; culo *Arg, fam*; fondillo *Cu*; fondongo *slang*; fundillo *Mex*; glúteo; nalga; olla *slang, Chicano*; pellín *m, Chicano*; petacas *Mex, Anat*; posaderas *f, pl*; posas *f, pl*; salvohonor *m, fam*; sentadera
button, botón *m*
button up, to, abotonar(se); abrochar(se)
buttonhole, ojal *m*
buzz, zumbido; **to get a** ~ agarrar onda; **to have a** ~ (*effect of a drug*) sonarse
buzz, to, zumbar
buzzed, to be, (*See high, to be; blasted, to be.*)
buzzing in the ears, zumbido de oídos

buzzer, chicharra *PR*
by hand, a mano
by-pass, derivación *f*; desviación *f*; cortocircuito; ~ (*coronary*) by-pass *m, Chicano*; puente coronario *m*; puente externo *m*; ~ operation operación de derivación *f*
by product, producto accesorio; subproducto

---

² This is new vocabulary, not necessarily listed nor yet recognized by the Royal Academy of Spanish Grammar. It is understood that this vocabulary is primarily slang. Unless otherwise indicated, the gender of nouns is assumed to be obvious.
³ For pronunciation purposes, the masculine definite and indefinite articles, *el* and *un*, not *la* or *una*, are used when the article immediately precedes the feminine singular noun which begins with stressed *a* or any other that begins with stressed *ha*.
⁴ This symptom is the result of eating *hot* foods.

C

cadaver, cadáver *m*
cadmium, cadmio; ~ **bromide** bromuro de cadmio; ~ **iodide** yoduro de cadmio; ~ **sulfate** sulfato de cadmio
caesarean, cesariano *adj*; cesáreo *adj*; cesárea *f*; ~ **delivery** parto cesáreo; parto por operación; ~ **section** operación cesárea *f*; sección cesárea *f*
cafeteria, cafetería
caffeine, cafeína
caftan, caftán *m*
cage, caja
caisson disease (*the bends*), enfermedad de los buzos *f*
cake, to, formar costra
caked breast, congestión mamaria *f, fam*; mastitis por estasis *f*
calamine, calamina
calcification, calcificación *f*
calcify, to, calcificar(se)
calcium, calcio; ~ **bisulfite** bisulfito de calcio; ~ **carbonate** carbonato de calcio; ~ **caseinate** caseinato de calcio; ~ **channel blocker** bloqueador de los canales de calcio *m*; ~ **gluconate** gluconato de calcio; ~ **sulfate** escayola; sulfato de calcio
calamity, guama *Col, Ven*
calculate, to, calcular
calculation, cálculo
calculus, cálculo
calf, (*pl, calves*) ~ (*animal*) ternera; ~ (*part of leg*) pantorrilla; camote *m, Guat*; chamorro *fam*; platanillo *fam*; ~ **bone** peroné *Anat, m*
calibrate, to, calibrar; ~ (*thermometer*) graduar
calibrator, calibrador *m*
calisthenics, calistenia; calisténica

call, visita; **on** ~ de guardia; **office** ~ visita al consultorio; **house** ~ visita al hogar
call, to, llamar; ~ (*housecall*) pasar visita
calliper, aparato ortopédico; compás *m*
callosity, callosidad *f*; dureza *Med*; duricia
calloused, calloso *adj*
callus, callo; callosidad *f*; **ensheathing** ~ callo envolvente
calm, ~ (*person*) tranquilo *adj*; ~ (*weather*) calmoso *adj*; ~ (*sensation*) calma
calm, to, calmar; ~ **down** calmarse; tranquilizarse
calmative, calmante *m*; sedante *m*
calmness, sosiego; tranquilidad *f*
caloric, calórico *m, adj*
calorie, caloría
camomile tea, agua³ de manzanilla *ethn*; té de manzanilla *m, ethn*
camp fever, tifus exantemático *m*; (*See fever, exanthematous and typhus, epidemic.*)
camphor, alcanfor *m*
can, bote *m*; lata; ~ (*usually for carrying milk*) purrón *m, PR*; ~ **opener** abrelatas *m, inv*
canal, canal *m*; conducto; **abdominal** ~ conducto inguinal; **alimentary** ~ conducto alimentario; tubo digestivo; **alveolar** ~ conducto dental; **auditory** ~ canal auditivo; **birth** ~ canal del parto; **bony** ~ **of the ear** conducto semicircular óseo; **cochlear** ~ conducto coclear; **Fallopian** ~ acueducto de Falopio; **interlobular biliary** ~ conducto biliar interlobulillar; **lacrimal** ~ canal lagrimal; **medullary** ~ cavidad

medular *f*; **nasal** ~ conducto nasal; **pulp** ~ conducto de la pulpa; **root** ~ conducto radicular; **semicircular** ~ conducto semicircular; **tympanic** ~ conducto timpánico

cancel, to, anular; cancelar

cancellous, esponjoso *adj*

cancer[4], cáncer[4] *m*; **breast** ~ cáncer de la mama *m, form*; cáncer del seno *m*; cáncer del pecho *m*; **lung** ~ cáncer del pulmón *m*; ~ **patient** canceroso *adj*; **prostate** ~ cáncer de la próstata; **to get** ~/**to have** ~ cancerarse

cancerous, canceroso *adj*; ~ **cell** célula cancerosa; ~ **tissue** tejido canceroso; ~ **tumor** tumor canceroso *m*; **to become** ~ cancerarse

candidate, candidato

candidiasis, candidiasis *f*

candle, vela; bujía; candela

candy, ~ (*barbiturates*) barbitúricos; ~ (*cocaine*)[6] carga[2]; coca; cocaína; nieve[2] *f*; perico[2] *Cu*; talco[2] *Tex, Cu*; ~ (*made with shredded coconut*) besito *PR*; ~ (*made of molasses and coconut*) mampostial *m, PR*; marrayo *PR*; ~ (*one piece of sweets*); dulce *m*; (*sweets*) dulces *m, pl*; bombón *m*

cane, báculo; bastón *m*; **walking** ~ bastón de paseo *m*

canker, llaga ulcerosa; ulceración bucal *f*; úlcera maligna; ~ **sore** afta[3]; angina herpética; llaga ulcerosa; pequeña úlcera en la boca; postemilla; úlcera gangrenosa; ulceración *f*

cannery, canería

cannula, cánula; **nasal** ~ cánula nasal

cap, ~ (*capsule*) cápsula; ~ (*drug abuse terms*) cachucha[2]; deque[2] *m*; gorra[2]; corona *Dent*; ~ (*head covering*) gorro; ~ (*of a bottle*) tapa; ~ (*of a needle*) protector *m*; **cervical** ~ capuchón cervical *m*;

gorro cervical; **safety** ~ tapa de seguridad

capable, capaz *adj*

capacity, capacidad *f*; **total lung** ~ capacidad pulmonar total

capillary, capilar *m*; capilaria; vaso capilar

capsule, cápsula

car sickness (*kinetosis*), cinesia; cinetosis *f*; mareo en un vehículo

carbohydrate, carbohidrato

carbon, carbono; ~ **dioxide** anhídrido carbónico; bióxido de carbono; dióxido de carbono; ~ **monoxide** monóxido de carbono; óxido de carbono; ~ **tetrachloride** tetracloruro de carbón; tetracloruro de carbono

carbonate, carbonato

carbuncle, ántrax *m*; carbunco

carcinoid, carcinoide *m, adj*

carcinoma, carcinoma *m*; **acute** ~ carcinoma agudo; **basal cell** ~ carcinoma basocelular; **small cell** ~ carcinoma de células pequeñas; **squamous cell** ~ carcinoma de células escamosas; carcinoma espinocelular

card, tarjeta

cardiac, cardíaco *adj*; cardiaco *adj*; ~ **arrest** fallo cardíaco; paro cardíaco; ~ **by-pass** circulación extracorpórea *f*; ~ **care** cuidado cardíaco; ~ **care unit/CCU** sala de cuidado cardíaco; ~ **chambers** cavidades cardíacas *f*; ~ **insufficiency** insuficiencia cardíaca; ~ **output** débito cardíaco; gasto cardíaco; ~ **problems** problemas cardíacos *m*; ~ **sphincter** esfínter del cardias *m*; ~ **standstill** paro cardíaco

cardiogenic, cardiogénico *adj*; cardiógeno *adj*

cardiogram, cardiograma *m*; **esophageal** ~ cardiograma esofágico

cardio-inhibitory, cardioinhibidor *adj*

cardiologist, cardiólogo

cardiology, cardiología

cardiomyopathy, cardiomiopatía; **alcoholic** ~ cardiomiopatía alcohólica; **dilated** ~ cardiomiopatía dilatada; **hypertrophic** ~ cardiomiopatía hipertrófica; **restrictive** ~ cardiomiopatía restrictiva

cardiopulmonary resuscitation/ CPR, reanimación cardiopulmonar *f*; resucitación cardiopulmonar/RCP *f*

cardiopulmonary resuscitator, resucitador cardiopulmonar *m*

cardioscope, cardioscopio

cardiovascular, cardiovascular *adj*; ~ **disease** enfermedad cardiovascular *f*; ~ **reactivity** reactividad cardiovascular *f*; ~ **system** aparato cardiovascular; sistema cardiovascular *m*

care, atención *f*; cuidado; **cardiac** ~ **unit/CCU** sala de cuidado cardíaco; **health** ~ atención médica *f*; **health ~ worker** trabajador de salud; **intensive** ~ cuidado intensivo; cuidado intenso; **medical** ~ ayuda médica; **prenatal** ~ atención prenatal *f*; cuidado prenatal; **primary** ~ atención del primer nivel *f*; atención primaria *f*; **to be under the ~ of** estar bajo el cuidado de; **to take ~ of** atender (ie) (a); **to take ~ of oneself** cuidarse

care for, to, cuidar (a)

carefree, despreocupado *adj*; paciente *adj, PR*

careful, cuidadoso *adj*; **to be (very)** ~ tener (mucho) cuidado

carefully, con cuidado *prep phr*; cuidadosamente *adv*

caregiver, cuidador

careless (*neglected*), descuidado *adj*

carelessness, descuido

caress, to, amasar

caries, caries *f, inv*; cavidad dental *f*; diente podrido *m*

carotene, caroteno

carotid, carótida; carotídeo *adj*

carrier (**of disease**), portador (de enfermedad); portador de microbios; **active** ~ portador activo; **hemophiliac** ~ portadora hemofílica; ~ (**of**) vehículo (de) *Med*

carry, to, cargar; llevar; portar; ~ (*microbes*) tra(n)smitir *Med*; ~ **on a stretcher** llevar en camilla; ~ **out** llevar a cabo; ~ **over** transferir (ie); transportar

cartilage, cartílago; menisco; ~ **of the nose** ternilla *Cu, Mex, Nic*

cartilaginous, cartilaginoso *adj*; ternilloso *adj*

cartridge, ampolla

case, caso; ~ **fatality rate** mortalidad de una enfermedad *f*; ~ **history** historia clínica; **just in** ~ para estar seguro; por precaución; por si acaso; **in** ~ **of** en el caso de que; ~ **report** observación médica *f*; presentación de un caso clínico *f*

casein, caseína

cash, al contado; efectivo

cashier, cajera; ~**'s office/window** caja

cast, ~ (*cylinder*) cilindro; **blood** ~ cilindro sanguíneo; cilindro hemático; **fatty** ~ cilindro adiposo; cilindro grasoso; **pus** ~ cilindro purulento; **urinary** ~ cilindro urinario; ~ (*model*) modelo (dental); **diagnostic** ~ modelo de diagnóstico; **master** ~ modelo patrón; **positive** ~ modelo positivo; ~ (*slight squint*) ligero estrabismo; ~ (*for immobilizing broken limb*) enyesadura; escayola; vendaje enyesado *m*; yeso; **gypsum** ~ vendaje de yeso *m*; **walking** ~ enyesadura para caminar; **to put in a** ~ enyesar; poner en yeso

cast, to, ~ **a spell on** hechizar; ~ **off** descartar; desechar

casting, vaciado *Dent*; colado *Dent*; ~ **flask** caja para vaciado; mufla refractaria; ~ **ring** anillo para vaciado *Dent*; ~ **wax** cera para vaciado *Dent*

castor oil, aceite de castor *m*; aceite de ricino *m*

castrate, to, castrar

castration, castración *f*

casualties list, lista de accidentados

casualty, ~ (*person*) accidentado; víctima; ~ (*event*) accidente *m*; desastre *m*; muerte violenta *f*

CAT/computerized axial tomography, TAC/tomografía axial computarizada

catalyst, catalizador *m*

cataplasm, cataplasma

cataract, catarata; granizo; nube en el ojo *f*, *fam*; **adherent** ~ catarata adherente; **congenital** ~ catarata congénita; **diabetic** ~ catarata diabética; **incipient** ~ catarata incipiente; **immature** ~ catarata inmadura; **irradiation** ~ catarata por radiación; **juvenile** ~ catarata juvenil; **mature** ~ catarata madura; **milky** ~ catarata lechosa; **overripe** ~ catarata hipermadura; **primary** ~ catarata primaria; **ripe** ~ catarata madura

catarrh, catarro

catatonia, catatonía

catatonic, catatónico *adj*

catch, to, coger; ~ (*to get hooked*) (*on*) engancharse (en); ~ (*the voice*) quebrarse; ~ **a cold** coger un resfriado; ~ **a disease** agarrar; contraer una enfermedad; darle (a uno) una enfermedad; pegarle (a uno); ~/**come down with a disease** caer con algo; contagiarse de; ~ **fire** (*to burst into flames*) incendiarse; ~ **fire** (*to start burning*) encenderse; ~ **on** comprender; ~ **one's breath** agarrar aire; recobrar el aliento; tomar aire; ~ **someone doing something illegal or forbidden** mangar; ~ **up** poner al día

catching, contagioso *adj*; pegadizo *adj*, *Med*; pegajoso *adj*, *Med*

catching, to be, pegarse *Med*

categorization, clasificación *f*

categorize, to, clasificar

category, clase *f*

caterpillar, oruga

catgut, catgut *m*

catharsis, catársis *f*; purificación emocional *f*

cathartic, purga *Med*; purgante *m*

catheter, catéter *m*; drenaje *m*, *Chicano*; sonda; tubo; **dwelling** ~ catéter permanente; **elbowed** ~ sonda acodada; **flexible** ~ sonda flexible; **Foley** ~ sonda de Foley; **Hickman** ~ catéter de Hickman; **Tenckhoff** ~ catéter de Tenckhoff; **Texas** ~ sonda de Tejas; **two-way** ~ sonda de doble corriente

catheterization, cateterismo; sondaje *m*; sondeo; **cardiac** ~ cateterismo cardíaco; **duodenal** ~ sondaje duodenal; **esophageal** ~ sondaje esofágico; **gastric** ~ sondaje gástrico; **permanent** ~ cateterismo permanente; **tubal** ~ cateterismo tubárico; **vesical** ~ cateterismo vesical; sondaje ureteral; sondaje vesical

catheterize, to, cateterizar; sondear

caucasian, caucasiano *adj*

caudal, coccígeo *adj*

cause, causa; ~ **of death** causa de muerte

cause, to, causar; engendrar; ~ **vomiting** provocarse el vómito

cauterization, cauterización *f*

cauterize, to, cauterizar

cautious, cauteloso *adj*; prudente *adj*; apendejao *adj*, *PR*, *vulg*

cavity, (**dental**) ~ carie *f*, *inv*, *form*; cavidad (dental) *f*; diente cariado *m*; diente picado *m*; guijón *m*; picadura *fam*; ~ (*space*) cavidad *f*; **abdominal** ~ cavidad abdominal; **alveolar** ~ cavidad alveolar; **amniotic** ~ cavidad amniótica;

cranial ~ cavidad craneal; **epidural** ~ cavidad epidural; **lymph** ~ cavidad linfática *f*; **mastoid** ~ cavidad mastoidea; **nasal** ~ fosa nasal; **oral** ~ boca; **pelvic** ~ cavidad pélvica; **pericardial** ~ cavidad pericardíaca; **peritoneal** ~ cavidad peritoneal; **pleural** ~ cavidad pleural; **pulp** ~ cavidad pulpar; **thoracic** ~ cavidad torácica; **tympanic** ~ cavidad timpánica, caja del tímpano; **visceral** ~ cavidad esplácnica; cavidad visceral

CBC/complete blood count, recuento hemático completo; recuento sanguíneo completo

CC/chief complaint, queja principal; síntoma principal *m*

cc/cubic centimeter, cc/centímetro cúbico

CCU/coronary care unit, unidad de asistencia coronaria *f*; unidad de cuidado cardíaco *f*; sala de cuidado cardíaco

cecum, (*pl, ceca*) ciego; intestino ciego; fondo de saco

celiac disease, celíaca; celiaquía

cell, célula; **B** ~ célula B, célula beta; **blood** ~ glóbulo; célula sanguínea; **red blood** ~ glóbulo rojo; **white blood** ~ glóbulo blanco; **ciliated** ~ célula ciliada; **islet** ~ célula insular; **marrow** ~ célula medular; **nucleated** ~ célula nucleada; **plasma** ~ célula plasmática; **sickle** ~ célula falciforme; drepanocito; **squamous** ~ célula escamosa; **T** ~ célula T; ~ **tissue** tejido celular

cellular, celular *adj*; ~ **division** división celular *f*; división de células *f*; ~ **growth** crecimiento celular

cellulitis, celulitis *f*

cement, cemento; **tooth** ~ cemento dentario

cementum, cemento

center, centro; **day-care** ~ guardería infantil; **health care** ~ centro de salud

centigrade, centígrado

centimeter, centímetro; **cubic** ~ centímetro cúbico

centipede, centípedo; ciempiés, *m, inv*

central, central *adj*; ~ **console** consola central; ~ **line** catéter central *m*; ~ **nervous system** sistema nervioso central *m*

cephalic, cefálico *adj*

cerebellum, (*pl, cerebella*) cerebelo

cerebral, cerebral *adj*; ~ **cortex** corteza cerebral; materia gris *fam*; ~ **hemisphere** hemisferio cerebral; ~ **palsy** parálisis cerebral *f*; ~ **paralysis** parálisis cerebral *f*; ~ **vascular accident** derrame del cerebro *m*; embolio; estroc *m, Chicano*

cerebrospinal meningitis, meningitis cerebroespinal *f*; meningitis cerebrospinal *f*

cerebrovascular, cerebrovascular *adj*

cerebrum, cerebro; **anterior chamber of the** ~ cámara anterior del cerebro; **posterior chamber of the** ~ cámara posterior del cerebro

certain, cierto *adj*

certificate, certificado; acta[3]; partida; **baptismal** ~ partida de bautismo; **birth** ~ acta[3] de nacimiento; certificado de nacimiento; **marriage** ~ partida de matrimonio; ~ **of death** certificado de defunción; partida de defunción; ~ **of fitness** certificado de aptitud

certify, to, certificar

cerumen, cera del oído

cervical, cervical *adj*; ~ **cap** (*See cap, cervical.*)

cervix, cervix *f*; cerviz *f*; cuello de la matriz *fam*; cuello del útero; cuello uterino

Cesarean, (*See Caesarean.*)

cesium, cesio
chafe, rozadura
chafe, to, rozar(se); raer *Med*
chafing, piel roja *f*; rozadura; espejeras *f, pl, Cu*
chain, cadena; **~ reaction** reacción en cadena *f*
challenge injection, inyección de prueba *f*
chamber, cámara; cavidad *f*; **air ~** *Dent* cámara vacía; **~s of the eye** cámaras oculares; **~s of the heart** cámaras del corazón; **pulp ~** cámara pulpar *Dent*
chamberpot, orinal *m*; pava *Chi, Mex*; papagayo *Perú*; tiesto *Chi*
chance, casual *adj*; fortuito *adj*; **~** (*possibility*) probabilidad *f*; posibilidad *f*; **~ of survival** probabilidad de sobrevivir; posibilidad de supervivencia
chancre, chancro; **hard ~** chancro duro; **soft ~** chancro blando
chancroid, chancroide *f*
change, cambio; modificación *f*; **~ in appetite** cambio de apetito; **~ in libido** cambio en el libido; **~ in weight** cambio de peso; **~ of life** cambio de vida; menopausia
change, to, cambiar (de); **~** (*oneself*) cambiar(se); **~** (*to become*) transformarse
changing room, vestuario
channel, canal *m*; conducto; **auriculoventricular ~** conducto auriculoventricular
chap, to, agrietarse; partirse; **~ skin** rozarse; pasparse *SpAm*
chapped, agrietado *adj*; cuarteado *adj*; partido *adj*; rozado *adj*; **~ skin** paspa *Bol, Ec, Perú*; paspadura *Ríopl*
character, carácter *m*; **~ disorder** enfermedad del carácter *f*; enfermedad moral *f*; **dominant ~** carácter dominante; **primary sex ~** carácter sexual primario; **recessive ~** carácter recesivo;

secondary sex ~ carácter sexual secundario; **sex-linked ~** carácter ligado al sexo
characteristic, característico *adj*; característica
characterize, to, caracterizar
charcoal, carbón *m*; **activated ~** carbón activado
charge, cobro; costo; **itemized ~** cobro detallado; **no ~** sin cobro; **~ nurse** enfermera de cargo; enfermera de sección; **total ~/cost** monto; **~** (*responsibility*) cargo; **~** (*of a furnace, battery, etc.*) carga
charge, to, cobrar
charged up, to be[5] (*See high, to be, and blasted, to be.*)
charitable, caritativo *adj*
chart, cartelón *m*; diagrama *m*; gráfica; hoja clínica; tabla expediente; **eye ~** carta de examen visual; **Snellen ~** carta de Snellen; cartelón de Snellen; **temperature ~** gráfico de la temperatura
chat, to, paliquear; rapiar *Chicano*
chatter, to, (**teeth**), castañetear
check, cheque *m*; **~** (*test*) repaso; inspección *f*; **~** (*control*) control *m*
check-up, chequeo *Chicano*; chequeo general médico *Chicano*; reconocimiento médico; revisión médica *f*
cheek, **~** (*nerve*) fuerza de cara; **~** (*of buttock*) cacha; **~** (*part of face*) cachete *m, fam*; mejilla; **~** (*inside wall of mouth*) carrillo
cheekbone, hueso malar; pómulo *f*
cheerful, alegre *adj*
cheese, queso; **big ~ in dope ring** peje grande[2] *PR*
cheesy, caseoso *adj, vulg*
cheilitis, queilitis *f*
cheilosis (*sore at corner of mouth*), boquilla *fam*; queilosis *f, form*
chemical, químico *adj*; **~ changes** modificaciones químicas *f*; **~** sustancia química

chemistry, química; **applied** ~ química aplicada; **forensic** ~ química forense; **inorganic** ~ química mineral; **organic** ~ química orgánica; **physical** ~ química física

chemosis, quemosis *f*

chemosurgery, quimiocirugía

chemotherapy, quimioterapia

chest, pecho *fam*; tórax *m*, *form*; **barrel** ~ tórax en tonel; ~ **pains** dolores en el pecho *m*; ~ **surgery** cirugía torácica; ~ **trouble** pechuguera *Bol, Col, Mex*; ~ **wall** pared torácica *f*

chew, to, mascar; masticar

chewing gum, wad of, mascaura

chicken pox/chickenpox, bobas *fam*; peste cristal *f*, *fam*; tecunda *Mex*; varicela *form*; viruela de gallina *slang*; viruelas locas *Mex, CA, fam*; payuelas *f, pl*

chigger, nigua; pique *m*; ~ **flea** garrapata; güina *Mex*

chigoe, nigua; chigo; chigra; chinche *f*

chilblain, sabañón *m*

child, cabro *Chi*; chamaco *Mex*; chico *Cu, Pan*; cipote *El Sal*; guagua *PR*; niño; ñaño *Col, Perú*; patojo *CA, Col, Guat*; pebete *Ríopl*; pelado *Bol, Col, Pan*; pericote *m, Arg, Perú*; pibe, piba *m/f, Bol, Chi, Ríopl*; pirinola *Mex*; piscoiro *Chi*; poroto *Chi*; purrete *m, Ríopl*; semilla *Chi*; ~ **abuse** maltrato de los niños; ~ **approaching puberty** púber *m/f*; **badly behaved** ~ majadero *PR*; **homeless** ~ guacho *Chi, Perú, Ríopl*; **hyperactive** ~ jiribilla *PR*; **illegitimate** ~ guacho *Chi, Perú, Ríopl*; **little** ~ tripón *Mex*; **sickly** ~ zocato *Mex*

childbearing, gestación *f*; ~ **age** edad procreadora *f*

childbed fever, fiebre puerperal *f*; pasmo del parto

childbirth, alumbramiento; parto; **multiple** ~ parto múltiple; **natural** ~ parto natural; **premature** ~ parto prematuro

childhood, infancia; niñez *f*

childless, infecundo *adj*; sin hijos *prep phr*

chili pepper, ají *m*

chill, escalofrío; chucho *SpAm, Med*; pasmazón *m, Med, CA, Mex, PR*; resfriado; ~**s** calo(s) fríos *slang*; tiritones *m, pl*; ~**s and fever** fiebre intermitente *f*; **to have** ~**s** entrarle calores y fríos *fam*

chin, barba; barbilla; mentón *m*; piocha *fam*

chip, astilla; pedacito

chip, to, astillar(se); ~ (*to use narcotics frequently*) chipear[2]; chipiar[2]

chiropodist, callista *m/f*; pedicuro; podíatra *m/f*; podiatra *m/f*; podólogo; quiropodista *m/f*

chiropractor, quiropractor, -ra *m/f*; quiropráctico

chirospasm, quiroespasmo; quirospasmo

Chlamydia, Chlamidia

chloasma (*facial discoloration*; *mask of pregnancy*), cloasma *m*; mancha de la preñez; mancha del embarazo; paño

chloramphenicol, cloranfenicol *m*

chloride, cloruro

chlorinated, clorado *adj*

chlorination, cloración *f*

chlorine, cloro

chloroform, cloroformo

chloromycetin, cloromicetín *m*; cloromicetina *m*

chlorophyll, clorofila

chloroquine, cloroquina

chlorpropamide, clorpropamide

chocolate-colored, choco *adj, Bol, Col, Ec, Ríopl*; de color chocolate *prep phr*

choice, opción *f*

choke, to, atorarse; dar al galillo *slang*; ~ (*due to lack of air, fumes*) ahogarse; asfixiar(se); sofocar; ~ **on** (*food, etc.*) atragantarse

choking, ahogo; asfixia

cholangiogram, colangiograma *m*; colangiografía

cholangiography, colangiografía; **percutaneous transhepatic** ~/**PTC** colangiografía transhepática percutánea /CTP

cholecystectomy, colecistectomía

cholecystitis, bilis *f*; dolor de la vesícula biliar *m*; mal de hiel *m*

cholecystogram, colecistograma *m*

cholera, cólera *m*

cholesterol, colesterina; colesterol *m*; grasa en las venas *fam*; ~ **count** nivel de colesterol *m*; ~ **deposit** depósito de colesterol; ~ **level** tasa de colesterol; **to lower the** ~ **count** bajar el nivel del colesterol

choose, to, elegir (i); escoger; seleccionar

chondrosarcoma, condrosarcoma *m*

chorea, baile de San Guido *m*; baile de San Vito *m*; corea; mal de San Guido *m*; mal de San Vito *m*; **Huntington's** ~ corea de Huntington

chorioid/choroid, corioides *f, inv*; coroides *f, inv*

chorionic villi sampling/CVS, muestreo de la vellosidad coriónica

chromium, cromo

chromosome, cromosoma *m*; **sex** ~ cromosoma sexual

chronic, crónico *adj*; duradero *adj*; ~ **cystitis** cistitis crónica *f*; ~ **illness** enfermedad crónica *f*; ~ **respiratory disease** enfermedad crónica respiratoria

chronically, crónicamente *adv*

chubby, rechoncho *adj*; regordete *adj*

church, iglesia

chutzpah, fuerza de cara

cigar, cigarro puro; jumazo *PR*; puro *common*; tabaco *esp*. *Carib*; ~ **band** vitola; ~ **case** cigarrera; petaca; ~ **cutter** cortapuros

cigarette, cigarrillo; cigarro; pitillo *m, fam*; ~ **butt** bachicha[2] (*esp*. *mariguana*); tecla[2]; tecolota[2]; ~ **case** pitillera; ~ **holder** boquilla; ~ **lighter** encendedor *m*; mechero

circle, círculo; ~ (*under the eyes*) ojera

circuit, circuito; **open** ~ circuito abierto; **reflex** ~ circuito reflejo; **short** ~ circuito corto

circular, circular *f, adj*; ~ **of the umbilical cord** circular del cordón

circulate, to, circular

circulation, circulación *f*; **cross** ~ circulación cruzada; **fetal** ~ circulación fetal; **pulmonary** ~ circulación pulmonar; **systemic** ~ circulación mayor; circulación sistémica

circulatory, circulatorio *adj*; ~ (**hematologic**) **system** aparato circulatorio; aparato hematológico; sistema circulatorio *m*; sistema hematológico *m*

circumcise, to, circuncidar

circumcision, circuncisión *f*

cirrhosis, cirrosis *f*; ~ **of the liver** cirrosis del hígado; cirrosis hepática; ~ **of the lung** cirrosis pulmonar

citology, citología

citrate, citrato

citrus fruit, fruta cítrica

city, ciudad *f*

clammy skin, piel viscosa *f*

clamp, clamp *m*; pinza

clamp, to, pinzar

clap (*gonorrhea, slang*), gonorrea

clasp, gancho *Dent*; **bar** ~ gancho en barra *Dent*; ~ (*of hands*) apretón *m*

class, clase *f*

classification, clasificación *f*

claustrophobia, claustrofobia

clavicle, clavícula; (*See collar bone/clavicle.*)

claw, en garra

clay, arcilla; ~**-colored stools** heces depigmentadas *f*

clean, limpio *adj*; **to be ~ (of drugs)** andar derecho[2]; andar limpio[2]

clean, to, limpiar; ~ **oneself** limpiarse; ~ **up** hacer la limpieza; higienizar *SpAm*

cleaning, limpieza (*also Dent*)

cleanliness, aseo; limpieza

clear, claro *adj*; transparente *adj*; **to stand ~ of** apartarse de; mantenerse a distancia de

clear, to, ~ **one's throat** aclararse la voz; carraspear; ~ **up (an illness, rash, etc.)** resolverse (ue); ~ **up**[5] cortarse el vicio[2]; kikear[2] *Chicano*; quitear

clearance, aclaramiento; depuración *f*; **blood-urea ~** depuración ureica; **creatinine ~** depuración de creatinina

clearer, más gráfico *adj*; aclarador *adj*

cleft, hendidura *form*; ~ **lip** labio leporino; ~ **palate** boquineta *Chicano*; grietas en el paladar; hendidura palatina; paladar hendido *m*; paladar partido *m*

clench, to, (*fist*) apretar (ie) (los puños); empuñar *Chi*; ~ (*teeth*) morder (ue) (los dientes)

clenching, rechinamiento de dientes

clerk, dependiente *m/f*

click, chasquido

climax, to (*sexually*), acabar; venirse

climb up, to, subirse

cling to, to, agarrarse; ~ (*clothes*) pegarse *slang*

clinic, ~ (*private place of consultation*) clínica; ~ (*place for free medical assistance*) ambulatorio; dispensario

clinical, clínico *adj*; ~ **laboratory** laboratorio clínico; ~ **thermometer** termómetro clínico

clinician, clínico

clip, clip *m*; grapa

clipped speech, lenguaje titubeante *m*

clitoris, bolita *slang*; clítoris *m*, *form*

clock, reloj *m*; **alarm ~** despertador *m*; **around the ~** durante 24 horas; **biological ~** reloj biológico; **to sleep around the ~** dormir(ue) doce horas seguidas

clog, to, (*to block up*) atascar; ~ (*to hinder movement*) entorpecer; ~ **up** (*to become thick*) espesarse

close, (*near*) cercano *adj*; ~ **relative** pariente cercano *m*; ~ (*intimate*) estrecho *adj*; ~ **relationship** relación estrecha *f*; ~ (*detailed*) minucioso *adj*; ~ (*room ventilation*) mal ventilado *adj*; ~ (*weather*) bochornoso *adj*; ~**-knit** (*family, etc.*) unido *adj*; **to be ~ to each other** ser uña y carne

closed, cerrado *adj*; ~ **system** sistema cerrado *m*

closemouthed, discreto *adj*; callado *adj*

close-shaven, bien afeitado *adj*

close, to, cerrar (ie); ~ (*a wound*) cicatrizarse

clot, coágulo; cuajarón *m*; **blood ~** coágulo sanguíneo; ~ **reaction time** tiempo de retracción del coágulo

clot, to, cuajar

clothes hanger, gancho

clothing, ropa

clotting time, tiempo de coagulación

cloudiness, enturbiamiento; opacidad *f*; ~ **of urine** turbieza de la orina

clouding of consciousness, torpor mental *m*

clubfoot, pie zambo *m*; talipes *m*; corino *PR*

clubfooted, talipédico *adj*

clubhand, mano zampa *f*
clumsiness of gait, marcha torpe; marcha zafia
clumsy, torpe *adj*; incrúspido *adj, Col, Mex, Nic*; ~ (*in movement*) pesado *adj*; ~ **gait** marcha desgarbada
cluster headache, cefalea por acúmulos
clutz, to be a, tener un sapo en la mano *PR*
coagulant, coagulante *m, adj*
coagulation time, tiempo de coagulación
coal tar, brea de hulla; coaltar *m*
coarse, grueso *adj*
coast, to[5], (*See high, to be, and blasted, to be.*)
coat, capa *Anat*; membrana *Anat*; ~ (*overcoat*) abrigo; **white** ~ (*of a doctor, etc.*) bata
coated tongue, lengua saburral; lengua sucia
cobalt, cobalto
cocaine[6], cocaína; acelere[2]; aliviane[2]; alucine[2]; arponazo[2]; azúcar[2] *m*; blanca nieves[2] *f*; carga[2]; chutazo[2]; coca[2]; cocacola[2]; cocada[2]; cocazo[2]; coco[2]; coka[2]; cotorra[2]; cucharazo[2]; doña blanca[2]; glacis[2] *m*; knife[2] *m*; marizazo[2]; nice[2]; nieve[2] *f*; nose[2]; pase[2] *m*; pepsicola[2]; pericazo[2]; perico[2] *Cu, PR*; polvito[2]; polvo[2]; talco[2] *Tex, Cu*; tecata[2]
coccyx, cócciz *m, Chicano, fam*; colita *fam*; coxis *m*; rabadilla *fam*
cochlea, cóclea; (*See ear, inner.*)
cockroach, cucaracha
cocoa butter, manteca de cacao
coconut, coco; ~ **drink** coquito *PR*; **fibrous covering of** ~ cachipa; ~ **oil** aceite de coco *m*
cod liver oil, aceite de hígado de bacalao *m*; aceite de pescado *m*
code of ethics, código de ética
codeine[7], codeína
codfish, fried or fritter, bacalaito
coefficient, coeficiente *m*

coffee, café *m*; **bad** ~ café ralo *PR*; **black without sugar** ~ puya *PR*; ~ **grounds** café molido; posos de café; ~ **shop** café; **small cup of** ~ pocillo; **unsweetened** ~ café soso *PR*; **unsweetened** ~ **with some milk** café término *PR*
coffin, ataúd *m*
cognac, coñac *m*
cognition, percepción *f*
cohabitation, cohabitación *f*
cohesion, cohesión *f*
coil, (*birth control*) alambrito; aparatito; coil *m, Chicano*; tubo de plástico; (*See birth control.*) ~ (*electric*) carrete *m*; ~ (*of a snake*) anillo
coitus, coito; **extravaginal** ~ parapareunia; ~ **interruptus** coito interrumpido; interrupción de coito *f*; **normal** ~ eupareunia; **vaginal** ~ eupareunia
cold, ~ (*disease*) catarro *fam*; resfriado; resfrío; **bad** ~ monga *PR*; **common** ~ resfriado común; **head** ~/"stopped-up" **head** constipado; romadizo; **to have a** ~ tener catarro; tener un resfriado; **to catch a** ~ pescar una monga *PR*; resfriarse; ~ (*temperature*) frío *adj*; ~ **compress** compresa fría; ~ **extremities** extremidades frías *f*; ~ "in the womb" (*suggested cause of sterility*) frío en la matriz *ethn*; ~ **pack** compresa fría; emplasto frío; ~ **sore** fuego en la boca; fuego en los labios; herpes labial *m*; úlcera catarral; úlcera en los labios; ~ **sweats** sudores fríos *m*; **to be** ~ (*a person*) tener frío; **to be** ~ (*the weather*) hacer frío; **to have** ~ **extremities** tener enfriamiento de los pies (o las manos); tener los pies fríos (o las manos frías); ~ **turkey**[5] a la brava[2] *slang*; a lo bronco[2] *slang*; bruscamente *adv*
colectomy, colectomía

colic, cólico *m, adj*
colitis, colitis *f*; **ulcerative** ~ colitis ulcerosa
collagen, colágena; colágeno
collapse, colapso; **physical** ~ colapso físico
collapsing pulse, pulso colapsante
collapse, to, caerse; desplomarse; sufrir un colapso; ~ (*a lung*) colapsarse
collar, collar *m*; **cervical** ~ collar cervical; collarín *m*; ~ (*of clothing, etc.*) cuello
collar bone/clavicle, clavícula *form*; cuenca *Chicano*; hueso del cuello *fam*; puente *m, Col*
colloid, coloide *m*
colon, colon *m*; intestino mayor; **ascending** ~ colon ascendente; **descending** ~ colon descendente; **irritable** ~ colon inestable; colon irritable; **sigmoid** ~ colon sigmoideo; sigma cólico *m*; **spastic** ~ colon espástico
colonoscope, colonoscopio
colonoscopy, colonoscopia; colonoscopía
colony, colonia
color, color *m*; ~ **blind** daltónico *adj*; ~ **blindness** daltonismo *form*; (*See blindness, color.*)
colostomy, colostomía
colostrum, calostro
colposcopy, colposcopia; colposcopía
column, columna; fascículo; **fat** ~ columna adiposa; **respiratory** ~ fascículo solitario; **vertebral** ~ columna vertebral
coma, coma *m*; **alcoholic** ~ coma alcohólico; **diabetic** ~ coma diabético
comatose, comatoso *adj*
comb, peine *m*; **fine-toothed** ~ chino *Mex*
comb one's hair, to, peinarse
combat, to, combatir
come, to, venir; ~ (*sexual climax*); venirse *vulg*; ~ **and go** ir y venir;

~ **back** regresar; volver (ue); ~ **down** bajar(se); ~ **on** empezar (ie); ~ **to a head** (*an abscess*) supurar (un absceso)
comfort, comodidad *f*
comfort, to, consolar
comfortable, agradable *adj*; cómodo *adj*; confortable *adj*; decente *adj*
commisure, comisura
committee, comité *m*
commode, inodoro portátil
common-law marriage, to live with someone in, acortejar *PR*; casar(se) por detrás de la iglesia
communicable, contagioso *adj*; transmisible *adj*
communicate, to, comunicar; ~ **a disease** contagiar
communication, comunicación *f*
communicative, comunicativo *adj*
community, comunidad *f*; comunitario *adj*; ~ **hospital** hospital comunitario *m*; ~ **responsibility** responsabilidad de la comunidad *f*
company, compañía; **insurance** ~ compañía de seguro
compassion, compasión *f*
compatible, compatible *adj*
compelling urge, necesidad urgente *f*
compensate, to, compensar
compensation, compensación *f*; **broken** ~ compensación rota; descompensación *f*
compete, to, competir (i)
competence, competencia; suficiencia
competent, competente *adj*
complain (about/of), to, quejarse (de)
complaint, enfermedad *f*; queja; síntoma *m*; **chief** ~ queja principal; síntoma principal; **chronic** ~ alifafe *m, slang*; **summer** ~ enfermedad estival
complement, complemento

complete, completo *adj*; total *adj*
complex, complejo; **AIDS related** ~ (**ARC**) complejo relacionado con el SIDA; **inferiority** ~ complejo de inferioridad; **Oedipal** ~ complejo de Edipo
complexion, cutis *m*; piel *f, fam*; tez *f*
complexity, complejidad *f*
complicate, to, complicar
complicated, pelú *adj, PR*; **to become** ~ amogollar(se) *PR*
complication, accidente *m*; complicación *f*; secuela
component, componente *m*
compose, to, componer
compound, compuesto; **fatty** ~ compuesto graso; ~ **fracture** fractura complicada; (*See fracture, compound.*); (**un**)**saturated** ~ compuesto (in)saturado
comprehension, listening, comprensión auditiva *f*
comprehensive, exhaustivo *adj*
compress, cabezal *m, Med*; compresa *Med*; **hot** ~**es** aplicaciones calientes *f, pl*
compress, to, comprimir
compression, compresión *f*; ~ **of the brain** compresión del cerebro; **chest** ~**s** compresiones torácicas
compulsion, compulsión *f*
compulsive, compulsivo *adj*
compulsory, necesario *adj*; obligatorio *adj*
computer, computadora
conceal, to, esconder; ocultar
conceive, to, concebir (i)
concentrate, concentrado *Chem*
concentrate, to, concentrar(se); ~ **on** enfocar
concentration, concentración *f*; **hydrogen ion** ~ concentración de iones de hidrógeno
conception, concepción *f*; fecundación del huevo *f*
concerned, inquieto *adj*; preocupado *adj*

conclude, to, concluir
conclusion, conclusión *f*
concussion, concusión *f*; conmoción cerebral *f, Med*; golpe *m*; ~ **of the brain** concusión del cerebro; ~ **of the spine** concusión de la médula espinal
condensed milk, leche condensada *f*
condiment, condimento
condition, condición *f*; estado de salud; estado general; **in bad** ~ escasifoyao *adj, PR*; esguanimao *adj, PR*; esmamoniao *adj, PR*
conditioning, condicionamiento; **air** ~ condicionamiento del aire
condom, condón *m*; forro *Arg, vulg*; goma; hule *m, slang*; preservativo *slang*; profiláctico
conduct, disorderly, relajo
conduction, conducción *f*; **delayed** ~ conducción retardada
condyle, cóndilo
cone, cono; **arterial** ~ cono arterioso; ~ **of light** cono luminoso
cone-shaped, coniforme *adj*
confess, to, confesar (ie)
confidence, confianza
confine to, (*to restrict*) limitar; ~ (*to isolate*) confinar; ~ **in an institution** confinar en una institución
confined to bed, to be, estar encamado; tener que guardar cama
confinement, confinamiento; riesgo; ~ (*childbirth*) alumbramiento; cuarentena[8]; puerperio; sobreparto
conflict, conflicto
conflicting, contradictorio *adj*; contrario *adj*
confront, to, confrontar; enfrentar(se) con
confrontation, confrontación *f*
confuse, to, confundir
confused, confuso *adj*; patidifuso *adj, PR*; ~ / **out of touch with reality** desorientado *adj*; **to become** ~ confundirse

confusion, confusión *f*

congenital, congénito *adj*; ~ **anomaly** anomalía congénita; ~ **defect** defecto congénito; ~ **hip** cadera dislocada de nacimiento; ~ **malformation** defecto de nacimiento; deformación congénita *f*; deformidad congénita *f*; malformación congénita *f*

congested, (*stuffed up*) constipado *adj*; **to be** ~ estar congestionado *adj*; estar constipado *adj*; estar obstruido *adj*; tener la congestión; tener tapado (*los oídos, la nariz*)

congestion, constipado; congestión *f, fam*; resfrío *fam*; ~ **of the chest** ahoguijo; ahoguío

conical, cónico *adj*

conjugal, conyugal *adj*

conjunctiva, conjuntiva

conjunctivitis, (*pinkeye*) aire en el ojo *m, fam*; conjuntivitis *f*; conjuntivitis catarral aguda; mal de ojo *m, fam*; oftalmia contagiosa; tracoma *m*; **acute contagious** ~ conjuntivitis aguda contagiosa

connect, to, conectar; conexionar

connection, conexión *f*

connective, conectivo *adj*; ~ **tissue** tejido conjuntivo

conscience, conciencia

conscious, consciente *adj*; **to be** ~ volver (ue) en sí

consciousness, conocimiento *Med*; estado de conciencia; **to lose** ~ perder (ie) el conocimiento; perder (ie) la conciencia; **to regain** ~ volver (ue) en sí

consequence, consecuencia

consent, consentimiento

consent, to, consentir (ie); ~ **to** consentir (ie) en

conservative, conservativo *adj*

conserve, to, conservar

consideration, consideración *f*; **in** ~ **of** en consideración a; **under** ~ en cuestión

console, to, consolar (ue)

constant, constante *adj, f*

constipated, aliñado *adj*; estítico *adj, fam, El Sal*; estreñido *adj*; tapado *adj*; **to be** ~ trancarse *Chi, Mex, Ríopl*; **to become** ~ estreñirse

constipation, aliñamiento; constipación *f, fam*; constipación fecal *f*; coproestasis *m*; dispepsia *fam*; empacho *fam*; entablazón *f, Chicano*; estasis fecal *m*; estómago sucio; estreñimiento; prendimiento *Chi*; **spastic** ~ estreñimiento espasmódico; **to have** ~ estar duro *fam*; estar entripado *fam*

constituent, constituyente *m/f, adj*; ~ **elements** elementos constituyentes

constitute, to, componer; constituir

constrict, to, (*to compress*) oprimir; ~ (*to make narrower*) estrechar; ~ (*a vein*) estrangular

constriction, constricción *f*

constrictor, constrictor *m, adj*

consult, to, consultar

consultant, consultor, -ra *m/f*; especialista *m/f, Med*

consultation, consulta

consulting, consultor, *adj*; ~ **physician** médico consultor; médico de apelación

consume, to, consumir

consumption, consumo; consunción *f*; marasmo; tisis *f*; tuberculosis *f*; **galloping** ~ tisis galopante *f*

consumptive, consuntivo *adj*

contact, contacto; ~ **dermatitis** dermatitis por contacto *f*; **direct** ~ contacto directo; **immediate** ~ contacto inmediato; (**gas permeable**) (**hard**) (**soft**) ~ **lens** lente de contacto (poroso) (duro) (blando); lentilla *Spain*; pupilente *m*; ~ **of teeth** oclusión de los dientes *f*

contagion, contagio

contagious, contagioso *adj*; pegadizo *adj*; pasoso *adj*, *Ec*
contain, to, contener
container, (*receptacle*) recipiente *m*
contaminate, to, (*disease, environment*) contaminar
contaminated, to become, conta-
minarse
contamination, (*of a disease*) contagio; contaminación *f*
content, contenido *m*, *adj*; contento *adj*
context, contexto
contiguity, contigüidad *f*
continual, continuo *adj*
continue, to, continuar; seguir (i);
~ working seguir (i) trabajando
continuous, continuado *adj*; continuo *adj*; seguido *adj*; ~ clasp
gancho continuo *Dent*
continuously, continuamente *adv*
contour, contorno
contoured, contorneado *adj*
contraception, anticoncepción *f*;
contracepción *f*
contraceptive, anticonceptivo *m*,
adj; contraceptivo *m*, *adj*; (*See
birth control—contraceptive.*); ~
jelly gelatina anticonceptiva; ~
pills pastillas anticonceptivas
contract, to, contraer(se); ~ tuberculosis heticarse *PR*, *RD*
contracted, contraído *adj*
contraction, contracción *f*; automatic ventricular ~ contracción
ventricular automática; isometric ~ contracción isométrica;
isotonic ~ contracción isotónica; premature atrial ~ contracción auricular prematura;
premature ventricular ~ contracción ventricular prematura;
f; ~s (*labor pain*) contracciones
de la matriz *Obst*, *f*; contracciones uterinas *f*; dolores del
parto *m*, *fam*
contraindication, contraindicación *f*
contrast medium, medio de contraste

contribute, to, contribuir
contribution, contribución *f*
control, control *m*; regulación *f*;
birth ~ control de la natalidad;
regulación de la natalidad; (*See
birth control.*); reflex ~ regulación refleja
control, to, controlar; regular
controllable, controlable *adj*
contusion, contusión *f*; magulladura; moretón *m*
convalesce, to, convalecer; recobrarse
convalescence, convalecencia
convalescent, convaleciente *m/f*,
adj; ~ home hogar de convalecencia *m*; clínica de reposo
convenient, conveniente *adj*
convergence, convergencia
convert, to, convertir (ie)
convex, convexo *adj*
convolute, convoluto *adj*; retorci-
do *adj*
convolution, circunvolución *f*;
convolución *f*; occipitotemporal ~ lóbulo fusiforme; subtemporal ~ tercera circunvolución
temporal; superfrontal ~
primera circunvolución frontal
convulsion, ataque *m*, *fam*; convulsión *f*; ~s tiritones *m*, *fam*; ~ resulting from fever alferecía fam
cook, to, ~ (*food*) cocer (ue); ~
(*person*) cocinar
cooked, cocido *adj*
cool, fresco *adj*
cooling, enfriamiento
cooperate, to, cooperar
cooperative, cooperativo *adj*;
cooperativa
coordinate, to, coordinar
coordination, coordinación *f*; ~
problems trastornos de coordinación
cope, arco dental *Dent*
cope with, to, enfrentarse a; hacer
frente con
copper, cobre *m*; ~ sulfate sulfato
de cobre

coproculture, coprocultivo
Coramine, coramina
cord, cordón *m*; cuerda; **nerve ~** cordón nervioso; **spermatic ~** cordón espermático; **spinal ~** médula espinal; **umbilical ~** cordón del ombligo *m*; cordón umbilical *m*; **vocal ~** cuerda vocal
core, centro; núcleo
corn, ~ (*food*) maíz *m*; ~ **oil** aceite de maíz; ~ (*on foot*) callo; ~ **plaster** emplasto para callos; parche para callos *m*
cornea, córnea
corner of the mouth, comisura de los labios
corona, corona
coronary, coronario *adj*; ~ **thrombosis** trombosis coronaria *f*
coroner, médico forense
corporal, corporal *adj*
corpse, cadáver *m*; cuerpo *fam*; difunto *fam*; muerto *fam*
corpus luteum, cuerpo lúteo
corpuscle, corpúsculo; glóbulo; **blood ~** corpúsculo de la sangre; **red blood ~** corpúsculo rojo; eritrocito *form*; glóbulo rojo; **white blood ~** corpúsculo blanco; glóbulo blanco; leucocito *form*
correct, correcto *adj*
correct, to, ajustar; corregir (i)
corrective, correctivo *adj*; ~ **lenses** lentes correctivos *m*
correlation, correlación *f*
corrode, to, corroer
corrosion, corrosión *f*
corrosive, corrosivo *adj*
cortex, corteza
corticosteroid, corticosteroide *m*
cortisone, cortisona
corset, corsé *m*
cosmetic, cosmético *m, adj*
cosmetology, cosmetología
cosmic, cósmico *adj*; ~ **rays** rayos cósmicos
cost, gasto
cost, to, costar (ue)
Costa Rican, costarricense *m/f, adj*

cotton, algodón *m*; **absorbent ~** algodón absorbente; ~ **ball** bolita de algodón; torunda de algodón *Mex, CA*; **sterile ~** algodón estéril; ~ **swab** escobillón *m*; hisopillo; hisopo de algodón
cough, tos *f*; tosido *Chi, Guat, Mex*; ~ **drop** gota para la tos; pastilla para la tos; **dry ~** tos seca *f*; **hacking ~** tos fuerte *f*; **loose ~** tos húmeda *f*; ~ **lozenge** pastilla para la tos; trocisco para la tos; **productive ~** tos productiva; tos húmeda; **smoker's ~** tos por fumar; ~ **suppressant** béquico; calmante para la tos *m*; ~ **syrup** jarabe para la tos *m*; **wet ~** tos blanda; tos húmeda; **whooping ~** coqueluche *f*; tos ahogana *Mex*; tos convulsiva *f*; tos ferina *f*; tosferina; ~ **with phlegm** tos con flema; tos desgarrando
cough, to, toser; ~ **up** escupir; expectorar *form*; ~ **up phlegm** desgarrar *Chicano*; esgarrar
Coumadin, Cumadina
counselor, consejero
count, cuenta; recuento; **blood ~** recuento sanguíneo *fam*; (*See blood count.*); **differential blood ~** cuenta leucocitaria diferencial; **direct platelet ~** cuenta directa de plaquetas
count, to, contar (ue)
counter, over the, al contado
country, ~ (*nation*) país *m*; ~ (*rural, not city*) campo; ~ **doctor** médico rural
county, condado
couple, par *m*; **a ~ of** un par de
cousin, primo; **first ~** primo hermano
cover, cubierta; ~ (*lid*) tapa; ~ (*protection*) amparo
cover, to, cubrir; tapar; ~ **up** (*to conceal*) encubrir; ~ **up** (*to put on*) abrigarse
CPR/cardiopulmonary resuscitation, resucitación cardio-

pulmonar *f*; reanimación cardiopulmonar/RCP[11] *f*
crab louse, chato *slang*; ladilla
crack, ~ (*blow*) golpe *m*; ~ (*bone, teeth*) fisura; ~ (*cocaine*) crack *m*; ~ (*fissure*) grieta; raza; **nipple** ~ grieta del pezón; ~ (*in voice*) gallo; ~ (*on the skin*) quebraza; ~ (*slit*) raja; rendija
crack, to, ~ (*the skin*) agrietar(se); pasparse *SpAm*; ~ (*a bone*) astillar(se); ~ (*the voice*) cascar; ~ (*the knuckles*) crujir; ~ (*glass, etc.*) rajar; ~ **up** craquear(se) *Chicano*; tostar(se); volverse (ue) loco
cracked skin, piel agrietada *f*; paspa *Bol, Ec, Perú*; paspadura *Ríopl*; ~ **voice** voz bronca *f*
cracker, galleta
cradle, cuna; ~ **cap**, costra láctea
cramp, calambre *m*; dolor espasmódico *m*; espasmo; **abdominal** ~ cólico *fam*; dolores de estómago *m*, *pl*; dolor de panza *m*, *fam*; retorcijón *m*, *fam*; retortijón *m*; torsón *m*, *fam*; torzón *m*, *fam*; **cane-cutter's** ~ calambre de los cortadores de caña *m*; **charley horse** ~ rampa; **heat** ~ calambre por calor; calambre térmico *m*; **intermittent** ~ calambre intermitente; **menstrual** ~ calambre *m*; cólico menstrual; dolor de hijá *m*, *fam*; dolor del período *m*; dolor de la regla *m*, *fam*; dolor menstrual *m*; retorcijón *m*, *fam*; retortijón *m*, *fam*; **muscular** ~ calambre *m*; **occupational** ~ calambre profesional; **postpartum** ~ entuerto; **stomach** ~ torcijón cólico *m*, *Mex*; retortijón de tripas *m*; **violinist's** ~ calambre de los violinistas *m*; **writers'** ~ calambre de los escribientes
cranial, craneal *adj*; craneano *adj*
cranium, cráneo; **base of the** ~ base del cráneo *f*

craving, antojo
crawl, to, gatear; andar a tatas
craziness, locura
crazy, arrematao *adj*; chiflado *adj*; craqueao *adj*, *Chicano*; loco *adj*; loquillo *adj*; tostao *adj*; **to go** ~ enloquecer(se); volverse (ue) loco
CRD/chronic respiratory disease, enfermedad respiratoria crónica *f*
cream, crema
creamy, cremoso *adj*
creatine, creatina
creatinine, creatinina
credibility, credibilidad *f*
credit, on, a plazos
cremaster, cremáster *m*
cremasteric, cremastérico *adj*
cremation, cremación *f*
crematory, crematorio
crescent, creciente *m*, *adj*
crest, cresta
cretinism, cretinismo
crevice, grieta; hendidura; **gingival** ~ espacio subgingival
crib, camilla de niño; cuna; **warming** ~ armazón de calentamiento *f*; camilla calentadora de niño; estufa *fam*; incubadora; ~ **death/Sudden Infant Death Syndrome/SIDS** muerte en la cuna *f*; muerte súbita *f*; síndrome de muerte infantil repentina *m*
cribsheet, bate *m*
cripple, cojo *m*, *adj*; inválido *m*, *adj*; lisiado *m*, *adj*; tullido *m*, *adj*
cripple, to, incapacitar; lisiar; tullir
crippled, cojo *adj*; derrengado *adj*; empedido *adj*; imposibilitado *adj*, *Med*; lisiado *adj*; ñongo *Col*, *Ven*; tullido *adj*; ~ (*one-handed*) manco *adj*; ~ **in the foot** cojo *adj*
crisis, (*pl*, *crises*) crisis *f*, *inv*; **identity** ~ crisis de identidad; **midlife** ~ crisis de la edad madura

criterion, (*pl, criteria*) criterio
critical, crítico *adj*
croaker[9], **hungry**, matasanos avaricioso
crooked, torcido *adj*; chueco *adj*
cross, to get, estrillar *Perú, Ríopl*
cross-cultural, transcultural *adj*
cross-eye, estrabismo (convergente)
cross-eyed, bisojo *adj*; bizco *adj*; bizcorneado *adj, SD*; bizcorneto *Col, Mex*; ojituerto *adj*; turnio *adj*; **to look ~** mirar bizco; ponerse bizco; bizcornear *Cu, PR*
cross-eyes, bizquera
cross match, pruebas cruzadas
cross matching, pruebas sanguíneas cruzadas
cross match, to, cruzar la sangre *fam*; hacer prueba(s) cruzada(s)
Cross, Red, Cruz Roja *f*
cross-section, corte transversal *m*
crossed, cruzado *adj*
crotch, empeine *m, fam*; entrepierna; entrepiernas
croup, crup *m*; garrotillo; ronquera
crow's feet, patas de gallo
crown, corona; **acrylic jacket ~** corona acrílica *Dent*; **anatomical ~** corona anatómica; **jacket ~** corona en cáscara *Dent*; **porcelain jacket ~** corona de porcelana *Dent*; **~ of tooth** filete *m, Dent*; **~ of the head** mollera *Anat*
crown, to, coronar; estar coronando
crowning, coronamiento *Obst*
crucial, crucial *adj*
crush on, to have a, estar enamorado de; estar perdido por
crush, to, **~** (*to squash*) aplastar; **~** (*finger, foot, etc.*) machucar; **~** (*reduce to powder*) machacar; triturar; **~ into** amontonarse
crushed by, to be, (*overwhelmed*) anonadar
crushing, (*pain*) aplastante *adj*; opresivo *adj*

crust, costra
crutch, muleta; sobaquera *fam*
cry, **~** (*yell*) grito; **~ of pain** grito de dolor; **~** (*with tears*) llanto
cry, to, **~** (*to yell*) gritar; **~** (*with tears*) llorar; tirar moco *slang, Chicano*
cryogen, criógeno *m, adj*
cryosurgery, criocirugía
cryotherapy, crioterapia
crypt, cripta
crystal, cristal *m*; **blood ~s** cristales hemáticos
crystalline, cristalino
CSF/cerebrospinal fluid, LCR/líquido cefalorraquídeo
CT/computed tomography, TC/tomografía computada
Cuban, cubano *m, adj*
cubic centimeter, centímetro cúbico
cubicle, cubículo
cuddle, to, apestillar(se); tongonear *PR*
cuddling, ñoño
cuff, manguito; **rotator ~ of the shoulder** manguito rotador del hombro; **~** (*of pants*) doblez *m*
cult, culto
cultivation, cultivo
culture, cultura; (*micro*) **~** cultivo; **bacterial ~** cultivo bacteriano; **blood ~** hemocultivo; **~ medium** caldo de cultivo; medio de cultivo; **stool ~** coprocultivo; cultivo de materia fecal; **tissue ~** cultivo de tejidos; **urine ~** urocultivo
culture, to, cultivar
cumulative, acumulativo *adj*
cunnilingus, cunilinguo
cup, taza; ventosa *ethn*; **dry ~** ventosa seca *ethn*; **wet ~** ventosa húmeda *ethn*
cup, to, acopar *ethn*
cupful, taza
cupping[10], aplicación de ventosas *f, ethn*; **~ glass** ventosa *ethn*
curable, curable *adj*

curari, curare *m*

cure, cura; curación *f*; método curativo; remedio

cure-all, panacea

cure, to, aliviar; curar; ~ **from the evil eye** desaojar

cured, to be, curarse

curettage, curetaje *m*; legrado *fam*; raspado *fam*; **uterine** ~ vaciado uterino

curette, cuchilla cortante; cureta *form*; legra

curl, ~ (*of hair*) rizo; ~ (*of smoke, etc.*) espiral *f*

curl, to, ~ (*hair*) rizar; ~ (*paper, etc.*) arrollarse

curly, rizado *adj*; blondo *adj, Arg, Mex*; choco *adj, Chi, Ec*; churrusco *adj, Col, Pan*; ~-**haired** choco *adj, Chi, Ec*

current, corriente *f*; **alternating** ~ corriente alterna; corriente alternativa; **battery** ~ corriente galvánica; **centrifugal** ~ corriente centrífuga; **constant** ~ corriente continua; **direct** ~ corriente directa; **electrostatic** ~ corriente electrostática; **high-frequency** ~ corriente de alta frecuencia; **reversed** ~ corriente invertida; **sine wave** ~ corriente sinusoidal; **static** ~ corriente estática

curse, to have the (monthly), caer mala; dar la luna; tener la regla

curvature, curvatura; **greater** ~ **of stomach** curvatura mayor del estómago; **lesser** ~ **of stomach** curvatura menor del estómago; **spinal** ~ curvatura espinal

curve, curva; curvatura; **buccal** ~ curva bucal *Dent*; **compensating** ~ curva de compensación; **dental** ~ curva dental *Dent*; **growth** ~ curva de crecimiento; ~ **of occlusion** curva de oclusión *Dent*; **pulse** ~ curva del pulso; **temperature** ~ curva térmica; curva de la temperatura

cushion, ~ (*for sitting on, etc.*) almohada; almohadilla; ~ (*lining*) reborde *m, Dent, Med*; relieve *m, Dent, Med*; **coronary** ~ reborde coronario; **endocardial** ~ relieve endocárdico

cusp, cúspide *f*; **canine** ~ cúspide canina; ~ **angle** ángulo cuspídeo; ~ **height** altura cuspídea

cuspal interference, interferencia cuspídea

cuspid, colmillo *fam*; cuspídeo *adj*; diente canino *m*

cuspless teeth, dientes sin cúspides

custom, costumbre *f*

cut, cortada *f, SpAm*; ~ (*small wound*) cortadura; ~ (*incision*) corte *m*; ~ (*on the face*) chirlo; tajo; ~ (*gash*) herida; ~ **made into a vein** sangradura *Med*

cut, to, cortar; ~ (*an abscess*) abrir; ~ **down (on)** disminuir; tomar menos; ~ **down on smoking** fumar menos; gastar menos en cigarrillos; ~ **off** (*to amputate*) amputar; ~ **one's hair** cortarse el pelo; ~ **one's nails** cortarse las uñas; ~ **oneself** cortarse; ~ **open** abrir con un corte; sajar *Med*; ~ **out** suprimir; remover (ue) *Med*; resecar *Med*; ~ **teeth** dentar (ie); echar dientes; endentecer; salir dientes; ~ **up (a person) with a knife/switchblade** tajear

cutaneous, cutáneo *adj*

cutdown, ventostomía; **venous** ~ disección de una vena *f*

cute, chulo *adj, PR*; mono *adj*

cuticle, cutícula; **dental** ~ cutícula dental; **enamel** ~ cutícula del esmalte; ~ **of root sheath** cutícula de la vaina radicular

cutting, cortadura; ~ (*sharp*) cortante *adj*; ~ **edge** filo cortante

cyanide, cianuro

cyanosis, cianosis *f*; piel azulada *f, fam*

cyanotic, cianótico *adj*; amoratado *adj, fam*; morado *adj, fam*

cyclamate, ciclamato; **calcium** ~

ciclamato cálcico; **sodium** ~ ciclamato sódico

cycle, ciclo; **cardiac** ~ ciclo cardíaco; **life** ~ ciclo vital; **menstrual** ~ ciclo menstrual; **ovulatory** ~ ciclo ovulatorio; **reproductive** ~ ciclo reproductivo; ciclo reproductor

cyclic, cíclico *adj*

cyclical, cíclico *adj*

cylinder, **graduated**, probeta

cyst, abscesos *fam*; bolsas de pus *fam*; lupia; quiste *m*; **cutaneous** ~ quiste cutáneo; **distention** ~ quiste por distensión; **milk** ~ quiste láctico; **mucous** ~ quiste mucoso; **ovarian** ~ quiste ovárico; **periodontal** ~ quiste radicular; **sebaceous** ~ quiste sebáceo; **spermatic** ~ quiste espermático; espermatocele *m*

cystic, (*artery*, *duct*) cístico *adj*; quístico *adj*; ~ **fibrosis** fibrosis quística *f*

cystitis, cistitis *f*; infección de la vejiga *f*; **chronic** ~ cistitis crónica

cystocele, cistocele *m*

cystogram, cistograma *m*

cystography, cistografía

cystoscope, cistoscopio

cystoscopic, cistoscópico *adj*

cystoscopy, cistoscopia; cistoscopía

cytoblast, citoblasto

cytologist, citólogo

cytology, citología

cytoplasm, citoplasma *m*

cytosis, citosis *f*

---

[2] This is new vocabulary, not necessarily listed nor yet recognized by the Royal Academy of Spanish Grammar. It is understood that this vocabulary is primarily slang. Unless otherwise indicated, the gender of nouns is assumed to be obvious.

[3] For pronunciation purposes, the masculine definite and indefinite articles, *el* and *un*, not *la* or *una*, are used when the article immediately precedes the feminine singular noun which begins with stressed *a* or any other that begins with stressed *ha*.

[4] In rural areas, especially Mexico and Puerto Rico, peasants often call any serious skin disease, especially infected wounds or gangrene, *cancer*.

[5] Part of the Drug Abuse Vocabulary.

[6] The current English street terminology for *cocaine* includes: angel dust, Bernice gold dust, bernies, big C, blow, burese, C, candy, c-game, C & H, carrie, Cecil, Charlie, cholly, coca, coke, Corine, dream, dust, dynamite, flake, gin, girl, gold dust, happy dust, heaven dust, her, jelly, joy powder, King's habit, killer stuff, lady, lady snow, leaf, love affairs, M & C, Merck, nose, nose candy, nose powder, one & one, paradise, rich man's heroin, rock, schmeck, schoolboy code, sleigh ride, snow, snowbird, speedball, star dust, thing, white lady, white stuff, whiz bang.

[7] Street terminology generally uses "syrup" (terpinhydrate) and "terps" for *codeine*.

[8] This is the forty-day period following delivery during which there is a prolonged period in bed, much freedom from household responsibilities, and abstention from sexual intercourse.

[9] A croaker is a physician who dispenses prescriptions for drugs.

[10] *Cupping* is a folk remedy that is used for pains in the side of the abdomen which are thought to be caused by contact with cold air. The cure uses a wide-mouthed glass and a candle. It consists of warming the air in the glass with the candle and placing the glass over the affected abdominal area. It is thought that the cold air is sucked out by the glass, curing the patient.

[11] Use the Spanish pronunciation of these letters.

D

D & C/dilation and curettage, D y R/dilatación y raspado *f*; legrado *fam*; raspa *fam*; raspado diagnóstico *m*

dab, mancha; toque *m*

dab, to, dar unos toques de; golpear ligeramente

dacryagogue, dacriagogo *m, adj*; que provoca flujo de lágrimas

dacryocystis, dacriocisto

dacryocystitis, dacriocistitis *f*; infección de la bolsa de lágrimas *f*

dactylogram, dactilograma *m*; huellas digitales

dactyloscopy, dactiloscopia; examen de las huellas para la identificación de las personas *m*

D.A.H./disordered action of the heart, disfunción cardíaca *f*

daily, cotidiano *adj*; diario *adj*; por día *prep phr*; **~ schedule** programa diario *m*

dainty, delicado *adj*

dairy, lácteo *adj*

daltonism, daltonismo; (*See blindness, color.*)

damage, daño; lesión *f*

damage, to, dañar; hacer daño; lesionar; **~** (*eyesight*) deshacer

damp, húmedo *adj*; mojado *adj*

dampen, to, humedecer

dampness, humedad *f*

dance, danza; (*See chorea.*); **St. Anthony's ~** danza de San Antonio; **St. Guy's ~** danza de San Guido; **St. John's ~** danza de San Juan; **St. Vitus' ~** danza de San Vito

dancing disease, corea epidémica

dandruff, caspa

dandy fever, dengue *m*; (*See fever, breakbone.*)

danger, peligro; **~-light** señal (luminosa) de peligro *f*; **~ of miscarriage** peligro de aborto

dangerous, peligroso *adj*

dangle (one's legs), to, colgar (ue) (las piernas)

dark/(*in color, unilluminated*), oscuro *adj*; **~ field** fondo oscuro; **~ glasses** gafas ahumadas; **~** (*complexion*) moreno *adj*; **~ haired** moreno *adj*; **~ skinned** moreno *adj*

dashed line, línea discontinua

data, (*sg, datum*) datos *m, pl*

date, **~** (*calendar*) fecha; **~ of birth** fecha de nacimiento; **~** (*appointment*) cita

day, día *m*; **~ after tomorrow** pasado mañana; **~ before yesterday** anteayer; **~care center** guardería; **~-to-day** cotidiano *adj*; **every ~** todos los días; **every other ~** cada dos días; **~ nurse** enfermera de día; (*See nurse.*); **~ nursery** guardería infantil

day-dreamer, soñador, -ra *m/f*

day-dribbling, incontinencia urinaria durante el día

dayblindness, ceguera diurna

daydream, ensueño

daydream, to, imaginar; soñar despierto *adj*

daylight, luz del día *f*; **~-saving time** hora de verano

daze, aturdimiento; **in a ~** aturdido *adj*

daze, to, (*to stun*) aturdir

dazed, aturdido *adj*

dead, **~** (*inert*) inactivado *adj*; inerte *adj*; **~** (*not living*) muerto *m, adj*; extinto *adj, Chi, Mex, Ríopl, euph*; **~ body** cadáver *m*; **~-born** mortinato; nacido muerto; **~-end cycle** ciclo ciego; **~ limb** adormecimiento de los miembros; **~ person** difunto; **~ pulp** pulpa dental desvitalizada; ~ **space** espacio muerto

deaden the nerve, to, adormecer el nervio

deadliness, letalidad *f*

deaf, sordo *adj*; ~ **and dumb** sordomudo *adj*; opa *adj*, *Bol, Perú, Ríopl*; ~ **mute** sordomudo *m, adj*; **~mutism** sordomudez *f*; ~ **person** peña *Ec, Guat, PR*; sordo

deafen, to, ensordecer

deafness, ensordecimiento; sordera

death, defunción *f*; fallecimiento; muerte *f*; pelada *Chi, Cu, Ec*; **apparent** ~ muerte aparente; ~ **bed** lecho de muerte; lecho mortuorio; ~ **certificate** certificado de defunción; partida de defunción; **crib ~/SIDS** muerte súbita del lactante; muerte súbita en la cuna; muerte súbita infantil; **fetal** ~ muerte fetal; ~ **in the family** muerte de familiares; ~ **mask** máscara mortuoria; **proof of** ~ acta[3] de defunción; ~ **rate** índice de mortalidad *m*; mortalidad *f*; ~ **rattle** estertor agónico *m*; estertor de la muerte *m*; ~ **struggle** período agónico; ~ **wound** herida mortal

deathlike, cadavérico *adj*; letárgico *adj*

debility, debilidad *f*

debilitate, to, debilitar

debilitated, debilitado *adj*

debilitating, debilitante *adj*

debride, to, desbridar

debris, desecho; despojo; residuo

debubbler, desburbujeador *m*

decalcification, descalcificación *f*

decalcified, descalcificado *adj*

decalcify, to, descalcificar

decant, to, decantar

decapitate, to, decapitar

decapitation, decapitación *f*; decolación *f*; derotomía; embriotomía

decay, decaimiento; **caries** *Dent*; ~ (*rotting*) pudrición *f*

decay, to, decaer; degenerar; pudrir

decayed, podrido *adj*; pudrido *adj*; ~ (*teeth*) cariado *adj*

decease, fallecimiento; defunción *f*; muerte *f*

deceased, difunto *m, adj*; cadáver *m*; persona muerta; extinto *adj*, *Chi, Mex, Ríopl, euph*

deceitfulness, doblez *f*

deceleration, deceleración *f*

decerebration, descerebración *f*

dechloridation, descloruración *f*

decibel, decibel *m*

deciduous, deciduo *adj*; no permanente *adj*

decigram, decigramo

deciliter, decilitro

decimeter, decimetro

decoagulant, descoagulante *adj*

decoction, cocimiento; decocción *f*; infusión *f*

decompensation, descompensación *f*

decompression, descompresión *f*; ~ **sickness** enfermedad de los buceadores *f*; enfermedad por descompresión *f*; (*See the bends.*)

decongestant, descongestionante *m, adj*; descongestivo, *m, adj*

decongestive, descongestivo *adj*

decontamination, descontaminación *f*; ~ **station** estación de descontaminación *f*

decrease, disminución *f*

decrease, to, disminuir

decrepit, decrépito *adj*

decubation, decubación *f*; período en las enfermedades desde la desaparición de los síntomas hasta la curación completa

decubital ulcer, úlcera por decúbito

decubitus, decúbito

deep, profundo *adj*; ~ (*a wound*) penetrante *adj*; ~ **x-ray therapy** radioterapia profunda

deface, to, deformar; desfigurar; mutilar

defatted, desengrasado *adj*

defecate, to, defecar; eliminar; ensuciar; purgar

defecation, defecación *f, form*; **fragmentary ~** defecación fragmentaria

defect, defecto; imperfección *f*; falta; **atrial septal ~** comunicación interauricular *f*; **birth ~** defecto de nacimiento; **congenital ~** defecto congénito; **hearing ~s** defectos de la audición; defectos del oído; **speech ~s** defectos del habla; defectos del lenguaje; **ventricular septal ~** comunicación interventricular *f*; **visual ~s** defectos de la visión; defectos de la vista

defective, defectuoso *adj*; deficiente *adj*

defense, defensa; **~ mechanism** mecanismo de defensa

defibrillate, to, desfibrilar

defibrillation, desfibrilación *f*

defibrillator, defibrilador *m*; desfibrilador *m*

deficiency, carencia; defecto; deficiencia

deficient, deficiente *adj*

deficit, déficit *m*; **oxygen ~** déficit de oxígeno

definite, definitivo *adj*

deflate, to, deshinchar; desinflar; desviar

deflection, deflexión *f*

defloration, desfloración *f*; desvirgamiento

defluxion, deflujo

deform, to, ~ (*body*) deformar; **~** (*person*) afear; desfigurar

deformation, ~ (*of a body*) deformación *f*; deformidad *f*; **~** (*of people*) desfiguración *f*

deformed, contrahecho *adj*; eclipsado *adj, fam, SpAm*; inocente *adj, Mex*; **~** (*misshapen*) deforme *adj*; **~** (*ugly*) disforme *adj*; **~ child** engendro

deforming, deformante *adj*

deformity, deformidad *f*

deganglionate, to, desganglionar; extirpar un ganglio o ganglios

degas, to, desgasificar

degeneracy, degeneración *f*; degenerado; **inferior/superior ~** degenerado inferior/superior

degenerate, to, degenerar

degeneration, degeneración *f*

degenerative, degenerativo *adj*

degerm, to, desgerminar

degree, grado

dehumanizing, deshumanizante *adj*

dehumidification, deshumedecimiento

dehumidifier, deshumectante *adj*; deshumedecedor *m, adj*

dehumidify, to, deshumedecer

dehydrant, deshidratante *adj*

dehydrate, to, deshidratar

dehydrated, deshidratado *adj*

dehydration, desecación *f*; deshidratación *f*; **~ fever** fiebre de deshidratación *f*; fiebre de la sed *f, fam*

dehydrogenase, deshidrogenasa

dehypnotize, to, deshipnotizar

déjà, ya; **~ entendu** ya oído; **~ éprouve** ya probado; **~ vu** ya visto

dejected, decaído *adj*

delay, demora; **~** (*developmental*) retardo; retraso

delay, to, demorar; **~** (*developmentally*) retardar; retrasar

delayed, ~ delivery parto prolongado; **~ pain** dolor tardío *m*; **~ type reaction** reacción de tipo diferido *f*

deleterious, deletéreo *adj*; nocivo *adj*; pernicioso *adj*

deletion, supresión *f*

delicate, delicado *adj*; frágil *adj*

delinquency, delincuencia

delirious, delirante *adj*; **to be ~** delirar; desvariar *Med*

delirium, (*pl, deliria*) delirio; desvarío; devaneo *Med*; **acute ~** delirio agudo; **chronic alcoholic ~** delirio alcohólico crónico; **traumatic ~** delirio traumático

deliver, to, ~ (*a baby*) aliviarse *Chicano, Mex, fam*; dar a luz; parir; partear *Obst*; tener el niño; ~ (*someone of a baby*) asistir al parto; asistir un parto; atender (ie) (un parto); ayudar al parto

delivery, (*parturition*) parto; **abdominal** ~ parto abdominal; **breech** ~ extracción de nalgas *f*; **delayed** ~ parto prolongado; **forced** ~ parto forzado; **forceps** ~ extracción con fórceps *f*; ~ **of the placenta** expulsión de la placenta *f*; **premature** ~ parto prematuro; ~ **room** sala de partos; ~ **table** mesa del parto

delouse, to, despiojar; espulgar

delousing, despiojamiento

deltoid, deltoides *m*; ~ **muscle** músculo deltoide

delude, to, engañar

deluge, diluvio; inundación *f*

delusion, delirio; delusión *f*; engaño; ilusión *f*; **depressive** ~ delirio depresivo; ~ **of grandeur** delirio de grandeza; ~ **of negation** delirio de negación; ~ **of persecution** delirio de persecución; **systematized** ~ delirio sistematizado; **unsystematized** ~ delirio no sistematizado

delusional, delusorio *adj*

demagnetize, to, desmagnetizar

demanding, exigente *adj*

demarcation, demarcación *f*

demasculinization, desmasculinización *f*

demecarium bromide, bromuro de demecario

demented, demenciado *adj*; dementado *adj*; demente *adj*

dementia, demencia; **chronic** ~ demencia crónica; **epileptic** ~ demencia epiléptica; ~ **precox** demencia precox

demerol, demerol *m*; ~ **hydrochloride** Clorhidrato de Demerol

demineralization, desmineralización *f*

demise, fallecimiento

demography, demografía; **dynamic** ~ demografía dinámica; **static** ~ demografía estática

demonstrate, to, (*to show*) demostrar (ue)

demoniac, demoníaco *adj*

demoralization, desmoralización *f*

demoralize, to, desmoralizar

demoralized, to become, desmoralizarse; desanimarse

demoralizing, desmoralizador *adj*; desmoralizante *adj*

denatured, desnaturalizado *adj*

dengue, dengue *m*; fiebre rompehuesos *f*; ~ **fever** dengue *m*; fiebre roja *f*; fiebre rompehuesos *f*; (*See fever, dengue.*)

denial, negación *f*; rechazo

density, densidad *f*

dental, dental *adj*; ~ **artery** arteria dental; ~ **bridge** puente dental *m*; ~ **calculus** cálculo dental; sarro; ~ **drill** broca; fresa dental; taladro; torno; trépano; ~ **dysfunction** disfunción dental *f*; ~ **engineering** ingeniería dental; ~ **filling** empaste dental *m*; odontoplerosis *f*; ~ **floss** cordón dental *m*; hilo dental; seda encerada; ~ **forceps** gatillo; pinzas; tenazas de extracción; ~ **geriatrics** geriatría dental; ~ **hygienist** higienista dental *m/f*; ~ **impression** mordisco; ~ **mirror** espejo de dentista; espejo dental; ~ **nerve** nervio dental; ~ **office** clínica dental; ~ **plate** plancha *Dent*; ~ **practitioner** dentista *m/f*; ~ **prosthetic laboratory procedures** métodos de laboratorio para prótesis dental; ~ **vein** vena dental

dentifrice, dentífrico *m, adj*

dentin, dentina

dentine, dentina

dentinoma, dentinoma *m*

dentist, dentista *m/f*; odontólogo; ~**'s chair** silla de dentista;

~'s **office** consultorio del dentista; ~'s **operating equipment** grupo dental

dentistry, dentistería; estomatología; odontología *form*; **operative** ~ odontología operatoria; **preventive** ~ odontología preventiva; **prosthetic** ~ odontología prostética

dentition, dentición *f*; **artificial** ~ dentición artificial; dentadura artificial; **deciduous** ~ dentición caduca; **permanent** ~ dentición permanente; *(See secondary dentition.)*; **primary** ~ dentición primaria; primera dentición; **secondary** ~ dentición secundaria; segunda dentición

denture, dentadura (postiza); ~ **base** base de dentadura *f*; ~ **base foundation** soporte de la base de la dentadura; ~ **border** borde de dentadura *m*; **complete** ~ dentadura completa; ~ **cup** recipiente para guardar la dentadura *m*; ~ **curing** procesado de la dentadura; ~ **design** diseño de la dentadura; **distal extension partial** ~ dentadura parcial de extensión distal; **fixed partial** ~ dentadura parcial fija; **full** ~ dentadura (postiza) completa; **immediate insertion** ~ dentadura de inserción inmediata; ~ **impression surface** superficie de impresión de la dentadura *f*; ~ **occlusal surface** superficie oclusal de la dentadura *f*; **partial** ~ dentadura (postiza) parcial; **polished surface** ~ superficie pulida de la dentadura *f*; **removable partial** ~ dentadura parcial removible; ~ **retention** retención de la dentadura *f*; ~ **space** espacio de dentadura; ~ **stability** estabilidad de la dentadura *f*; ~ **supporting structures** estructuras de soporte de la dentadura

denucleated, desnucleado *adj*

deny, to, negar (ie)

deodorant, desodorante *m, adj*

deodorize, to, desodorizar

deodorizer, desodorante *m*

deoxidization, desoxidación *f*

deoxyribonuclease, desoxirribonucleasa

deoxyribonucleic, desoxirribonucleico *adj*; ~ **acid/DNA** ácido desoxirribonucleico/ADN o DNA

department, departamento; ~ **of welfare** departamento de bienestar

departure from normal, desviación de la normalidad *f*

dependence, dependencia; ~ (*drug*) farmacodependencia; toxicomanía

dependency, dependencia; ~ (*drug*) farmacodependencia

dependent, dependiente *m/f*

depilation, depilación *f*

depilatory, depilatorio *m, adj*

deplete, to, agotar; descongestionar *Med*

depletion, agotamiento; descongestión *Med, f*

depolarization, despolarización *f*

depolarize, to, despolarizar

deposit, (*sediment*) depósito; poso; sedimento

deposit, to, depositar(se)

depravation, depravación *f*

depraved, depravado *adj*

depress, to/press down, to, deprimir

depressant, calmante *m, adj*; debilitante *m, adj*; depresor *m*; deprimente *m, adj*; sedante *m, adj*

depressed, deprimido *adj*; hundido *adj*; **to get** ~ deprimirse

depressing, deprimente *adj*

depression, abatimiento; depresión *f*; **reactive** ~ depresión reactiva; **systolic** ~ depresión sistólica; **ventricular** ~ depresión ventricular

depressive, depresivo *adj*

depressor, depresor *m, adj, Med,*

Anat; **tongue** ~ bajalenguas *m,inv*; depresor; depresor de la lengua; depresor lingual; abatelenguas *m, inv, Mex*; paleta *fam*; pisalengua; (*See tongue depressor.*)

deprivation, carencia; privación *f*

deprive, to, privar

deproteinization, desproteinización *f*

depth, profundidad *f*; **focal ~** profundidad focal; **~ perception** (*stereopsis*) estereopsia *form*; percepción de la profundidad *f*; visión estereoscópica *f*; visión profunda *f*

deranged, trastornado *adj*

derangement, ~ (*disorder*) desarreglo; ~ (*breakdown*) trastorno mental *Med*

derivation, derivación *f*

derivative, derivativo *m, adj*

dermabrasion, dermabrasión *f*

dermatitis, dermatitis *f*; **allergic ~** dermatitis alérgica; **~ calorica** dermatitis calórica; **caterpillar ~** dermatitis por orugas; **contact ~** dermatitis por contacto; **diaper/napkin area ~** dermatitis amoniacal; **industrial ~** dermatitis industrial

dermatologist, dermatólogo

dermatology, dermatología

DES/diethylstilbestrol, DES[4]/dietilestilbestrol *m*

descendant, descendiente *m/f, adj*

descending, descendente *adj*

describe, to, describir

desensitization, desensibilización *f*

desensitize, to, desensibilizar

desiccant, desecante *m, adj*

desiccate, to, desecar

design, dibujo; esbozo

desire, deseo

desire (to), to, tener deseos (de)

desoxyephedrine, desoxiefedrina

desoxyribonuclease, desoxirribonucleasa

desoxyribonucleic, desoxirribonucleico *adj*; **~ acid/DNA** ácido desoxirribonucleico/ADN o DNA

desperate, desesperado *adj*; **to become ~** desesperarse

despondency, desánimo; desaliento; descorazonamiento

despondent, desanimado *adj*; desalentado *adj*; descorazonado *adj*

dessert, postre *m*

dessertspoonful, cucharada de postre (10 cc)

destroy, to, destruir

destroyed, destruido *adj*

destructive, destructivo *adj*

detached retina, retina desprendida

detachment, despegamiento; desprendimiento; **~ of retina** desprendimiento de la retina

detect, to, descubrir; detectar

detectable, perceptible *adj*

detection, detección *f*

detergent, detergente *m, adj*

deteriorate, to, ~ (*patient's condition*) empeorar(se); ~ (*to wear out*) deteriorarse

deterioration, ~ (*patient's condition*) empeoramiento; ~ (*wearing out*) deterioro

deteriorative, deteriorante *adj*

determinant, determinante *m, adj*

determination, determinación *f*; **sex ~** determinación del sexo

detoxicate, to, desintoxicar; destoxicar

detoxication, destoxicación *f*; **metabolic ~** destoxicación metabólica

detoxification, destoxicación *f*

detoxify, to, desintoxicar

detoxifying, desintoxicante *adj*; destoxificante *adj*

detrimental, nocivo *adj*; perjudicial *adj*

devastating, arrollador *adj*

develop, to, desarrollarse; **~ an x-ray** revelar una radiografía

development, desarrollo; **arrested ~** desarrollo detenido; **delayed ~** desarrollo tardío; **speech ~** desarrollo del habla; desarrollo del lenguage; **~ of an x-ray film** revelado de una radiografía; **~ (of**

an idea, theory, etc.) desenvolvimiento *adj*

deviation, aberración *f*; desviación *f*; **axis ~** desviación del eje eléctrico; **primary ~** desviación primaria; **secondary ~** desviación secundaria; **standard ~** desviación estándar; **strabismic ~** desviación estrábica

device, aparato; dispositivo; **intrauterine ~** aparato intrauterino; **sequential compression ~** aparato de compresión consecutiva

devils, (*seconals, barbiturates*) coloradas[2]; diablos[2]; rojas[2]

devital tooth, diente desvitalizado *m*

devitalization, desvitalización *f*

devitalize, to, desvitalizar

devitalized, desvitalizado *adj*

dexedrine/dexies/dextroamphetamine, dextroanfetamina; dexedrina

dextrin, dextrina

dextrinase, dextrinasa

dextrose, azúcar de uva *m*; dextrosa; glucosa

diabetes, diabetes *f, form*; diabetis *f*; azúcar en el orín *m*; **alimentary ~** diabetes alimentaria; diabetes debida al metabolismo defectuoso de los hidratos de carbono de los alimentos; **bronze ~** diabetes bronceada; **cerebral ~** diabetes cerebral; tipo de diabetes con presencia de cerebrosa en la orina en vez de glucosa; **enzymic ~** diabetes diastásica; **fat ~** diabetes lipógena; diabetes con obesidad; **gouty ~** diabetes gotosa; diabetes asociada con gota; **hunger ~** diabetes carencial *f*; **~ innocens** diabetes inocente; **~ insipidus** diabetes insípida *f*; poliuria esencial con polidipsia y polifagia; pérdida de fuerzas y emaciación, pero sin glucosuria;

~ mellitus diabetes mellitus *f*; diabetes sacarina *f*; trastorno del metabolismo de los hidratos de carbono caracterizado por hiperglucemia, glucosuria y perturbación del mecanismo de acción de la insulina; **pancreatic ~** diabetes pancreática; diabetes que guarda relación con enfermedad del páncreas; **puncture ~** diabetes por punción; **renal ~** diabetes renal; tipo de diabetes debida al funcionamiento anormal del riñón sin hiperglucemia; **steroid ~** diabetes esteroide; **temporary ~** diabetes temporal; **toxic ~** diabetes tóxica; **true ~** diabetes verdadera

diabetic, diabético *m, adj*; **~ needle** aguja de insulina; **~ sugar** dextrosa

diagnose, to, diagnosticar; hacer un diagnóstico

diagnosis, (*pl, diagnoses*) diagnosis *f, inv*; **~** (*of a disease*) diagnóstico

diagnostic, diagnóstico *m, adj*; **~** (*science*) diagnosis *f, inv*; **~** (*symptom*) síntoma *m*; **~ approach** marcha diagnóstica; **biological ~** diagnóstico biológico; **clinical ~** diagnóstico clínico; **differential ~** diagnóstico diferencial; **direct ~** diagnóstico directo; **~ by exclusion** diagnóstico por exclusión; **laboratory ~** diagnóstico de laboratorio; **pathologic ~** diagnóstico patológico; **physical ~** diagnóstico físico; **roentgen ~** diagnóstico roentgenológico; **serum ~** diagnóstico serológico; **topographic ~** diagnóstico topográfico; **~ workup** diagnóstico diferencial

diagnostician, diagnosticador, -ra *m/f*

diagram, diagrama *m*; representación esquemática *f*

dialysis, (*pl, dialyses*) diálisis *f, inv*; en diálisis; **peritoneal** ~ diálisis peritoneal

dialyzed, dializado *m, adj*

dialyzer, dializador *m*

diameter, diámetro; **cranial** ~ diámetro del cráneo; **pelvic** ~ diámetro de la pelvis

diapason, diapasón *m*; (*See tuning fork.*)

diaper, braga; pañal *m*; paño; pavico *Chicano*; sapeta *Chicano*; talega; zapeta *Chicano*; **cloth** ~ pañal de tela; **disposable** ~ pañal desechable; ~ **rash** chincual *m, Mex, Chicano*; dermatitis por pañal *f*; escaldadura (en los bebés); pañalitis *f*; salpullido

diaper, to, cambiar el pañal; proveer con pañal; renovar (ue) el pañal (de)

diaphoresis, diaforesis *f, form*; sudores a chorros *m, pl*

diaphragm, diafragma *m, Anat*; ~ (*birth control*) diafragma anticonceptivo *m*; diafragma contraceptivo *m*; (*See birth control.*)

diaphysary, diafisaria *adj*

diaphysis, diáfisis *f*

diarrhea, asientos *slang*; cagadera *Chicano, vulg*; cámara *slang*; chorrillo *slang*; chorro *slang*; churrias *f, pl, Col, Guat, RD*; corredera *Chicano*; cursera *slang*; diarrea; escurribanda *f, fam, Med*; estómago suelto; excremento suelto; obradera *Col, Guat, Pan*; soltura *Chicano*; soltura de vientre *Med*; turista *slang*; **dysenteric** ~ diarrea disenteriforme; **epidemic** ~ diarrea epidémica; **morning** ~ diarrea matinal; **summer** ~ diarrea estival; **traveler's** ~ diarrea del viajero; **watery** ~ diarrea líquida; **to have** ~ estar de vareta *Med, fam*; soltarse (ue) del estómago

diastem, diastema *Dent, m*

diastole, diástole *f*

diastolic, diastólico *adj*

diathermy, diatermia; **medical** ~ diatermia médica; **short wave** ~ diatermia de onda corta; **surgical** ~ diatermia quirúrgica; **ultrashort wave** ~ diatermia de onda ultracorta

die, ~ (*for minting, shaping*) molde *m*; ~ troquel *m, Dent*

die, to, (*to cease living*) fallecer; morir (ue); templarse *Ec, Guat, Hond*; ~ **in childbirth** morir (ue) de sobreparto

diet, dieta; régimen alimenticio *m*; **absolute** ~ dieta absoluta; **acid-ash** ~ dieta de residuo ácido; dieta que consiste en carne roja, pescado, huevos y cereales, sin queso ni leche y con poca fruta y verduras; **alkali-ash** ~ dieta de residuos alcalinos; dieta que consiste en fruta, verduras, y leche, con la restricción máxima posible de carnes, huevos y cereales; **bland** ~ dieta blanda; **dechlorinated** ~ dieta declorurada; **diabetic** ~ dieta diabética; **elimination** ~ dieta de eliminación; **high fat** ~ dieta rica en grasas; **kosher** ~ dieta que sigue las reglas dietéticas judías; **light** ~ dieta ligera; **liquid** ~ dieta de líquidos; **low residue** ~ dieta de escaso residuo; **salt-free** ~ dieta desclorurada; **to be on a** ~ estar a dieta; estar a régimen; **to follow a** ~ seguir (i) una dieta; **to put s.o. on a** ~ poner a dieta; poner a uno a régimen

dietary, dietético *adj*

dietetic, dietético *adj*

dietetics, dietética

dietician/dietitian, dietético; dietista *m/f*; dietetista *m/f*

diethylstilbestrol/DES, dietilestilbestrol/DES *m*

differential, ~ **blood count** cuenta sanguínea diferencial; fórmula hemática; ~ **count** hemograma *m*; ~ **leukocyte count** fórmula leucocitaria

differentiation, diferenciación *f*; **correlative** ~ diferenciación correlativa; **functional** ~ diferenciación funcional

difficulty, dificultad *f*; ~ **in** dificultad en; ~ **in breathing** opresión *f, Med*

diffusion, difusión *f*

digest, to, digerir (ie)

digestant, digestivo *adj*

digested, digerido *adj*

digestible, digerible *adj*; digestible *adj*

digestibility, digestibilidad *f*

digestion, digestión *f*; **biliary** ~ digestión biliar; **gastric** ~ digestión gástrica; **intestinal** ~ digestión intestinal; **pancreatic** ~ digestión pancreática; **primary** ~ digestión primaria; **salivary** ~ digestión salival; **secondary** ~ digestión secundaria

digestive, digestivo *adj*; ~ **system** aparato digestivo; sistema digestivo *m*; ~ **tube** tubo digestivo

digital computer, computador digital *m*

digitalin, digitalina

digitalis, digitalis *f*; digitalina

dilantin, dilantina

dilate, to, dilatar(se)

dilation, dilatación *f*; ~ **and curettage/D & C** dilatación y raspado; **digital** ~ dilatación digital; ~ **of the cervix** dilatación del cuello de la matriz; ~ **of the heart** dilatación del corazón; ~ **of the stomach** dilatación del estómago

dilator, dilatador *m*

diligent, diligente *adj*

dill, eneldo

dilute, to, diluir; aguar

dilution, dilución *f*

dim, ~ (*not bright*) oscuro *adj*; ~ (*blurred*) borroso *adj*; ~ (*distant*) lejano *adj*

dime[5], diez años de prisión[2]; diez dólares[2]; sinónimo para diez; ~ **bag**[5] (*envelope of heroin, cocaine, or marijuana*) paque de drogas *m*

diminish, to, disminuir(se)

dimple, hoyo *Carib, Ríopl*; hoyuelo

dinner, cena

diopter, dioptría

dioptric, dióptrico *adj*

dioxide, dióxido

dip, caída; depresión *f*; ~ **stick** tira reactiva; ~ **stick test** prueba de las tiras mojadas

diphenhydramine, difenhidramina

diphtheria, difteria; diteria *fam*; garrotillo; **calf** ~ difteria de los terneros; **cutaneous** ~ difteria cutánea; **laryngeal** ~ difteria laríngea; **pharyngeal** ~ difteria faríngea; **surgical** ~ difteria quirúrgica

diplegia, parálisis bilateral *f*

diplomate, diplomado *adj*

diplopia, diplopía *form*; visión doble *f*; vista doble

direction, dirección *f*; ~**s** instrucciones *f*

dirt, suciedad *f*

dirty, puerco *adj, fam*; sucio *adj*; inhumano *adj, Chi*; **to be** ~ estar caquis maquis *euph*; **to get** ~ ensuciarse

dirty, to, ensuciar

disability, inhabilidad *f*; invalidez *f*; incapacidad *f, Med*; **mental** ~ incapacidad mental; **physical** ~ incapacidad física

disable, to, ~ (*to incapacitate legally*) incapacitar (para); ~ (*to incapacitate mentally*) dejar mentalmente incapacitado *adj*; ~ (*to incapacitate physically*) dejar imposibilitado

disabled, incapacitado *adj*; tullido *adj*; imposibilitado *adj, Med*

disadvantage, desventaja

disagree with one, to, (*bad effect*) caerse mal; no sentarle (ie) bien a uno

disagreeable, antipático *adj*
disappointment, decepción *f*; desengaño; desilusión *f*
disaster, desastre *m*; guama *Col, Ven*
disc, disco; *(See disk.)*
discern, to, discernir (ie)
discharge, ~ (*fluid*) desagüe *m*; descarga; desecho; flujo; secreción *f*; supuración *f*; **bloody ~** derrame *m*; **neural ~** descarga nerviosa; **vaginal ~** flujo vaginal; **white ~** flores blancas *f, fam*; flujo blanco; ~ (*of gas*) escape *m*; ~ (*pus*) pus *m*; ~ (*of an employee*) despido; ~ (*from the hospital*) alta de un enfermo
discharge, to, ~ (*from the hospital*) dar de alta; ~ (*pus*) echar
discoloration, coloración anormal *f*
discomfort, ~ (*lack of comfort*) incomodidad *f*; ~ (*feeling of uneasiness*) malestar *m*; ~ (*physical pain*) molestia
discontinue, to, descontinuar; ~ (*a medication*) dejar de tomar; ~ (*a treatment*) suprimir (un tratamiento); suspender (un tratamiento)
discourage, to, desalentar (ie); desanimar; descorazonar
discouraged, to get/become, desalentarse (ie); desanimarse; descorazonarse
discovery, descubrimiento
disease, dolencia; enfermedad *f, form*; mal *m*; **acute ~** enfermedad aguda; **Alzheimer's ~** enfermedad de Alzheimer; **cat-scratch ~** enfermedad por arañaz o de gato; **celiac ~** enfermedad celíaca; **chronic ~** enfermedad crónica; **chronic obstructive pulmonary ~/COPD** enfermedad pulmonar obstructiva crónica/EPOC; **communicable ~** enfermedad comunicable; enfermedad transmisible; **connective tissue ~** enfermedad del tejido conjuntivo; **contagious ~** enfermedad contagiosa; **degenerative joint ~** enfermedad articular degenerativa; ~ **due to an act of witchcraft** enfermedad endañada *Chicano, Mex*; **fibrocystic ~** enfermedad fibroquística; ~ **of the bone** enfermedad fibroquística ósea; **fibrocystic ~ of pancreas** enfermedad fibroquística del páncreas; **foot-and-mouth ~** enfermedad glosopeda; **glycogen storage ~** enfermedad de almacenamiento de glucógeno; **hoof-and-mouth ~** enfermedad glosopeda; **hyaline membrane ~** enfermedad de membrana hialina; **industrial ~** enfermedad profesional; **infectious ~** enfermedad infecciosa; **interstitial lung ~** enfermedad intersticial pulmonar; **minimal change ~** enfermedad de lesiones mínimas; **Morton's ~** metatarsalgia; **notifiable ~** enfermedad de notificación *f*; ~ **of social pathology** enfermedad de carácter; enfermedad moral; **pelvic inflammatory ~/PID** enfermedad inflamatoria pélvica; infección pélvica *f*; **peripheral vascular ~** enfermedad vascular periférica; **reportable ~** enfermedad obligatoria; **rheumatic heart ~** cardiopatía reumática; **sexually transmitted ~/STD** enfermedad de transmisión sexual; enfermedad pasada sexualmente; enfermedad venérea; **sickle cell ~** drepanocitemia; enfermedad de células falciformes; (*See anemia, sickle cell.*); **skin ~** enfermedad dérmica; ~ **that is "going around"** enfermedad de andancia *Chicano*; enfermedad que anda *Chicano*; **venereal ~** enfermedad venérea; (*See venereal disease.*)
disfigured, desfigurado *adj*
disfigurement, deformación *f*; disfiguración *f*

disgorge, to, vomitar
disgust, asco
disgusting, repugnante *adj*; inhumano *adj, Chi*
dish, caja; disco; plato; **Petri ~** placa de Petri
dishcloth, estropajo
dishearten, to, desalentar (ie); desanimar; descorazonar
dishwasher, lavaplatos *m*
disillusion(ment), desilusión *f*
disinfect, to, desinfectar
disinfectant, desinfectante *m, adj*
disinfestation, desinfestación *f*
disinterment, desenterramiento; exhumación *f*
disjoint, to, dislocar
disk, disco; (*See disc.*); **blood ~** plaqueta; **calcified ~** disco calcificado; **dental ~** disco dental; **emery ~** disco de esmeril; **herniated ~** disco herniador; **intervertebral ~** disco intervertebral; **~ protrusion** hernia discal; **slipped ~** disco desplazado; disco intervertebral luxado; **space narrowing ~** pinzamiento del espacio discal
diskogram, discograma *m*
diskography, discografía
dislike, antipatía; aversión *f*
dislocate, to, desconcertar (ie) *Anat*; desconchabar *SpAm*; descoyuntar; desencajar *Anat*; dislocar(se); zafar(se) *Chicano, fam*; **~ a bone** recalcarse *SpAm*; **~ one's jaw** desencajarse la mandíbula; **~ one's shoulder** dislocarse el hombro
dislocated, dislocado *adj*; zafado *adj, SpAm*; **~/out of joint** descoyuntado *adj*
dislocation, desarticulación *f*; desplazamiento; luxación *f*; zafadura *Chicano, fam*; **~** (*of a jaw*) desencajamiento; **~** (*of a bone*) dislocación *f, form*; **compound ~** dislocación compuesta; **congenital ~** dislocación congénita;

~ fracture fractura y luxación; **habitual ~** dislocación iterativa; **traumatic ~** dislocación traumática
dislodge, to, (*to remove*) sacar
dismantle, to, desmantelar
dismay, desmayo; **~** (*discouragement*) desaliento
dismember, to, desmembrar
dismemberment, desmembramiento
dismiss, to, descartar; despedir (i); **~ from the hospital** dar de alta
disorder, ~ (*state of confusion*) desorden *m*; **~** (*ailment*) enfermedad *f*; trastorno; **nervous ~** trastorno nervioso; **personality ~** trastorno de la personalidad; **post-traumatic stress ~** trastorno del estrés postraumático; **psychological ~** desequilibrio *Med*; **sleep ~** trastorno del sueño
disorganization, desorganización *f*
disorientation, desorientación *f*
dispensary, dispensario
dispensation, dispensación *f*
dispense, to, dispensar
disperse, to, dispersar
displace, to, desplazar
displacement, descompostura; desplazamiento
disposable, desechable *adj*; disponible *adj*
disprove, to, refutar
dissect, to, disecar
dissecting, disecante *adj*; **~ aneurysm** aneurisma disecante *m*; **~ forceps** pinzas de disección; **~ hook** erina; **~ knife** escalpelo; **~ room** anfiteatro; sala de disección; **~ set** estuche de disección *m*
dissection, disección *f*; **blunt ~** disección roma; **cadaverous ~** disección cadavérica; **sharp ~** disección cortante
disseminate, to, diseminar(se)
disseminated, diseminado *adj*

dissimilation, desasimilación *f*
dissolve, to, disolver (ue)
dissolvent, disolvente *m, adj*
distal, distal *adj*; ~ **end** extremo distal *Dent*
distance, distancia; **focal** ~ distancia focal; **pupillary** ~ distancia pupilar
distend, to, (*skin*) distender (ie)
distention, distensión *f*
distil, to, destilar
distillate, destilado *adj*
distillation, destilación *f*; **dry** ~ destilación seca
distinguishing feature, característica distintiva
distobuccal, distobucal *adj, Dent*
distobucco-occlusal, distobuco-oclusal *adj, Dent*
distobuccopulpal, distobucopulpar *adj, Dent*
distocervical, distocervical *adj, Dent*
distogingival, distogingival *adj, Dent*
distolabial, distolabial *adj, Dent*
distolabioincisal, distolabioincisivo *adj, Dent*
distolingual, distolingual *adj, Dent*
distolinguoincisal, distolinguoincisivo *adj, Dent*
distolinguo-occlusal, distolinguoclusal *adj, Dent*
distolinguopulpal, distolinguopulpar *adj, Dent*
disto-occlusal, distooclusal *adj, Dent*
distopulpal, distopulpar *adj, Dent*
distopulpolabial, distopulpolabial *adj, Dent*
distopulpolingual, distopulpolingual *adj, Dent*
distortion, distorsión *f*
distracted, to be, andar volado *fam*
distractibility, distractibilidad *f*
distraction, distracción *f*
distress, ~(*afflicted*) aflicción *f*; ~ (*anguish*) angustia; congoja; ~ (*exhaustion*) agotamiento *Med*; ~ (*pain*) dolor *m*; malestar *m*; pena; sufrimiento
distress, to, ~ (*afflict*) afligir; ~ (*an-*

guish) angustiar; ~ (*to exhaust*) agotar *Med*
distressing, ~ (*grievous*) angustioso *adj*; ~ (*afflicting*) aflictivo *adj*; ~ (*painful*) penoso *adj*
distribution, distribución *f*
disturb, to, ~ (*to bother*) molestar; ~ (*to move out of order*) desordenar; ~ (*the peace*; *plans*) alterar; perturbar; ~ (*s.o.'s mind*) trastornar; ~ (*to worry*) preocupar
disturbance, ~ (*bother*) molestia; ~ (*worry*) preocupación *f*; ~ (*mental*) trastorno (mental); **sleep** ~ trastorno del sueño; ~ (*upset*) perturbación *f, Med*
disturbing, ~ (*annoying*) molesto *adj*; ~ (*mentally*) trastornante *adj*; ~ (*worrying*) preocupante *adj*
disuse, desuso; falta de uso; inactividad *f*
diuresis, (*pl, diureses*) diuresis *f*; **tubular** ~ diuresis tubular
diuretic, diurético *m, adj*; píldora diurética; **cardiac** ~ diurético cardíaco; **direct** ~ diurético directo; **indirect** ~ diurético indirecto; **mechanical** ~ diurético mecánico; **saline** ~ diurético salino
diurnal, diurno *adj*
diurnally, diariamente *adv*
divergence, divergencia; **negative vertical** ~ divergencia vertical negativa; **positive vertical** ~ divergencia vertical positiva
divergent, divergente *adj*
diverticulitis, colitis ulcerosa *f*; diverticulitis *f*
diverticulum, divertículo
divide, to, desmembrar; seccionar; separar
division, ~ (*branch*) rama; ~ (*section*) división *f*; sección *f*; (**in**)**direct cell** ~ división celular (in)directa; **multiplicative** ~ división multiplicativa
divorce, divorcio
divorce, to, divorciar

divorced, divorciado *adj*; **to get ~ (from)** divorciarse (de)

dizziness, desvanecimiento; mareo; tarantas *Chicano, Mex, Hond*; vahido; vértigo; **feeling of ~** atacado de vértigo

dizzy, atarantado *adj*; aturdido *adj*; desvanecido *adj*, *Med*; mareado *adj*; vertiginoso *adj*; **~ spell** vaguido; vahido; vapor *m*, *Med*; **to become ~** atarantarse; marearse; **to feel ~** estar mareado; tener vértigo; **to make ~** encalabrinar *Med*

DNA/de(s)oxyribonucleic acid, ADN/ácido desoxirribonucleico

do, to/make, to, hacer

DOA/dead on arrival, fallecido al llegar *adj*

docile, dócil *adj*

doctor, doctor, -ra *m/f*; médico; **~'s advice** consejo médico; **~'s bag** maletín *m*; **to be under ~'s care** seguir (i) un tratamiento médico; **family ~** médico de cabecera; médico de la familia; **~'s fee** honorarios médicos; **~'s office** consultorio; **~'s orders** órdenes médicas *f*; **~'s prescription** receta médica; **private ~** médico privado

doctor, to, (*to give medical attention to*) asistir; atender (ie); **~** (*a patient*) tomar medicinas

doctrine, doctrina

dog, perro

dominance, dominancia; **cerebral ~** dominancia cerebral; **lateral ~** dominancia lateral; **ocular ~** dominancia ocular

dominant, dominante *adj*

donate, to, (*blood*) donar; dar

donee, donatario

donor, dador *m*; donado *adj*; donador *m*, *adj*; donante *m/f*; **blood ~** donante de sangre; **general ~** donador general; **universal ~** donador universal

dope[5], nombre inglés para marigua-

na; droga; estupefaciente *m*; fármaco; narcótico *vulg*; **~ fiend** *fam* toxicómano *m/f*; **~ pusher** burro[2]; madre[2]; narcotraficante *m/f*; pusheador[2] *Chicano*

doper[5], mariguano[2]; moto[2]; quemón[2]; yesco[2]

dormant, durmiente *adj*; inactivo *adj*; latente *adj*

dorsal, dorsal *adj*

dosage, administración de un medicamento *f*; **~** (*determination*) dosificación *f*; **~** (*amount of medicine*) dosis *f*, *inv*; **lethal ~** dosis mortal

dose, medida; toma *Med*; **~** (*amount of medicine*) dosis *f*, *inv*; **average ~** dosis media; **booster ~** dosis de refuerzo; **daily ~** dosis diaria; **effective ~** dosis eficaz; **maintenance ~** dosis de sostén; **maximum ~** máxima dosis ; **maximum tolerated ~** máxima dosis tolerada *f*; **minimum ~** mínima dosis ; **optimum ~** dosis óptima

dose, to, administrar un medicamento (a); medicinar

dosis, dosis *f*, *inv*; **curativa ~** dosis curativa

dossier, expediente *m*

dotage, chochera; chochez *f*; debilidad senil *f*; **to be in one's ~** estar chocho *adj*

dotted line, línea de puntos

double, doble *adj*; **~ blind** doble ciega; **~-blind study** estudio doble a ciegas; **~ bond** doble enlace; **~ chin** papada; sotabarba; **~-chinned** papudo *adj*; **~-edged** de dos filos; **~ flap amputation** amputación a doble colgajo *f*; **~-jointed** con articulaciones dobles; **~ murmur** tono doble; **~ vision** visión doble *f*; vista doble

double, to, doblar; **~ up** (*from pain*) doblarse; **~ up with pain** devanarse de dolor *Cu, Guat, Mex*; **~ up in laughter** retorcerse (ue) de risa

doubling, duplicación *f*; doblez *m*; repliegue *m*

doubt, duda

doubt, to, dudar

douche, ducha; ducha interna; ducha vaginal; irrigación *f*; lavado interno; lavado vaginal

douche, to, ducharse

doughy, pastoso *adj*

Down's syndrome, mal de Down *m*; mongolismo

downer[5]/**downs**[5]/(*barbiturate*), tranquilizante *m*; calmante *m*; sedativo

downgrade, to, rebajar

downhearted, desalentado *adj*

downhill, to go, empeorar

downiness, vellosidad *f*

downstairs, abajo *adv*

doze, to, dormirse (ue); pescar *Col, Ríopl*

DPT/diphtheria-pertussis-tetanus, vacuna triple

draft, poción *f*

drag[5], (*puff of* [*marijuana*] *cigarette*) toque *m*

dragging pain, dolor dragante *m*; dolor opresivo *m*; dolor terebrante *m*; (*See pain.*)

drain, dren *m*; drenaje *m*; tubo de drenaje; **stab wound** ~ dren por contraabertura; dren por transfixión; ~ **tube** tubo de drenaje

drain, to, ~ (*an abscess*) drenar; ~ (*to empty*) vaciar; ~ (*pus, etc.*) salir

drainage, desagüe *m*; supuración *f*; ~ (*surgical*) drenaje *m*; **suction** ~ drenaje por aspiración

draining, drenante *adj*; **dripping** ~ escurrimiento

dram, dracma *m*

Dramamine, Dramamina *f*

drastic, drástico *adj*

draught, poción *f*; pócima; brebaje *m*

draw, to, ~ **an abscess** hacer madurar un absceso; ~ **blood** hacer sangrar; sacar sangre

drawer, cajón *m*; gaveta

drawing, dibujo; esbojo; esquema *m*

dream, sueño

dream (of), to, soñar (ue) (con); fantasear

dreamer, soñador, -ra *m/f*

dregs, sedimento

drench, to, (*to soak*) calar

drenched in blood, bañado en sangre *adj*

drenched to the skin, to be, estar calado hasta los huesos *adj*

drepanocyte, drepanocito *form*

drepanocytemia, anemia de hematíes falciformes; anemia drepanocítica; (*See anemia, sickle cell.*)

dress, to, ~ (*a wound*) vendar; ~ **oneself** vestirse (i)

dressing, ~ (*bandage*) apósito; compresa; cura; curación *f*; emplaste *m*; parche *m*; venda; vendaje *m*; **air** ~ cura abierta; **antiseptic** ~ cura antiséptica; **dry** ~ cura seca; **protective** ~ cura protectora; ~ **scissors** tijeras de vendaje; tijeras de cura; ~ (*edible*) relleno

DRG/diagnostically related group, GRD[4]/grupo relacionado diagnósticamente

dribble, to, gotear

drill, fresa; perforador *m*; taladro; torno; trépano; ~ **hole** agujero de trépano

drill, to, perforar; taladrar

drink, bebida

drink, to, beber; tomar; guarapear(se) *RD*; traguear *CR*; ~ **plenty of** beber mucho

drinker, bebedor, -ra *m/f*

drinking, ~ **fountain** fuente para beber *f*; fuente de agua potable *f*; ~ **test** prueba del glaucoma; ~ **water** agua[3] potable

drip, ~ (*drop*) gota; ~ **by drip** gota a gota; ~ **intravenous** gota a gota intravenosa; **postnasal** ~ escurrimiento postnasal; ~ (*a falling in drops*) goteo; ~ **apparatus** gotero

drip, to, gotear
dripping, que gotea *adj*; ~ **with per-spiration** bañado en sudor *adj*
drive, (*energy, impulse*) impulso; instinto; **sex** ~ impulso sexual
drive, to, manejar; conducir
drivel, ~ (*slobber of an adult*) baba; ~ (*foolishness*) tonterías
drivel, to, decir tonterías *fam*
drool, (*of a child*) baba
drool, to, babear
drooling, babeo
droop, ~ (*of eyelids*) caída; ~ (*of head*) inclinación *f*; ~ (*of shoulders*) encorvamiento
droop, to, ~ (*eyelids*) caerse; bajar; ~ (*head*) inclinar; ~ (*shoulders*) encorvar
drooping, ~ (*ears*) caído *adj*; gacho *adj*; ~ (*eyes*) bajado *adj*; ~ (*head*) inclinado *adj*; ~ (*shoulders*); caído *adj*
drop, gota *Med*; ~ (*in temperature*) baja; ~ (*in pressure, voltage, etc.*) bajada; ~ (*of blood, sweat, water, etc.*) gota; ~[5] *slang* entrega ; lugar donde se deja o se esconde una droga
drop, to, ~ (*the eyes, voice, etc.*) bajar, ~ (*a fever, temperature*) descender (ie); ~ (*to fall*) caerse; ~ **dead** caerse muerto *adj*; ~ **from exhaustion** caerse de cansancio; ~ **on one's knees** caer de rodillas; ~ (*to drip*) gotear; ~ **back into** retroceder
droplet, gotita
dropper, cuentagotas *m, inv*; **eye** ~ cuentagotas *m, inv*; gotero (para los ojos) *m, SpAm*
dropping, ~ (*fall*) caída; ~ (*of womb*) descendimiento
dropsical, hidrópico *adj*
dropsy, hidropesía *Med*; **acute anemic** ~ hidropesía anémica aguda; **cardiac** ~ hidropesía cardíaca; **cutaneous** ~ hidropesía cutánea; **tubal** ~ hidrosálpinx *m*; hidrosalpinge *m*

drosophila, drosofila
drown, to, ahogarse
drowning, ahogamiento; sumersión *f*
drowsiness, modorra; somnolencia; chavalongo *Arg, Chi*; perro *Col*; sopor *m, Med*; sueñera *SpAm*
drowsy, (*sleepy*) amodorrado *adj*; somnoliento *adj*; soñoliento *adj*
drug, ~ (*medicament*) fármaco; medicamento; medicina; ~ **acne** acné medicamentoso; ~ **fever** fiebre medicamentosa *f*; ~ **reaction** reacción medicamentosa *f*; ~ **therapy** tratamiento medicamentoso; **wonder** ~ droga milagrosa; ~ (*narcotic*) droga; estupefaciente *m*; narcótico; ~ **abuse** abuso de (las) drogas; abuso de los estupefacientes; ~ **addict** drogadicto; adicto a las drogas; ~ **addiction** dependencia farmacológica; habituamiento a las drogas; narcomanía; **antagonistic** ~ droga antagonista; ~ **habit** morfinomanía; toxicomanía; **habit-forming** ~ droga que produce hábito; **hallucinogenic** ~ alucinógeno; droga alucinadora; ~ **overdose** sobredosis de drogas *f*; ~ **supply** cachucha; ~ **traffic** venta y tráfico de drogas; ~ **withdrawal** desintoxicación *f*; supresión de un narcótico *f*; **to be on** ~**s** drogarse; ~ (*remedy*) remedio
drug, to, endrogar[2]
drugged, endrogado[2] *adj*; prendido[2] *adj*
druggist, boticario; farmacéutico
drugstore, botica; droguería *SpAm*; drugstore *m, Chicano*; farmacia *Chicano, Spain*
drum, tímpano *Anat*
drunk, alumbrado *adj, slang, Chicano*; bolo *adj, CA*; borracho *adj*; caneco *adj, Arg, Bol*; ebrio *adj*; embriagado *adj*; envinado *adj, Arg*; intoxicado *adj*; pisto *adj*; pitongo *adj, Chi*; rascado *adj*,

Ven; tacuache *adj*; tiberio *adj,
Guat, Mex*; tlacuache *adj*; tronado *adj*; **to be/to get ~** agarrarse
un peludo; agarrar una perica
Col, Ec, Pan; andar bombo *slang*;
andar eléctrico *slang*; andar en
la línea *slang*; andar loco *slang*;
chumarse *Ec, Ríopl*; coger una
borrachera;   emborracharse;
empedarse *Mex, Ríopl*; encalamocarse *Col, Ven*; estar chupado;
estar duro *Mex, Ur*; estar mediagua *slang*; estar tomado *SpAm*;
guarapear(se) *RD*; ponerse alto
fam; rajarse *PR*; rascar *slang,
SpAm*; socarse *CA*; tener una
tranca *SpAm*; tiznarse *Chi, Guat,
Mex*; traguear *Ven*; traguearse
CA, Col, Mex; trancarse *Cu, Ven*;
to get ~ (*on wine*) envinarse *Mex*

drunkard, trinco *Mex, PR*

drunken, cuete *adj*; **~ fit** borrachera; pítima

drunkenness, borrachera; chinga
Ven; chuma *Ec, Ríopl*; embriaguez *f*; tagarnina *Col, Guat,
Mex*; taranta *Mex*; tiempla *Chi*;
trinca *Cu, Mex, PR*

dry, **~** (*not wet*) seco *adj*; **~ blood**
sangre desecada *f*; **~ ice** nieve
carbónica *f*; **~ heaves** náusea sin
vomitar; **~ labor** parto seco; **~
mouth** sequedad de boca *f*; **~
rale** estertor seco *m*; **~ tap** punción diagnóstica que no con-
sigue extraer líquido a causa del
espesor de éste *f*; **~ weight** peso
en seco; **~** (*parched*) reseco *adj*

dry, to, secar

dryer, secador *m*; **clothes ~** secadora; **hair ~** secador de cabello/de
pelo; secador para el pelo

drying, desecante *adj*; secante *adj*

dryness, sequedad *f*; **~ of the skin**
resequedad de la piel *f*; se-
quedad de la piel

**D.S.C./Doctor of Surgical Chi-
ropody**, Doctor en Quiropodia
Quirúrgica

duct, tubo; **~ canal** canal *m, Anat*;
conducto *Anat*; trompa *Anat*;
acoustic ~ conducto meato auditivo external; **alimentary ~** conducto torácico; **alveolar ~**
conducto alveolar; **arterial ~**
conducto arterioso; **auditory ~**
conducto auditivo; **cochlear ~**
conducto coclear; **common bile
~** conducto colédoco; **ejaculatory ~** conducto eyaculador; **hepatic ~** conducto hepático; **left
lymphatic ~** conducto torácico;
right lymphatic ~ conducto linfático derecho; **nephric ~** uréter
m; **ovarian ~** conducto ovárico;
pancreatic ~ conducto pancreático; **prostatic ~s** conductos
prostáticos; **salivary ~s** conductos salivales; **tear ~** canal lagrimal; conducto lagrimal; vaso
Med

ductless, *Anat* endocrino *adj*; de
secreción interna; que no tiene
conducto excretor; **~ gland**
glándula de secreción interna;
glándula endocrina

dull, **~** (*color*) opaco; **~** (*intellectu-
ally*) estúpido *adj*; tonto *adj*; **~**
(*lackluster*) sin relieve *prep phr*;
~ (*lifeless*) sin vida *prep phr*; **~**
(*obtuse*) lerdo *adj*; torpe *adj*; **~**
(*sounds*) mate *adj*; **~** (*pain,
sounds*) sordo *adj*; **~** (*sense*) embotado *adj*; **~ sense of hearing**
duro de oído *adj*; **to have a ~
sense of hearing** ser duro de
oído; **~ voice** voz apagada

dull, to, **~** (*to lessen pain*) aliviar(se);
~ (*emotions*) enfriar(se); **~** (*senses*) embotar(se); **~** (*sounds*)
amortiguar(se); apagar

dullness, (*sound*) matidez *f*

dumb, (*not speaking*) mudo *adj*;
born ~ mudo de nacimiento

dumbbell, halterio; pesa

dumbness, mudez, *f, Med*

dump, to, (*to get rid of*) dompear[2]

duodenal, duodenal *adj*

duodenitis, duodenitis *f*
duodenum, duodeno
dura mater, duramadre *f*
durable, duradero *adj*
duration, duración *f*
dusk, (*twilight*) crepúsculo
dusk, at, al anochecer; al atardecer
dust, ~ (*powder*) polvo; ~~free libre de polvo *adj*; ~ (*ashes of dead person*) cenizas *f, pl*; ~ (*cocaine, PCP*) cucuy[2]; fencyclidina; líquido[2]; PCP[4]; polvo[2]
dust, to, (*powder*) espolvorear
duty, off ~ libre de servicio; **to be off** ~ no estar de servicio; **on** ~ de servicio; de turno; **to be on** ~ estar de servicio
D.V.M./Doctor of Veterinary Medicine, Doctor en Medicina Veterinaria
dwarf, enano
dwarfism, enanismo
dwelling catheter, catéter permanente *m*; (*See catheter.*)
dye, colorante *m*; tinte *m*; tintura; ~ **test** reacción de coloración *f*
dye, to, colorar; teñir (i)
dying, moribundo *adj*
dynamic, dinámico *adj*; ~ **relations** relaciones dinámicas *f, Dent*
dynamics, dinámica
dysentery, cursio *fam*; disentería; **amoebic** ~ disentería amebiana; disentería amibiana;

bacillary ~ disentería bacilar; **to have** ~ obrar con sangre
dysfunction, disfunción *f*
dyslexia, dislexia
dysmenorrhea, dismenorrea *form*; menstruación dolorosa *f*; **acquired** ~ dismenorrea adquirida; **inflammatory** ~ dismenorrea inflamatoria; **mechanical** ~ dismenorrea mecánica; **tubal** ~ dismenorrea tubárica
dyspareunia/painful coitus, dispareunia
dyspepsia, dispepsia *form*; estómago sucio; indigestión *f*; **acid** ~ dispepsia ácida; **flatulent** ~ dispepsia flatulenta; **gastric** ~ dispepsia gástrica; **reflex** ~ dispepsia refleja; **salivary** ~ dispepsia salival
dysphagia, dificultad al tragar *f*; disfagia *form*
dysplasia, displasia
dyspnea, dificultad al respirar *f*; disnea *form*; **cardiac** ~ disnea cardíaca; **exertional** ~ disnea de esfuerzo; **paroxysmal** ~ disnea paroxística; **renal** ~ disnea renal
dyspneic, corto de respiración *adj*
dystrophy, progressive muscular, distrofia muscular progresiva
dysuria, disuria *form*; dolor al orinar *m*

---

[2] This is new vocabulary, not necessarily listed nor yet recognized by the Royal Academy of Spanish Grammar. It is understood that this vocabulary is primarily slang. Unless otherwise indicated, the gender of nouns is assumed to be obvious.
[3] For pronunciation purposes, the masculine definite and indefinite articles, *el* and *un*, not *la* or *una*, are used when the article immediately precedes the feminine singular noun which begins with stressed *a* or any other that begins with stressed *ha*.
[4] Use the Spanish pronunciation of these letters.
[5] Part of the Drug Abuse Vocabulary.

E

E & H/environment and heredity, ambiente y herencia

each, cada; ~ **week** cada semana

EAHF/eczema, asthma, and hay fever, eczema, asma y fiebre del heno

ear (*outer portion*), oreja; ~ (*organ of hearing*), oído; **acute** ~ otitis media aguda *f*; **auditory** ~ auditivo *adj*; **buzzing of** ~**s** zumbido en los oídos; ~**-deafening** ensordecimiento; ~ **blockage** bloqueo de la trompa; ~ **cough** tos auricular *f*; ~**ache** dolor de oído *m*; dolor de sentidos *m, fam*; dolencia *fam*; ~ **drops** gotas óticas; ~**drum** (*tympanic membrane*) tímpano; tambor *m, Anat*; **perforated** ~ tambor roto; tímpano roto; ~ **dust** otoconio; ~ **infection** infección de los oídos *f*; **Eustachian tube** trompa de Eustaquio; **external** ~ aurícola; oído externo; oreja; pabellón externo de la oreja *m*; ~ **canal** canal de la oreja *m, fam*; conducto auditivo externo; ~ **lobe** lóbulo; pulpejo; **inner** ~ oído interno; **cochlea** caracol *m, fam*; cóclea *form*; **semicircular** ~ **canal**[4] conducto semicircular; ~ **memory** memoria auditiva; **middle** ~ oído medio; **anvil** (*incus*) yunque *m*; **hammer** (*malleus*) martillo; **stirrup** (*stapes*) estribo; ~**, nose and throat specialist** otorrinolaringólogo; ~**-piercing** (*sound*) ensordecimiento; ~ **pit** fístula congénita de la oreja; **saccule** sáculo; ~**scope** audioscopio; ~**-shattering** (*sound*) ensordecimiento; ~**trumpet** otoscopio; ~**wax** cera de los oídos; cerilla, cerumen *m*; **impacted** ~ tapón de cera *m*

early, precoz *adj*; temprano *adj*; ~ **birth** parto prematuro; ~ **detection** detección temprana *f*; ~ **syphilis** sífilis primaria *f*; ~ **treatment** tratamiento precoz

earnest, grave *adj*

earring, ~ (*close to earlobes*) arete *m*; pantalla *PR*; ~ (*dangling from earlobes*) pendiente *m*

earth, tierra

earwigs, tijeretas; tijerillas

ease, to, aliviar; mitigar; relajar; ~ **off/up** bajar

easily, fácilmente *adv*; con facilidad *prep phr*

easy, fácil *adj*; talao *adj, PR*; ~ (*life*) cómodo *adj*; ~ (*gullible*) fácil de engañar *adj*; ~ (*morals*) laxo *adj*; ~ (*punishment*) leve *adj*; ~ (*manner*) natural *adj*; ~ (*gentle*) suave *adj*; ~ (*conscience, mind*) tranquilo *adj*; **to take it** ~ cogerlo suave *PR*; tomárselo con calma

eat, to, comer; ~ **breakfast** desayunarse; ~ **dinner/supper** cenar; ~ **frugally** templarse en la comida; ~ **lunch** almorzar (ue); ~ **too much** comer demasiado; empancinar(se) *PR*

eatable, comestible *adj*

EB virus, virus de Epstein-Barr *m*

EBM (expressed breast milk), leche humana exprimida *f*

ebriety, embriaguez *f*

ebullient, hirviente *adj*

EBV/Epstein-Barr virus, virus de Epstein-Barr *m*

eccentric, excéntrico *adj*

ecchymosis, cardenal *m, fam*; equimosis *f*

ecchymotic mask syndrome, síndrome de asfixia traumática *m*

ECF/extracellular fluid, LEC/ líquido extracelular

ECG/electrocardiogram, electrocardiograma *m*; electrocardiografía

electrocardiographic pattern, trazado electrocardiográfico

echocardiogram, ecocardiograma *m*; ecocardiografía

echoencephalography, ecoencefalografía

eclampsia, eclampsia

eclipse blindness, ceguera por eclipse; retinitis solar *f*

ecology, ecología

economy, economía

ecosystem, ecosistema *m*

ecstasy, éxtasis *f*

ecstatic trance, trance histérico *m*

ECT/electroconvulsive therapy, electroshockterapia; terapia electroconvulsiva; terapia electrochoque

ectoderm, ectodermo

ectopia, ectopia; **~ of the testicles** ectopia testicular

ectopic, ectópico *adj*

ectoplasm, ectoplasma *m*

eczema, eccema *m/f*, [*Ú.m.c.m.*]; eczema *m/f*, [*Ú.m.c.m.*]; lepra *fam*; rezumamiento; **crackled ~** eccema fisurado; **dry ~** eccema seco; **infantile ~** eccema del lactante; eccema infantil; **moist ~** eccema húmedo; **seborrheic ~** eccema seborreico; **squamosum ~** eccema escamoso; **vaccination ~** eczema vacunado

E.D./effective dose, dosis eficaz *f*, *inv*; dosis efectiva *f*, *inv*

E.D.C./expected date of confinement, fecha calculada de parto

E.D.D./expected date of delivery, fecha esperada del parto

edema, edema *m*; hinchazón *f*; **acute pulmonary ~** edema agudo de pulmón; **angioneurotic ~** edema angioneurótico; **cardiac ~** edema cardiaco/cardía-co; **famine ~** edema de hambre; **pulmonary ~** edema pulmonar

edge, filo; borde *m*; margen *m*; **~-to-edge occlusion** oclusión borde a borde *f*

edged, afilado *adj*

edible, comestible *adj*

educate, to, educar

education, educación *f*; **health ~** educación para la salud

educational program, programa de instrucción *m*; programa educativo *m*

EEG/electroencephalogram, EEG/electroencefalograma *m*; (*brain wave test*)

eel worm, nematodo

EENT/eyes, ears, nose, and throat, ojos, oídos, nariz y garganta

efface, to, borrar; tachar

effacement, borradura; tachón *m*, *Med*

effect, efecto; **additive ~** efecto de sumación; **adverse ~** efecto adverso; **cumulative ~** efecto acumulativo; **side ~** efecto colateral; efecto secundario; **to have no ~** no dar resultado; **to take ~** surtir efecto

effective, efectivo *adj*; eficaz *adj*; útil *adj*

effeminate, afeminado *adj*; partido *adj*, *PR*; **~ male** plumero *PR*

effervescent, efervescente *adj*

efficiency, eficiencia

efficient, eficaz *adj*; eficiente *adj*

effleurage, forma de masaje en dirección de la corriente venosa

efflorescence, eflorencia *form*; erupción *f*; roncha

efflux, derrame *m*; flujo; salida

effluxion, efluxión *f*; expulsión del huevo, generalmente inadvertida, en los primeros días del embarazo *f*

effort, esfuerzo

effusion, derrame *m*; **hemorrhagic ~** derrame hemorrágico; **peri-**

cardial ~ derrame pericárdico; **pleural** ~ derrame pleural
efuniculate, sin cordón umbilical
e.g., por ejemplo
egg, huevo; **fried** ~ huevo frito; **hard-boiled** ~ huevo duro; **scrambled** ~ huevo revuelto; **~shell nail** uña en cáscara de huevo; **small** ~ (*of a parasite*) huevecillo; **soft-boiled** ~ huevo pasado por agua; ~ **white** clara de huevo; ~ **yolk** yema de(l) huevo; óvulo *Med*
eggshell, cáscara de huevo
ego, ego; ~ **enhancement** refuerzo del ego; ~ **libido** narcisismo
egocentric, egocéntrico *m, adj*
ejaculate, **to**, eyacular *form*; venirse *slang*
ejaculatio (praecox), eyaculación (precoz) *f*; eyaculación (prematura) *f*
ejection, excreción *f*; expulsión *f*; eyaculación *f*
EKG/electrocardiogram, electrocardiograma *m*; electrocardiografía
elapse, **to**, transcurrir
elastic, elástico *adj*; elástica *f, adj*
elasticity, elasticidad *f*
elbow, codo; **at one's** ~ al alcance de la mano; **baseball pitcher's** ~ codo de lanzador; ~ **grease** fuerza de puños; **miners'** ~ codo de los mineros; **tennis** ~ codo de tenis; **to be up to the ~s in work** estar agobiado de trabajo
elbow, **to**, dar un codazo
elbowed catheter, sonda biacodada
elder, ~ (*tree*) saúco; ~ (*age*) anciano *m, adj*; de más edad; mayor *adj*
elderly (man), anciano
elderly, **to be getting**, ir para viejo
elective, electivo *adj*
electric, eléctrico *adj*; ~ **cataract** catarata por fulguración; ~ **current** corriente eléctrica *f*; ~

eye célula fotoeléctrica; ~ **field** campo eléctrico; ~ **intensity** intensidad eléctrica *f*; ~ **polarity** polaridad eléctrica *f*; ~ **potential** potencial eléctrico *m*; ~ **shock** excitación eléctrica; ~ **socket** enchufe *m*; tomacorriente *f, SpAm*; ~ **valve** válvula
electrical, eléctrico *adj*; ~ **activity** actividad eléctrica *f*; ~ **burn** quemadura eléctrica; ~ **current** corriente *f*; ~ **ground(ing)** a tierra; ~ **lead wire** alambre de contacto *m*; ~ **outlet** salida; ~ **plug** clavija de contacto; enchufe *m*
electrician, electricista *m/f*
electricity, electricidad *f*; **dynamic** ~ electricidad dinámica; **galvanic** ~ electricidad galvánica; **static** ~ electricidad estática
electrify, **to**, electrificar
electro-analysis, electroanálisis *m, inv*
electrocardiogram, electrocardiograma *m*; electrocardiografía
electrocardiograph, electrocardiógrafo
electrocardiography, electrocardiografía
electrocautery, electrobisturí *m*
electrocoagulation, electrocoagulación *f*
electrocute, **to**, electrocutar
electrocution, electrocución *f*
electrode, electrodo; **depolarizing** ~ electrodo despolarizante; ~ **supporting-arm** brazo portaelectrodo; **therapeutic** ~ electrodo terapéutico
electrodiagnostic, electrodiagnóstico *m, adj*
electrodialysis, electrodiálisis *f*; electrólisis *f*
electroencephalogram, electroencefalograma *m*
electroencephalography, electroencefalografía
electrolyte, electrólito
electrolytic, electrolítico *adj*

electromagnet, electroimán *m*
electromagnetic, electromagnético *adj*
electromagnetism, electromagnetismo
electromyogram, electromiograma *m*
electromyography, electromiografía
electron, electrón *m*; ~ **beam** haz electrónico *m*; ~ **microscope** microscopio electrónico
electronic, electrónico *adj*; ~ **monitoring** monitoría electrónica
electronics, electrónica
electrophoresis, electroforesis *f*; ~ **on paper curtain** electroforesis en tira de papel; ~ **on starch block** electroforesis en bloques de almidón
electroplate, to, galvanizar
electroplating, galvanoplastia
electroshock, choque eléctrico *m*; electrochoque *m*; electroshock *m, Chicano*; ~ **therapy** terapéutica por electrochoque
electrosurgery, electrocirugía
electrotherapy, electroterapia
element, elemento; **anatomic** ~ elemento anatómico; **electronegative** ~ elemento electronegativo; **electropositive** ~ elemento electropositivo; **galvanic** ~ pila eléctrica; **morphological** ~ elemento morfológico; **tracer** ~ elemento trazador
elephantiasis, elefantiasis *f*; elefancía
elevate, to, ~ (*to raise*) elevar; ~ (*eyes, voice*) alzar
elevated, elevado *adj*
elevation, elevación *f*
elevator, ascensor *m*; ~ (*lift*) elevador *m, Dent*
eligible, elegible *adj*
eliminate, to, eliminar
elimination, eliminación *f*
elixir, elixir *m*
elongation, distensión *f*; elon-

gación *f*; **surgical** ~ **of the nerves** elongación quirúrgica de los nervios
emaciate, to, adelgazar; enflaquecer
emaciated, chupado *adj*; demacrado *adj*; flaco *adj*; severamente enflaquecido *adj*; ~ (*person*) deshecho *adj, Med*
emaciation, demacración *f*; desmedro *Med*; emaciación *f*; enflaquecimiento
emasculated, castrado *adj*; demasculinizado *adj*
emasculation, emasculación *f*; castración masculina *f*
embalm, to, embalsamar
embalming, embalsamamiento
embalment, embalsamamiento
embarrass, to, ~ (*to complicate*) complicar; ~ (*to disconcert*) turbar; ~ (*to hinder*) molestar; ~ (*to put in tight spot*) embarazar; ~ (*to cause to blush*) avergonzar; encaramar *Col, CR*
embarrassed, to be, avergonzarse; mortificarse *Mex, CA, Ven*; pasar vergüenza; sentirse (ie) molesto
embarrassed, to get, encaramarse *Col, CR*
embarrassing, embarazoso *adj*
embarrassment, vergüenza
embed, to, empotrar; sujetar
embody, to, incluir; incorporar
embolism, embolia; embolismo; **air** ~ embolia gaseosa; **cerebral** ~ embolia cerebral; **coronary** ~ embolia coronaria; **lymphogenous** ~ embolia linfática; **pulmonary** ~ embolia pulmonar; **retinal** ~ embolia de la retina; **retrograde** ~ embolia retrógrada
embolus, (*pl, emboli*) émbolo; **air** ~ émbolo de aire; **cancer** ~ émbolo canceroso; **fat** ~ émbolo de grasa; **obturating** ~ émbolo obturador; **straddling** ~ émbolo en silla de montar

embrace, abrazo
embrace, to, abrazar
embryo, embrión *m*
embryocardia, embriocardia
embryologic lumen, tubo ebriológico
embryologist, embriólogo
embryology, embriología
embryonic development, desarrollo del embrión; desarrollo embrionario
embryotherapy, embrioterapia
emend, to, corregir (i); enmendar (ie)
emergency, caso urgente; emergencia; urgencia; ~ **reaction** reacción de alarma *f*; ~ **room** sala de emergencia; sala de urgencia
emesis, emesis *f, adj*; ~ **basin** escupidera; riñonera; vasija para vomitar
emetic, emético *m, adj*; vomitivo *m, adj*; ~ **cough** tos emetizante *f*
EMG/electromyogram, EMG[5]/ electromiograma *m*; EMG[5]/ electromiografía
emission, (nocturnal), emisión (nocturna) *f*
emit, to, emitir
emollient, emoliente *m, adj*
emotion, emoción *f*
emotional, emocional *adj*; ~ **bond** unión emocional *f*; ~ **shock** choque emocional *m*; coraje *m, fam*; susto *m, fam*; ~ **stress** estrés emocional *Chicano*; ~ **tension syndrome of infants** síndrome de tensión emocional de la madre durante el embarazo *m*
empathy, empatía
emphasize, to, enfatizar *SpAm*; poner de relieve
emphysema, enfisema *m*; **alveolar** ~ enfisema alveolar; **compensatory** ~ enfisema suplementario; **pulmonary** ~ enfisema pulmonar; **surgical** ~ enfisema traumático

empiric, empírico *adj*
employees' health service, dispensario de empleados
employer, empleador, -ra *m/f*; jefe/jefa *m/f*; patrón, -na *m/f*
employment, empleo; trabajo
empoison, to, envenenar
empty, desocupado *adj*; vacío *adj*
empty (out), to, vaciar
EMS/emergency medical service, servicio médico de urgencia
emulsification, emulsificación *f*
emulsifier, emulsor *m, adj*
emulsify, to, emulsionar
emulsion, emulsión *f*
enamel, esmalte *m*; substancia adamantina; **mottled** ~ esmalte manchado; esmalte moteado
encapsulation, encapsulación *f*
encapsulated, encapsulado *adj*
encasing cell, célula de revestimiento
encephalalgia, dolor intenso, profundo de la cabeza *m*; encefalalgia *f, form*
encephalitis, encefalitis *f*; **acute disseminated** ~ encefalitis aguda diseminada *f*; **hemorragic** ~ encefalitis hemorrágica; **postvaccinalis** ~ encefalitis postinfectiva; **purulent** ~ encefalitis purulenta
encephalogram, encefalograma *m*
encephalography, encefalografía
encephalon, encéfalo
encephalomyelitis, encefalomielitis *f*
encephalopathy, encefalopatía
encircling, circundante *adj*
enclosed, encerrado *adj*
encourage, to, animar; dar ánimos
encrust, to, incrustar
encrusted tongue, lengua saburral
encysted, enquistado *adj*
end, fin *m*; ~ **product** producto de desecho; producto final
end, to, acabar; terminar
endanger, to, poner en peligro
endaortic, endaórtico *adj*

endarterectomy, endarterectomía
endemic, endémico *adj*
ending, terminación *f*; **nerve ~** terminación nerviosa *f*
endlobe, lóbulo terminal
endocardial ridges, crestas endocárdicas
endocarditis, endocarditis *f*; **acute bacterial ~** endocarditis bacteriana aguda; **fetal ~** endocarditis fetal; **infective ~** endocarditis infectiva; **malignant ~** endocarditis maligna; **septic ~** endocarditis séptica; **ulcerative ~** endocarditis ulcerosa; endocarditis ulcerativa
endocardium, endocardio
endocranium, duramadre encefálica *f*; endocráneo
endocrine, endocrino *adj*; **~ system** aparato endocrino; sistema endocrino *m*
endocrinologist, endocrinólogo
endocrinology, endocrinología
endoderm, endodermo
endodontist, endodontista *m/f*
endodontitis, endodontitis *f*; inflamación de la pulpa dental *f*
endometriosis, endometriosis *f*
endometritis, endometritis *f*; inflamación de la mucosa uterina *f*
endometrium, endometrio
endomyocardial, endomiocárdico *adj*
endorphin, endorfina
endoplasm, endoplasma *m*
endoscope, endoscopio
endoscopy, endoscopia; inspección directa de una cavidad o conducto del cuerpo por medio de instrumentos ópticos *f*
endostethoscope, endostetoscopio
endotracheal, endotraqueal *adj*
endow, to, dotar
end-plate, placa terminal
endurance, resistencia
endure, to, aguantar; soportar; sufrir
enema, ayuda; enema *m/f*,

[*Ú.m.c.f.*]; lavado; lavaje *m*, *Med*; lavativa *fam*; visitadora *SpAm*; visita *Perú*, *PR*; **~ bag** bolsa para enemas; **barium ~** enema de bario; enema opaca; **blind ~** enema ciega; **cleansing ~** enema de limpieza; **(double) contrast ~** enema de contraste (doble); **nutrient ~** enema nutritiva; **retention ~** enema de retención; **soapsuds ~** enema jabonosa; **~ syringe** jeringa de lavativa
energetic, enérgico *adj*
energy, energía; **chemical ~** energía química; **conservation of ~** conservación de la energía *f*; **kinetic ~** energía cinética; **nuclear ~** energía atómica; energía nuclear; **~ output** producción energética *f*; **radiant ~** energía radiante
enervate, to, desnervar
enervation, enervación *f*
enfeeble, to, debilitar
enfeebled, decrépito *adj*
engage, to, encajar
engagement, encajamiento (de la cabeza fetal) *Obst*
engender, to, engendrar
engineer, ingeniero
engineering, ingeniería; **genetic ~** ingeniería genética
engorge, to, engullir
engorged, ingurgitado *adj*; **~ nipple** pezón enlechado *m*
engorgement, estancamiento
enjoy, to, disfrutar con (*to possess health, etc.*); **~ oneself** divertirse (ie)
enlarge, to, **~** (*to make larger*) agrandar; **~** (*to make bigger*) ampliar; dilatar *Med*
enlarged heart, corazón grande *m*
enlarged kidney, nefromegalia
enlargement, agrandamiento; ampliación *f*; dilatación *f*; ensanchamiento; **~ of the veins** agrandamiento de las venas; venas agrandadas *fam*; várices *fam*

enough, bastante *adj*; suficiente *adj*
enormous, enorme *adj*
enrich, to, enriquecer
enriched, enriquecido *adj*
ENT/ear, nose, and throat, (*otorhinolaryngologist*) GNO⁵/ garganta, nariz, y oídos (*otorrinolaringólogo*); ~ **exam** examen otorrinolaringológico *m*
enter, to, ~ (*to go into*; *penetrate into*) entrar (en); penetrar (en); ~ (*go through*; *endure*) pasar (por); ~ (*to record*) registrar
enterectomy, enterectomía; resección de una parte de intestino *f*
enteric fever, fiebre tifoidea *f*
enteritis, enteritis *f*; **cicatrizing chronic** ~ enteritis cicatrizante crónica
enterologist, enterólogo *m*
enterology, enterología
enteropathy, enteropatía
entire, entero *adj*
entrails, entrañas; intestinos; vísceras
entrance, entrada
entropy, entropía
enucleate, to, extirpar
enucleation, enucleación *f*
enunciation, pronunciación *f*
envelope, ~ (*sheath*) envoltura (*membrana limitante de algunos virus*); ~ (*for letters*) sobre *m*
environment, ambiente *m*
environmental, ambiental *adj*
enzyme, enzima; jugo digestivo; **bacterial** ~ enzima bacteriana; **coagulating** ~ enzima coagulante; **inorganic** ~ enzima inorgánica
enzymic diabetes, diabetes diastásica *f*
eosinophil, eosinófilo
ephedrine, efedrina
ephemeral fever, fiebre de un día *f*, *fam*; fiebre fugaz *f*, *fam*
epiblast, epiblasto
epicanthus, epicanto

epicarditis, epicarditis *f*
epicardium, epicardio
epicondyle, epicóndilo
epicondylitis, humeral, (*tennis elbow*) **form** codo de tenis *fam*; epicondilalgia del húmero; epicondilitis humeral *f*, *form*
epidemic, epidemia; epidémico *adj*; peste *f*
epidemiologist, epidemiólogo
epidemiology, epidemiología
epidermal, epidérmico *adj*
epidermis, epidermis *f*
epididymis, epidídimo
epidural, epidural *adj*; ~ **injection** inyección epidural *f*
epigastric, epigástrico *adj*; ~ **fullness** plenitud epigástrica *f*; ~ **throbbing** latido epigástrico
epigastrium, boca del estómago
epiglottis, epiglotis *f*
epiglottitis, epiglotitis *f*
epilepsy, epilepsia *form*; enfermedad de San Valentín *f*; enfermedad lunática *f*; mal comicial *m*; mal caduco *m*; mal de Hércules *m*; mal de San Juan *m*; mal de San Pablo *m*; mal de San Pedro *m*; mal intelectual *m*; **abortive** ~ epilepsia abortiva; **autonomic diencephalic** ~ epilepsia autonómica diencefálica; **major** ~ gran mal *m*
epileptic, epiléptico *m, adj*; ~ **attack** ataque de epilepsia *m*; ataque epiléptico *m*; baile de zambito *m, fam*; convulsión *f*; ~ **seizure** crisis epiléptica *f, inv*
epinephrine, epinefrina
epiphysis (*bone head*), epífisis *f*
episiotomy, corte de las partes *m*; episiotomía; tajo *slang*
episode, episodio
epithelium, epitelio; **ciliated** ~ epitelio celiado; **columnar** ~ epitelio cilíndrico; **false** ~ epitelio falso; **squamous** ~ epitelio escamoso; **stratified** ~ epitelio estratificado

Epsom salt, sal de Epsom *f*; sal de higuera *f*; sulfato de magnesia

equation, ecuación *f*; **chemical ~** ecuación química

equator, ecuador *m*; **~ of the cell** ecuador de la célula; **~ of crystalline lens** ecuador del cristalino; **~ of the eyeball** ecuador del ojo

equilibrate, to, equilibrar

equilibration, equilibración *f*; **occlusal ~** equilibración oclusal

equilibrium, balance *m*; equilibrio; **acid-base ~** equilibrio acidobásico; **homeostatic ~** equilibrio homeostático; **physiologic ~** equilibrio fisiológico; **radioactive ~** equilibrio radioactivo

equipment, aparato; equipo

equivalent, equivalente *m*

eradiate, to, irradiar

eradicate, to, erradicar; extirpar

erect, ~ (*upright*) derecho *adj*; tieso *adj*

erectile, eréctil *adj*

erection, erección *f*; **to lose an ~** bajar(se) *vulg*

erode, to, corroer; disminuir por roce; erosionar(se)

erogenous, erógeno *adj*

erosion, erosión *f*; **cervical ~** erosión cervical

erotic, erótico *adj*

eroticism, eroticismo

erotism, erotismo

ERPF/effective renal plasma flow, flujo plasmático renal efectivo

erratic, errático *adj*

erroneous, erróneo *adj*

error, error *m*

eruption, erupción *f*; **drug ~** erupción por medicamentos; **~ of the skin** sampullido; sarpullido

erysipelas, erisipela *form*; dicipela *Chicano*; **coast ~** erisipela de la costa; **idiopathic ~** erisipela médica; **migrant ~** erisipela migratoria

erythema, eritema *m*; **endemic ~** eritema endémico; **infectiosum ~** eritema infeccioso; **inflammatory ~** eritema inflamatorio; **multiform ~** eritema multiforme; **nodosum (syphiliticum) ~** eritema nudoso (sifilítico)

erythroblast, eritroblasto; **basophilic ~** eritroblasto basófilo

erythroblastosis, eritroblastosis *f*

erythrocyte (*red blood cell*), eritrocito; glóbulo rojo; hematíe *m*; **achromic ~** eritrocito acrómico; **immature ~** eritrocito inmaduro

erythrodermia, eritrodermia

erythromycin, eritromicina

escape, ~ (*of gas, steam, etc.*) escape *m*; **ventricular ~** escape ventricular; **~** (*of liquid*) salida; **fire ~** escalera de incendios; **~ reaction** reacción de evitación *f*

escape, to, escaparse

esophageal, esofágico *adj*

esophagitis, esofagitis *f*; **peptic ~** esofagitis péptica; **reflux ~** esofagitis por reflujo

esophagology, esofagología

esophagoscope, esofagoscopio

esophagoscopy, esofagoscopia

esophagospasm, esofagospasmo; esofagismo

esophagus, esófago; boca del estómago *fam*; tragante *m, fam, Chicano*; tragadero *fam*; **~ thoracic inlet** hiato superior del esófago

esophoric, esofórico *adj*

ESP/extrasensory perception, percepción extrasensorial *f*

essence, esencia; **~ of peppermint** esencia de menta

essential, esencial *adj*; fundamental *adj*; necesario *adj*

EST/electroshock therapy, electroshockterapia *Chicano*; terapéutica por electrochoque

established, establecido *adj*

estimate, cálculo
esthetic, estético *adj*
estrangement, enajenación *f*; enajenamiento
estriol, estriol *m*
estrogen, estrógeno; ~ **replacement therapy** terapia sustitutoria con estrógeno
et al., y otros
ethanol, etanol *m*
ether, éter *m*; **anesthetic** ~ éter anestésico; **ethyl** ~ éter etílico
ethical, ético *adj*
ethics, ética; **medical** ~ ética médica; **professional** ~ ética profesional
ethnic, étnico *adj*
ethnography, etnografía
ethnology, etnología
ethyl, etilo; ~ **acetate** acetato de etilo; etilo acético; ~ **alcohol** alcohol etílico *m*; ~ **bromide** bromuro de etilo; éter bromhídrico *m*; ~ **chloride** cloruro de etilo; ~ **iodide** éter yodhídrico *m*; yoduro de etilo
ethylene, etileno
etiology, etiología
etiological, etiológico adj
EUA/exam under anesthesia, examen bajo anestesia *m*
eucalyptol, eucaliptol *m*
eucalyptus, eucalipto; ~ **leaves** hojas de eucalipto
eucalyptus oil, esencia de eucalipto
eugenics, eugenesia
eugenol, eugenol *m*, *Dent*
eunuch, eunuco
euphoria, euforia
Eustachian tube, trompa de Eustaquio
euthanasia, eutanasia
evacuate, to, evacuar
evacuation, evacuación *f*
evaluate, to, evaluar
evaluation, evaluación *f*
evanescent, que desaparece

evaporate, to, evaporarse
evaporated milk, leche evaporada *f*
evaporation, evaporación *f*
even, incluso *adv*; ~ (*number*) par *adj*; ~ (*placid*) apacible *adj*; ~ (*smooth*) liso *adj*; ~ (*uniform*) uniforme *adj*
event, episodio; proceso; suceso
eventually, con el tiempo
ever, alguna vez *adv*; jamás *adv*
eversion, eversión *f*
every, cada *adj*; ~ **other day** a días alternos; cada dos días; un día sí, otro no
everywhere, en todas partes; por todas partes
evidence, evidencia
evident, evidente *adj*
evil, ~ **eye** aojadura; mal ojo; **to cast the ~ eye on** aojar; **~-minded** malicioso *adj*; malintencionado *adj*; ~ **smelling** fétido *adj*; maloliente *adj*
evisceration, evisceración *f*
evolve, to, convertirse (ie); evolucionar; transformarse
evolution, evolución *f*
exacerbation, exacerbación *f*
exaggerated, exagerado *adj*
exaggeration, exageración *f*
exaltation, exaltación *f*
examination, chequeo *Chicano*; examen *m*; examinación *f*; exploración *f*; reconocimiento; revisión *f*; **breast** ~ examen de los senos; **eye** ~ examen visual; **medical** ~ examen médico; **pelvic** ~ examen ginecológico; revisión de sus partes; **physical** ~ examen físico; reconocimiento médico; **rectal** ~ tacto rectal
examine, to, examinar; reconocer *Med*; revisar
examiner, examinador, -ra *m/f*; **medical** ~ examinador médico
examining instruments, instrumentos de exploración

examining table, mesa de exploración

example, for, por ejemplo

exanguination, hemorragia

exanimation, desmayo; síncope *m*

exanthem, exantema *m*; **vesicular ~** exantema vesicular

exanthematous fever, fiebre exantemática *f*; tifus exantemático *m*

excavation, excavación *f*

excavator, excavador *m*; **dental ~** excavador dental

exceed, to, exceder

excellent, chévere *inter, adj, PR*; chuchín *adj, PR*; chula *adj, PR*; excelente *adj*

excess, exceso

excessive, excesivo *adj*

exchange, intercambio; **~ list** lista de intercambios; **~ of gases** intercambio de gases; **~ resins** resinas de intercambio; **~ transfusion** exanguinotransfusión *f*

exchangeable, intercambiable *adj*

exchanger, cambiador *m*, *adj*; **heat ~** cambiador de calor

excise, to, escindir; remover (ue) *Med*

excision, excisión *f*; **wound ~** excisión de heridas

excisional planes, planos de clivaje

excitability, excitabilidad *f*

excitant, excitante *adj*

excitation, **(direct)(indirect)** excitación (directa)(indirecta) *f*

excite, to, **~ (*to deeply move*)** emocionar; **~ (*to irritate*)** poner nervioso; **~ (*to upset*)** agitar; **~ sexually** bellacar(se) *slang*

excitement, excitación *f*; **~ (*disturbance*)** alboroto; **~ (*enthusiasm*)** entusiasmo

exciting, estimulante *adj*; **~ injection** inyección sensibilizante *f*

excrement, excremento; excreción *f*; materia fecal; miércoles *m, sg, euph*; ñisca *CA, Col*; ñola *Col, Guat*; ñusca *Col, Ec*

excretory pyelogram, pielograma excretorio *m*

excruciating pain, dolor agudísimo *m*

excuse, excusa; **~ me (*pardon*)** lo siento; perdón; **~ me (*permission*)** con permiso; **work ~** certificado para no trabajar; incapacidad de trabajo *f, Mex*

executive, ejecutivo *adj*; **~ group** grupo ejecutivo

exempt, to (*to release*), eximir

exercise, ejercicio; **active ~** ejercicio activo; **active resistive ~** ejercicio activo contra resistencia; **breathing ~** ejercicio respiratorio; **corrective ~** ejercicio terapéutico; **passive ~** ejercicio pasivo; **static ~** ejercicio estático

exercise, to, **~ (*authority, influence*)** ejercer; **~ (*a dog*)** sacar de paseo; **~ care** tener cuidado; **~ (*moderately*)** (one's body) hacer ejercicios (moderado) (con)

exert oneself, to, esforzarse (ue); hacer esfuerzos

exertion, **~ (*effort*)** esfuerzo; **~ (*strength*)** empleo

exertional dyspnea, disnea de esfuerzo

exhalation, exhalación *f*; espiración *f*

exhale, to, exhalar

exhaust, to, agotar; consumir; debilitar; depauperar *Med*; postrar *Med*

exhausted, agotado *adj*; **~ (*person*)** esmamoniao *adj, PR*; **to be ~** enjuañangarse *PR*; escasifoyarse *PR*; esmamoniarse *PR*; yonquearse *Chicano*; **to become ~** agotarse

exhausting, agotador *adj*

exhaustion, fatiga; agotamiento; depauperación *f, Med*; **heat ~** agotamiento por calor; **nervous ~** agotamiento nervioso; **to pant with ~** echar el bofe *PR*

exhumation, exhumación *f*

existence, existencia

exit, salida; **~ wound** punto de salida

exocrine, exocrino *adj*

exodontics, exodoncia (*trata de la extracción de los dientes*)

exodontist, exodontista *m/f*

exodontology, exodontología

exotic, exótico *adj*

expand, to, distender (ie); expandir

expander, expansor *m*; **plasma volume ~** expansor del plasma

expanding, expansivo *adj*; **~ lesion,** lesión expansiva *f*; **~ pulmonary cyst,** quiste pulmonar expansivo *m*

expect, to, esperar

expectant, expectante *adj*

expectation, expectación *f*; **~ of life** expectación de (la) vida

expecting, to be, estar con familia

expectorant, expectorante *m, adj*

expectorate, to, escupir; expectorar

expectoration, expectoración *f*

expel, to, expulsar; **~ anal gas** tirarse flato; ventosearse *Chicano*

expense, gasto

expensive, caro *adj*; costoso *adj*

experience, experiencia

experience, to, experimentar

experienced, experto *adj*; hábil *adj*

experiment, experimento

experimentation, experimentación *f*

expert, experto *m, adj*; perito *m, adj*

expiration, expiración *f*; **~ date** fecha de caducidad

expire, to, **~** (*to breathe out*) espirar; **~** (*to die*) expirar; fallecer; morir (ue)

explain, to, explicar

explanation, explicación *f*

exploration, exploración *f*

exploratory, exploratorio *adj*; explorador *adj, Surg*; **~ puncture** punción exploradora *f*

explore, to, explorar *Surg*

explorer, explorador *m*

expose, to, exponer; **to be ~d to** estar expuesto a; estar en contacto con

exposure, exposición *f*; **~ time** tiempo de exposición; tiempo de irradiación

express, to, expresar; **~** (*to press*) exprimir; **~ milk from the breast** sacar leche del pecho

expression, expresión *f*

expressionless face, cara inexpresiva

expulsion, expulsión *f*

expulsive pression, contracciones expulsivas *f*

exsanguinate, to, desangrarse

exsiccant drugs, medicamentos sicativos

exsiccate, to, resecar

extended labor, parto prolongado

extense, extenso *adj*

extension, extensión *f*; prolongación *f*

extensive, extenso *adj*

exterior, exterior *m, adj*

external, externo *adj*; **~ acoustic meatus** conducto auditivo externo; **for ~ application** tópico *adj, Med*

extirpation, extirpación *f*; **pulp ~** extirpación de la pulpa; pulpectomía

extract, extracto; **allergenic ~** extracto alergénico; **animal ~** extracto animal; **compound ~** extracto compuesto; **(pure) licorice root ~** extracto de raíz orozuz (puro); extracto de regaliz (puro); **(dry) liver ~** extracto (seco) de hígado; **(liquid) liver ~** extracto (líquido) de hígado; **parenteral liver ~** extracto de hígado para uso parenteral; **parathyroid ~** extracto de paratiroides; **pollen ~** extracto de polen

extract, to (*to remove, take out*), extraer; sacar

extraction, extracción *f*; sacada *Arg, Col, Perú*; sacadura *Chi, Col, Perú*; **breech ~** extracción de nalgas

extraneous, extraño *adj*

extraordinary, extraordinario *adj*; **~ measure** medida extraordinaria

extrapolate, to, extrapolar

extrasensory, extrasensorial *adj*

extrasystole, extrasístole *f*; **auricular ~** extrasístole auricular; **auriculoventricular ~** extrasístole auriculoventricular; **interpolated ~** extrasístole interpolada; **nodal ~** extrasístole nodal; **retrograde ~** extrasístole retrógrada; **ventricular ~** extrasístole ventricular

extrauterine, extrauterino *adj*

extreme, extremo *adj*; **~ unction** santos óleos

extremity, extremidad *f*; **lower/upper ~** extremidad inferior/superior

extricate, to, desenredar

extrinsic, extrínseco *adj*

extrovert, extrovertido *m, adj*

extubate, to, desintubar; extubar

extubation, desintubación *f*; extubación *f*

exuberant, exuberante *adj*

exudate, exudado *m*

exude, to, exudar; rezumar

eye, ojo; vista *fam*; **~ bath** baño ocular; **black ~** hematoma periorbitario debido a un traumatismo *m*; **bloodshot ~s** ojos inyectados (en sangre); **bulging ~s** ojotes *m, pl, CA, Col*; **~ chart** carta de examen visual; **corner of the ~** ángulo del ojo; **~ cup** copa ocular; lavaojos *m, inv*; ojera; **~ drops** colirio; gotas oftalmológicas; **~ (ophthalmo-** logical) **exam** examen oftalmológico *m*; **exciting ~** ojo excitante; **~ gnat** bobito; **monochromatic ~** ojo monocromático; **~ ointment** colirio graso; **parts of ~** partes del ojo *f, pl*; **aqueous humor** humor acuoso *m*; **chorioid** corioides *f, sg*; **cone** cono; **conjunctiva** conjuntiva; **cornea** córnea; **~ball** globo del ojo; globo ocular; tomate *m, slang, Chicano*; **~brow** ceja; **fovea centralis** fóvea central; **iris** iris *m*; **lachrymal** lacrimal *adj*; lagrimal *adj*; **~lash** pestaña; **~lid** párpado; **lens** cristalino; **pupil** niña del ojo; pupila; **retina** retina; **rod** bastoncillo; **sclera** esclerótica; **~ socket** cuenca de los ojos; órbita; **tear duct** conducto lagrimal; **tear sac** bolsa de lágrimas; **~ powder** colirio seco; **protruding ~s** guayabas *CR*; **rolling ~** nistagmo rotatorio; **~ salve** colirio; ungüento para los ojos; **~ shield** escudo ocular; ojeras; **~ sight** vista; **sympathizing ~** ojo simpatizante; **trichromatic ~** ojo tricromático; **watery ~s** ojos llorosos; **wink** guiño; **to have ~s bloodshot from smoking or drinking** tener los ojos a millón *PR*; tener los ojos de pescao de nevera; tener los ojos de un gato que lambe aceite *PR*

eyedropper (*medicine dropper*), cuentagotas *m, inv*; goteador *m*; gotero (para los ojos) *SpAm*

eyeglasses, anteojos *m, pl*; espejuelos *m, pl*; gafas *f, pl*; lentes *m, pl*; quevedos *m, pl*

eyeground, fondo del ojo

eyelid closure reflex, reflejo corneal

eyelid winking, parpadeo

eyepads, paños en los ojos; toallas en los ojos

eyepiece, ocular *m*

eyestrain, astenopía *form*; fatiga

ocular; ojos fatigados; vista cansada

eyetooth, canino; colmillo; diente canino

eyewear, lentes *m, pl*; **protective ~** lentes protectores

eyewitness, testigo ocular

---

[4] In Spanish *canal* is an open duct, *conducto* is closed.
[5] Use the Spanish pronunciation of these letters.

F

F.A.C.D./Fellow of the American College of Dentists, Miembro del Colegio Norteamericano de Odontólogos

face, cara; carátula *slang, Chicano*; rostro; **~ache** neuralgia facial; **~bow** arco facial *Dent*; **~ down** boca abajo; **~ form** forma facial *Dent*; **~ lift** estiramiento de la piel; estiramiento facial; operación facial de estética *f*; **~ up** boca arriba

face, to, enfrentar(se) con

facial, masaje facial *m*; **~ powder** polvo facial; **~ profile** perfil facial *m*; **~ tissues** kleenex *m*; pañuelos faciales; pañuelos de papel; servilletas faciales

facies, facies *m, inv*

F.A.C.P./Fellow of the American College of Physicians, Miembro del Colegio Norteamericano de Médicos

F.A.C.S./Fellow of the American College of Surgeons, Miembro del Colegio Norteamericano de Cirujanos

factor, factor *m*; **~s I, II, III, and IV in the clotting of blood** factores I, II, III, y IV de la coagulación de la sangre (*Son fibrinógeno, protrombina, tromboplastina y calcio, respectivamente.*); **~ VIII, in clotting of blood** (*antihemophilic factor A*) factor VIII de la coagulación de la sangre (*factor antihemofílico A*); **~ IX, in the clotting of blood** (*antihemophilic factor B*) factor IX de la coagulación de la sangre (*factor antihemofílico B*); **~ X, in the clotting of blood** factor X de la coagulación de la sangre (*fracción globulínica del plasma*); **~ XI, in the clotting of blood** (*plasma thromboplastic antecedent*) factor XI de la coagulación de la sangre (*antecedente tromboplástico plasmático*); **animal protein ~** factor proteína animal; **antihemophilic ~/AHF** factor antihemofílico; **antihemorrhagic ~** factor antihemorrágico (*Vitamina K*); **erythrocyte maturation ~** factor madurador de eritrocitos; **Rh ~** factor Rh; **risk ~** factor de riesgo

factory, fábrica

faculty, facultad *f*; **fusion ~** facultad de fusión; **germinative ~** facultad germinativa

fade, to, **~** (*colors when washed*) desteñir (i); **~** (*weaken*) debilitar; **~** (*pale*) palidecer

Fahrenheit thermometer, termómetro de Fahrenheit

fail, to, fallar; fracasar

failure, fallo; fracaso, omisión *f*; **~** (*organ*) insuficiencia; **heart ~** insuficiencia cardíaca; insuficiencia cardiaca; **kidney ~** insuficiencia renal; **respiratory ~** insuficiencia respiratoria

faint, débil *adj*; desvanecido *adj, Med*; desmayo; síncope *m*; sirimba *Cu*; vahído

faint, to, desmayarse; asombrar *CR*; **~** (*away*) desvanecerse *Med*

fainting fit, insulto *Arg, Ven*; repente *m, Mex*; sirimba *Cu*

fainting spell, desfallecimiento; desmayo; desvanecimiento; lipotimia; mareo *fam*; síncope *m*; vértigo; **~ during pregnancy** achaque *m, CR*

faintness, desfallecimiento; vapor *m, Med*

fair, **~** (*complexion*) blanco *adj*; claro *adj*; güero *adj, Mex, CA*; **~**

/**fair-haired** (*blond*) rubio *adj*; pelirubio *adj*; ~ (*just*) justo *adj*; ~ (*middling*) regular *adj*

faith, confianza, ~ **healer** curandero; ~ **healing** curanderismo

fall, caída; ~ (*of temperature, pressure*) baja

fall, to, caer(se); ~ (*temperature, fever, voice*) bajar(se); ~ **asleep** (*to doze off*) dormirse (ue); ~ **down** caerse; ~ **in a faint** caer desvanecido; ~ **sick** enfermarse

fallen fontanel, caída de la mollera *ethn*; fontanela caída *ethn*; mollera caída *ethn*

falling out, (*overdose of narcotics or sedatives*) durmiéndose a medias; durmiéndose[2]

falling sickness, epilepsia

Fallopian, Falopio; ~ **canal** acueducto de Falopio; ~ **tubes** oviductos de los mamíferos; trompas de Falopio; tubos; tubos falopios

fallout, lluvia radiactiva; residuos atmosféricos

false, falso *adj*; ~ **pains** parto falso

falsification, falsificación *f*

falter, to, balbucear; tartamudear

familial, familiar *adj*

familiar, conocido *adj*

family, familia; **degenerate** ~ familia degenerada; ~ **doctor/physician** médico de cabecera; ~ **history** historia familiar; ~ **member** familiar *m*; miembro de la familia; ~ **name** apellido; ~ **planning** planificación de la familia *f*; planificación familiar *f*; ~ **practice** medicina familiar; ~ **problem** problema familiar *m*; problema personal *m*; **racially mixed** ~ familia interracial; ~ **tree** árbol genealógico *m*

famine, hambre[3] *f*

famish, to, hacer padecer hambre

famished, to be, estar muerto de hambre *adj*

fang, colmillo

farsighted, hipermétrope *adj*; hiperópico *adj*; présbita *adj*

farsightedness, hipermetropía; hiperopía; presbicia; presbiopía; vista larga *fam*

fart, aire *m*; pedo *slang*; viento

fart, to, pederse *vulg*

fascia, (*pl, fasciae*) fascia; venda; vendaje *m*

fast, ~ (*abstinence*) ayuno; abstinencia; ~ (*speed*) rápido *adj*; ~ **heart beat** palpitación *f*

fast, to, ayunar

fasten, to, abrochar; atar

fasting, ayuno; ~ **blood sugar** glucemia en ayunas; ~ **condition** en ayunas; ~ **glucose** glucosa en ayunas

fat, ~ (*grease*) grasa; ~ **cell** célula grasa; ~ **in the veins** colesterol *m*; grasa en las venas; **diet rich in** ~ dieta grasosa; ~ (*lard*) manteca; ~ (*obese*) gordo *adj*; grueso *adj*; obeso *adj*; guatón *adj*, *Arg*, *Chi*, *Perú*; ~ (*obesity*) gordura; **to grow** ~ engordar

fatal, ~ (*accident*) mortal *adj*; ~ (*very serious*) fatal *adj*; ~ **outcome** desenlace fatal *m*

fatality rate, índice de mortalidad *m*

fate, ~ (*luck*) destino; suerte *f*; ~ (*death*) muerte *f*

father, padre *m*; papá *m*

father, to, engendrar

fatherhood, paternidad *f*

father-in-law, suegro

fatigue, (*weariness*) cansancio; fatiga; decaimiento *fam*; pesadez *f*, *fam*; flojera *fam*; **unexplained** ~ fatiga sin causa

fatigue, to, (*to tire out*) cansar; fatigar; estar desgonzado *fam*; estar rendido *fam*

fatigued, agotado

fatten, to, engordar

fatty, grasoso *adj*; sebáceo *adj*; ~ **acid** ácido graso

fauces, fauces *f, pl*

favor, favor *m*

fear, miedo; temor *m*; **generalized** ~ alarma generalizada;
morbid ~ temor morboso
fear, to, temer; tener miedo
fearful, miedoso *adj*
feather, pluma
features, características físicas;
facciones *f*; rasgos
febrile, febril *adj*
feces, aguas mayores *fam*; caca
slang; cagada *vulg*; cámara; deposiciones *f*; evacuación del
vientre *f*; excremento; heces fecales *f*, *pl*; materia fecal; miércoles *m*, *sg*, *euph*; mierda *vulg*;
pase del cuerpo *m*
fee, recompensa
feeble, débil *adj*; endeble *adj*,
Med; enfermizo *adj*; ñango *adj*,
Mex; pachaco *adj*, *CA*; revejido
adj, *Col*; telenque *adj*, *Chi*; ~
minded imbécil *Med*, *adj*; ~
mindedness debilidad mental
f; deficiencia mental; **to grow** ~
deshacerse *Med*
feed, to, alimentar; dar de comer
feedback, autorregulación *f*;
retroacción *f*
feeding, alimentación *f*; **artificial**
~ alimentación artificial; **breast**
~ alimentación al seno; ~ **by**
tube alimentación por sonda; ~
tube tubo nutricio
feel, to, ~ (for) (*to touch*) palpar; ~
(*to regret*; *to touch*) sentir (ie); ~
(*emotion/pain*; *health*) sentirse
(ie); ~ (*to touch manually*) tentar
(ie); tocar; ~ **like** tener ganas
(de); ~ **nothing** no sentir (ie) nada
feeling, ~ (*palpation*) palpación *f*;
~ (*sensation*) sensación *f*; ~ (*sentiment*) sentimiento; ~ (*sensitivity*) sensibilidad *f*
fellatio, felación *f*; felatorismo
felon, panadizo
female, hembra
femoral, femoral *adj*; ~ **hernia**
hernia crural

femur, fémur *m*
ferment, fermento
ferment, to, fermentar; hacer fermentar
fermentation, fermentación *f*
ferrous sulfate, sulfato ferroso
fertile, fértil *adj*
fertilization, fecundación *f*; fertilización *f*
fester, llaga; úlcera superficial
fester, to, enconarse; ulcerarse
festering, ulceroso *adj*
fetal, fetal *adj*; ~ **heart tone** latido
del corazón fetal; tono cardíaco
fetal; ~ **wastage** pérdidas fetales
fetishism, fetichismo
fetoscope, estetoscopio fetal; fetoscopio
fetus, feto
fever[4], fiebre *f*; calentura[4] *fam*;
chavalongo *Arg*, *Chi*; chucho
SpAm, *Med*; temperatura; **acute
infectious adenitis** ~ fiebre ganglionar; **blackwater** ~ malaria; ~
blister herpe[5] febril *m/f*
[*Ú.m.e.p.*]; herpes labial *m/f*;
llaga de fiebre; vesículas de la
fiebre; **breakbone** ~ dengue *m*;
fiebre rompehuesos; **catheter** ~
fiebre producida por infección;
childbed ~ fiebre puerperal;
Colorado tick ~ fiebre
tra(n)smitida por garrapatas;
fiebre de Colorado; **continued** ~
fiebre continua; **enteric** ~ fiebre
entérica; fiebre tifoidea; fiebre
paratifoidea; **ephemeral** ~
fiebre fugaz *fam*; fiebre de un
día *fam*; fiebre efímera; **exanthematous** ~ fiebre exantemática; tifus exantemático *m*;
glandular ~ amigdalitis *f*; fiebre
glandular; **hay** ~ alergia; catarro
constipado *Chicano*; fiebre
de(l) heno; jey fíver *m/f*, *Chicano*; **hospital** ~ fiebre de los
hospitales; **intermittent** ~ fiebre
intermitente; **malarial** ~ chucho *Arg*, *Chi*; fiebre palúdica;

Malta ~ brucelosis *f*; fiebre ondulante; fiebre de Malta; **marsh** ~ malaria; paludismo; **Mediterranean** ~ fiebre del Mediterráneo; **neurogenic** ~ fiebre neurogénica; **paratyphoid** ~ fiebre paratífica; fiebre paratifoidea; **parrot** ~ fiebre de las cotorras; enfermedad de los papagayos *f*; **rabbit** ~ fiebre de conejo; **rat-bite** ~ fiebre por mordedura de rata; sodoku *m*; **relapsing** ~ fiebre intermitente; fiebre recurrente; **remittent** ~ fiebre remitente; **rheumatic** ~ fiebre reumática; **Rocky Mountain** ~ fiebre de las Montañas Rocosas; maculosa de las Montañas Rocosas; **sandfly** ~ flebótomo; **scarlet** ~ (fiebre) escarlatina; **slight** ~ destemplanza; **spotted** ~ fiebre manchada; fiebre purpúrea (de las Montañas Rocosas); fiebre punticular; tifus exantemático *m*; tifus epidémico *m*; **thermic** ~ fiebre térmica; **three-day** ~ dengue *m*; fiebre rompehuesos; flebótomo; **tick** ~ fiebre de las Montañas Rocosas; **trench** ~ fiebre de las trincheras; fiebre de los cinco días; **typhoid** ~ fiebre tifoidea; tifus abdominal *m*; **typhus** ~ tifo; tifus *m*; tifus exantemático *m*; úrzula *Chicano*; **undulant** ~ fiebre ondulante; **valley** ~ (*coccidioidomycosis*) fiebre del valle; **yellow** ~ fiebre amarilla; fiebre tropical; tifo de América; tifus icteroides *m*; vómito negro

feverish, destemplado *adj*, *Med*

fiancé, novio

fiancée, novia

fiber, fibra; **elastic** ~ fibra elástica; **motor** ~ fibra motriz; **muscle** ~ fibra muscular; **nerve** ~ fibra nerviosa

fiberoptic, de fibra óptica

fibril, fibrina

fibrillation, fibrilación *f*; **atrial** ~ fibrilación auricular; **auricular** ~ fibrilación auricular; **ventricular** ~ fibrilación ventricular

fibrin, fibrina

fibrinogen, fibrinógeno

fibrocystic, fibrocístico *adj*; fibroquístico *adj*; ~ **disease of bone** enfermedad fibroquística ósea *f*; ~ **disease of pancreas** enfermedad fibroquística del páncreas *f*

fibroid, fibroide *m*, *adj*; fibroideo *adj*

fibroma, fibroma *m*

fibrous tumor, fibroma *m*; tumor fibroso *m*

fibula, peroné *m*; fíbula

fibular, peroneo *adj*; peroneal *adj*; fibular *adj*

field, campo; **auditory** ~ campo auditivo; ~ **of consciousness** campo de la conciencia; ~ **of fixation** campo de fijación; **magnetic** ~ campo magnético; ~ **of a microscope** campo del microscopio; ~ **of vision** campo visual; **electrical** ~ campo eléctrico visual; **overshot** ~ campo visual excedido

fight, lucha

fight, to, luchar; ~ **the disease** capear; soportar bien la enfermedad

figure, figura; ~ (*de una mujer*) talle *m*, *Anat*

filament, filamento

file, ~ (*archive*) archivo; ~ (*dossier*) expediente *m*; ~ (*folder*) carpeta; ~ (*tool*) lima; **card index** ~ fichero; **to be on** ~ estar archivado *adj*

file, to, ~ (*a record, chart*) archivar; ~ **down** limar

filings, limaduras

fill, to, llenar; ~ **a prescription** (*patient*) llenar una receta; hacer una receta; ~ **a prescription** (*pharmacist*) preparar una receta; despachar una receta; ~ (*a tooth*) empastar *form, Dent*; emplomar *Dent, Arg*; obturar *form, Dent*; rellenar *Dent*; tapar *Dent*; ~ **with gold** orificar *Dent*; ~ **out** (*to gain weight*) aumentar de peso; ~ **out a form** llenar una planilla; llenar un formulario

filled tooth, diente relleno

filling, ~ (*of tooth*) empastadura *Dent*; empaste *m, Dent*; emplomadura *Dent, Arg*; tapadura *Dent*; **temporary** ~ empaque *m, Dent, Chicano*; empaste provisional *Dent*; empaste temporal *Dent*; ~ (*stuffing—food*) relleno; ~ (*adj*) que llena mucho

filling, to do a, empastar

film, película; **fixed blood** ~ película de sangre fijada; ~ **of blood** extensión de sangre *f*; ~ (*x-ray*) placa; radiografía; ~ (*thin layer*) capa; ~ (*on surface of liquid*) tela; ~ (*in the eye*) nube *f*; ~ (*on teeth*) sarro

film, to, filmar; ~ **with** cubrir con (*una película, capa*); ~ **with** (*something*) cubrirse de (*una tela, nube, etc.*); ~ **with tears** arrasarse (los ojos) de lágrimas

filter, filtro; **intermittent sand** ~ filtro intermitente de arena; **percolating** ~ filtro percolador; **slow sand** ~ filtro lento de arena; **trickling** ~ filtro por escurrimiento

filter, to, destilar; filtrar

filtering scar, cicatriz filtrante *f*

filth, porquería

filthy, asqueroso *adj*

filtrate, filtrado; líquido filtrado

filtrate, to, filtrar

filtration, destilación *f*; filtración *f*

finances, recursos

financial, financiero *adj*

find, to, descubrir; encontrar (ue); hallar; ~ **it difficult to breathe** sentir (ie) opresión; ~ **out** averiguar; descubrir; saber

finding, descubrimiento; hallazgo; resultado

fine, fino *adj*; ~ **catgut** catgut fino *m*; ~**toothed comb** peine espeso *m*; ~**toothed forceps**, pinzas de dientes finos

finger, dedo; **baseball** ~ dedo de beisbolista; **clubbed** ~ dedo en maza; ~ **cot** dedo de hule; **dead** ~ dedo muerto; **fleshy tip of the** ~ yema; **fore**~ dedo índice; **hangnail on the** ~ padrastro; **index** ~ índice *m*; **knuckle of** ~ nudillo; **little** ~ meñique *m*; **mallet** ~ dedo en martillo; **middle** ~ dedo del medio; dedo del corazón; ~**nail** uña; **ring** ~ dedo anular; **tip of the** ~ punta del dedo; yema del dedo; **trigger** ~ dedo en gatillo; **webbed** ~ dedo palmado; **thumb** dedo gordo; pulgar *m*; **ball of** ~ pulpejo

fingerprint, impresión digital *f*; huella *fam*; huella dactilar; huella digital

fingerprint, to, tomar las huellas digitales a

finish, to, terminar; acabar

fire, fuego; incendio; ~ **extinguisher** extintor de incendios *m*

first, primero *adj*; ~ **aid** cura de urgencia; primera ayuda; primeros auxilios *m, pl*; ~ **aid bandage** vendaje provisional *m*; ~ **aid kit** botiquín de primeros auxilios *m*; botiquín de urgencia *m*; equipo de primeros auxilios; ~ **aid packet** paquete de vendas *m*; ~ **aid post** puesto de socorro; ~ **aid treatment** tratamiento de urgencia; ~**born** primogénito; ~ **cousin** primo hermano; ~ **name** primer nombre *m*; ~ **stage** primer período de dilatación

fish, ~ (*in water*) pez *m*; ~ (*food*) pescado; ~ **bone** espina

fish, to, pescar

fission, fisión *f*; **binary** ~ fisión binaria; **nuclear** ~ fisión nuclear

fissure, abertura; cisura; fisura; grieta; partidura; raza; **anal** ~ cisura del ano; **auricular** ~ fisura auricular

fist, puño; ñeque *m*, *Ec*; **tight** ~ puño apretado; **to make a** ~ hacer un puño

fistula, fístula; **blind** ~ fístula ciega; **rectovaginal** ~ fístula rectovaginal; **urinary** ~ fístula urinaria

fit, arrebato; ataque *m*; convulsión *f*; paroxismo; ~[6] (*outfit/tools necessary for injection of drugs: needle syringe (eyedropper and rubber bulb), cooker, cotton, matches, tie off*) equipo hipodérmico; estuche *m*; herramienta[2]; herre[2] *f*; R[2] *f*; ~ **of anger** viaraza *Col*, *Guat*, *Ríopl*; ~ **of coughing** quinta de tos

fit, to, ~ (*glasses, shoes*) ajustar; ~ (*in*) encajar

fitness, aptitud *f*; ~ (*good health*) buena salud *f*

fitting surface, superficie de ajuste *f*, *Dent*

fix[6], (*an IV injection of drugs*) abuja[2]; abujazo[2]; cura[2]; filerazo[2]; gallazo[2]

fix, to, arreglar; componer; ~ (*eyes*) clavar; ~[6] (*to inject drugs*) clavarse[2]; componerse[2]; curarse[2]; filerearse[2]; jincarse[2]; picarse[2]; rayarse[2]; shootear[2]; ~ **up**[6] (*to heat and mix heroin*) arreglar; cuquear[2]

fixation, fijación *f*; **obsessive** ~ fijación obsesiva

fixative, fijador *m*, *adj*

fixing solution, solución fijadora *f*

flabbiness, blanducho; flac(c)idez *f*

flabby, blando de carnes *adj*; flác(c)ido *adj*; flojo *adj*; ~ **muscles** músculos flácidos

flaccid, flác(c)ido *adj*

flagellation, flagelación *f*

flail joint, articulación de movimiento anormal *f*

flake, (*scale of skin*) escama

flake, to, (*skin*) descamar

flaky, escamoso *adj*

flame, llama; ~ **burn** quemadura por llama; **capillary** ~s llamas capilares

flammable, inflamable *adj*

flange, aleta *Dent*; **buccal** ~ aleta bucal *Dent*; **denture** ~ aleta de dentadura *Dent*; **labial** ~ aleta labial *Dent*

flank, costado; ~ (*loin*) ijada; ijar *m*; ~ **pain** dolor del costado; mal de ijar *m*; dolor de ijar *m*, *fam*; puntada *fam*

flannel, flanela

flap, colgajo; ~ **amputation** amputación a colgajos *f*; **skin** ~ colgajo cutáneo

flapless amputation, amputación sin colgajo *f*

flapping sound, ruido de bandera

flare up, ~ (*new outbreak of epidemic*) recrudecimiento; ~ (*of an epidemic*) declaración *f*; reactivación *f*

flare up, to, ~ (*to worsen*) agravar(se); ~ (*an epidemic*) declararse; ~ (*to arouse; to burn*) encenderse (ie); ~ (*in anger*) encolerizarse

flash, sofoco; bochorno; **hot** ~es sofocos de calor; bochornos; calofrío; calores *m*, *pl*

flashing, to be[7], oler (ue) cola

flask, frasco; mufla *Dent*; ~ **closure** oclusión de la mufla *f*; **trial** ~ **closure** oclusión de prueba de la mufla *f*

flat, horizontal *adj*; plano *adj*; ~ **bosomed** con el pecho aplanado *prep phr*; ~ **foot** pie plano *m*; planovegus *m*

flatulence, flatulencia; reventazón *f*, *Mex*

flatus, aire *m*; flato; pedo *slang*; ventosidad *f*; viento

flatworm, platelminto

flavor, sabor *m*; **cherry** ~(**ed**) sabor a cereza; **mint** ~(**ed**) sabor a menta; sabor de menta; **orange**

~(**ed**) sabor a naranja; **pleasant** ~(**ed**) un sabor agradable

flea, pulga

fleabite, salpullido

fleeting, fugaz *adj*; pasajero *adj*; momentáneo *adj*; transitorio *adj*

flesh, carne *f*; ~ **and blood** carne y hueso; ~ **wound** herida superficial

flex, to, doblar(se); encorvar(se) (ue)

flexible, flexible *adj*

flexion, flexión *f*

flip, to, *slang* volverse (ue) loco

floater, (*in the eye*) estrellita *fam*; mancha volante; mosca volante; partícula flotante

floating, flotante *adj*; ~ **kidney** riñón flotante *m*; ~ **rib** costilla flotante

floating[6], **to be**, *slang* (*See high, to be; blasted, to be.*)

flooding, inundación *f*; hemorragia uterina

floor, ~ (*flooring*) suelo; ~ (*of a building*) piso; ~ **of the pelvis** ligamento transverso de la pelvis

floppy, flác(c)ido *adj*; flojo *adj*; hipotónico *adj*; que se cae

florid, florido *adj*

flour, harina

flow, flujo; **blood** ~ flujo sanguíneo; circulación *f*; **renal blood** ~ flujo sanguíneo renal; **renal plasma** ~ flujo plasmático renal; ~ (*of tears*) torrente *m*

flow, to, fluir; ~ (*menstrual*) bajar la regla; ~ (*blood in body*) circular; ~ (*tears; blood of a wound*) correr

flowchart, organigrama *m*

flower, flor *f*

flu, gripa; gripe *f*; influenza; trancazo *fam*, *Med*; **Asiatic** ~ gripe asiática; influenza asiática

fluctuate, to, fluctuar

fluctuation, fluctuación *f*

fluent, to be ~ **in English** dominar el inglés; hablar el inglés con soltura; **to speak** ~ **Spanish** hablar un español bueno

fluently, ~ (*in speaking*) con soltura; **to speak Spanish** ~ hablar español con soltura; ~ (*in writing*) con fluidez; **to write Spanish** ~ escribir el español con fluidez

fluid, fluido *m*, *adj*; líquido; **amniotic** ~ líquido amniótico; **cerebrospinal** ~/**CSF** líquido cefalorraquídeo/LCR[9]; líquido cerebrospinal; ~ **diet** dieta hídrica; ~ **level** nivel líquido *m*; **pleural** ~ líquido pleural; **seminal** ~ líquido seminal; semen *m*; **synovial liquid** líquido sinovial; sinovia

fluke, duela; **intestinal** ~ duela intestinal; **liver** ~ duela hepática; **lung** ~ duela pulmonar

fluorescent, fluorescente *adj*

fluoridation, fluoración *f*; fluoridación *f*; fluorización *f*

fluoridization, (*See fluoridation.*)

fluoride, fluoruro

fluorine, flúor *m*

fluoroscope, fluoroscopio

fluoroscopy, fluoroscopia

flush, ~ (*embarrassment*; *red color*) rubor *m*; **atropine** ~ rubor atropínico; **breast** ~ rubor mamario; ~ (*illness*, *fever*) sofoco ; **hot** ~ sofoco de calor

flush, to, ruborizar(se); tener sofocos; ~ **the toilet** tirar la cadena; ~ **with anger** ponerse rojo de ira *adj*

flushed, enrojecido *adj*

flushes, oleadas de calor

flutter, flúter *m*; aleteo; ~ (*of eyelids*) parpadeo; pestañeo; ~ (*of heart*) palpitación *f*; ~ (*of pulse*) pulsación irregular *f*

flutter, to, ~ (*eyelids*) parpadear; ~ (*heart*) palpitar; ~ (*pulse*) latir irregularmente

fly, ~ (*insect*) mosca; **cattle** ~ tábano; ~ (*slang*: *zipper*) bragueta

fly, to, volar (ue)
flying saucers[6], *slang* (*morning glory seeds*) semillas de dondiego de día[2]; dompedro[2]
foam, espuma
foamy, espumoso *adj*
focus, (*pl, foci*) foco
focus, to, enfocar la vista
fog, niebla
fogging, enturbiamiento
foggy, brumoso *adj*
fold, arruga; doblez *m*; pliegue *m*; **gastropancreatic** ~ ligamento gastropancreático; **genital** ~ pliegue genital; **lateral umbilical** ~ pliegue umbilical lateral; **skin** ~ pliegue cutáneo
fold, to, doblar; ~ **one's arms** cruzar los brazos; ~ **one's hands** cruzar las manos
folic acid, ácido fólico
folk illness, enfermedad casera *f*
follicle, folículo; **grafian** ~ folículo de De Graaf; **hair** ~ folículo piloso; **ovarian** ~ folículo ovárico; ~ **stimulating hormone** hormona folículo-estimulante; hormona foliculoestimulante
folliculitis, foliculitis *f*
follow, to, seguir (i); siguetear *Perú*; ~ (*to practice a profession*) ejercer; ~ (*to look after a patient*) atender (ie)
follow-up, observación *f*; ~ **care** atención médica subsecuente *f*; cuidados posthospitalarios; tratamiento complementario
foment, fomento
fomentation, fomentación *f*
fondle, to, acariciar
fontanelle, fontanela; mollera; **fallen** ~ caída de la mollera *ethn*; fontanela caída *ethn*; mollera caída *ethn*
food, alimento; comida; **baby** ~ comida para niños; ~ **poisoning** intoxicación alimenticia *f*
foolishness, tontería
foot, pie *m*; **athlete's** ~ infección de serpigo *f*; pie de atleta; ~ **and mouth disease** glosopeda; (*See disease, foot and mouth.*); ~ **powder** polvo para los pies; **sole of the** ~ planta del pie
footwear, calzado
foramen, foramen *m*
force, fuerza; **catabolic** ~ fuerza catabólica; **reserve** ~ fuerza radical; **vital** ~ fuerza vital
force, to, forzar (ue)
forceps, fórceps *m*; hierros; tenazas; gatillo *Dent*; fórceps *m*, *Obst*; ~ **assisted delivery** alumbramiento con fórceps; parto con fórceps; (**surgical**) ~ pinzas *Surg*; **dressing** ~ pinzas de curación; **hemostatic** ~ pinzas hemostáticas; **hooked** ~ pinzas de garfios; **suture** ~ pinzas de sutura; **torsion** ~ pinzas de torsión
forearm, antebrazo
forefather, progenitor *m*
forefinger, dedo índice
forehead, frente *f*
foreign body, cuerpo extraño
forensic, forense *adj*; ~ **medicine** medicina legal; ~ **physician** (*coroner*) médico forense
foresee, to, prever
foreskin, prepucio
forget, to, olvidar; olvidarse de
forgetful, olvidadizo *adj*
fork, tenedor *m*; ~ **test** prueba del diapasón
forked, bifurcado *adj*
form, ~ (*shape, nature*) forma; ~ (*document*) formulario; **medical** ~ hoja clínica
formaldehyde, formaldehido
formation, formación *f*
formula, fórmula; **blood** ~ fórmula hemática; **chemical** ~ fórmula química; **dental** ~ fórmula dental; **empirical** ~ fórmula empírica
fornicate, to, fornicar *form*; (tener ayuntamiento carnal fuera del matrimonio)

fornix, fórnix *m*
fortify, to, fortalecer; fortificar
fortifying, fortificante *adj*
fortuitous, fortuito *adj*
forty days following parturition, cuarentena[8]
fossa, (*pl, fossae*) fosa
foster, ~ **child** hijo de leche; ~ **home** hogar adoptivo *m*; ~ **mother** ama[3] de leche; madre adoptiva *f*
foul, fétido *adj*; ~ **breath** fetidez de aliento *f*; ~**smelling** apestoso *adj*
fountain, fuente *f*; **drinking** ~ fuente de agua potable; fuente para beber
fourth stage, postparto
fovea, fosa pequeña; fosita; fóvea *form*; ~ **centralis** fóvea central
fracture, fractura; quebradura de huesos; quebrantamiento; hueso quebrado *fam*; **avulsion** ~ fractura por arrancamiento; **butterfly** ~ fractura en mariposa; **buttonhole** ~ fractura en ojal; **closed** ~ fractura cerrada; **comminuted** ~ fractura conminuta; **complete** ~ fractura completa; **complicated** ~ fractura complicada; **compound** ~ fractura complicada; fractura compuesta; fractura abierta; **compression** ~ fractura por compresión; **depressed** ~ fractura con hundimiento; fractura desviada; **green stick** ~ fractura en rama verde; fractura en tallo verde; **hairline** ~ fisura; **impacted** ~ fractura con impacto; fractura impactada; fractura empotrada; **incomplete** ~ fractura incompleta; **multiple** ~ fractura múltiple; **oblique** ~ fractura oblicua; **open** ~ fractura abierta; **pathologic** ~ fractura patológica; **perforating** ~ fractura perforante; **serious** ~ fractura mayor; **simple** ~ fractura simple; **skull** ~ fractura del cráneo; **spiral** ~ fractura espiral; fractura espiroidea; **spontaneous** ~ fractura espontánea; **stress** ~ fractura por esfuerzo; **supracondylar** ~ fractura supracondílea; **torsion** ~ fractura por torsión; **transcondylar** ~ fractura transcondílea
fracture, to, fracturar(se); quebrar(se) *fam*
fragile, frágil *adj*; deleznable *adj*; ~ (*health*) delicado *adj*
fragility, fragilidad *f*; ~ **of the blood** fragilidad de la sangre; **hereditary** ~ **of bone** fragilidad de los huesos
fragment, fragmento
fragmentation, fragmentación *f*; ~ **of myocardium** fragmentación del miocardio
frail, débil *adj*; endeble *adj*, *Med*; enteco *adj*; frágil *adj*; quebradizo *adj*
frame, ~ (*of bed, etc.*) armadura; ~ (*of building, machine, etc.*) armazón *f*; **quadriplegic standing** ~ armazón para cuadripléjicos; ~ (*in filmstrips, T.V.*) imagen *f*; ~ (*of glasses*) montura; portalentes *m, inv*; ~ (*of picture, door, window*) marco; ~ (*stature*) esqueleto; estatura; ~ **of reference** punto de referencia
framework, estructura; armazón *f*; esqueleto *Dent*; **within the** ~ **of** en el marco de *prep*
frantic, frenético *adj*
freak out[6], **to**, *slang*, (*See* **high, to be; blasted, to be.**)
freckled, (*person*) saraviado *adj*, *Col*
freckles, efélides *f, pl, form*; pecas
free, ~ (*which costs nothing*) gratis *adj*; ~ (*loose*) suelto *adj*; ~ **will** libre albedrío
freeze, to, congelar; helar (ie)
freeze dried, congelado en seco *adj*

freeze drying, secado al frío
freezing point, punto de congelación
frenetic, frenético *adj*
frenum (*of the tongue*), frenillo
frenzied, enloquecido *adj*
frenzy, frenesí *m*
frequency, frecuencia; **audio ~** frecuencia audible; **~ distribution** distribución de frecuencia *f*
frequent, frecuente *adj*
frequently, frecuentemente *adv*; con frecuencia
fresh, fresco *adj*; **~ air** aire fresco *m*; aire puro *m*; **~ milk** leche fresca de vaca *f*; **~ water** agua³ dulce *f*
friction, fricción *f*; **~ murmur** ruido de roce; **~ rub** roce por fricción *m*
fried, frito *adj*
friend, amigo
fright, susto
frighten, to, asustar
frightened, asustado *adj*; to **become ~** asustarse
frightening, aterrorizador *adj*
frigid, frígido *adj*
frigidity, frigidez *f*; frío en la matriz
fringe, franja
frog, rana; **to have a ~ in one's throat** tener carraspera
from the waist up, de la cintura para arriba *prep phr*
from the waist down, de la cintura para abajo *prep phr*
front desk, recepción *f*
frontal, frontal *adj*
frost, escarcha
frostbite, congelación *f*; daño sufrido por causa de la helada; heladura
frosted glass, cristal opalino *m*
frothy, espumoso *adj*
frown, ceño
frown, to, fruncir el ceño
frozen, congelado *adj*; helado *adj*; paralizado *adj*; bloqueado *adj*; **~ section** corte por congelación *m*;

~ to the bone transido de frío *adj*
fructose, fructosa
fruit, fruta
fruitful, fecundo *adj*
frustration, frustración *f*
fry, to, freír (i)
FSH/follicle stimulating hormone hormona folículo-estimulante; hormona foliculoestimulante
fugitive, fugaz *adj*
full, completo *adj*; lleno *adj*; **~-blown** completamente desarrollado *adj*; **~-blown** (*referring to symptom*) florido *adj*; **~-blown picture** cuadro florido; **~ mouth x-ray** radiografía de toda la boca; **~-size(d)** de tamaño natural; **~ term** a término
fumes, humo; vapor *m*
fumigate, fumigar
fumigation, fumigación *f*
fun, to have, divertirse (ie)
function, función *f*
functional, funcional; **~ disease** enfermedad funcional *f*
fundus, fondo
funduscope, funduscopio
funeral, entierro; **~ home** funeraria; **~ wake** vela *CA, RD*; velorio *SpAm*
fungicide, fungicida *m, adj*
fungus, (*pl, fungi*) hongo; **athlete's foot** infección de serpigo *f*; pie de atleta *m*; **~ infection** infección de hongos *f*; **moniliasis** boquera; candidiasis *f*; moniliasis *f*; muguet *m/f*; **ringworm/tinea** culebrilla; empeine *m*; serpigo; sisote *m*, *Chicano*; tiña; **tinea corporis** jiotes *f*, *fam*
funnel, embudo; en embudo *adj*
funny, gracioso *adj*
F.U.O./fever of undetermined origin, fiebre de origen desconocido *f*
fur, **~** (*pelt*) piel *f*; **~** (*on tongue*) saburra; sarro

furious, furioso *adj*; china *adj*, *CA*, *Cu*

furniture polish, pulimento para muebles

furor, furor *m*

furred, saburral *adj*

furrow, surco; pliegue *m*

furry tongue, lengua saburral

furuncle, furúnculo; grano enterrado

fury, cólera; furor *m*; rabia

fuse, to, (*broken bones*) soldarse *Med*

fusion, fusión *f*; **binocular ~** fusión de las imágenes dobles

future, futuro *m*, *adj*

fuzzy, velloso *adj*

---

[2] This is new vocabulary, not necessarily listed nor yet recognized by the Royal Academy of Spanish Grammar. It is understood that this vocabulary is primarily slang. Unless otherwise indicated, the gender of nouns is assumed to be obvious.

[3] For pronunciation purposes, the masculine definite and indefinite articles, *el* and *un*, not *la* or *una*, are used when the article immediately precedes the feminine singular noun which begins with stressed *a* or any other that begins with stressed *ha*.

[4] The word *fiebre* is a more common choice of terms than *calentura*. *Calentura* is the word of choice when fever is sudden or especially high. *Calentura* is used especially by Mexican–Americans. For other Spanish speakers it often has sexual connotations. *Fiebre*, or *fever*, technically refers to an elevation of body temperature to a point higher than normal. In rural areas of Mexico, *fiebre* refers to a number of illnesses that cause a rise in body temperature: malaria, typhoid fever, typhus, pneumonia, rheumatic fever, postpartum fever, and brucellosis. *Fiebre* is generally used to refer to a specific disease, i.e., *fiebre reumática*—rheumatic fever. See David Werner, *Donde no hay doctor*, pp. 26–27, 4th ed. México: Editorial Pax–México, 1980.

[5] This word is often used in the plural form.

[6] Part of the Drug Abuse Vocabulary.

[7] A flash is the euphoric initial reaction to IV narcotics.

[8] This is the forty-day period following delivery during which there is a prolonged period in bed, much freedom from household responsibilities, and abstention from sexual intercourse.

[9] Use the Spanish pronunciation of these letters.

G

gadget, simiñoco *PR*

gag reflex, reflejo faríngeo

gag, to, ~ (*nauseate*) dar náuseas; sentir (ie) bascas; ~ (*prevent from speaking*) amordazar; ~ (**retch**) tener náuseas; **to make** ~ provocar náuseas

gain, aumento; ganancia

gain, to, aumentar; ganar; ~ **weight** aumentar de peso

gait, marcha; porte *m*; **antalgic** ~ marcha antálgica; **paralytic** ~ marcha paralítica; **spastic** ~ marcha espasmódica

gall, bilis *f*; hiel *f*; yel *f*, *Chicano*

gallbladder, vejiga de la bilis; vesícula biliar; ~ **attack** ataque vesicular *m*; derrame de bilis *m*; dolor de la vesícula *m*; ~ **disease** colecistopatía; mal de hiel *m*; bilis *f*; ~ **disorder** malestares de la vesícula biliar *m*; **fish-scale** ~ vesícula biliar en escama de pescado; **sandpaper** ~ vesícula biliar en papel de lija; **strawberry** ~ vesícula biliar en fresa

gallery[6], (*place to take drugs*) galería[2]

gallon, galón *m*

gallop, ~ *Med* ruido de galope

gallstone, cálculo biliar; cálculo en la vejiga; colelitiasis *f*; piedra en la vejiga; piedra en la yel *Chicano*; ~ **operation** talla *Med*

galvanic, galvánico *adj*

game, pley *m*, *Chicano*

gamete, gameto

gamma globulin, gamaglobulina; globulina gamma

gang, (*street*) ganga *PR*, *Chicano*; pandilla

ganglion, ganglio; **cardiac** ~ ganglio cardíaco; **ciliary** ~ ganglio ciliar; **compound palmar** ~ ganglio compuesto palmar; **dia-**phragmaticum ~ ganglio diafragmático; **facial** ~ ganglio geniculado; **inferior cervical** ~ ganglio cervical inferior; **inferior vagus** ~ ganglio inferior del vago; **jugular** ~ ganglio yugular; **lenticular** ~ ganglio lenticular; **middle cervical** ~ ganglio cervical medio; **otic** ~ ganglio ótico; **petrous** ~ ganglio petroso; **phrenic** ~ ganglio frénico; **sphenopalatine** ~ ganglio esfenopalatino; **spiral** ~ ganglio espiral; **splanchnic** ~ ganglio esplácnico; **stellate** ~ ganglio estrellado; **submandibular** ~ ganglio submandibular; **superior cervical** ~ ganglio cervical superior; **superior mesenteric** ~ ganglio mesentérico superior; **superior** ~ **of vagus** ganglio superior del vago; **trigeminal** ~ ganglio trigémino

ganglioglioma, ganglioglioma *m*

gangrene, cangrena; gangrena; **diabetic** ~ gangrena diabética; **dry** ~ gangrena seca; **gas** ~ gangrena gaseosa; **hospital** ~ gangrena hospitalaria; **moist** ~ gangrena húmeda; **senile** ~ gangrena senil; **spontaneous** ~ gangrena espontánea

gangrenous, gangrenoso *adj*

gap, ~ (*opening*) abertura; ~ (*breach*) brecha; ~ (*cavity*) hueco; ~ (*of time*) intervalo; **auscultatory** ~ intervalo auscultatorio; ~ (*diastem*) mella *Dent*; ~ **in the teeth** mella dentaria; ~**-toothed** mellado *adj, Dent*

garbage, basura; ~ **can** cubo de la basura; zafacón *m, PR*

gargle, gárgara; ~ (*liquid*) gargarismo

gargle, to, gargarizar; hacer buches (de sal) *fam*; hacer gárgaras
gargling, gárgaras; gargarismo
garlic, ajo
garrot, garrote *m*
gas, gas *m*; **arterial blood ~es** gases arteriales; **~ bacilli** bacilo gaseoso; **coal ~** gas de hulla; **ethylene sewer ~** gas oleificante; **~ exchange** recambio gaseoso; **~ gangrene** gangrena gaseosa; **inert ~** gas inerte; **marsh ~** gas de los pantanos; **natural ~** gas natural; **tear ~** gas lacrimógeno; **~ (*nitrous oxide*)** gas exhilarante *m, slang*; gas hilarante *m, slang*; óxido nitroso; **~ (*flatus*)** aire *m, slang*; pedo *slang*; viento *slang*
gas, to have, tener gas
gas, to pass, pasar gas; tirar gases; tirar vientos
gash, cuchillada
gash, to, acuchillar
gasoline, gasolina
gasp, **~ (*before dying*)** boqueada; **~ (*difficulty in breathing*)** jadeo
gasp, to, **~ (*make sound before dying*)** boquear; **~ (*pant*)** jadear; **~ for air** hacer esfuerzos para respirar
gastight, hermético *adj*
gastric, gástrico *adj*; **~ content** contenido gástrico; **~ juice** jugo gástrico
gastritis, gastritis *f*
gastroduodenal, gastroduodenal *adj*
gastroenteritis, gastroenteritis *f*; **acute infectious ~** gastroenteritis infecciosa aguda; **hemorrhagic ~** gastroenteritis hemorrágica
gastroenterologist, gastroenterólogo
gastroenterology, gastroenterología
gastrointestinal system, aparato gastrointestinal; sistema gastrointestinal *m*
gastrology, gastrología
gastrorrhea, gastrorrea; secreción excesiva de moco o jugo gástrico *f*

gastroscope, gastroscopio
gastroscopy, gastroscopia; endoscopia gástrica
gather together, to, reunir
gathering, absceso
gauge, **~ (*meter, caliber*)** calibrador *m*; indicador *m*; **catheter ~** calibrador de sondas; **~ (*demonstration*)** indicación *f*; muestra
gauge, to, **~ (*to measure*)** medir (i); **~ (*to assess*)** determinar
gaunt, flaco *adj*
gauze, gasa; **absorbable ~** gasa absorbible; **absorbent ~** gasa absorbente; **antiseptic ~** gasa antiséptica; **~ pad** apósito; **~ roll** rollo de gasa; **sterile absorbent ~** gasa absorbente estéril; **~ swab** compresa de gasa
gay, entendido *m, adj, fam*; en el ambiente *prep phr, PR*; del ambiente *adj, PR*; **~ female** tortillera *PR, vulg*; **~ male** mariposa *vulg*; pájaro *fam*
gel, gel *m*; **~ foam** esponja de gelatina
gelatin, gelatina; **medicinal ~** gelatina medicinal
gelatinize, to, gelatinificar
gelatinous, gelatinoso *adj*
gelfoam, esponja de gelatina; gelfoam *Chicano*
gender, género
gene, gen *m*; **dominant ~** gen dominante; **recessive ~** gen recesivo; **sex-linked ~** gen ligado al sexo
general, general *m/f, adj*; **~ donor of blood** donante universal de sangre *m/f*; **~ condition** estado general; **~ duty nurse** enfermera general; **~ practitioner/ GP** médico general; medico de familia
generalize, to, generalizar
generate, to, generar
generation, generación *f*; **alternate ~** generación alternante;

spontaneous ~ generación espontánea

generic, genérico *adj*

genetic, genético *adj*; ~ **code** código genético; ~ **counselor** asesor genético *m*; ~ **disease** enfermedad genética *f*; ~ **engineering** ingeniería genética; ~ **factor** factor genético *m*

geneticist, genetista *m/f*

genetics, genética

genital, genital *adj*; ~ **herpes** herpe(s)⁴ genital *m/f*

genitals, órganos genitales; partes *f*, *slang*; partes ocultas *f*, *slang*; partes privadas *f*, *slang*; vergüenzas *f*, *pl*; verijas *f*, *pl*

genitalia, genitales *m*, *pl*

genitourinary, genitourinario *adj*; ~ **disease** enfermedad genitourinaria *f*; ~ **system** aparato genitourinario; sistema genitourinario *m*

gentian violet, violeta de genciana

gentle, apacible *adj*; cuidadoso *adj*; suave *adj*

genius, genio

geomedicine, geomedicina

geriatric, geriátrico *adj*

geriatrician, geriatra *m/f*, *adj*

geriatrics, geriatría

germ, germen *m*; microbio; ~ **free** aséptico *adj*; libre de gérmenes *adj*; **wheat** ~ germen de trigo

German measles, alfombría *Chicano*; alfombrilla *Chicano*; fiebre de tres días *f*; rubéola⁵; sarampión alemán *m*; sarampión bastardo *m*; sarampión de tres días *m*

germicidal, germicida *adj*

germicide, germicida *m*, *adj*

germination, germinación *f*

gerodontics, gerodoncia *Dent*

gerodontist, gerodontista *m/f*, *Dent*

gerontologist, gerontólogo

gerontology, gerontología

gestation, gestación *f*; gravidez *f*

gestational, gestacional *adj*

gesture, ademán *m*; gesto

get, to, conseguir (i); obtener; ~ **a disease** pegarle (a uno); ~ **along** ir *Med*; ~ **angry** enfadarse; enojarse; ~ **around on one's own** desplazarse; ~ **better** mejorar(se); ~ **close** acercarse; ~ **down**⁶ (*to acquire drugs*) tomar drogas; usar drogas; ~ **down** (*to go down stairs, etc.*) bajar; ~ **down** (*to swallow*) tragar; ~ **dressed** vestirse (i); ~ **drunk** ajumar(se); guayar(se); templarse *Col*, *Perú*, *PR*; (*See drunk, to be/get.*); ~ **goose bumps** enchinarse la piel; ponerse chinito *adj*; ~ **in the groove** ponerse al tanto²; ~ **larger** engrandecerse; hacerse más grande; ~ **mad** enfadarse; enfogonarse *PR*; enojarse; (*See mad.*); ~ **one's hair cut** pelarse; ~ **out** salir; ~ **out of joint** desconcertar (ie) *Anat*; ~ **over an illness** recobrarse; recuperarse; reponerse de una enfermedad; ~ **over** pasarse; ~ **scared** asustarse; ~ **sick** empacharse *PR*; enfermarse; ~ **smaller** disminuirse; ~ **up** levantarse; ~ **up on the table** subir a la mesa; ~ **used to** acostumbrarse; ~ **well** aliviarse; sanarse; ~ **worse** agravarse; empeorarse; ~ **worse again** reagudizarse *Med*

GH/growth hormone, hormona de crecimiento

ghetto, gueto *PR*, *Chicano*

GI/gastrointestinal, gastrointestinal *adj*

giant, gigante *m*, *adj*; ~ **cell sarcoma** sarcoma de células gigantes *m*

giddiness, desvanecimiento; mareo; vahido; vértigo

giddy, desvanecido *adj*, *Med*; mareado *adj*; vertiginoso *adj*; **to make** ~ encalabrinar *Med*

giggle, to, reírse (i) por nada

giggle micturition, micción al reírse *f*

gin, ginebra

ginger, jengibre *m*; ~ **ale** gaseosa de jengibre; ginger ale *m*

gingiva, (*pl, gingivae*) gingiva *Dent*; encía *Dent*; **alveolar** ~ gingiva alveolar; **buccal** ~ gingiva bucal; **labial** ~ gingiva labial; **lingual** ~ gingiva lingual

gingival, gingival *adj, Dent*; ~ **contour** contorno gingival *Dent*; ~ **retraction** retracción gingival *f, Dent*

gingivitis, gingivitis *f*; **acute necrotizing ulcerative** ~ gingivitis ulcerosa necrosante aguda; **suppurative marginal** ~ gingivitis marginal supurativa

gingivolabial, gingivolabial *adj, Dent*

girdle, cintura; faja; **pelvic** ~ cintura pélvica; **shoulder** ~ cintura escapular; **thoracic** ~ cintura torácica

girdle, to, ceñir (i)

girl, chamaca *Mex*; muchacha; niña; (*See child and kid.*); **large young** ~ potranca *PR*

give, to, dar; ~ (*to administer*) poner; ~ (*to donate*) donar; ~ (*to infect*) contagiar; pegar; ~ **an injection** poner una inyección; ~ **birth** alumbrar; dar a luz; parir; sanar *Chicano*; ~ **it a chance** dar lugar a; dar una oportunidad; ~ **off** (*a smell, gas, etc.*) despedir (i); ~ **off** (*a sound*) emitir; ~ **out** distribuir; ~ **s.o. a cold** resfriar a uno *Med*; ~ **stitches** dar puntadas; dar puntos; ~ **up** (*to renounce*) renunciar; ~ **up** (*to stop*) abandonar; dejar de (+ *infinitive*); ~ **up on** (*a patient*) desahuciar (a un enfermo); ~ **way** (*to yield*) ceder

giving (*of medication*), administración (de un medicamento) *f*

glacial, glacial *adj*

glad (**to**), **to be**, alegrarse (de)

glance, ojeada; vistazo

gland, glándula; **accessory** ~ glándula accesoria; **adrenal** ~ glándula adrenal; glándula suprarrenal; **buccal** ~ glándula bucal; **carotid** ~ glándula carotídea; glándula carótidea; **Cowper's** ~ glándula de Cowper; **duodenal** ~ glándula duodenal; **endocrine** ~ glándula endocrina; **excretory** ~ glándula excretoria; glándula excretora; **exocrine** ~ glándula exocrina; glándula de secreción externa; **intestinal** ~ glándula intestinal; **lacrimal** ~ glándula lagrimal; **lymph** ~ glándula linfática; **mammary** ~ glándula mamaria; **nasal** ~ glándula nasal; **parathyroid** ~ glándula paratiroide; glándula paratiroides; **parotid** ~ glándula parotídea; glándula parótida; **pineal** ~ glándula pineal; **pituitary** ~ glándula pituitaria; **prostate** ~ glándula de la próstata; glándula prostática; próstata; **salivary** ~ glándula salival; glándula salivar; **sebaceous** ~ glándula sebácea; **sore** ~ glándula inflamada; **swollen** ~ **in groin** encordio; incordio; **sublingual** ~ glándula sublingual; **submandibular** ~ glándula submandibular; **submaxillary** ~ glándula submaxilar; **sudoriferous** ~ glándula sudorípara; **sudoriparous** ~ glándula sudorípara; **suprarenal** ~ glándula suprarrenal; **sweat** ~ glándula sudorípara; **thymus** ~ glándula timo; **thyroid** ~ glándula tiroide; glándula tiroides; tiroides, *m/f*, [*Ú.m.c.m.*], *inv*

glanders, muermo

glandular, glandular *adj*

glans, (*penis*) bálano; cabeza *slang*; glande *m*

glare, ~ (*angry look*) mirada airada; mirada feroz; ~ (*strong light*) luz brillante *f*; luz deslumbrante *f*

glare, to, ~ (*to stare angrily*) mirar airadamente; ~ (*to shine*) brillar; ~ (*to be extremely obvious*) saltar a la vista

glass, ~ *(substance)* vidrio; ~ (*drinking container*) vaso; ~ (*pane*) cristal *m*; ~ **case** estuche *m*; funda de gafas; ~ **cup** ventosa; **drinking** ~ vaso; ~ **eye** ojo de vidrio; ~ **eyes**[6] (*drug addict*) (*See addict* [*drug*].)

glasses, anteojos *m, pl*; espejuelos *m, pl, Cu*; gafas *f, pl*; lentes *m, pl, Mex*; **sun** ~ gafas de sol

glaucoma, glaucoma *m*

globulin, globulina; **gamma** ~ gamaglobulina; globulina gamma

gloomy, melancólico *adj*; sombrío *adj*

glossoscopy, examen de la lengua *m*

glossy, lustroso *adj*

glottis, glotis *f*

glove, guante *m*; **rubber** ~**s** guantes de goma; **sterile** ~**s** guantes estériles; **surgical** ~**s** guantes quirúrgicos

glow, incandescencia

glucagon, glucagón *m*

glucatonia, glucatonia

glucokinetic, glucocinético *adj*; (*que mantiene el nivel del azúcar sanguíneo*)

glucose, glucosa; ~ **monitor** aparato para medir la glucosa; ~ **water** agua[3] con azúcar *f*

glucoside, glucósido

glucosin, glucosina

glucosuria, (*See glycosuria.*)

glue, goma; ~[6] cola *slang*; ~ **sniffer** glufo[2]; güelepega[2] *PR*

glue, to, pegar

gluey, ~ (*sticky*) pegajoso *adj*; viscoso *adj*; ~[6] *slang* drogadicto a cola[2]

glum, sombrío *adj*; triste *adj*

glutamine, glutamina

gluteal region, glúteo; región glútea *f*

glutin, glutina

glycerine, glicerina; glicerol *m*

glycerol, glicerol *m*

glycine, glicina

glycogen, glucógeno; glicógeno; **hepatic** ~ glucógeno hepático; **tissue** ~ glucógeno tisular

glycogenase, glucogenasa

glycol, glicol *m*

glycolysis, (*pl, glycolyses*) glucólisis *f, inv*

glycometabolic, glucometabólico *adj*; (*concerniente al metabolismo de los azúcares*)

glycoprotein, glucoproteína *m/f*

glycose, (*See glucose.*)

glycoside, glucósido; **cardiac** ~ glucósido cardíaco

glycosuria, glucosuria; **alimentary** ~ glucosuria alimentaria; **digestive** ~ glucosuria digestiva; **emotional** ~ glucosuria emocional; **epinephrine** ~ glucosuria adrenalínica; **non-diabetic** ~ glucosuria no diabética; **pituitary** ~ glucosuria hipofisaria; **renal** ~ glucosuria renal; **toxic** ~ glucosuria tóxica

gnarl, to, gruñir; rechinar los dientes

gnashing of the teeth, rechinamiento de los dientes

gnat, guasana; jején *m*; maje *m, PR*; mime *m, PR*

gnawing pain, dolor mordiente *m*

GnRH/gonadotropin-releasing hormone, hormona liberadora de gonadotropinas

go, to, ir; ~ (*to break*) romperse; ~ (*to lose*) perder (ie); ~ **after** seguir (i); ~ **against** ir en contra de; ~ **away** (*to leave*) irse; ~ **away** (*to disappear*) desaparecer; ~ **back** regresar; ~ **berserk** andar volado *fam*; ~ **crazy** volverse (ue) loco; ~ **down in the birth canal** encajarse; ~ **down on someone** tragar *vulg*; ~ **down** (*temperature*) bajar; ~ **down with** (*an illness*) caer enfermo de; ~ **downhill** agravarse; ~ **grey**

encanecer; ~ **in** (*to enter*) entrar (en); ~ **into hysterics** ponerse histérico; ~ **into mourning** ponerse de luto; ~ **out** (*matches, light, etc.*) apagarse; ~ **soft** (*erection*) bajar(se) *vulg*; ~ **through** (*to undergo*) pasar por; sufrir; ~ **through with** llevar a cabo; ~ **to bed** acostarse (ue); ~ **to sleep** dormirse (ue); ~ **to the bathroom** ir al baño; ~ **up** subir

goad, to, ~ (*to needle*) incitar; provocar; aguijar *PR*; puyar *CA, PR*

goal, fin *m*; hito; meta; objetivo

goat, cabra

goatpox, viruela caprina

godchild, ahijado

godfather, padrino

goiter, bocio; buche *m, slang*; canana *SpAm*; chorcha *CA*; estruma *m*; güegüecho *m, CA, Mex*; orejón *m, Col*; papo *Med*; struma; **aberrant** ~ bocio aberrante; **cystic** ~ bocio quístico; bocio cístico; **fibrous** ~ bocio fibroso; **nodular** ~ bocio nodular; **simple** ~ bocio simple; **substernal** ~ bocio retrosternal; **suffering from a** ~ güegüecho *adj, CA, Mex*; **suffocative** ~ bocio sofocante; **toxic** ~ bocio tóxico

gold, oro

golden, dorado *adj*

golfer's arm, hombro doloroso de los golfistas

golfer's elbow, codo de golf

gonad, gónada

gonadal, gonadal *adj*

gonadokinetic, gonadocinético *adj*

gonadotropin, gonadotropina; **chorionic** ~ gonadotropina coriónica; **human chorionic** ~/**HCG** gonadotropina coriónica humana; **pituitary** ~ gonadotropina hipofisaria; ~ **-releasing hormone** hormona liberadora de gonadotropinas

goniometer, goniómetro

gonococcus, (*pl, gonococci*) gonococo

gonorrhea, blenorragia; chorro *fam*; gonorrea; purgación *f, slang*

gonorrheal, gonorreico *adj*

good, ~ bueno *adj*; ~ **risk patient** paciente con buen estado general *m/f*; paciente con escaso riesgo *m/f*; bien *m, adv*; **for your own** ~ por su propio bien

goof off, to, *slang* mangonear *PR*; miquear *Chicano*

goofballs[6], (*sedatives, especially barbiturates*) cápsulas de drogas

goose, ganso; **to get** ~ **bumps** enchinarse la piel; ponerse chinito *adj*; ~**flesh** (*pl, goose pimples*) carne de gallina *f*; piel de gallina; **to get** ~ **flesh/pimples** escarapelarse *Mex, Perú*

gorge, fauces *f, pl*

gorged, bimba *adj*; como goma que vá para Ponce *adj, PR*; pimpo *adj*

gouge, gubia

gout, gota; podagra; **articular** ~ gota articular (*ataca a las articulaciones*); **masked** ~ gota latente; **misplaced** ~ gota metastática; gota retrógrada; gota retropulsa; **poor man's** ~ gota de los pobres; **retrocedent** ~ gota retropulsa

gouty, gotoso *adj*

government, gobierno; ~ **subsidy** mantengo *fam*

gown, bata

GP/general practitioner, practicante general *m/f*; (*See general practitioner.*)

grab, to, agarrar(se) de

gradient, gradiente *m*; **atrioventricular** ~ gradiente auriculoventricular; **mitral** ~ gradiente mitral; **ventricular** ~ gradiente ventricular

gradual, gradual *adj*

graduate, graduado *m, adj*; ~ **nurse** enfermera diplomada

graduated, graduado *adj*

graft, ~ (*skin*) injerto *Med*; **animal** ~ injerto animal; **autodermic** ~ injerto autoepidérmico; injerto epidérmico de la piel del mismo paciente; **autoplastic** ~ injerto autoplástico; injerto autógeno; injerto tomado del cuerpo del propio paciente; **bone** ~ injerto óseo; **free** ~ injerto libre; **full-thickness** ~ injerto cutáneo; injerto dermoepidérmico; **split-skin** ~ injerto laminar; injerto cutáneo parcial; injerto de espesor parcial; **thyroid** ~ injerto tiroideo; **tube** ~ injerto tubular; **tunnel** ~ injerto tubular

graft (**in**, **into**, **on**, **onto**), **to**, injertar (en)

grafting, aplicación de un injerto *f*

grain, grano

grainy, granular *adj*

gram, gramo; ~**-negative** gramnegativo *adj*; ~**-positive** grampositivo *adj*

grand mal, gran mal *m*

grandfather, abue *m*, *Chicano*; abuelo

grandson, nieto

grant, ~ (*money donated*) subvención *f*; ~ (*scholarship*) beca

granular, granular *adj*

granulation, granulación *f*

granule, gránulo; **basophil** ~ gránulo basófilo; **eosinophil** ~ gránulo eosinófilo; **neutrophil** ~ gránulo neutrófilo

granulocyte, granulocito

granulocytosis, granulocitosis *f*

granuloma, granuloma *m*; **benign** ~ **of thyroid** granuloma benigno de tiroides; **infectious** ~ granuloma infeccioso; **lipoid** ~ granuloma lipoideo; **ulcerating** ~ **of the pudenda** granuloma ulcerativo de los genitales

granulomatosis, granulomatosis *f*; **lipoid** ~ granulomatosis lipoide; **malignant** ~ granulomatosis maligna; enfermedad de Hodgkin *f*

granulomatous, granulomatoso *adj*

grape sugar, dextrosa

graph, gráfica; gráfico

graphite, grafito

graphospasm, (*writers' cramp*) grafospasmo; calambre de los escritores *m*

grasp, to, agarrarse

grasping reflex, reflejo de prehensión

grass, hierba; ~[6] zacate[2] *m*; (*See marijuana.*); **bag of** ~ funda *PR*; ~ **snake** serpiente del pasto *m*

grate, to, frotar

gratification, gratificación *f*

grave, grave *adj*

gravel, arenilla

gravida, grávida; mujer preñada

gravidic, gravídico *adj* (*relativo al embarazo o a la mujer preñada*)

gravidity, gravidez *f*; preñez *f*

gravity, gravedad *f*, *Phys*, *Med*; **of uncertain** ~ de prognóstico reservado; **specific** ~ gravedad específica

gravy[6], (*a mixture of blood and heroin*) salsa[2]

gray/grey, gris *adj*; ~ **hair** cana(s); ~ **haired** canoso *adj*; ~ **matter** substancia gris

graze, ~ (*sore place*) rozadura *Med*; rozón *m*; ~ (*scrape*) abrasíon *f*

graze, to, ~ (*to scrape skin*) raspar; ~ (*to chafe, rub gently*) raer *Med*; rozar *Med*

grease, grasa

grease, to, engrasar

greasy, grasoso *adj*

great, grande *adj*; ~ **cardiac vein** vena coronaria magna; ~ **saphenous vein** vena safena interna; ~ **grandfather** bisabuelo; ~ **grandson** biznieto; ~ **great grandfather** tatarabuelo; ~ **great grandson** tataranieto

green, verde *m*, *adj*

greenish, verdoso *adj*

greet, to, saludar

greeting, saludo

grey, gris *adj*; (*See gray.*); ~ **hair**

cana(s); ~ **haired** canoso *adj*; ~
matter substancia gris; **to turn** ~
volverse (ue) gris
grey, to, encanecer
grief, aflicción *f*; pesadumbre *f*;
pena
grieve, to, afligirse
grimace, mueca
grimace, to, hacer una mueca
grind, to, ~ (*mill*) moler (ue); ~
(*crush*) triturar; ~ (*sharpen*)
afilar; ~ (*teeth*) hacer rechinar
(los dientes); ~ (*oppress*) oprimir
grip, (*pain*) punzada de dolor
grip, to, (*grasp, to*) agarrar(se)
grippe, gripa; gripe *f*
grit one's teeth, to, ~ (*to grate*)
rechinar los dientes; ~ (*in determination*) apretar (ie) los dientes
groan, (*moan*) gemido; quejido
groan, to, ~ (*to moan*) gemir (i);
quejarse; ~ (*to grumble*) gruñir;
~ (*to creak*) crujir
groin, aldilla *fam*; empeine[7]; ingle *f*
groove, surco; hendidura; canal[8] *m*;
alveololingual ~ surco alveololingual; **anterior interventricular** ~
surco interventricular anterior;
anterior paramedian ~ surco paramedio anterior de la médula espinal; **auricular** ~ hendidura
auricular; **basilar** ~ canal basilar;
bicipital ~ surco bicipital; **genital** ~
surco genital; **infra-orbital** ~ hendidura infraorbital; **medullary** ~
surco medular; **meningeal** ~ hendidura meníngea; **mylohyoid** ~
hendidura milohioidea; **nasal** ~
hendidura nasal; **nuchal** ~ hendidura de la nuca; **obturator** ~
hendidura del obturador; **occipital** ~ hendidura occipital; **olfactory** ~ hendidura del olfatorio;
peroneal ~ hendidura peroneal;
popliteal ~ hendidura poplítea;
posterior interventricular ~ surco
interventricular posterior; **posteri-
or paramedian** ~ surco paramedio
posterior de la médula espinal;

primitive dental ~ surco dental
primitivo; **sigmoid** ~ hendidura
sigmoidea; **subclavian** ~ canal del
subclavio; **subcostal** ~ canal costal
grooved, acanalado *adj*
grope, to, andar a tientas; ~ **for**
buscar a tientas
gross, ~ (*twelve dozen*) gruesa; ~
(*fat; thick*) grueso *adj*; ~ (*glaring*)
craso *adj*; ~ **ignorance** ignorancia crasa; ~ (*indecent*) indecente
adj; ~ (*unrefined; vulgar*) grosero
adj; ~ **examination** examen
macroscópico *m*; ~ (*weight*) bruto *adj*; ~ **weight** peso bruto
grouch, (*grumbling individual*) cascarrabias *m/f, inv*; refunfuñón,
-ñona *m/f*
grouch, to, ~ (*to complain*) quejarse; refunfuñar; ~ (*to be bad-
tempered*) estar de mal humor
grouchy, ~ (*grumbling*) refunfuñón *adj*; ~ (*bad-tempered*)
malhumorado *adj*
ground chalk in water, creta pulvorizada en agua
group, grupo; **blood** ~ grupo sanguíneo; ~ **insurance** seguro
colectivo; ~ **practice/G.P.** P.G.[9]
f; práctica de un grupo ; ~**specific** específico de grupo; ~
therapy terapia en grupo
grow, to, ~ (*to develop*) desarrollarse; ~ (*to increase in size*) crecer; ~ **dark** oscurecer; ~ **old**
envejecer(se); ~ **out a culture**
aislar en cultivos bacterianos; ~
out of (*a habit*) perder (ie) una
costumbre; ~ **out of** (*an illness*)
curar espontáneamente una
enfermedad; ~ **out of** (*clothes*)
quedársele pequeño; ~ **up**
madurar
growing, ~ (*increasing*) creciente
adj; en aumento; ~ **pain** dolor
del crecimiento *m*; ~ (*child*)
crecedero *adj*
growl, gruñido
growl, to, gruñir

growth, crecimiento; **new ~** crecimiento nuevo; **~ retardation** retardación de crecimiento *f*; **~ spurt** estirón *m*; **~ (*tumor*)** bulto; excrecencia; tlacote *m*, *Mex*; tumor *m*

growth, to reach full, alcanzar su pleno desarrollo

grumble, to, ~ (*to moan*) refunfuñar; **~ (at/about)** (*to complain*) quejarse (de)

grunt, (*sound*) gruñido; pujido

g.u./genitourinary, genitourinario *adj*

guaiacol, guayacol *m*

guarantee, to, garantizar

guard closely, to, vigilar de cerca

guarded, **(prognosis)**, (pronóstico) reservado

guardian, guardián, -iana *m/f*

guidance, guía

guide, guía

guideline, ~ (*directive*) directriz *f*; **~ (*model*)** pauta

guilt, culpa; **~ feelings** sentimiento de culpabilidad

guiltiness, culpabilidad *f*

guinea pig, cobayo

gullet, gaznate *m*; boca del estómago; esófago

gulp, ~ (*drink*) trago; **~ (*of food*)** bocado; **~ (*of anxiety*)** nudo en la garganta; **~ (*sip*)** sorbo

gulp, to, tragar; **~ down** engullir; **~ for breath** respirar hondo

gum, goma, **~ (*chewing gum*)** chicle *m*; **~ (*glue*)** pegamento; **~ (*of the eyes—rheum*)** legaña; **~ (*of mouth*)** encía; **~ contour** (*See gingival contour.*); **sore ~s** encías dolorosas

gumboil, flemón (dentario) *m*; absceso gingival; postemilla *SpAm*

gun[6], **~ (*drug abuse terms*)** equipo hipodérmico; estuche[2] *m*; herramienta[2]; herre[2] *f*; pistola[2]; R[2] *f*

gunshot, tiro; **~ wound** herida de bala; herida por bala

gurgle, to, gorgotear

gurgling, gorgoteo

gush, (*of fluid*) chorro

gust, ráfaga

gustatory, gustatorio *adj*

guts, *fam* entrañas *f*, *pl*; intestinos *m*, *pl*; tripas *f*, *pl*; **blind ~** intestino ciego

gutta-percha, gutapercha

guy, effeminate ~ plumero *PR*; *fam*; chillo *fam*; chingón *fam*; macho *PR*, *fam*; **sexually aggressive and active ~** cabro *fam*; cerebrito *PR*, *fam*; chillo *fam*; chingón *fam*; macho *PR*, *fam*; **well-dressed, well-educated ~** tipo *fam*; tiro *fam*

gymnastics, gimnasia; **occular ~** gimnasia ocular; **vocal ~** gimnasia vocal

gynecologic, ginecológico *adj*

gynecological, ginecológico *adj*; **~ floor** piso ginecológico

gynecologist, especialista en señoras *m/f*, *fam*; ginecólogo

gynecology, ginecología

---

[2] This is new vocabulary, not necessarily listed nor yet recognized by the Royal Academy of Spanish Grammar. It is understood that this vocabulary is primarily slang. Unless otherwise indicated, the gender of nouns is assumed to be obvious.

[3] For pronunciation purposes, the masculine definite and indefinite articles, *el* and *un*, not *la* or *una*, are used when the article immediately precedes the feminine singular noun which begins with stressed *a* or any other that begins with stressed *ha*.

[4] This word is often used in the plural form.

[5] In Spanish-speaking countries, especially in Mexico, *rubella*, or *German measles*, is called *rubeola*. To be certain, therefore, as to which disease a patient has/has had, it is advisable to inquire about the symptoms rather than ask the name of the disease.

[6] Part of the Drug Abuse Vocabulary.

[7] Multiple meanings of *empeine* include groin, instep, and ringworm.

[8] In Spanish *canal* is an open duct, *conducto* is closed.

[9] Use the Spanish pronunciation of these letters.

H

H[7] (*heroin*)[4], azúcar *m*, *Arizona*, *Texas*; caballo[2]; carga[2]; chiva[2]; cohete[2] *m*; heroína *form*

habit, adicción *f*; drogadicción *f*; farmacodependencia; hábito; habituación *f*; toxicomanía; ~ (*custom*) costumbre *f*; **bad ~** (*vice*) vicio; **~-forming drug** medicamento que produce habituamiento

hack, tos seca *f*

hacking cough, tos seca *f*; tosecilla

haggard, ojeroso *adj*

hair, cabello *fam*; chimpa *Chicano*; greñas *fam*; pelo; ~ (*of body, esp. pubic*) vello; ~ (*of head*) cabello(s); **(premature) gray ~** canas (verdes) *f, pl*; **curl of ~** chino *Chicano*; rizo; tirabuzón *m*; **curly ~** pelo crespo; pelo rizado; **having long, dirty ~** como pepa jobo *PR phr*; **kinky ~** pelo grifo *Chicano*; pelo pasudo; **pubic ~** pelitos *pl*, *Chicano*; pelo púbico; pendejos *fam, slang, Arg*; vello púbico; **~ shaft** tallo del pelo; **straight ~** pelo liso; **wavy ~** pelo quebrado

hairball, tricobezoar *m*

haircut, corte de pelo *m*; pelada *SpAm*; **in need of a ~** pelú *PR*, *adj*; **to get a ~** cortarse el pelo; **to have a ~** peluquearse *SpAm*

hairiness, hirsutismo

hairless, calvo *adj*; depilado *adj*

hairline, línea capilar

hairlip, culco; fañoso

hairnet, redecilla; invisible *m, Mex*

hairpin, horquilla; invisible *m, Arg*

hairy, hirsuto *adj*; peludo *adj*; pelú *adj*; piloso *adj*; tarántula *adj*, *Chicano*; velloso *adj*; **~ tongue** lengua vellosa

half, medio *adj*; mitad *f*; **~ asleep** medio dormido *adj*

half-life, vida media; semidesintegración *f*

halitosis, aliento feo; halitosis *f*; mal aliento

hall, pasillo; ~ (*entrance area*) vestíbulo; ~ (*huge room*) salón *m*

hallmark, característica; signo característico

hallucinate, to, alucinar

hallucination, alucinación *f*; visión *f*; **auditory ~** alucinación auditiva; **depressive ~** alucinación depresiva; **gustatory ~** alucinación gustativa; **olfactory ~** alucinación olfativa; **reflex ~** alucinación refleja; **stump ~** alucinación del muñón; **tactile ~** alucinación táctil; **visual ~** alucinación visual

hallucinatory, alucinatorio *adj*

hallucinogen, alucinante *adj*; alucinógeno; droga alucinadora

hallway, pasillo

halogen, halógeno *m, adj*

halothane, halotano

halter, cabestrillo

ham, (*back of the thigh*) corva

hamburger, hamburguesa

hammer, martillo

hammertoe, dedo gordo en martillo

hams, ~ *fam* nalgas; trasero

hamster, criceto

hamstring, tendón de la corva *m*; tendón (del hueso) poplíteo *m*; **inner ~** tendones internos de la corva; **~ muscles** músculos del jarrete; músculos posteriores del muslo; **outer ~** tendón externo de la corva; **to ~** (*to sever the hamstring*) cortar el tendón de la corva; desjarretar

hand, mano *f*; **back of the ~** dorso de la mano; **claw ~** mano en garra; **palm of the ~** palma de la mano

handcart, carretilla

handful, puñado

handgrip, asidero; **~** *(of racquet, club)* mango; **~**(*of cycle*) puño

handicap, impedimento; incapacidad *f*

handicapped, incapacitado *adj*

handkerchief, pañuelo

handle, asa; mango; **~ around waistline** (*love handle*) chicho; **to ~** manejar

hand-out, mantengo

hands and knees, on, a gatas

handsome, guapo *adj*

hang, to, colgar (ue); **~** (*by the neck*) ahorcar; **~ around** janguear *Chicano*; **~ around low-class places** cucarachear *Chicano*

hanger, gancho; **~** (*clothes rack*) perchero; **~** (*clothes*) percha

hanging, ahorcadura; ahorcamiento

hangnail, cutícula desgarrada; padastro *fam*; repelo *Anat*

hangover, depresión nerviosa al pasar los efectos de un barbitúrico *f*; cruda *fam*; quemao *fam*; malestar postalcohólico *m*; **to have a ~** andar crudo; estar crudo

Hansen's disease, lepra

happen, to, ocurrir; pasar; suceder

happiness, felicidad *f*

happy, contento *adj*; feliz *adj*

harass, to, chavar(se); jorobar; pejigar

hard, indurado *adj*; **~** (*consistency*) duro *adj*; **~** (*difficult*) difícil *adj*; **~** (*muscle*) firme *adj*; **~** (*rule*) inflexible *adj*; **~** (*tissue*) escleroso *adj*; **~ feeling** resentimiento; **~ headed** (*tough-minded*) testarudo *adj*; **~ measles** (*rubeola*) sarampión malo *m*; **~ of hearing** corto de oído; duro de oído; medio sordo; parcialmente sordo; **~ palate** paladar duro *m*; paladar óseo *m*

harden, to, endurecer

hardening, endurecimiento

hardness, dureza; **permanent ~** dureza permanente; **temporary ~** dureza temporal

hardship, sufrimiento

hard-working, diligente *adj*

harelip, boquineta *m, Chicano*; cheuto *adj, Chi*; comido de la luna *fam*; jane *adj, Hond*; labihendido; labio cucho *Chicano*; labio leporino

harm, daño; mal *m*

harm, to, dañar; injuriar; **~ oneself** dañarse; hacerse daño; **~** (*eyesight*) deshacer

harmful, dañino *adj*; dañoso *adj*; nocivo *adj*; **~ habit** costumbre dañina *f*

harmless, inocuo *adj*; inofensivo *adj*

harsh, áspero *adj*; **~ raucous sound** ronquido

harshness, aspereza

hash[7]**,** *slang* (**hashish**) hachich *m*; hachis *m*; haschich *m*; mafú *m*, (*uncommon*)

hasten, to, darse prisa

hat, sombrero

hate, odio; **to ~** odiar

have, to, ~ (*aux. verb*) haber; **~** (*to possess*) tener; **~ a bowel movement** mover (ue) el vientre; hacer caca *slang, juv.*; **~ a good time** divertirse (ie); pachangiar *fam*; relajar(se) *fam*; vacilar *fam*; **~ dinner** cenar; **~ lunch** almorzar (ue); **~ to** (*must*) tener que (+ *infinitive*); **~ to do with** tratarse de

havoc, estragos *m, pl*

hawk nose, de nariz aguileña *prep phr*

hay fever, fiebre del heno *f*; jey fiver *m/f, Chicano*; pituita *PR*

hazard, peligro; riesgo; **to ~** (*endanger*) arriesgar; correr riesgo; poner en peligro; **to ~** (*a guess*) aventurar

hazardous, peligroso *adj*

haziness, opacidad *f*

HCG/human chorionic gonadotropin, GCH[8]/gonadotropina coriónica humana

HDL/high density lipoprotein, LAD[8]/lipoproteína de alta densidad

head, cabeza *Anat*; cráneo; catrueca *fam*; chola *fam*; coco *fam*; chaveta *fam*; chompeta *fam*; paguacha *Anat, fam*; ~ (*of an abscess*) centro; **bald** ~ pelada *Chi, Ríopl*; ~ (*of bed, table*) cabecera; ~ **circumference** perímetro cefálico; ~ **cold** resfrío; resfriado; romadizo; ~ **down** cabeza en declive; ~ **first** de cabeza; ~ **nurse** enfermera jefe; enfermera mayor; jefa de enfermeras; ~ **of hair** cabellera; ~ **of household** jefe de la casa *m*; jefe de la familia *m*; ~ **presentation** presentación cefálica *f*; presentación de la cabeza *f*; ~**rest** apoyo de la cabeza; ~**rolling** rotación de la cabeza *f*; **to come to a ~** (*an abscess*) madurar

headache, cajetuda *Chicano*; cefalalgia *form*; cefalea *form*; dolor de cabeza *m*; jaqueca; zangarri(an)a; **anemic** ~ dolor de cabeza anémico; **cluster** ~ dolor de cabeza en grupos; **congestive** ~ dolor de cabeza congestivo; **histamine** ~ dolor de cabeza histamínico; **migraine** ~ jaqueca; migraña; **puncture** ~ dolor de cabeza por punción; **reflex** ~ dolor de cabeza reflejo; **tension** ~ dolor de cabeza por tensión; **vascular** ~ dolor de cabeza vascular

headband, cinta (para la cabeza); venda (para la cabeza)

headboard, cabecera

heading, encabezamiento; título

headrest, apoyo para la cabeza

headstrong teenager, mosalbete *m/f*

heal, to, curar; sanar; sanarse; ~ (**up**) cicatrizarse; encarnar *Med*; ~ **superficially** sobresanar *Med*

healer, curador *m*; curandero

healing, curación *f*; **folk** ~ curanderismo; ~ **power** virtud curativa *f*

health, ~ (*of a person*) salud *f*; ~ (*public*) sanidad *f*; higiene *f*; **broken** ~ quebranto; salud quebrantada; ~ **center** (*usually government sponsored*) centro de salud; ~ **certificate** certificado médico; ~ **counseling** consejos acerca de la salud; ~ **department** centro de salud; departamento de salubridad; departamento de salud; **mental** ~ **department** departamento de enfermedades mentales; **public** ~ **department** departamento de salud pública; ~ **education** educación higiénica *f*; instrucción higiénica *f*; ~ **insurance** seguro médico; ~ **maintenance organization** organización del mantenimiento de la salud *f*; ~ **measures** medidas sanitarias; ~ **officer** inspector, -ra de sanidad *m/f*; **public** ~ salubridad pública *f*; sanidad pública *f*; **state of** ~ estado de salud; ~ **statistics** salubridad *f*; **to be in bad/poor** ~ estar mal de salud; **to be brimming with** ~ vender salud; **to be in good** ~ estar bien de salud; gastar salud; gozar de buena salud; **to be in perfect** ~ no doler (ue) ni una uña *PR*; **to give s.o. back his/her** ~ devolverle (ue) la salud a uno; **to improve one's** ~ mejorar de salud; **to recover one's** ~ recobrar la salud; **to take care of one's** ~ mirar por su salud

healthcare, atención médica *f*; servicios médicos

healthiness, salubridad *f*

healthy, sano *adj, Med*; saludable *adj, Med*

heaping teaspoon, cucharadita colmada

hear, to, oír

hearing, audición *f*; oído; sentido; oír *m*; ~ **aid** aparato auditivo; aparato para la sordera; audífono; audiófono; otófono; prótesis acústica *f*; prótesis auditiva *f*

heart, corazón *m*; **apex of the ~** punta del corazón; **athletic ~** corazón atlético; ~ **attack** ataque *m, fam*; ataque al corazón; ataque cardíaco; ataque del corazón; infarto; infarto del corazón; mal del corazón *m, fam*; ~ **blockage** bloqueo cardíaco; bloqueo del corazón; ~ **bypass** derivación del flujo coronario *f*; **congenital ~ defect** defecto congénito del corazón; ~ **disease** cardiopatías; enfermedad cardíaca *f*; enfermedad del corazón *f*; mal del corazón *m*; ~ **failure** fallo del corazón; colapso cardíaco; insuficiencia cardíaca; paro cardíaco; paro del corazón; **backward ~ failure** insuficiencia cardíaca retrógrada; **congestive ~ failure** insuficiencia cardíaca congestiva; **forward ~ failure** insuficiencia cardíaca anterógrada; **left ventricular ~ failure** insuficiencia cardíaca ventricular izquierda; **right ventricular ~ failure** insuficiencia cardíaca ventricular derecha; **fatty ~** corazón graso; **fibroid ~** corazón fibroide; **irritable ~** corazón irritable; ~ **murmur** murmullo; soplo *fam*; ~ **problems** enfermedad del corazón *f*; ~ **sac** pericardio; ~ **stoppage** bloqueo cardíaco; ~ **tracing** electrocardiograma *m*; ~ **valve** válvula del corazón; ~**auricle** aurícula; ~**ventricle** ventrículo

heartache, aflicción *f*; angustia; congoja

heartbeat, latido (cardíaco); latido del corazón; palpitación *f*; **irregular ~** (*arrhythmia*) arritmia; latido irregular; palpitación irregular; **rapid ~**

(*tachycardia*) palpitación rápida; taquicardia; **rhythmical ~** palpitación rítmica; **slow ~** palpitación lenta

heartburn, acedía; acedías *fam*; acidez (estomacal) *f*; agriera *SpAm*; agruras (del estómago) *fam*; ardor del estómago *m*; ardor epigástrico *m*; cardialgia; dolor de aire en el estómago *m, fam*; gastralgia; hervedera *PR*; pirosis *f*

heartfelt, hondo *adj*

heart-lung, cardiorespiratorio *adj*

heat, ~ (*warmth*) calor *m*; ~ **apoplexy** calor apoplético; fiebre térmica *f*; golpe de calor *m*; insolación *f*; **atomic ~** calor atómico; **body ~** calor equilibrado *cult*; **conductive ~** calor de conducción; **convective ~** calor de convección; **dry ~** calor seco; ~ **exhaustion** agotamiento por calor; **radiant ~** calor radiante; ~ **resistant** resistente al calor *adj*; **steamy ~** vaporizo *Mex, PR*; **stroke** fiebre térmica *f*; golpe de calor *m*; insolación *f*; ~ **therapy** termoterapia; tratamiento térmico; ~ (*heating system*) calefacción *f*; **to ~ (up)** calentar (ie)

heating pad, electric, almohadilla caliente eléctrica; cojín eléctrico *m*

heaviness, pesadez *f*

heavy, pesado *adj*

heavyset, corpulento *adj*; rechoncho *adj*

heel, calcañar *m, Anat*; talón *m, Anat*; zancajo *Anat*; ~ (*of foot, sock, stocking, shoe*) talón *m, Anat*; ~ (*on sole of shoe*) tacón *m*; **high ~** tacón alto; ~ **tap** reflejo aquíleo; ~ **walking** marcha sobre los talones

height, (*of person*) altura; estatura; talle *m*; **of average ~** de talle mediano; **sitting ~** altura en posición sentada; **standing ~** altura en posición de pie

helium, helio
helix, hélix *m*
helminth, helminto
help, asistencia; auxilio; ayuda; socorro; **immediate** ~ socorro inmediato
help, to, ayudar ~ (*esp. in distress*) auxiliar; socorrer; ~ (*pain*) aliviar
hem, (*sewing*) doblez *m*
hemangioma, hemangioma *m*; **capillary** ~ hemangioma capilar; **cavernous** ~ hemangioma cavernoso
hematic, hemático *adj*; relativo a la sangre *adj*
hematoblast, hematoblasto
hematocrit, hematócrito
hematologist, hematólogo
hematology, análisis de la sangre *m, inv*; hematología
hematoma, hematoma *m*; chichón *m, fam*; **aneurysmal** ~ hematoma aneurismático; **dural** ~ hematoma dural; **pelvic** ~ hematoma pélvico; **subdural** ~ hematoma subdural
hematuria, hematuria; sangre en la orina *f*
hemiplegia, hemiplejía; parálisis de un lado del cuerpo
hemisphere, hemisferio; **dominant** ~ hemisferio dominante
hemodialysis, hemodiálisis *f*
hemoglobin, hemoglobina; **inactive** ~ hemoglobina inactiva; **oxidized** ~ hemoglobina oxigenada; **reduced** ~ hemoglobina reducida
hemolysis, hemólisis *f*
hemolytic, hemolítico *adj*
hemophilia, hemofilia; hematofilia; hemorrafilia; enfermedad hemática *f*; **hereditary** ~ hemofilia hereditaria; **sporadic** ~ hemofilia esporádica
hemophiliac, hemofílico *m, adj*
hemophilic, hemofílico *adj*
hemorrhage, desangramiento; hemorragia; morragia *Chicano*; sangramiento; sangrado *fam*; **arterial** ~ hemorragia arterial; **cerebral** ~ hemorragia cerebral; **concealed** ~ hemorragia oculta; **essential** ~ hemorragia espontánea; **external** ~ hemorragia externa; **internal** ~ hemorragia interna; **postpartum** ~ hemorragia puerperal; **primary** ~ hemorragia primaria; **pulmonary** ~ hemorragia pulmonar; **recurring** ~ hemorragia recurrente; **renal** ~ hemorragia renal; **secondary** ~ hemorragia secundaria; **spontaneous** ~ hemorragia espontánea; **subarachnoid** ~ hemorragia subaracnoidea; **unavoidable** ~ hemorragia inevitable; **venous** ~ hemorragia venosa; **to** ~ salir sangre; sangrar; tener sangramiento *fam*
hemorrhagic, hemorrágico *adj*
hemorrhaging, hemorragia
hemorrhoids, almorranas *fam*; hemorroide *f*; hemorroides *f, pl*
hemorrhoidal, hemorroidal *adj*
hemostat, pinza hemostática; hemostato; hemóstato *m, adj*
hemostatic, hemostático *m, adj*
heparin, heparina
heparinize, to, heparinizar
hepatic, hepático *adj*
hepatitis, fiebre *f, fam, Mex*; hepatitis *f*; inflamación del hígado *f*; **infectious** ~ hepatitis infecciosa; **transfusion** ~ hepatitis por transfusión; **viral** ~ hepatitis viral
herb, baqueña *PR*; hierba; recao *PR*; yerba; ~ **bath** baño aromático; ~ **shop** botánica
herbaceous, herbáceo *adj*
herbal, herbario *adj*
herbalist, botánico; herbolario
herbicide, herbicida *m*; matayerbas *m, inv*
hereditary, hereditario *adj*; ~ **de-**

fects defectos hereditarios; ~ **disease** enfermedad hereditaria *f*
heredity, herencia
hernia, desaldillado *fam, Mex*; destripado *slang*; hernia; pagua *Chi*; potra *Med*; potro *SpAm, Med*; quebradura; relajado; relajadura *Mex*; rotura *fam*; **abdominal** ~ hernia abdominal; **acquired** ~ hernia adquirida; **concealed** ~ hernia oculta; **congenital** ~ hernia congénita; **cystic** ~ hernia cística; **direct** ~ hernia inguinal directa; hernia inguinal interna; **encysted** ~ hernia enquistada; **epigastric** ~ hernia epigástrica; **femoral** ~ hernia femoral; **hiatal** ~ hernia hiatal; **hiatus** ~ hernia hiatal; **indirect** ~ hernia inguinal externa; hernia inguinal indirecta; hernia inguinal oblicua; **inguinal** ~ hernia inguinal; quebradura en la ingle; bubonocele *m*; **intermuscular** ~ hernia intermuscular; **interstitial** ~ hernia intersticial; ~ **of the bladder** hernia vesical; **retrograde** ~ hernia retrógrada; **sliding** ~ hernia por deslizamiento; **strangulating** ~ hernia estrangulada; **umbilical** ~ hernia del ombligo; hernia umbilical; ombligo salido *slang*; ombligón *m, slang*
heroin[4], heroína *form*; adormidera[2]; achivia[2]; amor[2] *m*; ardor[2] *m*; arpon[2] *m*; arponazo[2]; azúcar[2] *m*; azufre[2] *m*; bandillera[2]; blanca[2]; blanco[2]; borra blanca[2]; caca[2]; caballo[2]; cagada *vulg*[2]; carga[2]; cáscara[2]; chiva[2]; chutazo[2]; cohete[2] *m*; cristales[2] *m*; cura[2]; dama blanca[2]; estofa *PR*; gato[2]; golpe[2] *m*; goma[2]; H[2] *f*; helena[2]; heroica[2]; la cosa[2]; la duna[2]; lenguazo[2]; manteca[2]; nieve[2] *f*; papel[2] *m*; papelito[2]; pasta[2]; pericazo[2]; piquete[2] *m*; polvo[2]; polvo amargo[2]; polvo blanco[2]; stufa[2]; tecata[2]; **bad** ~

manteca; ~ **capsule** cachucha[2]; capa[2]; gorra[2]; timba[2]; **a fix of** ~ cantazo; ~ (*prison code*) jacket *m*; ~ (*a hit from sniffing heroin*) pase *m*; ~ **pusher** traquetero; ~ **user** (*addict*) teco[2]; tecato[2]
herpes, herpes[5] *m/f*; zoster *m, fam*; fuegos *m, pl, fam*; ampollas *f, pl, fam*; ~ **facialis** herpes facial; ~ **febrilis** herpes febril; ~ **genitalis** herpes genital; ~ **menstrualis** herpes menstrual; ~ **simplex** herpes simple; ~ **virus**, virus herpético *m*; ~ **zoster** zoster *f*
herpetic, herpético *adj*
hesitate, to, vacilar
heterosexual, heterosexual *m/f, adj*
hex, (*jinx*) mal de ojo *m*; mal puesto *m*; maleficio; **to** ~ embrujar; hacer un mal
hiatal, hiatal *adj*
hiatus, hiato; ~ **hernia** hernia hiatal
hibernating, hibernante *adj*
hiccough, **hiccup**, hipo; hipsus *m*; **to have the** ~**s** tener hipo
hiccough, **to**/**to hiccup**, hipar; hipear *Mex*; hipiar *Mex*
hickey, chupón *m*
hide, cuero
hide, to, esconderse
hideous, horrible *adj*
high, alto *adj*; ~ **arched foot** pie hueco *m*; ~ **cholesterol** colesterol elevado *m*; ~ **from glue sniffing**[7] glufo[2] *adj*; ~ **from sniffing paint thinner**[7] tiniado[2] *adj*; ~ **on**[7] (*marijuana*; *turned on*) motiado[2] *adj*; **anything that prolongs a** ~[7] curita; ~ **on**[7] (*narcotics*) alivianado[2] *adj*; caballón[2] *adj*; curao[2] *adj*; drogado *adj*; embarsado[2] *adj*; embetunado[2] *adj*; embollado[2] *adj*; espaseao[2] *adj*, *Chicano, PR*; loco[2] *adj*; locote[2] *adj*; nota[2] *f*; petardo[2] *f*, (*less common*) sonado[2] *adj*; sonámbulo[2] *adj*; **extremely** ~ bombiao[2] *adj*; cañinga de mono[2] *PR*; embetunado[2] *adj*;

volcao[2] *adj*; ~ **on pills**[7] píldoro[2] *adj*; ~ **pitched** agudo *adj*; de tono agudo; de tono alto; ~ **voice** voz aguda *f*; ~ **tone deafness** sordera para los sonidos altos; ~ **triglycerides** triglicéridos elevados; ~ **up** muy alto *adj*; ~ **water pants** brincacharcos *m, pl*; **to be** ~[7] andar botando[2]; andar elevado a-mil[2]; andar hasta las manos[2]; andar hasta las manitas[2]; andar hypo[2]; andar loco[2]; andar locote[2]; andar pasado[2]; andar prendido[2]; andar servido[2]; andar subido amil[2]; **to get** ~[7] agarrar onda[2]; andar botando[2]; andar hypo[2]; andar loco[2]; andar locote[2]; andar pasado[2]; andar prendido[2]; andar servido[2]; embollarse[2]; sonarse[2]

hinder, to, obstaculizar; obstruir

hip, cadera *Anat*; cuadril *m, Mex, Chicano*; ~ **bone** hueso coxal; hueso de la cadera; ~ **flask** caneca; ~ **joint** articulación coxofemoral *f*; articulación de la cadera *f*; ~ **measurement** perímetro de caderas

hippocratic, hipocrático *adj*; ~ **Oath** juramento hipocrático

hircus, pelo axilar; pelo de la axila

hiss, ~ (*of disapproval; steam, gas*) silbido; ~ (*to call attention*) siseo; **to** ~ silbar; sisear

histamine, histamina

histeria, histerismo

histidine, histidina

histologist, histólogo

histology, histología

history, historia; **family** ~ historia de la familia; **medical** ~ historia clínica

hit, ~ (*attack*) ataque *m*; ~ (*blow*) golpe *m*; guantón *m, SpAm*; ~ (*good guess*) acierto; ~ (*shot*) tiro; ~ (*success*) éxito; sensación *f*; ~ (*with bomb, shell, etc.*) impacto; ~ **of cocaine or heroin**[7] cantazo[2]; pase[2] *m*; ~ **of marijuana**[7] jalá[2];

jalaita[2]; pase[2] *m*; toque[2] *m*; ~ **or miss** al azar *prep phr*

hit, to, ~ (*to collide with*) chocar con; dar contra; ~ (*to damage*) hacer daño a; dañar; afectar; ~ (*to find, reach*) llegar a; alcanzar; ~ (*to overtake*) sobrecoger; ~ (*to strike*) golpear; pegar; ~ **oneself** golpearse; ~ (*a target*) alcanzar; dar en; ~ (*to wound*) herir (ie); ~ **up**[7] clavarse[2]; componerse[2]; curarse[2]; filerearse[2]; jincarse[2]; picarse[2]; rayarse[2]; shootear[2]

HIV/Human Immunodeficiency Virus, VIH[8]/Virus de (la) Inmunodeficiencia Humana *m*

hives, granos *m, pl, fam*; ronchas, roñas *f, pl, fam*; salpullidos *m, pl, fam*; urticaria

H.M.O./health maintenance organization, O.M.S.[8]/organización para el mantenimiento de la salud *f*

hoarse, afónico *adj*; ronco *adj*; **chronically** ~ carrasposo *adj*; **to be** ~ carraspear; estar afónico *fam*; estar ronco *fam*; ronquear

hoarseness, carraspera *fam*; pechuguera *Bol, Col, Mex*; ronquera; tajada *Med*

hobble, to, renguear

hobby, pasatiempo

hodgepodge, burundanga

hold of, to keep ~ no soltar (ue); **to lose** ~ soltar (ue); **to relax one's** ~ aflojar la mano; **to take** ~ coger

hold, to, ~ (*an object*) tener; ~ (*to fasten*) sujetar; ~ (*to grasp*) agarrar; ~ (*to keep*) guardar; ~ **onto** agarrarse; ~ **away from** separar; ~ **back** (*emotions, etc.*) contener; ~ **back** (*truth*) ocultar; ~ **down** sujetar; ~ **one's breath** aguantar la respiración; contener la respiración; retener el aliento; sostener la respiración; ~ **one's nose** taparse la nariz; ~ **up** (*payments*) suspender; ~ **up** (*to lift up*) levantar

hole, agujero; orificio; ~ (*meatus*) hoyito; ~ **in the ground** joyanco; ~**d up in one's house** añiao *adj*; encuevao *adj*

hollow, hueco *adj*; ~ **needle** aguja hueca; ~ **sound** sonido hueco; ~ (*eyes, chest, cheeks*) hundido *adj*; ~ **cheeked** de mejillas hundidas; ~ **chested** de pecho hundido; ~ **eyed** de ojos hundidos; ~ (*voice*) cavernoso *adj*; ~ (*empty*) vacío *adj*; ~ **stomach** estómago vacío; ~ **eyed** (*from illness, fatigue*) ojeroso *adj*

home, casa; domicilio; hogar *m*; **at** ~ en casa; ~ **cure** curación casera *f*; ~ **health agency** agencia de salud doméstica; ~ **health services** servicios domiciliarios de salud; **old people's** ~ residencia para ancianos; residencia para jubilados; ~ **remedy** remedio casero; **to be away from** ~ **a lot** no parar la pata *PR*

homeless, sin hogar *prep phr*; guacho *adj*, *Chi, Perú, Ríopl*

homeopath, homeópata *m/f*

homeopathic, homeópata *adj*; homeopático *adj*

homeopathist, homeópata *m/f*

homeopathy, homeopatía

homesick, to be, sentir (ie) nostalgia

homesickness, añoranza; nostalgia

homicide, homicidio

homosexual, homosexual *m/f*, *adj*; **to be** ~ cambiar(se) los cables *PR*; **to have the looks of a** ~ tener sello *PR*

honey, miel *f*

hoof it, to, (*to go on foot*) camonear

hook, ~ (*on a dress*) corchete *m*; ~ (*for holding, lifting*) gancho; garfio; ~ (*for hanging clothes*) percha; **to** ~ **on narcotics**[7] prender[2]

hooked, (*hook-shaped*) ganchudo *adj*; ~ **nose** de nariz aguileña *prep phr*; nariz ganchuda *f*; ~-

forceps pinza de garfios; ~ **on drugs**[7] adicto (a las drogas) *adj*; prendido[2] *esp. Mex, adj*

hookworm, uncinaria

hooky, to play, ir a comer jobos *fam*

hop, to, saltar

hope, esperanza; **to** ~ (**for**) esperar

hopeless, desesperado *adj*; sin esperanza *prep phr*; ~ **case** caso desesperado

hormonal, hormonal *adj*

hormone, hormón *m*; hormona; **adrenocorticotropic/ACTH** ~ hormona adrenocorticotrópica; **adrenotropic/ATH** ~ hormona adrenotrópica; **chondrotropic** ~ hormona condrotrópica; hormona del crecimiento; **follicle** ~ hormona folicular; **follicle-stimulating** ~ **/FSH** hormona foliculoestimulante; hormona estimulante del folículo; **gonadotropin-releasing** ~ hormona liberadora de gonadotropinas; **growth** ~ hormona del crecimiento; **luteinizing** ~ **/LH** hormona luteinizante; **ovarian** ~ hormona ovárica; **parathyroid** ~ **/PTH** hormona paratiroidea; **thyroid** ~ hormona tiroidea; **thyroid-stimulating** ~ **/TSH** hormona estimulante del tiroides; ~ **treatment** tratamiento hormonal

horn, cuerno

hornet, avispón *m*

horniness, bellaquera *vulg*

horny, (*sexual*) bellaco *adj, vulg*; enfermo *adj, vulg*; **to make** ~ bellacar *vulg*

horseshoe, herradura; ~ **kidney** riñón en herradura *m*; ~ **placenta** placenta en herradura

hose, ~ (*stocking*) medias; **panty** ~ medias pantalón; pantimedias; ~ (*tube*) manguera

hospice, hospicio

hospital, hospital *m*; nosocomio

Chicano; ~ **administration** administración del hospital *f*; **bad** ~ matadero; ~ **care** cuidado en el hospital; **community** ~ hospital de la comunidad; **county** ~ hospital del condado; ~ **for the insane** asilo de dementes; asilo de locos; manicomio; ~ **for the poor** hospicio; **mental** ~ hospital psiquiátrico; **private** ~ hospital privado; **public** ~ hospital público; **Veteran's Administration** ~ hospital para veteranos

hospitalization, hospitalización *f*; ~ **insurance** seguro de hospitalización

hospitalize, to, internar; encamar *CA, Mex*

hospitalized, hospitalizado *adj*; internado *adj*

host, huésped *m*; ~ **cell** célula huésped

hot, ~ (*spicy*) picante *adj*; ~ (*temperature; sexually*) caliente *adj*; ~ **abscess** absceso caliente; ~ **coffee** café caliente *m*; ~ **blooded** ardiente *adj*; ~ **flashes** bochornos; calofrío *m, Chicano*; calores *m, fam*; fogajes *m, PR*; llamaradas; sofocones *m, fam*; ~ **gangrene** gangrena infecciosa; ~ **shot** ([*often fatal*] *overdose*) dosis excesiva *f*; sobredosis *f*; sobredosis tóxica *f*; ~ **water bag** bolsa de agua caliente; ~ **wet compress** fomentos de agua caliente; **to be** ~ (*weather*) hacer calor; **to be** ~ (*people*) tener calor; **to feel** ~ sentir(se) (ie) caluroso; sentir(se) (ie) sofocado

hour, hora; **office** ~**s** horas de consulta; **visiting** ~**s** horas de visita

hourly, a cada hora

house, casa; ~ **dust** polvo de la casa; ~ **of correction** reformatorio; ~ **physician** médico de hospital; ~ **staff** personal médico *m*; ~ **surgeon** cirujano asistente; médico interno; **to** ~ internar[6]

housemaid knee, bursitis prerrotuliana *f*; inflamación de la rodilla *f*; mal de monja *m*; rodilla de monja

housewife, ama[3] de casa

how?, ¿cómo?; ~ **long?** ¿cuánto tiempo?; ~ **many?** ¿cuántos?; ~ **much?** ¿cuánto?

howl, ~ (*of a crying child*) berrido; ~ (*of wind*) rugido; ~ (*of laughter*) carcajada; ~ (*of pain*) alarido

howl, to, (*like a crying child*) berrear; ~ (*with pain*) dar alaridos (de dolor); **to** ~ (*the wind*) rugir; **to** ~ **with anger** bufar de cólera; **to** ~ **with laughter** reír (i) a carcajadas

HPI/history of present illness, historia de la actual enfermedad

HPN/hypertension, hipertensión *f*

HPV/human papilloma virus, virus de(l) papilloma humano *m*

H.R./heart rate, frecuencia cardíaca

h.s./hora somni/at bedtime, a la hora de acostarse *prep phr*

Ht/total hypermetropia, Ht/hipermetropía total

hue, ~ (*color*) tinte *m*; ~ (*shade*) matiz *m*

hued, colorado *adj*; **yellow** ~ de color amarillo *prep phr*

huff, to be in a ~, estar enojado *adj*; haberse picado *adj;* **to go off in a** ~ picarse

huffy, enojadizo *adj*

hug, abrazo; **to** ~ abrazar

hum, ~ (*of a machine, bees, etc.*) zumbido; ~ (*of a song*) tarareo; **to** ~ (*song*) zumbar; ~ (*a child to sleep*) arrullar; ~ (*a tune*) tararear

human, humano *m, adj*; ~ **being** ser humano *m*; ~ **Immunodeficiency Virus/HIV** Virus de (la) Inmunodeficiencia Humana/VIH[8] *m*; ~ **nature** naturaleza humana; ~ **papilloma virus** virus de(l) papilloma humano *m*

humanized, humanizado *adj*

humble, humilde *adj*

humerus, húmero

humid, húmedo *adj*

humidification, humectación *f*; humedecimiento

humidified, humedecido *adj*

humidifier, humectador *m*; humedecedor *m, adj*

humidity, humedad *f*; **absolute ~** humedad absoluta; **relative ~** humedad relativa

humming, **~** (*of engine, bees, etc.*) zumbido; **~** (*murmur*) murmullo; **~-top murmur** murmullo venoso; **~** (*a tune*) tarareo

humor, humor *m*; **aqueous ~** humor acuoso; **crystalline ~** humor cristalino; **vitreous ~** cuerpo vitreo; humor vitreo

hump, joroba; paguacha *Chi, Anat*; petaca *CA, Anat*

humpback, **~** (*back*) corcova; joroba; **~** (*person*) corcovado; jorobado

humpbacked, corcovado *adj*; jorobado *adj*

hunch, **~** (*hump*) corcova; joroba; **~** (*intuition*) idea; **to ~ one's back** encorvarse

hunchbacked, petacudo *adj, Guat*; tempozonte *adj, Mex*

hunched up, to sit, estar sentado con el cuerpo encorvado

hunger, hambre[3] *f*; **air ~** disnea paroxística *form*; falta de aire; **~ diabetes** diabetes carencial *f*; **~ edema** edema carencial *m*; edema de hambre *m*; **hormone ~** hambre[3] hormónica; **~ pain** contracción de hambre *f*; dolor por hambre *m*; **~ pang** latido; **~ swelling** edema de hambre *m*

hungover, crudo *Mex, adj*; **to be ~** estar crudo *Mex*; estar de goma *CA*; tener una cruda *Mex*; tener una resaca

hungry, hambriento *adj*; **extremely ~** esmayao *adj*; estragao *adj*; estrasijao *adj*; **to be (very) ~** tener (mucha) hambre

hurl, to, arrojar; tirar

hurry, to, apresurarse

hurt, coco *fam*; herida; lastimadura; **to get ~** (*to be wounded*) ser herido *adj*

hurt, to, **~** (*to ache*) doler (ue); **~** (*to cause pain*) causar dolor; **~** (*to cause bodily injury*) hacer daño; lastimar; **~** (*to injure*) lesionar; **~** (*to wound*) herir (ie); **to get ~** hacerse daño; lastimarse

husband, esposo; marido

huskily, (*voice*) con voz ronca *adv*

huskiness, ronquera; enroquecimiento

husky, **~** (*voice*) ronco *adj*; **~** (*strong*) fuerte *adj*

HW/housewife, ama[3] de casa

HWS/hot water soluble, soluble en agua caliente *adj*

Hx/history, historia

hybrid, híbrido *m, adj*

hydatid, hidátide *f*

hydride, hidruro

hydralazine hydrochloride, clorhidrato de hidralacina

hydrocarbon, hidrocarburo

hydrocele, hidrocele *m/f*, [*Ú.m.c.m.*]; líquido en el escroto *fam*; **cervical ~** hidrocele cervical; **congenital ~** hidrocele congénito; **encysted ~** hidrocele enquistado

hydrocephalus, agua[3] en los sesos *f*; hidrocéfalo; **acute ~** hidrocéfalo adquirido; **communicating ~** hidrocéfalo comunicante

hydrocephaly, hidrocefalia

hydrochloric, clorhídrico *adj*; **~ acid** ácido clorhídrico

hydrochloride, clorhidrato; **thiamine ~** clorhidrato de tiamina

hydrocortisone, hidrocortisona

hydrocyanic, cianhídrico *adj*

hydrodynamic, hidrodinámico *adj*

hydrodynamics, (*science*) hidrodinámica

hydroelectric, hidroeléctrico *adj*

hydroelectricity, hidroelectricidad *f*

hydrofluoric acid, ácido fluorhídrico

hydrogen, hidrógeno; ~ **chloride** hidrocloruro; **double weigh** ~ hidrógeno pesado; ~ **ion** hidrogenión *m*; ~ **peroxide** agua[3] oxigenada; peróxido de hidrógeno *form*; ~ **sulfide** sulfuro de hidrógeno

hydrogenate, to, hidrogenar

hydrolysis, hidrólisis *f*

hydromassage, hidromasaje *m*

hydrometer, hidrómetro

hydrophobia, hidrofobia; rabia *fam*

hydrophobic, hidrófobo *adj*

hygiene, higiene *f*; **oral** ~ aseo bucal

hygienic, higiénico *adj*

hygienist, higienista *m/f*

hymen, himen *m*; doncellez *f*, *Anat*

hype[7], (*an addict who uses subcutaneous injections*) adicto[2]; adicto a drogas[2]; drogadicto[2]; tecato[2]

hyperacidity, hiperacidez *f*

hyperactive, avancino *adj*; hiperactivo *adj*; ~ **child** jiribilla

hyperactivity, hiperactividad *f*

hyperbaric, hiperbárico *adj*; ~ **chamber** cámara hiperbárica

hyperflexion, hiperflexión *f*

hyperglycemia, hiperglucemia; hiperglicemia

hyperkeratosis, hiperqueratosis *f*

hyperketonuria, hipercetonuria *f*, *form*; exceso de cetonas en la orina

hyperlipidemia, hiperlipidemia

hypermetabolism, hipermetabolismo

hyperparathyroid, hiperparatiroideo *adj*

hyperparathyroidism, hiperparatiroidismo; hiperparotidia

hyperparotidism, hiperparotidia; hiperparotidismo

hyperpiesia, hiperpiesia *form*; hipertensión *f*

hyperplasia, hiperplasia

hypersensibility, hipersensibilidad *f*

hypersensitive, hipersensible *adj*

hypertension, (*high blood pressure*) alta presión *f*; hipertensión *f*; hipertensión arterial *f*; presión arterial alta *f*; presión alta *f*, *fam*; tensión alta *f*, *fam*; tensión arterial elevada *f*; **benign** ~ hipertensión benigna; **essential** ~ hipertensión esencial; **malignant** ~ hipertensión maligna; **pale** ~ hipertensión pálida; **portal** ~ hipertensión portal; **pulmonary** ~ hipertensión pulmonar; **renal** ~ hipertensión renal; **vascular** ~ hipertensión vascular

hypertensive, hipertenso *adj*

hyperthermal, hipertérmico *adj*

hyperthermia, hipertermia

hyperthyroid, hipertiroideo *adj*

hyperthyroidism, hipertiroidismo; **masked** ~ hipertiroidismo enmascarado; hipertiroidismo oculto

hypertonia, hipertonía

hypertonic, hipertónico *adj*

hypertrophic, hipertrófico *adj*

hypertrophy, hipertrofia; **adaptive** ~ hipertrofia de adaptación; **benign prostatic** ~ hipertrofia prostática benigna; **compensatory** ~ hipertrofia compensadora; **complementary** ~ hipertrofia complementaria; **simulated** ~ hipertrofia simulada

hyperventilate, to, respirar demasiado rápido

hyperventilation, hiperventilación *f*; susto con resuello duro *fam*

hyphemia, hemorragia detrás de la córnea; hifemia

hypnosis, hipnosis *f*; hipnotismo

hypnotic, hipnótico *m*, *adj*

hypnotism, hipnotismo; mesmerismo

hypnotist, hipnotista *m/f*; hipnotizador, -ra *m/f*

hypnotize, to, hipnotizar

hypo[7], **to lay the**, (*See bang, to.*)

hypoactivity, hipoactividad *f*

hypoallergenic, hipoalergénico *adj*
hypochondriac, adolorado *m*, *adj*, *Chicano*; adolorido *m*, *adj*, *Chicano*; hipocóndrico *m*, *adj*; hipocondríaco *m*, *adj*; hipocondriaco *m*, *adj*
hypocondria, hipocondría
hypodermic, hipodérmico *adj*; ~ **injection** inyección hipodérmica *f*; ~ **needle** aguja hipodérmica; ~ **needle used to inject drugs**[7] jaipo[2]; ~ **syringe** jeringuilla hipodérmica
hypodermis, hipodermis *f*
hypogastric, hipogástrico *adj*
hypogenetic, hipogenético *adj*
hypoglottis, hipoglotis *f*
hypoglycemia, hipoglicemia; hipoglucemia
hypoglycemic, hipoglucémico *adj*; hipoglicémico *adj*
hypometabolic state, estado hipometabólico
hypometabolism, hipometabolismo
hypoparathyroidism, hipoparatiroidismo; hipoparatiroidia
hypopyon, pus detrás de la córnea *m;* hipopión *m*

hypotension, (*low blood pressure*) hipotensión arterial *f*; presión arterial baja *f*
hypothyroid, hipotiroideo *adj*
hypothyroidism, hipotiroidismo
hypoxia, hipoxia
hypoxic, hipóxico *adj*
hysterectomy, extirpación de la matriz *f*; histerectomía; **abdominal** ~ histerectomía abdominal; **cesarean** ~ histerectomía cesárea; **radical** ~ histerectomía radical; **subtotal** ~ histerectomía subtotal; **vaginal** ~ histerectomía vaginal
hysteria, histeria; histerismo; ataque de nervios *m*, *fam*; **anxiety** ~ histeria de ansiedad
hysteric, histérico *adj*; ~ **pregnancy** embarazo falso
hysterical, histérico *adj*
hysterics, histeria; histerismo; crisis de histeria *f*, *inv*; ataque de nervios *m*, *fam*; ataque histérico *m*; **to go into** ~ ponerse histérico *adj*

---

[2] This is new vocabulary, not necessarily listed nor yet recognized by the Royal Academy of Spanish Grammar. It is understood that this vocabulary is primarily slang. Unless otherwise indicated, the gender of nouns is assumed to be obvious.

[3] For pronunciation purposes, the masculine definite and indefinite articles, *el* and *un*, not *la* or *una*, are used when the article immediately precedes the feminine singular noun which begins with stressed *a* or any other that begins with stressed *ha*.

[4] Currently the English street terminology for *heroin* includes: a-bomb, big H, blanks, boss, boy, brother, brown, ca-ca, caballo, carga, C & H, China white, Chinese red, chiva, cobics, crap, dogie, doojee, doojie, dope, duji, dynamite, dyno, eighth, Frisco speedball, girl, goods, gravy, H, hairy, hard stuff, harry, H-caps, Henry, him, hochs, horse, joy powder, junk, ka-ka, killer stuff, lemonade, love affairs, Mexican brown, Mexican horse, Mexican mud, noise, peg, poison, scag, scar, schmeck, shit, skag, smack, smeck, snow, speedball, stuff, sugar, tecata, thing, TNT, white junk, white lady, white stuff, whiz bang.

[5] This word is often used in the plural form.

[6] *Internar* also means to commit to a mental institution.

[7] Part of the Drug Abuse Vocabulary.

[8] Use the Spanish pronunciation of these letters.

I

ibuprofen, ibuprofén *m*

ice, hielo; ~ **bag** bolsa de hielo; bolsa de caucho para hielo; ~ **box** nevera; ~ **chips** pedacitos de hielo; ~ **cream** helado; nieve *f, Mex*; mantecado; ~ **habit**[6] *slang* uso irregular de drogas; ~ **cube** cubito de hielo; ~ **cube tray** bandeja para los cubitos de hielo; **dry** ~ hielo seco; nieve carbónica *f*; ~ **pack** aplicación de hielo empaquetado *f*

iced, helado *adj*

ichthyol, ictiol *m*

ICSH/interstitial cell stimulating hormone, hormona estimulante de las células intersticiales

icy, gélido *adj*; helado *adj*

idea, idea; noción *f*; **compulsive** ~ idea compulsiva; **dominant** ~ idea dominante; **fixed** ~ idea fija; **referential** ~ idea de referencia

ideal, ideal *m, adj*

identical, idéntico *adj*

identification, identificación *f*; ~ **bracelet** brazalete para identificación *m*

identify, to, identificar; ~ **with** identificarse con

identity, identidad *f*; ~ **crisis** crisis de identidad *f, inv*

idiocy, idiotez *f*

idiom, idioma *m*; lenguaje *m*

idiopathy, idiopatía

idiosyncrasy, idiosincrasia; **occupational** ~ deformación profesional *f*

idiosyncratic, idiosincrásico *adj*

idiot, idiota *m/f*

idiotic, idiota *adj*; ñango *adj, PR*; ñangue *adj, PR*

idioventricular, idioventricular *adj*

idle, desocupado *adj*

idle, to, ~ (*to be at leisure*) estar ocioso; ~ (*to be lazy*) holgazanear; ~ (*machine, engine*) funcionar en vacío

idler, güelegüele *m/f, PR*

ignorance, ignorancia

ileitis, ileítis *f*

ileum, íleon *m*

ileus, íleo

iliac, ilíaco *adj*

ilium, hueso ilíaco; ilion *m*

ill, doliente *adj, Med*; enfermo *adj*; ingerido *adj, Col, Mex, Ven*; malo *adj*; mal *adv*; ~ **health** mala salud *f*; **seriously** ~ grave *adj*; **to be taken** ~ caerse enfermo; ponerse enfermo; **to become** ~ indisponerse *Med*; **to feel** ~ encontrarse (ue) mal; sentirse (ie) mal; **to feel slightly** ~ sentirse indispuesto; **to make** ~ indisponer *Med*

illegality, ilegalidad *f*

illegitimacy, ilegitimidad *f*

illegitimate, ilegítimo *adj*

illicit, to do something, bretear *PR*

illiteracy, analfabetismo

illiterate, analfabeto *m, adj*

illness, enfermedad *f*; mal *m*; padecimiento; **acute** ~ enfermedad aguda *f*; **chronic** ~ enfermedad crónica *f*; **contagious** ~ enfermedad contagiosa *f*; enfermedad transmisible *f*; **mental** ~ enfermedad mental *f*; **minor** ~ enfermedad leve *f*; **organic** ~ enfermedad orgánica *f*; **serious** ~ enfermedad grave *f*; **tropical** ~ enfermedad tropical *f*; **to recover from a long** ~ salir de una larga enfermedad

illumination, iluminación *f*

illusion, ilusión *f*

image, imagen *f*; **acoustic** ~ imagen acústica; ~ **enhancement agent** agente que intensifica las imágenes *m*; **inverted** ~ imagen invertida; **mirror** ~ imagen en espejo; **sensory** ~ imagen sensorial

imaginary, imaginario *adj*

imagine, to, imaginarse

imbalance, desequilibrio

imbecile, imbécil *m/f, adj*

imbed, to, encajar; enclavar

immaculate, inmaculado *adj*

immature, inmaduro *adj*

immediate, inmediato *adj*

immediately, inmediatamente *adv*; en seguida

immersion, inmersión *f*

immigrate, to, inmigrar

imminent, inminente *adj*

immigrant, inmigrante *m/f*

immobile, inmóvil *adj*

immobility, inmovilidad *f*

immobilization, inmovilización *f*

immobilize, to, inmovilizar

immodest, ~ (*not humble*) inmodesto *adj*; ~ (*indecent*) impúdico *adj*; ~ (*bold*) desvergonzado *adj*

immodesty, ~ (*lack of modesty*) inmodestia; ~ (*indecency*) impudor *m*; ~ (*boldness*) desvergüenza

immune, inmune *adj*; inmunológico *adj*; ~ **system** sistema inmune *m*

immunity, inmunidad *f*; **acquired** ~ inmunidad adquirida; **active** ~ inmunidad activa; **antibacterial** ~ inmunidad antibacteriana; **artificial** ~ inmunidad artificial; **congenital** ~ inmunidad congénita; **intrauterine** ~ inmunidad placentaria; **species** ~ inmunidad racial; **specific** ~ inmunidad específica

immunization, (*vaccine*) inmunización *f, inv*; vacuna; **booster dose** dosis de refuerzo *f, inv*; dósis de refuerzo *f, inv*; **Schick test** prueba de Schick

immunize, to, inmunizar; vacunar

immunocharacter, inmunocarácter *m*

immunocompetent, inmunocompetente *adj*

immunodeficiency, inmunodeficiencia

immunodepressed, inmunodeprimido *adj*

immunogenetics, inmunogenética

immunologic/immunological, inmunológico *adj*

immunologist, inmunólogo

immunology, inmunología

immunosuppressant, inmunosupresor *m*

immunosuppression, inmunosupresión *f*

immunotherapy, inmunoterapia

immunotoxin, inmunotoxina

immunotransfusion, inmunotransfusión *f*

impact, choque *m*

impacted, impactado *adj*; ~ **tooth** diente incluido *m*; diente retenido *m*

impaction, impacción *f*; impacto

impairment, incapacidad *f*

impalpable, impalpable *adj*

impatient, impaciente *adj*

impecunious, pobre *adj*

impede, to, impedir (i)

impediment, impedimento; **speech** ~ defecto del habla

impel, to, impulsar

impending, inminente *adj*

imperative, ~ (*urgent*) imperioso *adj*; ~ (*necessary*) indispensable *adj*

imperfect, defectuoso *adj*; imperfecto *adj*

imperfection, small, chivo *PR*

impertinent, impertinente *adj*

impervious, ~ (*impenetrable*) impenetrable *adj*; ~ (*insensitive*) insensible *adj*

impetigo, erupción cutánea *f*; impétigo

impetus, (*force*) ímpetu *m*

implant, implantación *f*; injerto
implant, to, implantar(se); injertar
implement, to, implementar
implementation, implementación *f*
implicit, implícito *adj*
implore, to, suplicar
imploring, suplicante *adj*
imply, to, implicar; significar
impolite, mal educado *adj*
importance, importancia
important, importante *adj*
impose, to, imponer
impotence, impotencia
impotent, impotente *adj*; ~ **person** plasta *vulg, PR*; **to be sexually ~** esñemar(se) *PR*
impregnate, to, fecundizar; fertilizar; impregnar
impression, impresión *f*
improbable, improbable *adj*
improve, to, mejorar; perfeccionar; ~ (*to get better*) mejorarse
imprudent, imprudente *adj*
impudent, desvergonzado *adj*; impudente *adj*
impulse, impulso
impulsive, impulsivo *adj*
impurity, impureza
in, en; dentro de; ~ **a hurry** de prisa; ~ **case of** en caso de (que); **~-date medication** fármaco no caducado *f*; ~ **transit**[6] tripeando[2]; **to be ~ need** andar enfermo
inability to pay, incapacidad financiera *f*
inaccurate, ~ (*not accurate*) inexacto *adj*; ~ (*in error*) incorrecto *adj*
inactivate, to, inactivar
inactive, inactivo *adj*
inactivity, inactividad *f*
inadequacy, ~ (*unsuitability*) inadecuación *f*; ~ (*insufficiency*) insuficiencia
inadvisability of treatment, contraindicación de tratamiento *f*
inanimate, inanimado *adj*

inappropriate, inadecuado *adj*; inapropiado *adj*
inarticulate, inarticulado *adj*; ~ **with grief** voz embargada por el dolor *f*
inattentive, poco atento *adj*; **to be ~** eslembarse *PR*
in-between meals, entre comidas
inborn, congénito *adj*; innato *adj*; ~ **reflex** reflejo innato; reflejo no condicionado
incapable, incapaz *adj*
incapacity, incapacidad *f*
incapacitating, incapacitante *adj*
incarceration, incarceración *f*
incest, incesto
inch, pulgada
incidence, incidencia; ~ (*of a disease*) extensión *f*
incident, incidente *m*
incised wound, herida incisa
incision, cortada; incisión *f*
incisive, incisivo *adj*
incisor, incisivo; **central ~** incisivo central; **lateral ~** incisivo lateral
inclination, inclinación *f*; ~ **of the pelvis** inclinación de la pelvis
include, to, incluir
incoherence, incoherencia
incoherent, incoherente *adj*
income, ingresos
incompatibility, incompatibilidad *f*; **chemical ~** incompatibilidad química; **physiologic ~** incompatibilidad fisiológica; **therapeutic ~** incompatibilidad terapéutica
incompatible, incompatible *adj*
incompetence, incompetencia; inhabilidad *f*; insuficiencia; ~ **of the cardiac valves** insuficiencia de las válvulas cardíacas
incompetent, incompetente *adj*
incomprehensible, incomprensible *adj*
incontinence, incontinencia; **fecal ~** incontinencia fecal; **over-**

flow ~ incontinencia por rebosamiento; **stress** ~ incontinencia de esfuerzo; **urinary** ~ incontinencia urinaria

incontinent, incontinente *adj*

increase, aumento

increase, to, aumentar; ~ (*to persist*) (*fever*) cargar la calentura *Chicano*

increased reflex, reflejo exagerado

incredible, increíble *adj*

incrust, to, incrustar

incrustation, encostración *f*

incubation period, período de incubación

incubator, estufa; incubadora

incurable, incurable *adj*; insanable *adj*

incus, yunque *m*

indecisive, aplatanao *adj, PR*

indecisiveness, indecisión *f*

index, (dedo) índice *m*

indicate, to, indicar

indication, indicación *f*

indicator, indicador *m*

indigestion, dispepsia; embargo *Med;* estómago sucio *Chicano*; indigestión *f*; insulto *Chicano, Mex, Nic*; jaleo *PR*; mala digestión *f*; **acid** ~ indigestión ácida; **fat** ~ indigestión grasa; **gastric** ~ indigestión gástrica; **nervous** ~ indigestión nerviosa; **to get/have** ~ empacharse *Med*; **to give** ~ **to** empachar *Med*

indisposed, indispuesto *adj, Med*; destemplado *adj, Med*

indisposition, malestar *m*

individual, individuo; individual *adj*

indolent, indolente *adj*

indomethacin, indometacina

induce labor, to, provocar el parto

induced delivery, parto provocado

induced labor, parto inducido

indulge, to, mimar; ~ **someone** tongonear *PR*

induration, bolita; endurecimiento

indwelling, permanente *adj*

inebriate, to, embriagar

inebriation, embriaguez *f*

inertia, inercia

infancy, infancia

infant, criatura; infante *m/f*; lactante *m/f*; nena; nene *m*

infantile paralysis/polio (myelitis), parálisis infantil *f*; polio (mielitis) *f*

infarct, infarto

infarction, infarto; **anemic** ~ infarto anémico; **hemorrhagic** ~ infarto hemorrágico; **intestinal** ~ infarto intestinal; **myocardiac** ~ infarto miocardíaco; **myocardial** ~ infarto cardíaco; **pulmonary** ~ infarto pulmonar; **renal** ~ infarto renal; **splenic** ~ infarto esplénico

infatuated, enchulao *adj, PR*; **to become** ~ enchularse *PR*

infect, to, contagiar; infectar; lacrar *Med*; tra(n)smitir *Med*; ~ **with** pegar *Med*

infected, infectado *adj*; ~ (*una herida*) pasmado *adj, SpAm*; **to become** ~ (**with**) infectarse (de)

infection, infección *f*; pasmo; **airborne** ~ infección aérógena; **contact** ~ infección directa; **focal** ~ infección focal; (**upper**) **respiratory tract** ~ infección de las vías respiratorias (superiores); **urinary tract** ~ infección del tracto urinario

infectious, infeccioso *adj*; pegadizo *adj, Med*; pegajoso *adj, Med*; (**any**) ~ **disease**, peste *f, Ríopl*; ~ **period**, (*of a disease*) pega *Chi*

inferior, inferior *adj*

inferiority complex, complejo de inferioridad

infertile, capón *adj, Chicano*; estéril *adj*; infértil *adj*

infest, to, infestar; **to get infested with bugs** enchincharse *Guat, Mex, Perú, PR*

infestation, infestación *f*
infiltrate, infiltrado *m*, *adj*
infirm, enfermizo *adj*; canijo *adj*;
~ (*physically weak*) débil *adj*
infirmary, enfermería
infirmity, ~ (*illness*) achaque *m*;
enfermedad *f*; ~ (*weakness*) debilidad *f*
inflame, to, inflamar; irritar
inflamed, inflamado *adj*; enconado *Med*; to become ~ enardecerse *Med*
inflammation, encono; inflamación *f*; acute ~ inflamación
aguda; chronic ~ inflamación
crónica; ~ of the eyes (*caused
by snow glare*) surumpe *m*, *Bol*,
Perú; productive ~ inflamación
productiva; ~ of the throat garrotillo
inflammatory, inflamatorio *adj*
inflexible, inflexible *adj*
influence, pala *PR* (*lit. shovel; fig.
connections with people who have it*)
influenza, gripa; gripe *f*; influenza; monga *PR*
inform, to, ~ (*to communicate*) informar; ~ (*to tell*) avisar
information, información *f*
informed, to keep someone, tener a alguien al corriente
infrared, infrarrojo *adj*
infuse, to, hacer una infusión de
infusion, infusión *f*; infuso; tisana; meat ~ caldo de carne;
saline ~ infusión salina
ingest, to, ingerir (ie); injerir (ie);
~ narcotic pills[6] pildorear(se)[2];
pildoriar(se)[2]
ingestion, ingestión *f*
ingredient, ingrediente *m*
ingrown toenail, uña encarnada;
uña enterrada; uñero
inguinal region, aldilla; ingle *f*
inhalant, inhalante[2]
inhalation, inhalación *f*; inspiración *f*; vahos *m*, *pl*, *Med*; vaporizo *Med*, *Mex*, *PR*; by ~ por

inhalación; por vapor; ~ therapy terapia de inhalación
inhale, to, inspirar; sorber por las
narices *Med*; ~ (*air*) inhalar; ~
(*to breathe in*) aspirar; ~ (*tobacco smoke*) tragar; sequiar *Arg*; ~
glue[6] aspirar cola[2]; inhalar cola[2]; respirar cola[2]
inhaler, aerosol *m*; inhalador *m*,
adj; metered dose ~ aerosol
dosificador; ~[6] inhalador (dispositivo)[2]
inherent, inherente *adj*
inheritance, herencia; sex-linked
~ herencia cruzada
inherited, heredado *adj*; hereditario *adj*
inhibited, cohibido *adj*; to feel ~
estar cohibido; inhibirse
inhibition, inhibición *f*
inhibitor, inhibidor *m*
inhuman, inhumano *adj*
initial, inicial *adj*; ~ contact contacto inicial; ~ radiation radiación inicial *f*; ~ stage of the
illness etapa inicial de la enfermedad
initiate, to, iniciar
inject (oneself), to, inyectar(se);
~ oneself with drugs[6] clavarse[2];
componerse[2]; curarse[2]; darse
un piquete[2]; filerearse[2]; inyectarse[2]; jincarse[2]; picarse[2]; rayarse[2]; shootear[2]
injectable, inyectable *adj*
injected, inyectado *adj*
injection, chot *m*, *Chicano*; indección *f*, *Chicano*; inyección *f*; ~[6]
(*of a narcotic substance*) abuja[2];
abujazo[2]; piquete[2] *m*; hypodermic ~ inyección hipodérmica;
intracardiac ~ inyección intracardíaca; intracutaneous ~
inyección intracutánea; intradermic ~ inyección intradérmica; intramuscular ~ inyección
intramuscular; intravenous ~
inyección endovenosa; inyec-

ción intravenosa; **preparatory ~** inyección preparante; **subcutaneous ~** inyección subcutánea; **to give oneself an ~** hacerse inyección; ponerse inyección; **to give s.o. an ~** pincharle a uno *Med, fam*

injure, to, agraviar; hacer daño; herir (ie); injuriar; lastimar; lesionar; **~ the health of** lacrar *Med*

injured, herido *adj*; lisiado *adj*; **to be ~** lesionarse

injurious, dañino *adj*; dañoso *adj*

injury, coco *fam*; herida; lastimadura; lesión *f*

ink, tinta

inlay, empaste *m, Dent*; incrustación *f, Dent*; obturación *f, Dent*; orificación *f, Dent*

inner ear, oído interno

innervation, inervación *f*

innocent murmur, soplo funcional

inoculate, to, inocular

inoculation, inoculación *f*; **protective ~** inoculación protectora

inoffensive, inofensivo *adj*

inoperable, inoperable *adj*; intratable *adj*

inorganic, inorgánico *adj*

inpatient, enfermo hospitalizado

inquest, indagación *f*; pesquisa

inquiry, indagación *f*

insane, demente *adj*; loco *adj*

insanity, demencia; enajenación mental *f*; insania; locura; **manic-depressive ~** locura de doble forma; maniamelancolía; sicosis maniacodepresiva *f, inv*

insect, (type of) albayalde *m* (*one of two common, small Puerto Rican ants, also known as* hormiguilla brava: *very aggressive, lives outside, often near trees, its bite stings.*); boba *PR*; gongolí *m, PR* (*a millipede that rolls into a coil when touched, does not bite, also known as*

gongulén.); gongulén *m, PR* (*syn. for gongolí*); hormiguilla brava *PR* (*See albayalde.*); maje *m, PR* (*a very small biting gnat, commonly found mainly in humid areas near beach; its stings have an effect for anywhere between a few hours and a few days, depending on the victim's sensitivity; same as* mime; *in United States and Canada they are called* noseeums.); mime *m, PR* (*See maja.*); plumilla (*a Caribbean area caterpillar, has long white hairs and brittle spines that may burn human skin on contact— either mildly or severely; the larval form of a moth that feeds on leaves, esp. citrus.*); **~ bite** picadura de insecto; piquete de insecto *m*; **~ repellent** loción contra los insectos *f*; repelente de insectos *m*

insecticide, insecticida *m, adj*

insecure, inseguro *adj*

insecurity, inseguridad *f*

inseminate, to, engendrar

insemination, inseminación *f*; **artificial ~** inseminación artificial

insensibility, insensibilización *f*

insert, to, insertar; introducir; meter; poner(se)

inside (of), dentro de *prep*

inside, interior *m, adj*

insides, tripa(s) *Anat*

insidious, insidioso *adj*

insight, autocrítica

insincerity, doblez *f*

insole, (for shoes) plantilla

insomnia, insomnio; pérdida del sueño

inspection, inspección *f*

instable, inestable *adj*

instability, inestabilidad *f*

instep, (of foot) empeine[4] *m*

instinct, instinto; **herd ~** instinto de rebaño

instinctive, instintivo

institution, institución *f*

institutionalized, ingresado en una institución *adj*; internado *adj*
instruction, instrucción *f*
instrument, sharp-edged, instrumento afilado
insufficiency, insuficiencia; **acute circulatory ~** insuficiencia circulatoria aguda; **aortic ~** insuficiencia aórtica; **coronary ~** insuficiencia coronaria; **hepatic ~** insuficiencia hepática; **mitral ~** insuficiencia mitral; **pancreatic ~** insuficiencia pancreática; **renal ~** insuficiencia renal; **venous ~** insuficiencia venosa
insufficient, insuficiente *adj*
insufflation, tubal, insuflación endotimpánica *f*; insuflación tubárica *f*
insulin, insulina; insulínico *adj*; **~ reaction** reacción a la insulina; **~shock therapy**, insulinoshockterapia
insulinase, insulinasa
insult, insulto
insurance, seguro; **~ company** compañía aseguradora; compañía de seguros; **fully comprehensive ~** seguro a todo riesgo; **~ policy** póliza de seguros; **~ premium** prima de seguro; **to take out ~** hacerse un seguro
insure, to, asegurar
intake, ingestión *f*; ingreso; **~** (*of air*) entrada; **~** (*of food*) ración *f*; **~** (*of water*) toma; **caloric ~** ingestión calórica; **fluid ~** ingestión de líquidos
intellectual slowness, torpeza intelectual
intelligence, inteligencia; **~ quotient/IQ** cociente de inteligencia *m*
intelligent, inteligente *adj*
intelligible, inteligible *adj*
intend to, to, pensar (ie) (+ *infinitive*)
intense, intenso *adj*
intensify, to, intensificar

intensive care, cuidado intensivo; servicio de cuidados intensivos; vigencia intensiva; **~ care unit/I.C.U.** unidad de cuidados intensivos *f*; unidad de vigencia intensiva U.V.I.[7] (*See cardiac care unit and CCU.*); **~ therapy** terapia intensiva
intention, intención *f*
intentional, intencional *adj*
interaction, interacción *f*
intercostal, intercostal *adj*
intercourse, sexual, contacto sexual; relación sexual *f*; trato carnal; trato sexual; **to have ~** juntarse
interdependence, interdependencia
interest, interés *m*;
interest, to, ~ interesar
interested, interesado *adj*; **to be ~ in** estar interesado en
interface, interfase *f*
interfere, to, interferir (ie); obstaculizar
interference, interferencia; intervención *f*; obstrucción *f*, *SpAm*; **viral ~** interferencia viral
interferon, interferón *m*
intermediary, intermediario *m, adj*
intermediate, intermediario *m, adj*
interment, inhumación *f*
intermittent, intermitente *adj*; que va y viene *adj phr*
intern, interno; interno del hospital; médico interno; médico practicante
internal, interno *adj*
internally, internamente *adv*; por vía interna *prep phr*
internist, internista *m/f*
internship, internado
interosseous, interóseo *adj*
interpret, to, interpretar
interpretation, interpretación *f*
interpreter, intérprete *m/f*
interrupt, to, interrumpir
interrupted, interrumpido *adj*; **~ sutures** sutura de puntos separados

interrupter, interruptor *m*
interstitial, intersticial *adj*; ~ **cell stimulating hormone** hormona estimulante de las células intersticiales
interstitialoma, intersticialoma *m*
interval, intervalo
intervene, to, intervenir
intervention, intervención *f*
interview, entrevista
intestinal, intestinal *adj*; **occlusion** ~ oclusión intestinal *f*
intestine, intestino; **large** ~ intestino grueso; intestino mayor; **small** ~ intestino delgado; delgado *Anat, fam*
intimacy, intimidad *f*
intimate, íntimo *adj*
intimidate, to, intimidar
intolerance, intolerancia
intoxicated, ajumao *adj*; borracho *adj*; embriago *adj*; embriagado *adj*; guayao *adj*, *PR*; jalao *adj*; rajao *adj*; ~ (*severely*) jendío *adj*, *PR*; volcao *adj*, *PR*; ~ (*slightly*) picao *adj*, *PR*
intoxication, embriaguez *f*; intoxicación *f*
intradermal, intradérmico *adj*
intradermoreaction, intradermorreacción *f*
intraocular, intraocular *adj*
intrauterine device/IUD, aparato intrauterino; dispositivo intrauterino/DIU *m*; ~ **loop** espiral intrauterino *m*
intravascular, intravascular *adj*
intravenous, (*See I.V.*); intravenoso *adj*; ~ **feeding** alimentación por vía intravenosa *f*; ~ **injection** inyección intravenosa *f*
intrinsic, intrínseco *adj*
introduce, to, presentar; ~ (*something into*) introducir; ~ **a question** (*to bring up*) abordar un tema
introvert, introvertido *m, adj*
introverted, introvertido *adj*

intubate, to, intubar
intubation, intubación *f*
intussusception, intususcepción *f*
in utero, dentro del útero *prep phr*
invade, to, invadir
invagination, invaginación *f*; **intestinal** ~ invaginación intestinal; **uterine** ~ invaginación uterina
invalid, inválido *m, adj*
invaluable, de valor incalculable *prep phr*
invasion, invasión *f*
invasive, invasor *adj*
invasiveness, capacidad invasora *f*; invasibilidad *f*
invertebrate, invertebrado *m, adj*
investigate, to, investigar; ~ (*to examine*) examinar
investigator, investigador, -ra *m/f*
in vitro, dentro de un vaso de vidrio *prep phr*
in vivo, en el cuerpo vivo *prep phr*
involuntarily, involuntariamente *adv*; sin querer *prep phr*
involuntary, involuntario *adj*
involve, to, ~ (*to concern*) concernir (ie); ~ (*to imply*) suponer; ~ (*to require*) requerir (ie)
inward, hacia (a)dentro *adv*
iodine, yodo; ~ **number** índice de yodo *m*; ~ **water** agua³ yodurada *f*
iodize, to, yodurar
ion, ión *m*; ~ **exchange** intercambio de iones; intercambio iónico
ionize, to, ionizar
ionizing, ionizante *adj*
IOP/intraocular pressure, presión intraocular *f*
I.P.A./individual practice association, A.P.I.⁷/ asociación de práctica individual *f*
ipecac, syrup of, jarabe de ipecacuana *m*
IQ, cociente de inteligencia *m*
iris, iris *m*
irksome, molesto *adj*

iron, (*metal*) hierro; **available** ~ hierro utilizable; ~ **deficiency** ferropenia; ~ **anemia** anemia ferropriva; anemia perniciosa; ~ **lung** pulmón de acero *m*; pulmotor *m*; ~ **water** agua[3] ferruginosa; ~ (*for pressing clothes*) plancha; **to** ~ (*to press clothes*) planchar

irradiate, to, irradiar

irradiation, irradiación *f*

irregular, irregular *adj*; ~ **heart rhythms** trastornos del ritmo cardíaco

irrelevant, sin importancia *prep phr*

irresponsible, irresponsable *adj*

irreversible, irreversible *adj*

irrigate, to, irrigar

irrigation, irrigación *f*

irrigator, irrigador *m*

irritable, irritable *adj*; **to become** ~ entorunarse *PR*

irritability, bilis[5] *f*; irritabilidad *f*; ~ **of the bladder** irritabilidad vesical; **nervous** ~ irritabilidad nerviosa

irritant, irritante *adj*; agente irritante *m*

irritate, to, irritar; ~ (*to bother, annoy*) chavar(se); hinchar *fig*; ~ (*to bother, pester*) pejigar *PR*; ~ (*a wound*) enconar; ~ (*organ, skin*) irritar

irritated, to become, irritarse

irritating, irritador *adj*; irritante *adj*; ~ (*annoying*) molesto *adj*

irritation, irritación *f*

ischemia, isquemia

ischemic, isquémico *adj*

ischialgia, isquialgia

ischiatic, isquiático *adj*

ischiocavernous, isquiocavernoso *adj*

ischiococcygeus, isquiocoxígeo *adj*

ischiofemoral, isquiofemoral *adj*

ischium, isquion *m*

ischuria, iscuria

island, isla; ~**s of Langerhans** islas de Langerhans; islotes de Langerhans *m*

islet, islote *m*

isolate, to, aislar; apartar

isolation, aislamiento; aislamiento por cuarentena; ~ **unit** unidad de aislamiento *f*

isomer, isómero

isometric, isométrico *adj*

isoproterenol, isoproterenol *m*

isotope, isótopo; **radioactive** ~ isótopo radiactivo; **stable** ~ isótopo estable

isotopic, isotópico *adj*

issue, ~ (*of blood, liquid*) derrame *m*; ~ (*question under discussion*) problema *m*; **side** ~ cuestión secundaria *f*; **to raise the** ~ (**of**) plantear el problema (de); **to avoid the** ~ andar con rodeos; **to take** ~ (**with**) estar en desacuerdo (con)

issue, to, ~ (*a certificate, etc.*) expedir (i); ~ (*to distribute*) distribuir; ~ (*to give; to order*) dar; ~ (*to publish*) publicar; ~ **forth** (*blood, liquid*) brotar; ~ **from** descender (ie) de

issuer, emisor *m*

isthmus, istmo; ~ **of the eustachian tube** istmo de la trompa de Eustaquio

itch, ~ (*desire*) ganas *f, pl*; ~ (*scabies*) sarna; ~ (*sensation*) comezón *f*; hormigas *Med*; picazón *f*; picor *m*; piquiña *PR*; prurito; **barbers'** ~ tiña de la barba; **jock** ~ tiña crural; **to** ~ (*to irritate*) picar; tener comezón; tener picazón; **to** ~ (*to smart*) dar picor

itching, escozor *m*; picazón *m, fam*; picor *m*; prurito; ~ **sensation** rasquera

itchy, picante *adj*; que pican *adj phr*

IV/intravenous solution, solución endovenosa *f*; suero glucosado; suero por la vena; suerofisiológico

IVT/intravenous transfusion, transfusión intravenosa *f*

ivory, marfil *m*

IVP/intravenous pyelogram, pielograma intravenoso/PIV *m*

ivy, hiedra; yedra; **poison ~** chechén *m*; hiedra venenosa; zumaque venenoso *m*

---

[2] This is new vocabulary, not necessarily listed nor yet recognized by the Royal Academy of Spanish Grammar. It is understood that this vocabulary is primarily slang. Unless otherwise indicated, the gender of nouns is assumed to be obvious.

[3] For pronunciation purposes, the masculine definite and indefinite articles, *el* and *un*, not *la* and *una*, are used when the article immediately precedes the feminine singular noun which begins with stressed *a* or any other that begins with stressed *ha*.

[4] Multiple meanings of this Spanish word include this as well as *groin, ringworm,* and *tinea.*

[5] This "disease" has nothing to do with bile.

[6] Part of the Drug Abuse Vocabulary

[7] Use the Spanish pronunciation of these letters.

J

jab, ~ (*a prick*) puyón *m*, *Col*, *Guat*, *PR*; ~ (*a stab*) pinchazo; puntazo *SpAm*; ~ (*from a needle*) *fam* inyección *f*; pinchazo; ~ (*with an elbow*) codazo

jab, to, ~ (*with an elbow*) dar un codazo a; ~ (*with the fist*) dar un puñetazo a; ~ (*with a needle*) pinchar; ~ (*to prick*) puyar *SpAm* (*See inject oneself with drugs, to*).

jack off, to,[4] *slang* (*See inject oneself with drugs, to.*)

jacket, chaqueta; saco; camisa; chamarra *Mex*; corsé *m/f*; ~ (*of a book*) sobrecubierta; ~ (*of a record, disk*) forro; ~ (*of a man's suit*) saco; ~ (*of a woman's suit*) chaqueta; **plaster-of-paris** ~ corsé enyesado *m*; **porcelain** ~ **crown** corona en cáscara de porcelana *Dent*; **strait** ~ camisa de fuerza

jag, ~ (*of a break*) mella; ~ (*serration*) diente *m*; **to have a** ~ **on** *slang* estar borracho *adj*

jag, to, mellar; dentar (ie)

jagged, ~ (*gapped-toothed*) dentado *adj*; mellado *adj*; **to be** ~ **up** (*under the influence of drugs*)[4] *slang* (*See blasted, to be.*)

jar, cubeta; envase *m*; frasco; jarra

jargon, jerga

jaundice, derrame biliar *m*; ictericia *form*; piel amarilla *f*; **acute febrile** ~ ictericia infecciosa aguda; **homologous serum** ~ ictericia por suero homólogo; **infectious** ~ ictericia infecciosa aguda; **obstructive** ~ ictericia obstructiva; **toxic** ~ ictericia toxémica; **urobilin** ~ ictericia urobilínica

jaundiced, ictérico *adj*

jaw, ~ (*usually of animals*) quijada; ~ (*of people*) mandíbula; ~ *slang* quijada; **broken** ~ mandíbula rota; quijada rota; **crackling** ~ mandíbula crujiente; **lower** ~ maxilar inferior *m*; mandíbula; ~ **malposition** malposición mandibular *f*; ~ **movement** movimiento mandibular; ~ **relation** relación mandibular *f*; **upper** ~ maxilar superior *m*

jawbone, mandíbula; maxilar *m*; varilla *Anat*

jealous, celoso *adj*; envidioso *adj*; suspicaz *adj*

jejunal, yeyunal *adj*

jejunitis, yeyunitis *f*

jejunum, yeyuno

jelly, jalea; **cardiac** ~ jalea cardíaca; **contraceptive** ~ jalea anticoncepcional; **glycerin** ~ jalea glicerinada

jellyfish, medusa

jerk, ~ (*sudden shove*) empujón *m*; ~ (*reflex action*) espasmo; **reflex** ~ espasmo; ~ (*sudden movement, shake*) contracción súbita *f*; sacudida; **Achilles** ~ sacudida de Aquiles; **ankle** ~ sacudida del tobillo; **by** ~s a sacudidas; **crossed** ~ sacudida cruzada; **jaw** ~ sacudida maxilar; **knee** ~ sacudida de la rodilla; **tendon** ~ sacudida tendinosa; ~ (*sudden tug, pull*) tirón *m*

jerk, to, ~ (*to give a sharp pull*) dar un tirón a; ~ (*to move by tugging*) mover (ue) a tirones; ~ (*to shake*) dar una sacudida a; sacudir; ~ **off**[4] *slang* (*See inject oneself with drugs, to.*)

jerking movements, contracciones espasmódicas *f*

jerky, ~ (*movement*) espasmódico *adj*; nervioso *adj*; ~ **pulse** pulso saltón; ~ **respiration** respiración entrecortada *f*; resspiración interrumpida *f*

jet, ~ (*gas burner*) mechero; ~ (*of blood, steam, water, etc.*) chorro

jewelry, joyas

jigger, nigua

jiggle, to, menear(se)

jitteriness, nerviosismo

jive stick,[4] (*marijuana cigarette*) ~ leño[2]; charuto[2]; cigarro de mariguana[1]; frajo (de seda)[2]; leñito[2]; pito[2]

job, empleo; trabajo

jock(ey) itch, eczema marginado *m*; tiña crural *fam*; tiña inguinal *fam*

jockstrap, suspensorio

jog, (*a run*) trote corto *m*; **to give someone's memory a** ~ refrescarle la memoria a alguien

jog, to, andar a trote corto; trotar

jogger, trotador, -ra *m/f*

join, to, juntar; unir

joining enzyme, enzima de unión

joint, ~ (*articulation*) articulación *f*, Anat; coyuntura *esp. CA, Mex*; hueso *CA, Mex, fam*; **ball-and-socket** ~ articulación esférica; **hip** ~ articulación de la articulación coxofemoral; **immovable** ~ articulación inmóvil; **irritable** ~ articulación irritable; ~ **pain** dolor articular *m*; ~[4] *slang*, (*marijuana cigarette*) charuto[2]; cigarro de mariguana[1]; frajo (de seda)[2]; leño[2]; pito[2]; ~[4] (*of a narcotic cigarette*) abuja[2]; ~ **account** cuenta en común; ~ **property** propiedad indivisa *f*; ~ **responsibility** responsabilidad solidaria *f*

joke, chiste *m*; **as a** ~ en broma *prep phr*

jolly, ~ (*jovial*) alegre *adj*; ~ (*slightly inebriated*) piripi *adj*; ~ (*entertaining*) divertido *adj*

jolly pop, to, (*to use drugs infrequently*)[4], chipear[2]; chipiar[2]

jolt, ~ (*jerk*) sacudida; ~ (*fright*) susto

jolt, to, ~ (*to give a shove*) dar un empujón a; ~ **someone back to reality** hacer que uno vuelva bruscamente a la realidad

jowl, ~ (*double chin*) sotabarba; ~ (*cheek*) carrillo

joy pop, to, (*to use drugs infrequently*)[4] *slang* chipear[2]; chipiar[2]

jugal bone, hueso malar

jugomaxillary, maxilomalar *adj*

jugular, yugular *adj*; vena yugular

juice, jugo; zumo; **cranberry** ~ jugo de arándano; **fruit** ~ jugo de fruta; **gastric** ~ jugo gástrico; **grapefruit** ~ jugo de toronja; **intestinal** ~ jugo intestinal; **lemon** ~ jugo de limón; **orange** ~ jugo de naranja; jugo de china; **pancreatic** ~ jugo pancreático; **prune** ~ jugo de ciruela pasa; **tomato** ~ jugo de tomate

juicy, jugoso *adj*

jump, to, saltar; brincar

junction, unión *f*

junk,[4] (*heroin, vulg*) heroína

junkie (*narcotic addict*)[4] *slang*, adicto; adicto a drogas; drogadicto; morfinómano[2]; tecato[2]; toxicómano[2]; yeso[2]

juvenile, juvenil *adj*

juxta-articular, yustaarticular *adj*

juxtaposition, yustaposición *f*

---

[1] I have followed the spelling given in the *Diccionario de la lengua española*, RAE, 21st edition, 1990. Spanish does recognize variations using *j* and *h*.

[2] This is new vocabulary, not necessarily listed nor yet recognized by the Royal Academy of Spanish Grammar. It is understood that this vocabulary is primarily slang. Unless otherwise indicated, the gender of nouns is assumed to be obvious.

[4] Part of the Drug Abuse Vocabulary.

kaluresis, caluresis *f*; aumento de la excreción urinaria de potasio

Kaposi's disease, enfermedad de Kaposi *f*

Kaposi's sarcoma, sarcoma de Kaposi *m*

karyotyping, análisis cromosómico *m*; determinación del cariotipo *f*

KE/kinetic energy, energía cinética

keel, quilla; **~-shaped** aquillado *adj*

keen, perspicaz *adj*; agudo *adj*

keep, to, guardar; mantener; ~ **alive** mantener con vida; mantener en vida; ~ **in bed** quedarse en cama; ~ **medicines away from kids** poner las medicinas fuera del alcance de los niños; ~ **to one's bed** guardar cama; ~ **to** (*to restrict o.s.*) limitarse a

kefir, kefir *m*

keloid, queloide *m*; **acne** ~ acné *f*

keratalgia, queratalgia *form*; dolor corneal *m*

keratin, queratina

keratitis, queratitis *f*

keratoconjunctivitis, queratoconjuntivitis *f*; inflamación de la córnea y la conjuntiva *f*

keratohypopyon, queratohipopión *m*

keratoma, queratoma *m*, *form*; callosidad *f*

keratoscopy, queratoscopia

keratotomy, queratotomía; **radial** ~ queratotomía radiada

kerosene, keroseno; querosén *m*

ketoacidosis, cetoacidosis *f*

ketogenic, cetógeno *adj*

ketone, cetona

ketolysis, cetólisis *f*

ketonuria, cetonuria

ketosis, cetosis *f*; quetosis *f*

ketosuria, cetosuria; presencia de cetosa en la orina; quetosuria

ketotic, cetónico *adj*

key, ~ (*code*) clave *f*; ~ (*lock*) llave *f*; **tooth** ~ llave dental *Dent*; ~ (*typewriter, computer, etc.*) tecla

kick, patada

kick, to, ~ (*a person*) dar un puntapié; dar una patada; ~ (*an animal*) dar de coces a; dar una coz; ~ (*a gun, etc.*) dar un culatazo; ~ **one's legs** mover (ue) las piernas; pernear; ~ **the habit**[4] cortarse el vicio; kikear[2]; quitear[2]

kid, (*child*) chiquillo; niño; cabro *Chi*; chamaco *Mex*; chaval, -la *m/f*; chico *Pan, Cu*; cipote *m, El Sal*; guagua *m/f, PR*; patojo *Guat*; pelado *Col*; pibe, -ba *m/f, Arg, Bol, Chi, Ríopl*

kidnapping, rapto; secuestro

kidney, riñón *m*; **arteriosclerotic** ~ riñón arteriosclerótico; **artificial** ~ riñón artificial; **atrophic** ~ riñón atrófico; **cirrhotic** ~ riñón cirrótico; **cystic** ~ riñón quístico; ~ **disease** mal de riñón *m*; enfermedad de los riñones *f*; **doughnut** ~ riñón anular; **enlargement of the** ~ agrandamiento del riñón; ~ **failure** insuficiencia renal; **floating** ~ riñón ectópico; riñón flotante; **fused** ~ riñón único por fusión; **horseshoe** ~ riñón en herradura; ~ **infection** infección de los riñones *f*; **pelvic** ~ riñón pélvico; **polycystic** ~ riñón poliquístico; **~-shaped** arriñonado *adj*; ~ **stone** cálculo en el riñón; cálculo renal; cálculo urinario; piedra en los riñones;

piedra nefrítica; **supernumerary** ~ riñón supernumerario; ~ **transplant** trasplante de riñón *m*

kill, to, ~ (*machine, etc.*) inactivar; limpiar el pico *PR*; ~ (*to slaughter*) matar; ~ (*sound, light, fire*) amortiguar

kilocalorie, kilocaloría

kilogram, kilogramo

kilohertz, kilohercio

kiloliter, kilolitro

kilometer, kilómetro

kilowatt, kilovatio; ~**-hour** kilovatios-hora *m, pl*

kin, parientes *m, pl*; **next of** ~ pariente más cercano

kind, amable *adj*; tipo; género; clase de *f*

kinematics, cinemática

kinesitherapist, quinesioterapeuta *m/f*

kinesitherapy, quinesiterapia

kinesthesia, cinestesia; sentido muscular

kinetosis, cinetosis *f*

kink, (*in hair*) rizo

kink, to, ~ (*hair*) rizarse; ~ (*to twist*) retorcer(ue)

kinky, (*hair*) churrusco *adj, Col, Pan*

kit, botiquín *m*; estuche *m*; **emergency** ~ botiquín de emergencia; **first aid** ~ botiquín de primeros auxilios; equipo de urgencia; ~ *slang* (*See fit.*)

kite, chiringa; **to be higher than a** ~[4] estar a millón[2]; estar más jalao que un timbre de guagua *PR*; tener una nota[2]

kitten, gatito

k.j./knee jerk, reflejo rotuliano

Kleenex, kleenex *m*; pañuelo de papel

kleptomania, cleptomanía

kleptomaniac, cleptómano

Klinefelter's syndrome, síndrome de Klinefelter *m*

knead, to, amasar

kneading, amasadura; amasamiento

knee, rodilla; **back of the** ~ corva; flexura de la pierna; ~ **bandage** rodillera; ~**-bend(ing)** inflexión de las rodillas *f*; ~ **joint** articulación de la rodilla *f*; **locked** ~ rodilla bloqueada

kneecap, (*patella*) choquezuela; hueso de la rodilla; rótula

kneel, to, arrodillarse; hincarse

knife, cuchillo; **endotherm** ~ cuchillo eléctrico; **pocket** ~ cuchilla; ~ **sharpener** (aparato) afilador *m*; **switchblade** ~ gurbia *PR*; sevillana

knit, to, (*bones*) soldarse

knitting (**of a fracture**), consolidación (de una fractura) *f*

knob, protuberancia; bulto; **door** ~ pomo

knock, choque *m*; **pericardial** ~ choque pericárdico; ~**-kneed** chueco *adj, SpAm*; ñangado *adj, Cu*

knock, to, ~ (*to hit*) golpear; pegar; ~ **out some teeth** partirse unos dientes; ~ **up** *euph* dejar embarazada

knockout drops,[4] narcótico *sg*

knot, nudo; **double** ~ nudo doble; **surgeons'** ~ nudo de cirujano; ~ (*of nerves*) haz *m*; ~ (*type of tissue swelling*) bolas *f, pl, Chicano*; **to get tied up in** ~**s** enmarañarse

knot, to, anudar

knotted suture, sutura abotonada

know, to, ~ (*know facts, how to*) saber; ~ (*be acquainted with people, places*) conocer

knowledge, conocimiento

knowledgeable, erudito *adj*; alumbrao *adj, PR*

knuckle, nudillo

kosher meat, carne de animal sacrificado según la ley judía *f*

K.U.B./kidney, ureter, bladder, riñón, uréter, vejiga

kwashiorkor, cuasiorcor *m*; kwashiorkor *m*; desnutrición húmeda
f
kyllosis, quilosis *f*; cilosis *f*; temblor de párpado *m*, *Sp*, *SpAm*;
pie zambo *m*, *Arg*

kyphosis, cifosis *f*; curvatura anormal con prominencia dorsal de
la columna vertebral

---

[2] This is new vocabulary, not necessarily listed nor yet recognized by the Royal Academy of Spanish Grammar. It is understood that this vocabulary is primarily slang.
Unless otherwise indicated, the gender of nouns is assumed to be obvious.
[4] Part of the Drug Abuse Vocabulary.

label, etiqueta
label, to, marcar
labia, (*sg, labium*) labios; ~ **majora**
labios mayores; ~ **minora** labios
menores
labial, labial *adj*
labio-alveolar, labioalveolar *adj*
labiodental, labiodental *adj*
lability, (*emotional instability*) labilidad del humor *f*
labium, (*pl, labia*) labio
labor, labor *f*; parto *Obst*; trabajo
de parto *Obst*; **artificial** ~ parto
artificial; ~ **bed** cama de partos;
complicated ~ parto complicado; **dry** ~ parto seco; **false** ~
parto falso; **first stage of** ~
primer período del parto; **immature** ~ parto inmaduro; **induced** ~ parto inducido;
instrumental ~ parto instrumental; **mimetic** ~ parto falso;
multiple ~ parto múltiple; ~
pains dolores de parto *m*; **podalic** ~ parto podálico; **premature** ~ parto prematuro;
habitual premature ~ parto prematuro habitual; **prolonged** ~
parto prolongado; ~ **room** sala
de partos; sala prenatal; **second
stage of** ~ segundo período del
parto; **spontaneous** ~ parto
espontáneo; **third stage of** ~
tercer período del parto;
woman in ~ parturienta *f*; **to be
in** ~ enfermarse *Chicano*; estar
de parto; **to have a difficult** ~
tener un parto difícil
laboratory, laboratorio; ~ **facilities** instalaciones de laboratorio *f*; recursos de laboratorio; ~
finding hallazgo de laboratorio; resultado del análisis; ~
technician laboratorista *m/f*;

técnico de laboratorio; ~ **test**
análisis de laboratorio *m, inv*
labored, dificultoso *adj*; ~ **breathing** respiración jadeante *f*; ~
respiration disnea; respiración
laboriosa *f*
laborious, trabajoso *adj*
labyrinth, laberinto; oído interno;
membranous ~ laberinto membranoso
labyrinthitis, laberintitis *f*; otitis
interna
labyrinthosis, laberintosis *f*
lacerate, to, desgarrar; lacerar
lacerated, lacerado *adj*; desgarrado *adj*; ~ **wound** herida lacerada
laceration, cortada; desgarradura; laceración *f*; **perineal** ~s
desgarros perineales
lack, carencia; deficiencia; falta; ~
of confidence falta de confianza; ~ **of control** falta de control;
~ **of credibility** falta de credibilidad; ~ **of exercise** falta de
ejercicio
lack, to, faltar
lacking, defectivo *adj*; ~ **a fin-
ger/hand** tuco *SpAm, adj*
lachrymal, lagrimal *adj*
lactagogue, lactagogo
lactase, lactasa
lactate, lactato
lactate, to, lactar; salirle leche
fam; secretar leche
lactation, lactancia; lactación *f*
lactic, láctico *adj*; ~ **acid** ácido láctico; ~ **dehydrogenase** deshidro-
genasa láctica; ~ **ferments**
fermentos lácticos
lactodensimeter, lactodensímetro
lactoscope, lactoscopio
lactose, (*used to cut heroin*) lactosa;
azúcar de leche *m/f* [*Ú.m.c.s.f.*]
en sing; [*Ú.c.s.m.*] *en pl*

lacuna, laguna; **absorption** ~ laguna de absorción; **blood** ~ laguna sanguínea

lady, dama; señora

lag, período de latencia; retraso

laid up, to be, estar incapacitado; guardar cama

lamb, cordero

lame, cojo *adj*; derrengado *adj*; lisiado *adj*; rengo *adj*; chueco *adj*, *Col*; patojo *adj*, *SpAm*

lameness, cojera

lamina, lámina

laminectomy, laminectomía

lamp, lámpara; **arc** ~ lámpara de arco; **mercury vapor** ~ lámpara de vapores de mercurio; **quartz** ~ lámpara de cuarzo

lance, to, abrir con bisturí; sajar *Med*

lancet, sangradera *Med*

landmarks, marcas; puntos de referencia

languidness, languidez *f*

languish, to, languidecer

languishment, postración *f*

languor, (*interest*) decaimiento

lank, ~ (*cheeks*) hundido *adj*; ~ (*gawky*) desmadejado *adj*; ~ (*hair*) lacio *adj*; ~ (*tall and thin*) larguirucho *adj*; ~ (*thin*) delgado *adj*; flaco *adj*

lankiness, ~ (*gawkiness*) desmadejamiento; ~ (*thinness*) flacura

lanolin, lanolina

lap, regazo *Anat*; ~ (*sports term*) vuelta

lap, to, ~ (*to drink quickly and noisily*) sober; ~ (*to enjoy*) disfrutar con

laparoscopy, laparoscopia

laparotomy, laparotomía

lapse, lapso

lapse, to, ~ (*to err*) caer en el error; ~ **into silence** quedarse callado; ~ **into unconsciousness** perder(ie) el conocimiento

lard, manteca

large, corpulento *adj*; grande *adj*;

~ **bowel** intestino grueso; ~ **cell nucleus** núcleo ambiguo; ~ **intestine** intestino grueso

laryngeal, laríngeo *adj*

laryngectomy, laringectomía

laryngitis, laringitis *f*

laryngoscope, laringoscopio

laryngoscopy, laringoscopia

larynx, laringe *f*

laser, láser *m*; rayo láser

lash, ~ (*blow with the whip*) azote *m*; ~ (*eyelash*) pestaña

last, ~ **name** apellido; ~ **rites** santos óleos; ~ **sleep** último sueño; ~ **week** la semana pasada; ~ (*of a shoe*) horma

last, to, aguantar; durar; ~ **a long time** perdurar

lasting, duradero *adj*; profundo *adj*; ~ (*fear, etc.*) constante *adj*; ~ (*strong*) resistente *adj*

late, tarde *adv*; tardío *adj*; ~ **in life** a una edad avanzada; ~ (*after appointed time*) con retraso; ~ (*deceased*) difunto *adj*; fallecido *adj*; ~ (*delayed*) retrasado *adj*; ~ (*delivery*) atrasado *adj*; ~ (*development, etc.*) tardío *adj*; ~ (*recent*) reciente *adj*; **to be** ~ (*a person*) llegar tarde; ~ (*a train, plane, etc.*) llevar retraso; ~ **in** tardar en (+ *infinitive*); **to stay up** ~ quedarse levantado hasta muy tarde

latent, latente *adj*; ~ (*defect, quality*) oculto *adj*

later, más tarde *adv*

lateral view, proyección lateral *f*; vista lateral

latex, látex *m*

lather, (*soap*) espuma; jabonadura

latrine, excusado; retrete *m*

laugh, risa; **loud** ~ carcajada

laugh, to, reír (i); reírse (i); **to give a forced** ~ reír (i) con risa de conejo; ~ **until one's sides ache** reír (i) a mandíbula batiente

laughing, risueño *adj*; ~ **gas** gas hilarante *m*

laughter, risa

launder, to, lavar (y planchar)

laundry, ~ (*clean*) ropa limpia; ~ (*dirty*) ropa sucia; ~ (*place*) lavandería

lavage, irrigación *f*; lavado; ~ (*of a stomach, etc.*) lavado; **bronchoalveolar** ~ lavado broncoalveolar; **gastric** ~ lavado gástrico; **intestinal** ~ lavado intestinal; **peritoneal** ~ lavado peritoneal; **pleural** ~ lavado pleural

lavatory, ~ (*basin*) lavabo; lavamanos *m, inv*; lavatorio; ~ (*restroom*) baño; excusado; retrete *m*; servicio

lavender, espliego

law, ley *f*

lawsuit, pleito

lawyer, abogado; licenciado *Mex*

lax, ~ (*bowels*) flojo *adj*; suelto *adj*; ~ (*discipline*) laxo *adj*; ~ (*flesh*) flácido *adj*; ~ (*untensed*) flojo *adj*

laxative, laxante *m*; laxativo; purgante *m*

lay, lego *adj*; popular *adj*

lay, to, poner; ~ **down**; ~ (*to establish*) establecer; ~ (*to put to bed*) acostar (ue); ~ **out** (*to present*) presentar; ~ **up** (*to confine to bed*) obligar a guardar cama; ~ (*to make ill*) enfermar

layer, capa; estrato; **germ** ~ capa germinal; **nerve fiber** ~ capa de fibras nerviosas; ~ **of rods and cones** capa de conos y bastones

layer, to, formar capas

layette, canastilla de niño

layout, *slang* (*See fit.*)

lazy, ~ (*indolent*) indolente *adj*; ~ (*idle*) holgazán *adj*; perezoso *adj*; petacón, petacona *adj, Col*

lazy eye (*amblyopia*), ambliopía

LDL/low density lipoprotein, LBD[4]/lipoproteína de baja densidad

lead (*metal*), plomo; ~ **acetate** acetato de plomo; ~ **apron** delantal de plomo *m*; ~ **poisoning** intoxicación saturnina *f*; saturnismo; ~ **screen** pantalla de plomo

lead, ~ (*register*) derivación *f*; **esophageal** ~**s** derivaciones esofágicas; **precordial** ~**s** derivaciones precordiales; **unipolar limb** ~**s** derivaciones unipolares de los miembros

leading, ~ **case** caso precedente; ~ **cause** causa inmediata; ~ **practitioner** clínico principal

leak, rezumamiento; ~ (*of gas*) escape *m*; ~ (*of water*) gotera; ~ (*of gas, or liquid*) fuga

leak, to, derramar

lean, ~ (*face*) enjuto *adj*; ~ (*person*) delgado *adj*; flaco *adj*; ~ (*meat*) magro *adj*

lean, to, inclinar(se); ~ **upon to** apoyarse en; ~ **forward** inclinarse; ~ **against** apoyarse contra; ~ **one's head back** echar la cabeza hacia atrás; ~ **out of** asomarse a

lean-to, cobertizo

leap, salto

leap up, to, pegar un salto

learn, to, aprender

learning, aprendizaje *m*; ~ **disability** impedimento en el aprendizaje; ~ **center** centro de aprendizaje

leather, cuero; piel *f*

leathery, (*skin*) curtido

leave, to, (*to go away*) salir (de); jalarse *PR*

lecithin, lecitina

LED/lupus erythematosus disseminata, LED[4]/lupus eritematoso diseminado *m*

leech, ventosa; ~ (*clinging person*) lapa; ~ (*parasite*) sanguijuela

left, izquierdo *adj*; ~ **heart** corazón arterial; ~ **hand** izquierda *f*; izquierdo *adj*; ~ **hand side** izquierda *f*; ~**-handed** izquierdo *adj*; zurdo *adj*; ~**-handedness** zurdería; ~ **side** izquierda *f*; **to be on the** ~ **of** estar a la izquierda; **to keep** (**to the**) ~ seguir (i) por la izquierda; **to the** ~ a la izquierda *prep phr*

leftovers, sobras

leg, pierna; **calf of the** ~ canilla; chamorro *Chicano*; pantorrilla; ~ **injury** traumatismo de la pierna; ~ **movement** movimiento de la pierna; ~ **rest** soporte de piernas *m*; **to be on one's last** ~ estar en las últimas; **to get back on one's** ~ recobrar la salud; **to stretch one's** ~ desentumecerse las piernas

leggings (*surgical stockings*), medias compresivas

legitimate, legítimo *adj*

legroom, sitio para las piernas

legume, legumbre *f*

leishmaniasis, leishmaniasis *f*; roncha hulera; roncha mala

leisure, ocio

length, longitud *f*; largo; **along the whole** ~ **of** a lo largo de todo *prep phr*; **crown-heel** ~ longitud vértex-talón; **crown-rump** ~ longitud vértex-rabadilla; ~ (*of time*) duración *f*; espacio; extensión *f*; ~ **of pregnancy/LOP** duración del embarazo; ~ **of hospital stay** tiempo de internamiento; ~ **of time required to do sth** el tiempo requerido para hacer algo; **for what** ~ **of time?** ¿durante cuánto tiempo?; **to go to the** ~ **of** llegar hasta el extremo de; **to walk the** ~ **of** recorrer

lengthen, to, alargar; prolongarse

lengthwise, a lo largo *adv*; longitudinalmente *adv*

leniency, indulgencia

lenient, indulgente *adj*

lens, lente *m/f*, [*Ú.m.c.m.*]; ~ (*part of eye*) cristalino *Anat*; **artificial** ~ cristalino artificial; **bifocal** ~ lente bifocal; **cataract** ~ lente de catarata; **concave** ~ lente cóncava; **contact** ~ lente de contacto; lentilla *Spain*; pupilente *m*; **gas permeable contact** ~ lente poroso; **hard contact** ~ lente de contacto duro; **soft contact** ~ lente de contacto blando; **convex** ~ lente convexa *f*; ~ **implantation** lentes intraoculares; **magnifying** ~ lente de aumento; lupa; **toric** ~ lente tórica *f*; **trifocal** ~ lente trifocal

Lent, Cuaresma *f*

lenticula, lente pequeño

lentil, lenteja

leper, leproso; lazarino

leprosy, lazarín *m*; lepra; mal de Hansen *m*; mal de San Lázaro *m*

leprous, lazariento *adj*, *Arg, Mex, Nic*

leptomeninges, leptomeninges *f*

leptospirosis, leptospirosis *f*

lesbian, lesbiana *f*, *adj*

lesbianism, lesbianismo; lesbismo

lesion, lesión *f*; **degenerative** ~ lesión degenerativa; **gross** ~ lesión macroscópica; **minute** ~ lesión microscópica; **oral** ~ afta; boquera; perleche *f*; pupa; **precancerous** ~ lesión precancerosa; **primary** ~ lesión primaria; **skin** ~ grano; **structural** ~ lesión estructural; **systemic** ~ lesión sistematizada; **total** ~ lesión total; **toxic** ~ lesión tóxica; **vascular** ~ lesión vascular

less, menos *adj, adv*

lessen, to, disminuir; reducir

lesson, lección *f*

let, to, dejar; permitir; ~ **bleed** hacer una sangría; hacer sangrar; sangrar; **to be** ~ **down** llevarse un chasco; ~ **go of** soltar (ue)

letdown, bajón *m*; chasco

lethal, mortal *adj*; ~ (*Med*) letal *adj*; ~ **dose** dosis mortal *f, inv*; ~ **wound** herida mortal

lethargic, aletargado *adj*; letárgico *adj*

lethargy, aletargamiento; estupor *m*; letargia; letargo

lettuce, lechuga
leuconychia, manchas blancas en la uña
leukanemia, leucanemia
leukemia, cáncer de la sangre *m*; leucemia; **acute** ~ leucemia aguda; **aplastic** ~ leucemia aplástica; **basophilic** ~ leucemia basófila; **granulocytic** ~ leucemia granulocítica; **hepatic** ~ leucemia hepática; **lymphatic** ~ leucemia linfática; **lymphoblastic** ~ leucemia linfoblástica; (**acute**) **lymphocytic** ~ leucemia linfocítica (aguda); **lymphogenous** ~ leucemia linfógena; (**chronic**) **lymphoid** ~ leucemia linfoide (crónica); **myeloblastic** ~ leucemia mieloblástica; **myelocytic** ~ leucemia mielocítica; (**chronic**) **myelogenous** ~ leucemia mielógena (crónica); (**chronic**) **myeloid** ~ leucemia mieloide (crónica); **plasma-cell** ~ leucemia de células plasmáticas; **temporary** ~ leucemia transitoria; **undifferentiated cell** ~ leucemia de células indiferenciadas
leukemic, leucémico *adj*
leukemoid, leucemoide *adj*; ~ **reaction** reacción leucemoide *f*
leukoblast, leucoblasto; **granular** ~ leucoblasto granular
leukocytes, (*white blood cells*) glóbulos blancos de la sangre; leucocitos; **acidophil** ~ leucocito acidófilo; **agranular** ~ leucocito agranulocito; **basophil** ~ leucocito basófilo; **granular** ~ leucocito granuloso; **lymphoid** ~ leucocito linfoide; leucocito sin gránulos; **neutrophil** ~ leucocito neutrófilo; **polymorphonuclear** ~ leucocito polimorfonuclear
leukocytosis, leucocitosis *f*
leukoplakia, leucoplaquia
leukoplasia, leucoplasia

leukorrhea, flujo vaginal blancuzco; leucorrea; pérdidas blancas *fam*; **periodic** ~ leucorrea periódica
level, al ras (de) *prep*; al nivel de *prep*; **at eye** ~ a la altura del ojo; **at ground** ~ a ras de tierra; ~ (*instrument; height*) nivel *m*; ~ (*index*) índice *m*; **alcohol** ~ **in the blood** índice de alcohol en la sangre; **noise** ~ intensidad del ruido *f*; ~ (*flat*) raso *adj*; ~ **teaspoon** cucharadita rasa
lever, palanca
lewd, obsceno *adj*
lewdness, obscenidad *f*
L.F.D./least fatal dose, dosis letal mínima *f, inv*
LH/luteinizing hormone, hormona luteinizante
liability, ~ (*drawback*) inconveniente *m*; ~ (*legal responsibility*) responsabilidad *f*; ~ (*propensity*) tendencia
liable to catch cold, propenso a constiparse *adj*
liar, mentiroso
liberty, to be at, estar autorizado; ~ (*to be at leisure*) estar desocupado
libido, libido; **bisexual** ~ libido bisexual
lice, piojos; **crab** ~ ladillas
license, licencia; permiso
lichen, liquen *m*; ~ **planus** liquen plano
lick, to, lamer
licorice, regaliz *m*
lid, ~ (*of eye*) **eye** ~ párpado *Anat*; ~ (*cover*) tapa
lidocaine, lidocaína
lie, mentira; ~ situación *Obst, f*; **longitudinal** ~ situación longitudinal; **oblique** ~ situación oblicua; **transverse** ~ situación transversa
lie, to ~ (*to tell a falsehood*) mentir (ie); ~ **down** acostarse (ue); ~ **in** (*due to childbirth*) estar de parto;

~ **in** (*to stay in bed*) quedarse en la cama

life, vida; ~ **expectancy** esperanza de vida; expectativa de vida; ~ **force** fuerza vital; ~ **history** ciclo biológico; ~ **insurance** seguro de vida; aseguranza *Chicano*; ~ **preserver** salvavidas *m, inv*; ~ **span** duración de vida *f*; longevidad *f*; ~ **style** modo de vivir; ~ **support device** aparato para prolongar la vida; **to bring (back) to** ~ resucitar

lifeguard, bañero

lifeless, exánime *adj*; sin vida *prep phr*

lifelessness, falta de animación

lift, ~ (*raising*) levantamiento; elevación *f*; ~ (*in heel of a shoe*) tapa; ~ (*fig. mental state*) exaltación *f*; ~ (*upward support*) empuje *m*; **face** ~ estiramiento facial; **to have a face** ~ estirarle a alguien la piel de la cara; **to give s.o. a** ~ (*a ride*) llevar en coche; **to give s.o. a** ~ (*mental*) levantar el ánimo; reanimar

lift, to, ~ (*to raise*) alzar; levantar; ~ (*to pick up*) coger

ligament, ligamento; **accessory** ~ ligamento accesorio

ligamentum, vendaje *m*; ligamenta; ~ **accesoria plantaria** ligamenta accesoria plantaria; ligamentos plantares accesorios de las articulaciones metatarsofalángicas; ~ **arteriosum arteriae pulmonalis** ligamento arterial; ~ **flava** ligamenta flava; ~ **nuchae** ligamento cervical posterior; ~ **teres** ligamento redondo; ~ **venosum** conducto venoso

ligate, to, ligar; aplicar una ligadura

ligation, ligadura; **tubal** ~ amarre de las trompas *m, fam*

ligature, ligadura

light, luz *f*; ~ **bath** baño de luz; **di-fused** ~ luz difusa; **neon** ~ luz neón; **polarized** ~ luz polarizada; ~ **stroke** golpe de luz *m*; ~ (*brightness*) brillo; ~ (*disease*) leve *adj*; ~ (*flame*) fuego; ~ (*lamp*) luz *f*; lámpara; **overhead** ~ lámpara de techo; ~ (*street*) farol *m*; ~ (*not serious*) leve *adj*; ~ (*color, weight*) ligero *adj*; ~ **complexion** tez blonda *f*; **pilot** ~ piloto; **point of** ~ punto luminoso; ~ **source** fuente luminosa *f*; ~ **therapy** fototerapia; **to shine a** ~ **on something** enfocar

light, to, ~ (*to turn on*) encender (ie); ~ **up** iluminarse

light-footed, de paso ligero *prep phr*

light-headed, ~ (*from drink*) mareado *adj*; ~ (*scatterbrained*) casquivano *adj, fam*

light-headedness, sensación de desmayo *f*

lightening, (*childbirth*) aligeramiento

lightning, relámpago; ~ **spasm** espasmo centelleante

like, to, (*to be pleasing to*) gustarle a uno

like this, así *adv*

limb, extremidad *f*; miembro; **phantom** ~ miembro fantasma

limber, ~ (*person*) ágil *adj*; ~ (*thing*) flexible *adj*

limbus, limbo

lime, ~ **cal** *Chem, f*; **chlorinated** ~ cal clorurada; **soda** ~ cal sodada; **sulfurated** ~ cal sulfurada; ~ (*fruit*) lima

limit, límite *m*; **assimilation** ~ límite de asimilación; **saturation** ~ límite de saturación

limitation, limitación *f*; restricción *f*

limited, limitado *adj*; restricto *adj*; ~ **activity** actividad limitada *f*; ~ **autopsy** autopsia parcial

limiting, limitante *adj*; restrictivo *adj*; ~ **case** caso límite

limp, ~ (*floppy*) fláccido *adj*; flácido

adj; fofo *adj*; ~ (*lameness*) cojera; renguera *SpAm*; renqueo; ~ (*weak*) débil *adj*; debilitado *adj*

limp, to, (*to hobble*) cojear; dar cojetadas; renguear *SpAm*; renquear

limping, renguera *SpAm*

limpness, flaccidez *f*

lindane, lindano

linden tea, té de flores de tilo *m*

line, línea; **abdominal** ~ línea abdominal; **absorption** ~ línea de absorción; **cleavage** ~s línea de hendidura; **curved** ~ línea curva; **magnetic** ~s **of force** líneas de fuerza magnética; **oblique** ~ línea oblicua; ~ **of occlusion** línea de oclusión; ~ **of sight** línea visual; ~ (*feature*) rasgo; ~ (*of people*) cola; ~ (*by pen, pencil*) raya; ~ (*row*) fila; ~ (*wrinkle*) arruga

line, to, ~ (*to sheathe*) revestir (i); **to ~ up** alinear

lineage, linaje *m*

linear, lineal *adj*; ~ **equation** ecuación lineal *f*; ~ **fracture** fractura lineal

lingering, ~ (*illness*) crónico *adj*; ~ (*smell*) persistente *adj*; ~ (*death*) lento *adj*

lingual, lingual *adj*; ~ **swelling** protuberancia lingual *Dent*

liniment, linimento

lining, forro

link, enlace *m*

link, to, enlazar; unir

linkage, enlace *m*

linked, unido *adj*; ligado *adj*

linseed, linaza

lint, hilas *f, pl*

lip, labio; ~ (*of a wound*) borde *m*; **cleft** ~ labio hendido; labio leporino; **lower** ~ labio inferior; ~ **reading** labiolectura; **upper** ~ labio superior; **to bite one's** ~ morderse (ue) los labios; **to screw up/seal one's** ~s apretar (ie) los labios; **to smack one's** ~s relamerse

lipectomy, lipectomía

lipemia, lipemia *m*

lipid, lípido

lipidemia, lipidemia

lipoid, lipoide *m*; lipoideo *adj*

lipoma, lipoma *m*

lipoprotein, lipoproteína; **high density** ~/**HDL** lipoproteína de alta densidad/LAD⁴; **low density** ~/**LDL** lipoproteína de baja densidad/LBD⁴

liposarcoma, liposarcoma *m*

liposoluble, liposoluble *adj*

liposuction, liposucción *f*

lipped, thin-, de labios finos *prep phr*

lipstick, pintura de labios

liquefy, to, licuefacer; licuar

liquid, líquido *m, adj*; ~ **nitrogen** nitrógeno líquido; ~ **retention** retención de líquidos *f*

liquor, licor *m*

lisp, ~ (*of a child*) balbuceo; ~ (*speech defect*) ceceo; ~ (*stammer*) tartamudeo

lisp, to, balbucear; cecear

list, lista; **casualty** ~ lista de accidentados

list, to, pasar revista

listen (to), to, escuchar; ~ **one's lungs** escucharle los pulmones

listless, ~ (*lacking energy*) decaído *adj*; ~ (*uninterested*) apático *adj*

listlessness, apatía

liter, litro

lithium, litio

lithotomy, litotomía

lithotripsy, litotripsia

litmus paper, papel de tornasol *m*

litter, ~ (*disorder*) desorden *m*; ~ (*rubbish*) basura; ~ (*stretcher*) camilla; ~ **bearer** camillero

little, ~ (*amount*) poco *m, adj, adv*; ~ (*in distance*) corto *adj*; ~ (*size*) pequeño *adj*; ~ **finger** meñique *m*

live, vivo *adj*; ~ **birth** nacimiento con vida

live, to, vivir

liveborn, nacido vivo *adj*

lived, short-, de breve vida *prep phr*
liveliness, vivacidad *f*
liven up, to, animar(se)
liver, hígado; hepático *adj*; pana *Chi*; ~ circulation circulación hepática *f*; cirrhosis of ~ cirrosis hepática *f*; ~ complaint enfermedad del hígado *f*; enlargement of ~ agrandamiento del hígado; ~ extract extracto de hígado; dry ~ extract extracto seco de hígado; liquid ~ extract extracto líquido de hígado; ~ failure insuficiencia hepática; fatty ~ hígado adiposo; ~ function tests pruebas funcionales del hígado; ~ spots manchas hepáticas
livid, furioso *adj*
living, vida; viviente *adj*; vivo *adj*; ~ cell célula viviente; cost of ~ costo de vida; ~ conditions condiciones de vida *f*; ~ expenses gastos de mantenimiento; ~ will declaration declaración de voluntad de vida *f*
load, ~ (*burden*) carga; ~ (*fig*: *weight*) peso; ~ of narcotics carga²; ~ test prueba de sobrecarga; ~-carrying capacity capacidad de carga *f*
loaded, to be, (*See blasted, to be.*)
loaded, to get, agarrar onda²; sonarse²
loading dose, dosis inicial *f*
loan, préstamo
loan, to, prestar
loath, reacio *adj*; to be ~ to estar poco dispuesto a
loathe, to, aborrecer
lobar, lobar *adj*
lobby, salón principal *m*; vestíbulo; zaguán *m*
lobe, lóbulo; middle ~ syndrome síndrome del lóbulo medio del pulmón *m*; occipital ~ lóbulo occipital
lobectomy, lobectomía; complete ~ lobectomía completa; left

lower ~ lobectomía izquierda anterior; partial ~ lobectomía parcial
lobotomy, lobotomía
lobster, langosta
lobule, lobulillo; lóbulo pequeño
local, local *adj*; tópico *adj*, *Med*; ~ anesthesia anestesia local; ~ recurrence reaparición local *f*
localization, localización *f*; selective ~ localización electiva
localize, to, localizar
locate, to, (*to look for and discover*) localizar
located, situado *adj*
locator, localizador *m*
lochia, desecho; flujo; loquios
lock jaw/lockjaw, pasmo seco; tétano; espasmo masticatorio; pasmazón *m*, *Med*, *CA*, *Mex*, *PR*; pasmo *Med*; tétano; trismo
loculus, lóculo
logaphasia, logafasia
loin, fosa lumbar; ijada
lonely, to feel, sentirse (ie) solo
long, largo *adj*; extenso *adj*; prolongado *adj*; ~-acting de acción prolongada *prep phr*; ~ ago antaño *adv*; ~-sighted (*farsighted*) présbita *adj*, *Med*; ~-standing de larga duración *prep phr*; crónica *adj*; ~-term a largo plazo *prep phr*; ~-term results, resultados a largo plazo
longevity, duración larga de la vida *f*; longevidad *f*
longing, anhelo
longitudinal, longitudinal *adj*
look, to, ~ after ocuparse de; ~ (at) (*to watch*) mirar; ~ at (*to examine*) examinar; ~ at in great detail deletrear *Chi*; ~ away apartar la mirada; ~ back mirar hacia atrás; ~ (*appear*) bad (*person*) tener mala cara; ~ (*appear*) bad (*things*) tener mal aspecto; ~ down (*to lower one's eyes*) bajar la mirada; bajar los ojos; mirar hacia abajo; ~ for buscar; ~ ill pare-

cer enfermo *adj*; ~ **into** interiorizar *SpAm*; ~ **out for** (*to be careful*) tener cuidado con; ~ **out for** (*pay attention to*) estar atento *adj*; ~ **out of** asomarse a; ~ **over** (*look at superficially*) echar una ojeada a; ~ (*appear*) well (*person*) tener buena cara; ~ (*appear*) well (*things*) tener buen aspecto; ~ **up** mirar hacia arriba

loop, asa; ~ (*IUD*) lazo

loose, suelto; churriento *adj*, *SpAm*, *Med*; ~ (*untied*) desatado *adj*; ~ (*not fitting tightly*) holgado *adj*; ~ **bandage** venda floja; ~ **bowels** diarrea; excremento suelto; soltura; ~ **cough** tos húmeda *f*; ~ **definition** definición poco exacta *f*; ~ **skin** piel flácida *f*; piel laxa *f*; ~ **tongue** lengua desatada; ~ **tooth** diente que se mueve *m*; diente flojo *m*; ~ **translation** traducción libre *f*

loosen, to, aflojar; ~ **up** (*bowels*) descargarse; ~ **up** (*cough*) aliviarse; ~ **up** (*muscles*) desentumecer

lose, to, perder (ie); ~ **consciousness** perder (ie) el conocimiento; perder (ie) la conciencia; ~ **one's hair** pelarse; ~ **one's health** desmejorarse *Med*; ~ **one's teeth** mellar; ~ **the feeling in an ankle** relajarse un tobillo *Med*; ~ **weight** adelgazar; bajar de peso; perder (ie) peso

loss, pérdida; ~ **of appetite** pérdida de apetito; ~ **of balance** pérdida de equilibrio; ~ **of blood** pérdida de sangre; ~ **of consciousness** pérdida de conocimiento; ~ **of hair** lauca *Chi*; ~ **of memory** pérdida de memoria; amnesia; ~ **of muscle tone** pérdida de la tonicidad muscular; ~ **of sleep** pérdida de sueño; ~ **of weight** pérdida de peso

lotion, crema; loción *f*; **calamine** ~ loción de calamina; **hand** ~ crema para las manos; **suntan** ~ loción bronceadora; crema para el sol

loud, ruidoso *adj*

loud-speaker, altavoz *m*

lounge, salón de entrada *m*; **doctors'** ~ sala de los médicos

louse, (*insect*) piojo; **body** ~ piojo del cuerpo; **crab** ~ ladilla; **head** ~ piojo de la cabeza

lovastatin, lovastatina

low, bajo *adj*; ~ (*in spirits*) abatido *adj*; ~ **back pain** lumbago; ~ **birth weight** peso de nacimiento bajo; ~ **fat diet** régimen pobre en grasas *m*; ~ **magnification** pequeña amplificación *f*; ~ **-grade fever** fiebre moderada *f*; ~**-pitched** tono grave

lower, (*physically*) inferior *adj*

lower, to, bajar; ~ **the cholesterol count** bajar el nivel del colesterol

lozenge, comprimido; pastilla; pastilla de chupar; trocisco

LSD/lysergic acid diethylamide[5, 6], dietilamida del ácido lisérgico; aceite[2]; aceitunas[2]; acelide[2]; ácido lisérgico[2]; ácido(s)[2]; ALD[2]; alucinantes[2]; avándaro[2]; azúcar[2]; blanco de España[2]; bomba[2]; café[2]; cápsulas[2]; chochos[2]; cohete[2]; colorines[2]; cristales[2]; DAL *f*; diablos[2]; divina[2]; droga LSD; dulces[2]; onda[2]; gis[2]; grasas[2]; la salud[2]; lluvia de estrellas[2]; mica[2]; mureler[2]; nave[2]; orange[2]; papel[2]; paper[2]; piedrita de la luna[2]; pit[2]; purple haze[2]; staturnos[2]; sugar[2]; sunshine[2]; tacatosa[2]; terrones[2]; trip[2]; viaje en las nubes[2]; viaje[2]; white[2]

LSH/lutein stimulating hormone, hormona luteinizante

lubricant, lubricante *m*; lubricativo *adj*

lubricate, to, lubricar

lucid, lúcido *adj*

lucidity, lucidez *f*

lues, lúes *f*
lukewarm, templado *adj*; tibio *adj*
lumbago, lumbago; ischemic ~ lumbago isquémico
lumboarthrosis, lumboartrosis *f*
lumbodorsal, lumbodorsal *adj*
lumbosacral, lumbosacro *adj*
lumbricide, lumbricida *m*, *adj*
lump, bola; bolita; borujo; dureza; endurecimiento; hinchazón *f*; protuberancia; tolondro *Med*; tumorcito; large ~ borujón *m*; ~ (*bruise*) chichón *m*; ~ on head chichón *m*; pisporr(i)a *Chicano*; ~ (*swelling*) bulto; protuberancia
lumpectomy, lumpectomía
lunatic, lunático *m*, *adj*
lunch, almuerzo; comida *Mex*; to have ~ almorzar (ue)
lung, bofe *m*, *Chicano*, *SpAm*; pulmón *m*; ~ capacity volumen pulmonar *m*; collapsed ~ colapso de pulmón; ~ disease neumopatía; ~ elasticity elasticidad pulmonar *f*; iron ~ pulmón de acero; pulmotor *m*; ~ specialist neumólogo
lupous/lupus, luposo
lupus, lupus *m*; discoid ~ erythematosus lupus eritematoso discoide; disseminatus ~ erythematosus lupus eritematoso

generalizado; systemic ~ erythematosus lupus eritematoso generalizado; lupus eritematoso diseminado
luteal, lúteo *adj*
lutein, luteína
luteinizing hormone, hormona luteinizante
luxation, dislocación *f*; luxación *f*
lye, lejía
lying-in, puerperio; sobreparto; ~ period período puerperal
lymph, linfa; ~ duct vaso linfático; vaso quilífero; ~ glands glándulas linfáticas; ~ node ganglio linfático; nódulo linfático; nudo linfático *fam*
lymphatic, linfático *adj*
lymphoblast, linfoblasto
lymphocyte, linfocito
lymphogranuloma venereum/ LGV, bubones (tropicales) *m*; linfogranuloma venéreo *m*
lymphogranulomatosis/ Hodgkin's Disease, enfermedad de Hodgkin *f*; linfogranulomatosis *f*
lymphoid, linfoide *adj*
lymphoma, linfoma *m*
lysergic acid diethylamide/LSD[5], dietilamida del ácido lisérgico
lysine, lisina

---

[2] This is new vocabulary, not necessarily listed nor yet recognized by the Royal Academy of Spanish Grammar. It is understood that this vocabulary is primarily slang. Unless otherwise indicated, the gender of nouns is assumed to be obvious.

[4] Use the Spanish pronunciation of these letters.

[5] Current English street terminology for *LSD* includes: acid, barrels, (the) beast, big D, blue acid, blue cheer, blue heavens, blue mist, blue sky, blue tab, blue wedge, brown dots, California sunshine, cherry dome, cherry top, (the) chief, chocolate chips, Christmas acid, clear-light, coffee, contact lens, crackers, crystals, cube, cupcakes, deeda, dome, dots, double dimples, electric kool-aid, fifty, flats, gammon, (the) Ghost, grape parfait, grays, green barrels, (the) hawk, haze, heavenly blue, hit, instant Zen, L, LSD 25, Lucy in the sky (with diamonds), lysergide, mellow yellows, micro dots, mikes, mind detergent, oranges, orange mushrooms, orange sunshine, orange wedge, Owsley's acid, Ozzie's stuff, paper acid, peace, peace acid, peace pills, pearly gates, pellets, pink wedge, product IV, psychedelic, purple barrels, purple dome, purple dots, purple haze, purple microdots, purple ozoline, purple wedge, royal blue, smears, squirrels, Stanley's stuff, strawberry field, sunshine, tabs, ticket, trips, turtle, twenty-five, wedge, white lightning, window pane (paine), yellow dimples.

[6] Part of the Drug Abuse Vocabulary.

M

mace, macis *f*
macerate, to, macerar
maceration, maceración *f*
machine, máquina; aparato; **ultrasonic ~** máquina ultrasónica
machinery,[8] (*See fit.*)
macrobiotic, macrobiótico *adj*
macrocephalia, macrocefalia
macrocosm, macrocosmo
macrocyte, macrocito
macrodontia, macrodoncia *Dent*
macrophage, macrófago
macroscopic, macroscópico *adj*
macula, mácula; mancha; **~ densa** mácula densa; **~ lutea** mácula lútea; fovea centralis
mad, **~** (*angry*) enojado *adj*; furioso *adj*; **to get ~** (*angry*) encandilarse *PR*; enchismarse *PR*; enfadarse; enfogonarse *PR*; enojarse; entorunarse; ponerse furioso; **~** (*crazy*, *insane*) demente *adj*; loco *adj*; maníaco *adj*; **to go ~** (*insane*) enloquecer; volverse (ue) loco; **~** (*foolish*) insensato *adj*
made, hecho *adj*
madhouse, manicomio
madness, locura; manía
magazine, revista
maggot, gusano; **~** (*larva*) cresa; larva
magic mushrooms,[8] (*psilocybin*) *slang* hongos
magnesia, magnesia; **milk of ~** leche de magnesia *f*
magnesium, magnesio; **~ carbonate** carbonato de magnesio; **~ stearate** estearato de magnesio; **~ sulfate** sulfato de magnesio
magnet, imán *m*; **horseshoe ~** imán en herradura
magnetic, magnético *adj*; **~ field** campo magnético; **~ resonance**

imaging/MRI imágenes hechas por resonancia magnética *f*, *pl*; imágenes por resonancia magnética *f*, *pl*; resonancia magnética nuclear
magnetism, magnetismo
magnetize, to, magnetizar
magnetotherapy, magnetoterapia
magnification, magnificación *f*
magnifier, amplificador *m*
magnify, to, amplificar; aumentar
magnifying, de aumento *prep phr*; **~ glass** lupa; **~ lens** lente de aumento *f*
maid, criada
maidenhood, virginidad *f*; doncellez *f*, *Anat*
maiden name, nombre de soltera *m*
mail, correo
mail a letter, to, echar una carta en el correo
mailman, cartero
maim, to, estropear; lisiar; mutilar; tullir; **~** (*a limb*) lisiar
maimed, baldado *adj*; inválido *adj*; lisiado *adj*; manco *adj*; maneco *Arg*, *Mex*, *PR*; sucho *adj*, *Arg*, *Ec*; tuco *SpAm*, *adj*; tullido *adj*
main, principal *adj*; **~ pulmonary artery** arteria pulmonar principal
mainline, to,[8] *slang* inyectar drogas directamente en la vena principal del brazo
mainliner,[8] *slang* jaipa[2]; jaipo[2]
maintain, to, mantener
maintaining, mantenimiento
maintenance, mantenimiento; sostén *m*; **~ dose** dosis de mantenimiento *f*, *inv*; dosis de sostén *f*, *inv*
majority, mayoría

make, (*brand*) marca
make, to, hacer; ~ **a date** hacer cita; ~ **a fist** cerrar (ie) el puño ; ~ **an appointment** hacer turno; ~ **believe** fingir; suponer; ~ **better** aliviar; ~ **certain of** asegurarse de; ~ **difficult** dificultar; ~ **fun of** burlarse de; ~ **impossible** imposibilitar; ~ **mistakes** hacer errores; ~ **sense** tener sentido; ~ **up** (*a loss*) compensar; ~ **up** (*a prescription*) preparar; ~ **up** (*lost ground*) recuperar; ~ **worse** empeorar
makeup, ~ (*cosmetics*) cosméticos; maquillaje *m*; **to put on** ~ maquillarse; ~ (*nature*) carácter *m*; modo de ser; temperamento; ~ (*structure*) constitución *f*
make up, to, (*apply cosmetics*) maquillar
malabsorption, malabsorción *f*
maladjusted, inadaptado *adj*
maladjustment, desajuste *m*; inadaptación *f*
malady, dolencia; enfermedad *f*; mal *m*
malaise, destemplanza; indisposición *f*; mal *m*; malestar *m*
malar bone, pómulo
malaria, fiebre palúdica *f*; frío *SpAm*; malaria; paludismo; **autochthonous** ~ paludismo autóctono; **to catch** ~ achucharse *Ríopl*; **to have** ~ estar achuchado *Ríopl*
malarial, palúdico *adj*, *Med*
malariologist, mariólogo; paludólogo
malariology, malariología; paludología
malariotherapy, malarioterapia
maldevelopment, desarrollo anómalo
maldigestion, digestión difícil *f*
male, macho *m*, *adj*; masculino *adj*; pantalón *m*, *Ec*, *Perú*; varón *m*, *adj*; ~ **nurse** enfermero; ~ **hormone** hormona masculina

malformation, deformación *f*; malformación *f*
malfunction, funcionamiento defectuoso; malfuncionamiento
malfunction, to, malfuncionar
malice, malicia
malicious, malicioso *adj*
malignancy, enfermedad maligna *f*; malignidad *f*; tumor maligno *m*
malignant, maligno *adj*; ~ **disease** cáncer *m*; enfermedad cancerosa *f*; neoplasia; ~ **melanoma** melanoma maligno *m*; ~ **neuroblastoma of the sympathicus** neuroblastoma maligno del simpático *m*; simpaticoblastoma *m*; ~ **tumor** tumor maligno
malinger, to, fingirse enfermo
malleolus, maléolo
malleus, martillo
malnourished, desnutrido *adj*; mal asistido *adj*, *fam*; mal nutrido *adj*
malnutrition, desnutrición *f*; distrofia *f*; mala alimentación *f*; malnutrición *f*; nutrición defectuosa *f*; **kwashiorkor** kwashiorkor *m*; mala alimentación mojada *f*; niño rojo *fam*, *Costa de Oro*; **marasmus** mala alimentación seca *f*; marasmo
malocclusion, maloclusión *f*
malpractice, impericia; malpraxis *f*; negligencia médica; práctica inhábil; práctica impropia
maltase, maltasa
malt sugar, maltosa
mamma, mama; **supernumerary** ~ mama supernumeraria
mammalian, mamífero *m*, *adj*
mammary, mamario *adj*; ~ **gland** mama; glándulas mamarias; ~ **hypertrophy** (*barymazia*) barimastia
mammillary, mamilar *adj*
mammography, mamografía
mammogram, mamografía; mamograma *m*
mammoplasty, mamoplastia

man, hombre *m*; señor *m*; pantalón *m*, *Ec*, *Perú*

manage to, ~ (*an undertaking*) dirigir; ~ (*property*) administrar

management, conducto a seguir; tratamiento; ~ (*board of directors*) directiva; ~ (*of people, tools, etc.*) manejo; ~ (*skill*) habilidad *f*; ~ **of health services** gerencia de servicios médicos

mandible, mandíbula

mandibular, mandibular *adj*; ~ **glide** deslizamiento mandibular

mandibulopharyngeal, maxilofaríngeo *adj*; mandibulofaríngeo *adj*

maneuver, maniobra

manganese, manganeso

mange, roña; sarna

mangle, to, ~ (*a word*) deformar; ~ (*to cut; to hack*) despedazar

manhood, virilidad *f*

mania, manía; **acute hallucinatory** ~ manía aguda alucinatoria; **dancing** ~ manía danzante; **hysterical** ~ manía histérica; **puerperal** ~ manía puerperal

maniac, maníaco *adj*

manic depression, manía depresiva

manic-depressive, maníaco-depresivo *adj*; ~ **insanity** locura maníaco-depresiva; ~ **psychosis** (p)sicosis[9] maníaco-depresiva *f*

manicure, manicura

manicure, to,[8] (*clean and prepare marijuana for rolling into cigarettes*) *slang* limpiar (*mariguana*[1])

manifest, to, manifestar (ie)

manifestation, manifestación *f*

manipulation, manipulación *f*; ~ **therapy** quiropraxia *f*

manner, carácter *m*; comportamiento; manera; trato; **in this** ~ de esta manera *prep phr*

mannish, hombruno *adj*

manoeuver, maniobra

mantle, manto; palio; **nail** ~ manto de la uña

manual, manual *m*, *adj*

marasmus, marasmo

marble, mármol *m*

marbles, canicas

marbled skin, piel marmórea *f*

margarine, margarina

margin, borde *m*; margen *m*; **ciliary** ~ borde ciliar; **gingival** ~ borde gingival; **pupillary** ~ borde pupilar

marijuana[4], achicalada[2]; alfalfa[2]; amapola (*term used in prison*); bacha[2]; bailarina[2]; café[2]; campechana verde[2]; canabis; cáñamo[2]; carrujo[2]; cartucho[2]; chara[2]; chester[2]; chíchara[2]; chiclona[2]; chira[2]; chupe[2]; churus[2]; clorofila[2]; cochornis[2]; coffee[2]; coliflor tostada[2]; colombiana[2]; cosa[2]; cris[2]; dama de la ardiente cabellera[2]; de la buena[2]; de la verde[2]; diosa verde[2]; doña diabla[2]; doña Juanita[2]; doñajuanita[2]; doradilla[2]; epazote[2] *m*; fina esmeralda[2]; fitoca[2]; flauta[2]; flor de Juana[2]; frajo[2]; ganga[2]; ganja[2]; gavos[2]; golden[2]; grass[2]; griefo[2]; grifa[2]; grifo[2]; grilla[2]; guato[2]; güera[2]; habanita[2]; hashi[2]; hierba[2]; hoja verde[2]; huato[2]; índice[2]; jani[2]; Jefferson[2]; joint[2]; Juana[2]; Juanita[2]; Kris Kras[2]; la verde[2]; lucas[2]; macoña[2]; mafú[2]; mafufa[2]; maloja[2] *PR*; mani[2]; Margarita[2]; mari[2]; María Juanita[2]; María[2]; Mariana[2]; marifinga[2]; mariguana[1]; marihuana[1]; marijuana[1]; marinola[2]; mariola[2]; marquita[2]; Mary Jane[2]; Mary Popins[2]; meserole[2]; monstruo verde[2]; monte[2]; mora[2]; mostaza[2]; mota[2]; motor de chorro[2]; nalga de ángel[2]; orégano chino[2]; oro verde[2]; panetela[2]; pasto[2]; pastura[2]; pepita verde[2]; petate del soldado[2]; petate[2]; pitillo[2]; pito[2]; pochola[2]; pod[2]; polillo[2]; pot[2]; queta[2]; rollo[2]; tabaco (*common*); tabacón *m*, *Mex*; tacote *m*, *Mex*; té[2]; toque[2]; trueno verde[2]; tromadora^2; verdosa^2; yedo^2; yerba^2 (*very common*); yerba de oro^2; yerba del diablo^2; yerba santa^2; yerba verde^2; yerbabuena^2; yesca^2; zacate^2 (*low-grade variety*); zacate inglés^2; ~ **cigarette** frajo de seda^2; leñito^2; **to smoke** ~ (*See smoke marijuana, to.*); ~ **smoker** yesco^2; ~ **user** grifo^2; mariguano^1; marihuano^1; marijuano^1; moto^2; quemón^2; yesco^2

marital, marital *adj*; matrimonial *adj*; conyugal *adj*; ~ **status** estado civil; ~ **syphilis** sífilis conyugal *f*

mark, (*left by illness*) lacra *Med*; ~ (*trace*) huella; ~ (*brand*) marca; ~ (*of smallpox*) picadura; ~ **left by a lash** ramalazo; **marks**^{8} *slang* (*See tracks.*)

mark, to, señalar; ~ (*clothes*) marcar; ~ (*by smallpox*) picar; tener la cara picada de viruelas

marked, acusado *adj*; marcado *adj*; notable *adj*; ~ **difference** diferencia pronunciada

maroon, marrón *adj*; rojo obscuro *adj*

marriage, casamiento; matrimonio

married, casado *adj*; ~ **life** vida matrimonial; vida conyugal

marrow, médula; **bone** ~ médula ósea; ~ **puncture** punción de la médula ósea *f*; ~ **transplant**, trasplante de la médula *m*

marsh fever, malaria; paludismo

marsh gas, gas de los pantanos *m*; metano

marvelous, maravilloso *adj*

masculine, masculino *adj*; ~ **sterility** esterilidad masculina *f*

masculinity, masculinismo

mash, to, machucar

mask, máscara; mascarilla; **death** ~ mascarilla mortuoria; **ecchymotic** ~ máscara equimótica; **gas** ~ máscara antigás; ~ **of pregnancy** cloasma *m*; máscara gravídica; máscara del embarazo; **oxygen** ~

mascarilla de oxígeno; **surgical** ~ cubre-bocas/cubrebocas *m, inv*

mask, to, enmascarar; poner una mascarilla a

masked, enmascarado *adj*

masochism, masoquismo

masochist, masoquista *m/f*

mass, masa; ~ **immunization** inmunización masiva *f*; ~ **meeting** mitín popular *m, Chicano*; ~ **psychosis** psicosis de masas *f*; **to be a ~ of bruises** ser un puro cardena *fig*; **to be a ~ of nerves** ser un manojo de nervios *fig*

Mass, misa

massage, masaje *m*; **auditory** ~ masaje auditivo; **electrovibratory** ~ masaje electrovibratorio; **external cardiac** ~ masaje cardiaco externo; masaje cardíaco externo

massage, to, dar masajes (a); sobar

massive, masivo *adj*; ~ **hemorrhage** hemorragia masiva

massiveness, solidez *f*

mastectomy, mastectomía

master, to, dominar

masticate, to, masticar

mastitis, mastitis *f*; **cystic** ~ mastitis cística

mastoid, mastoideo *adj*; mastoides *f, adj*; ~ **antrum** antro mastoideo; cavidades mastoideas *f*; ~ **cells** células mastoideas; ~ **process** apófisis mastoides *f*; apófisis del hueso temporal *f*; proceso mastoideo

mastoidectomy, mastoidectomía

mastoiditis, mastoiditis *f*

masturbate, to, masturbar(se); hacerse la casqueta *Chicano*; puñetar *vulg*

masturbation, masturbación *f*; casqueta *Chicano*; puñetazo *vulg, Mex*

match, cerilla; fósforo; ~ (*sth that burns*)/~ (*persons or things exactly alike*) igual *m*; ~ (*couple*) pareja

match, to, ~ (*to catch up*) emparejar; ~ (*to compare*) equiparar; ~ (*blood, tissue, etc.*) ser compatible con

matching, prueba de compatibilidad

material, material *m*; **dental** ~ material dental; **restorative** ~s materiales restauradores

maternal, maternal *adj*; ~-**fetal exchange** intercambio materno-fetal; ~ **welfare** bienestar materno *m*

maternity, de maternidad *adj*; maternidad *f*; ~ **clothes** ropa de maternidad; ~ **floor** piso de maternidad; ~ **hospital** casa de maternidad; ~ **ward** sala de maternidad

matrix, ~ (*wonb*) mátriz *f*, *Anat*; útero

matter, ~ (*affair*) asunto; cuestión *f*; ~ (*discharge*) pus *m*; ~ (*substance*) materia; material *f*; **grey** ~ materia gris; **white** ~ materia blanca; **what's the** ~ ¿qué le pasa?; ¿qué tiene?

mattress, colchón *m*; **air** ~ colchón de aire *m*; colchón de viento *m*

maturation, maduración *f*

mature, maduro *adj*

mature, to, madurar

maturity, madurez *f*; edad madura *f*

maxilla, (*pl, maxillae*) maxilar *m*

maxillar, maxillary, maxilar *adj*

maxillofacial, maxilofacial *adj*

maxillolabial, maxilolabial *adj*

maximum tolerated dose/**M.T.D.**, dosis tolerada máxima *f*, *inv*

mayonnaise, mayonesa

M.D., médico

MDR/**minimum daily requirements**, requerimientos diarios mínimos

meager, escaso *adj*

meal, comida; **balanced** ~ comida balanceada

Meals on Wheels, comidas llevadas al domicilio

mean deviation, desviación media *f*

meaning, significado

measles, granuja *slang*; morbilia; sarampión *m*; sarampión malo *m*; tapetillo de los niños *fam*; **bastard** ~ (*See rubella.*); **German** ~ (*See German measles.*); **live** ~ **virus vaccine** vacuna antisarampión de virus vivo

measure, medida

measure, to, estimar; medir (i)

measurement, medida

measuring, ~ **cup** taza de medir; ~ **glass** copa graduada; ~ **tape** cinta métrica

meat, carne *f*

meats, organ, vísceras

meatus, meato

mechanic, mecánico

mechanical, mecánico *adj*

mechanism, mecanismo; **defense** ~ mecanismo de defensa; **escape** ~ mecanismo de escape

meconium, meconio

medial, interno *adj*

median, mediano *adj*; ~ **lethal dose** dosis fatal media *f*, *inv*; dosis letal media *f*, *inv*; ~ **nerve** nervio mediano

mediate, to, mediar

mediator, mediador

Medicaid, Medicaid *m*; Asistencia Médica

medical, médico *adj*; facultativo *adj*; ~ **advice** consejo médico; ~ **adviser** consejero médico; ~ **attention**/**care** asistencia médica; ~ **bulletin** parte facultativo *m*; ~ **card** ficha médica; ~ **certificate** certificado médico; ~ **consultant** médico consultor; médico de apelación; médico de consulta; ~ **corps** servicio de sanidad; ~ **diagnosis** dictamen médico *m*; ~ **doctor** médico; doctor en medicina; ~ **duty** deber médico *m*; servicio médico de guardia; ~ **ethics** ética medica; ~ **examination** examen médico *Chicano*; reconocimiento médico; ~

examiner médico forense; médico que emite informes (para una compañía de seguros); ~ **facility** facilidad médica *f*; clínica; hospital *m*; ~ **group** grupo médico; ~ **history** hoja clínica; ~ **jurisprudence** medicina legal; ~ **laboratory** laboratorio médico; ~ **orderly** enfermero; ~ **personnel** personal médico *m*; ~ **prescription** receta médica; receta facultativa; ~ **procedures** procedimientos médicos; ~ **record** (*of patient*) expediente del paciente *m*; ~ **records** registros médicos; ~ **records** (*department*) departamento de archivo clínico; ~ **report** dictamen facultativo *m*; ~ **school** facultad de medicina *f*; ~ **science** ciencia médica; ~ **staff** cuadro médico; cuadro facultativo; ~ **student** estudiante de medicina *m/f*; ~ **treatment** tratamiento médico; ~ (*school, student, etc.*) de medicina; ~ **book** libro de medicina; ~ **student** estudiante de medicina *m/f*

Medicare, Medicare *m*

medicate, to, medicar; medicinar

medicated, medicinal *adj*; ~ **bath** baño medicinal; baño medicamentoso

medication, medicación *f*; medicamento; medicina; **conservative** ~ medicación conservadora; **substitutive** ~ medicación derivativa

medicinal, medicinal *adj*; ~ **beer** cerveza medicinal; ~ **distilled water** agua[3] destilada medicamentosa; hidrolato; ~ **oil** oleólico; ~ **rash** dermatitis medicamentosa *f*; ~ **water solution** hidrolado

medicine, droga; medicamento; medicina; médico *adj*; remedio; ~ **cabinet** despensa *Chicano*; ~ **chest** botiquín *m*; **clinical** ~ medicina clínica; **community** ~ medicina comunal; ~ **dropper** cuentagotas *m, inv*; **environmental** ~ medicina ecológica; **experimental** ~ medicina experimental; **family** ~ medicina familiar; **folk** ~ curanderismo; **forensic** ~ medicina forense; medicina legal; ~ **form** forma medicamentosa; **geriatric** ~ medicina geriátrica; **homeopathic** ~ medicina homeopática; **internal** ~ medicina interna; **nuclear** ~ medicina nuclear; **occupational** ~ medicina ocupacional; **operative** ~ medicina operatoria; **patent** ~ medicina de la farmacia; medicina de la botica; medicina patentada; medicina registrada; específico *m, Med*; patente *m, Cu*; **preventive** ~ medicina preventiva; **psychosomatic** ~ medicina psicosomática[9]; **socialized** ~ medicina socializada; **sports** ~ medicina deportiva; **tropical** ~ medicina tropical; medicina colonial; **veterinary** ~ (medicina) veterinaria

medicolegal, medicolegal *adj*

meditate, to, meditar

medium, mediano *adj*; medio; **clearing** ~ medio aclarante; **contrast** ~ medio de contraste; **culture** ~ medios de cultivo; **nutrient** ~ medio nutritivo

medley, mezcla

medulla, médula; ~ **dorsalis** médula espinal; ~ **oblongata** bulbo raquídeo; médula oblonga(da); ~ **ossium** (*bone marrow*) médula ósea; ~ **spinal(is)** médula espinal; ~ **suprarenal** médula suprarrenal

meek, dócil *adj*; manso *adj*

meet, to, ~ (*debt*) costear; ~ (*to encounter*) encontrar(se) (ue) (con); reunirse (con); ~ (*to make acquaintance of*) conocer; ~ (*obligations*) cumplir con; ~ (*to see*) ver

meeting, encuentro; reunión *f*
megadose, megadosis *f, inv*
megalomania, megalomanía
megavitamin, megavitamina
melancholia, melancolía; **agitated**
~ melancolía agitada
melancholy, melancólico *adj*;
melancolía
melanin, melanina
melanoma, melanoma *m*
melt, to, ~ (*to make liquid*) derretir
(i); ~ (*to dissolve*) disolver (ue)
melting point, punto de fusión
melting-pot, crisol *m*
**member of police narcotics
squad**, narco[2]
membrane, membrana; tela; **hyaline** ~ membrana hialina; **mucous** ~ membrana mucosa;
perineal ~ membrana perineal;
permeable ~ membrana permeable; **placental** ~ membrana de la
placenta; **semipermeable** ~
membrana semipermeable;
serous ~ membrana serosa; **tympanic** ~ membrana timpánica
memorize, to, memorizar
memory, memoria; **long-term** ~
memoria remota; ~ **loss** amnesia; pérdida de memoria; **short-
term** ~ memoria inmediata;
memoria reciente
menarchal, menárquico *adj*
menarche, menarca; menarquia;
menarquía; primera regla
mend, to, componer(se); reparar
mendable, reparable *adj*
Mendel's laws, leyes de Mendel *f,
pl*
Ménière's disease, enfermedad
de Ménière *f*; vértigo
meningeal, meníngeo *adj*
meninges, meninges *f, pl*
meningitis, meningitis *f*; (**acute**)
aseptic ~ meningitis aséptica
(aguda); **cerebral** ~ meningitis
cerebral; **cerebrospinal** ~ meningitis cerebrospinal; **lymphocytic**
~ meningitis linfocítica; **spinal** ~

meningitis espinal; **tubercular** ~
meningitis tuberculosa
meningococcus, meningococo
meniscus, menisco
menopausal, menopáusico *adj*
menopause, cambio de vida; climatérico; menopausia
menorrhagia, menorragia; reglas
muy abundantes
menorrhalgia, menorralgia; hiper-
menorrea; menstruación dolorosa *f*
menses, menstruación *f*; menstruo *sg*; reglas
menstrual, menstrual *adj*; ~ **cycle**
ciclo menstrual; ~ **discharge**
desecho; ~ **disorder** trastorno
menstrual; ~ **flow** flujo menstrual; ~ **period** menstruación *f*;
período menstrual; regla
menstruate, to, estar enferma *fam*;
estar indispuesta; estar mala;
estar mala de la luna; estar
mala de la garra; menstruar;
perder (ie) sangre; reglar; tener el mes; tener la garra
menstruation, achaque *m, fam*; administración *f, Mex*; costumbre
f; enferma *euph*; luna *Chicano*;
menstruación *f* (*general term*);
mes *m*; período *fam*; regla *Mex,
PR*; tiempo del mes *fam*; **difficult** ~ dismenorrea
mental, mental *adj*; ~ **age** edad
mental *f*; ~ **deficiency** retraso
mental; ~ **derangement** enajenación mental *f*; ~ **disease** enfermedad emocional *f*; enfermedad
mental *f*; ~ **disorder** trastorno
mental; enajenación mental *f*; ~
disturbance trastorno mental;
taranta *CR, Ec*; ~ **health** salud
mental *f*; ~ **health department**
departamento de enfermedades
mentales; ~ **health program** programa de salud mental *m*; ~ **hygiene** higiene mental *f*; ~ **illness**
enfermedad mental *f*; ~ **problems** problemas mentales *m*; ~

retardation retardación *f*; retardo; retardo mental; retraso mental; debilidad mental *f*; ~ **state** estado mental; ~ **strain** agotamiento mental; esfuerzo mental; ~ **test** examen de capacidad mental *m*; **unbalanced** ~ **condition** desequilibrio *Med*
mentality, mentalidad *f*
mentally, mentalmente *adv*; ~ **ill** alienado *m. adj*; ~ **retarded**, inocente *adj, euph*; retardado *adj*; simple *adj, euph*; ~ **unbalanced person**, perturbado
menthol, mentol *m*
mentholatum, mentolato *Chicano*
mention, mención *f*
mention, to, mencionar
mentum, mentón *m*; barbilla
menu, menú *m*
merciful, misericordioso *adj*
merciless, despiadado *adj*
Mercurochrome, mercurocromo
mercury, mercurio
mercy, misericordia; ~ **death/killing** eutanasia
merge, to, unir
meridian, meridiano; ~ **of the cornea** meridiano de la córnea; ~ **of the eye** meridiano del ojo
Merthiolate, mertiolato
mescaline[5], mescalina; peyote *m, fam*
mesenteric, mesentérico *adj*
mesenteritis, mesenteritis *f*
mesentery, mesenterio
mesh, malla; ~**-graft** injerto en malla; ~ (*reticulum*) retícula
mesial, mesial *adj*; orientado hacia el centro
mesiobuccal, mesiobucal *adj*
mesiobucco-occlusal, mesiobucooclusal *adj*
mesiobuccopulpal, mesiobucopulpar *adj*
mesiocervical, mesiocervical *adj*
mesiogingival, mesiogingival *adj*
mesio-incisal, mesioincisivo *adj*
mesiolabial, mesiolabial *adj*

mesiolingual, mesiolingual *adj*
mesiolinguo-occlusal, mesiolinguoclusal *adj*
mesio-occlusal, mesioclusal *adj*
mesio-occlusodistal/M.O.D., mesioclusodistal *adj*
mesiopulpal, mesiopulpar *adj*
mesiopulpolabial, mesiopulpolabial *adj*
mesiopulpolingual, mesiopulpolingual *adj*
mesmerize, to, hipnotizar
mesocardium, mesocardio
mesoderm, mesodermo
mesogastrium, mesogastrio
mess, ~ (*disorderly state*) desorden *m*; **to make a** ~ (*to disarrange*) desordenar; ~ (*jam, muddle*) lío; **to get into a** ~ meterse en un lío; ~ (*something dirty*) porquería; **to make a** ~ (*to dirty*) ensuciar
message, mensaje *m*; recado
messenger RNA, ARN mensajero
mestizo with Chinese blood, injerto *Perú*
metabolic, metabólico *adj*; ~ **arthropathy** artropatías metabólicas; ~ **rate** índice metabólico *m*; intensidad del metabolismo basal *f*
metabolism, metabolismo; **basal** ~ metabolismo basal; **constructive** ~ (*anabolism*) anabolismo; metabolismo constructivo; asimilación *f*; **destructive** ~ (*catabolism*) catabolismo; desasimilación *f*; metabolismo destructivo; **endogenous** ~ metabolismo endógeno; **exogenous** ~ metabolismo exógeno
metacarpal, metarcarpiano *m, adj*; ~ **bones** huesos metacarpianos
metacarpus, metacarpo
metacycline, metaciclina
metal, metal *m*; **alkali** ~ metal alcalino; ~ **base** base metálica *f*
metallergy, metalergia
metallic tinkling, sonido metálico
metamorphosis, metamorfosis *f, inv*

metampicillin, metampicilina
metaphase, metafase *f*
metaphysis, metáfisis *f*
metastasis, metástasis *f*
metastasize, to, dar metástasis; metastatizar
metatarsal, metatarsiano *adj*
metatarsalgia, metatarsalgia
metatarsus, metatarso
meteorism, meteorismo
meter, metro
methadone, metadona
methane, metano *Chem*
methanol, metanol *m*
method, método; **birth control ~** método anticonceptivo; (*See birth control.*); **~ for creatinine** método para creatinina; **rhythm ~** método de ritmo
methodology, metodología
methyl, metilo; metílico *adj*; **~ alcohol** alcohol metílico *m*; **~ chloride** cloruro de metilo; **~ ether** éter de metilo *m*
meticulous, meticuloso *adj*
metric, métrico *adj*; **~ system** sistema métrico *m*
metrodynia, metrodinia
metrorrhagia, metrorragia; hemorragia uterina sin relación menstrual; pérdidas rojas
metrosalpingitis, metrosalpingitis *f*
MI/myocardial infarct, infarto miocárdico
miasma, miasma *m*
microbacterium, microbacteria
microbe, microbio; microorganismo
microbial, microbiano *adj*
microbiology, microbiología
microcardia, pequeñez del corazón *f*
microfiche, microficha
microfilm, microfilme *m*
microgram, microgramo
micron, micrón *m*
microorganism, microorganismo
microscope, microscopio; **binocular ~** microscopio binocular;

compound ~ microscopio compuesto; **electron ~** microscopio electrónico; **fluorescence/fluorescent ~** microscopio de fluorescencia; **phase difference ~** microscopio de fase; **~ slide** portaobjetos *m, inv*
microscopic section, corte microscópico *m*
microscopy, microscopia
microsection, microsección *f*
microsurgery, microcirugía
microtome, micrótomo
microwave, microonda
micturate, to, orinar
midbrain, cerebro medio; mesencéfalo
middle, medio *m, adj*; **~ age** edad madura *f*; **~-aged** de mediana edad; **around the ~** (*waist*) alrededor de la cintura; **~ ear** oído medio; **~ finger** dedo del corazón; dedo medio; **~ lobe syndrome** síndrome del lóbulo medio del pulmón *m*; **~ name** segundo nombre *m*; **~-sized** (*person*) de mediana estatura; **~-sized** (*thing*) de tamaño mediano
midget, enano
midgut, intestino medio
midline, línea media
midnight, medianoche *f*
mid-pelvic plane, estrecho medio de la pelvis
midstream, **~ jet of urine** orina de la mitad de la micción; **~ specimen** muestra de orina recogida a mitad de la micción
midwife, comadrona, comadrón; partera, partero; **~** (*empiric, untrained*) comadrona; **~** (*licensed, trained*) partera; **~** (*quack*) rinconera; **~** (*untrained*) facultativa
midwifery, obstetricia; tocología
migraine, jaqueca; hemicránea; migraña; zangarri(an)a
migrating abscess, absceso migrante

migration, migración *f*
mild, leve *adj*; ligero *adj*; ~ **sedative** sedante ligero; ~ **streptococcus** estreptococo leve; ~ (*disease*, *illness*) benigno *adj*; ~ **disorder** enfermedad benigna *f*;~ (*food*, *drink*) flojo *adj*; ~ (*medicine*, *tobacco*, *etc.*) suave *adj*
mildew, moho; ~ (*on vine*) mildeu *m*; mildiu *m*; ~ (*on plant*) añublo
mildew, to, enmohecerse
mildly, ~ (*lightly*, *slightly*) ligeramente *adv*; ~ (*softly*) suavemente *adv*
milk, leche *f*; milque *f*, *Chicano*; ~ **abscess** absceso de la mama; **breast** ~ leche materna; **chocolate** ~ leche con chocolate; **condensed** ~ leche condensada; **cow's** ~ leche de vaca; ~ **crust** costra láctea; ~ **diet** dieta láctea; ~ **duct** conducto galactóforo; conducto mamario; **evaporated** ~ leche evaporizada; **fortified** ~ leche fortificada; **goat's** ~ leche de cabra; **homogenized** ~ leche homogeneizada; **low fat** ~ leche baja en grasa; **mother's breast** ~ leche materna; ~ **of magnesia** leche de magnesia; **pasteurized** ~ leche pasteurizada; **powdered** ~ leche en polvo; ~ **product** producto lácteo; ~ **protein** proteína de la leche; **raw** ~ leche sin procesar; leche bronca *Mex*; **skim** ~ leche descremada; leche desnatada; **skimmed** ~ leche desnatada; **sour** ~ leche agria; **sterilized** ~ leche esterilizada; ~ **teeth** dientes caducos *m*; dientes de leche *m*; ~ **testing** examen de leche *m*; **whole** ~ leche entera
milk, to, ordeñar
milking, ordeño
milky, lácteo *adj*; lechoso *adj*; ~ **cataract** catarata hipermadura
milligram, miligramo
milliliter, mililitro

millimeter, milímetro
mimetic labor, parto falso
mince one's words, not to, no tener pelos en la lengua
mince, to, (*meat*) picar
mind, mente *f*; **conscious** ~ mente consciente; ~ (*memory*) memoria; ~ (*intelligence*) inteligencia; ~ (*sanity*) juicio; **in one's right** ~ en su sano juicio; **peace of** ~ tranquilidad de espíritu *f*; **sound in** ~ cuerdo *adj*; **state of** ~ estado de ánimo; **to be out of one's** ~ haber perdido el juicio; **to take a great weight off one's** ~ quitarle a alguien un peso de encima
mind, to, ~ (*to take care of*) cuidar; ~ (*to worry about*) preocuparse por
mineral, mineral *m*; ~ **oil** aceite mineral *m*; ~ **salt** sales minerales *f*; ~ **supplements** suplementos minerales; ~ **water** agua[3] mineral
minimize, to, reducir al mínimo
minimum, mínimo; ~ **effective dose** dosis efectiva mínima *f*, *inv*; ~ **lethal dose** dosis letal mínima *f*, *inv*; ~ **wage** salario mínimo
minister, ministro; pastor *m*
minor, ~ (*age*, *size*) menor *m/f*, *adj*; ~ (*secondary*) secundario *adj*; ~ (*slight*) leve *adj*; ~ (*small*) menudo *adj*
mint, hierbabuena; yerbabuena; ~ **leaves** hojas de yerbabuena
minute, ~ (*precise*) minucioso *adj*; ~ (*part of a degree*; *time*) minuto
miocardia, miocardia
miosis/myosis, miosis *f*
miracle, milagro
miraculous, milagroso *adj*
mirage, espejismo
mirror, espejo; **dental** ~ odontoscopio; **head** ~ espejo frontal; ~ **writing** escritura como en un espejo; escritura en espejo
misalignment, error de alineación *m*

misanthrope, misántropo *m, adj*
misanthropy, misantropía
misbehave, to, portarse mal
misbehaved, mal criado *adj*
miscalculate, hacer un error
miscalculation, error de cálculo *m*
miscarriage, aborto; aborto accidental; aborto natural; mal parto; malparto; parto malogrado
miscarry, to, abortar
mischief, travesura
mischievous, travieso *adj*
misdiagnosis, diagnóstico equivocado
misery, ~ (*misfortune*) desgracia; ~ (*pain, suffering*) sufrimiento; ~ (*poverty*) pobreza
misfit, mal adaptado *adj*
misformed, malformativo *adj*
misinform, to, dar información errónea
misinformed, mal informado *adj*
misjudge, to, tener una opinión errónea
mishap, accidente *m*
mismatched blood transfusion, transfusión de sangre incompatible *f*
misogynous, misógino *adj*
misogyny, misoginia
misplaced gout, gota metastática; gota retrógrada
miss, to, ~ (*a person*) echar de menos; extrañar; ~ (*an appointment*) faltar; ~ (*a dose of something*) dejar de tomar; ~ (*to overlook*) perder (ie)
missing, ~ (*absent*) ausente *adj*; ~ **tooth** diente ausente *m*; ~ (*disappeared*) desaparecido *adj*; ~ (*lost*) perdido *adj*; **to be** ~ faltar
mistake, error *m*
mistaken (about), to be, equivocarse (acerca de); rajarse *Arg, Col*
mistletoe, muérdago
mistrust, ~ (*lack of confidence*) desconfianza; ~ (*suspicion*) recelo
mistrust, to, desconfiar de

misunderstand, to, comprender mal
misunderstanding, equivocación *f*
misuse, abuso; maluso
mite, (*insect*) acárido; ácaro
mitigate, to, mitigar
mitochondria, mitocondria; condriosoma *m*
mitosis, mitosis *f*
mitral, mitral *adj*; ~ **lesion** lesión mitral *f*; ~ **regurgitation** regurgitación mitral *f*; ~ **stenosis**, estenosis mitral *f*; ~ **valve** válvula mitral; ~ **valve insufficiency** insuficiencia de la válvula mitral; ~ **valve prolapse/MVP** prolapso de la válvula mitral; cierre defectuoso de la válvula mitral *m*
mix, to, mezclar; ~ (*cement, flour, etc.*) amasar; ~ (*drinks*) preparar; ~ (*several ingredients*) mezclar
mixed, mixto *adj*
mixture, mezcla; mixtura
ml/milliliter, mililitro
moan, ~ (*complaint*) queja; protesta; ~ (*groan*) gemido; quejadera *Col, Mex*; quejido; quejumbre *f*
moan, to, ~ (*to complain*) quejarse (de); ~ (*to groan*) gemir (i)
moaning, ~ (*complaining*) quejoso *adj*; ~ (*groaning*) que gime
mobile, móvil *adj*
mobility, movilidad *f*
mobilization, movilización *f*
mobilize, to, movilizar
mock angina, angina de pecho refleja
M.O.D./mesio-occlusodistal, mesioclusodistal *adj*
mode, moda
moderate, moderado *adj*; ~ **physical exercise** ejercicio físico moderado
moderation, moderación *f*
modern, moderno *adj*
modest, modesto *adj*
modesty, pudor *m*
modification, modificación *f*
modify, to, modificar

moist, húmedo *adj*
moisten, to, humedecer; mojar
moisture, (*dampness*) humedad *f*
moisturize, to, humedecer
moisturizing, hidratante *adj*; ~
    cream crema hidratante
molar, diente molar *m*; molar *m*;
    muela; impacted ~ molar im-
    pactado; sixth-year ~ primera
    muela permanente; third molar
    (*See tooth, wisdom.*); twelfth-year
    ~ segunda muela permanente
mold, ~ (*fungus*) moho; ~ (*hollow
    container*) molde *m*
mold, to, ~ (*to grow fungus*) enmo-
    hecerse; ~ (*to shape*) moldear
mole, ~ (*birthmark*) lunar *m*; man-
    cha; ~ (*uterine mass*) mola; cys-
    tic ~ mola cística; fleshy ~ mola
    carnosa; invasive ~ mola ma-
    ligna; ~ (*nevus*) nevo; common
    ~ nevo intradérmico; hairy ~
    nevo piloso; pigmented ~ nevo
    pigmentario
molecular biology, biología mole-
    cular
molecule, molécula
molt, to, mudar
mom, mamá
moment, momento
money, dinero
mongolism, mongolismo
mongoloid, mongoloide *adj*
Monilia, Monilia
moniliasis, algodoncillo; boquera;
    candidiasis *f*; moniliasis *f*;
    muguet *m*
monitor, monitor *m*; cardiac ~
    monitor cardíaco; fetal heart ~
    monitor cardíaco fetal; Holter
    ~ monitor cardíaco portátil
monitor, to, monitorizar
monitoring, control del ritmo
    cardíaco *m*; monitoreo; moni-
    toría; observación continuada
    f; blood pressure ~ monitoría
    de la presión arterial; cardiac ~
    monitoría cardíaca; fetal heart
    ~ monitoría del corazón fetal

monoblast, monoblasto
monocytic, monocítico *adj*
mononucleosis, mononucleosis *f*;
    infectious ~ mononucleosis agu-
    da *f*; mononucleosis infecciosa *f*
monosodium   glutamate/MSG,
    glutamato monosódico
month, mes *m*
monthly, al mes *adv*; mensual-
    mente *adv*; por meses *adv*
mood, estado de ánimo; humor
    m; ~ elevator estimulante *m*; to
    be in a bad ~ estar con la
    viaraza *Col, Guat, Ríopl*; estar de
    chicha *CA, Ec*
moral, moraleja; moral *adj*; ~ de-
    cision decisión moral *f*; ~ in-
    sanity depravación mental *f*
morale, moral *f*
morbid, morboso *adj*; patológico
    adj
morbidity, morbilidad *f*, *Med*;
    morbosidad; ~ rate, índice de
    morbilidad *m*
morbilli (measles), morbilia; sa-
    rampión *m*
more, más; ~ or less más o menos
morgue, depósito de cadáveres;
    morgue *f*, *Chicano*; necrocomio
morning, mañana; ~ glory seeds[6,8]
    semillas de dondiego del día[2];
    dompedro[2]; good ~ buenos
    días *m, pl*; ~ sickness achaques
    mañaneros *m*; ansias matutinas;
    enfermedad matutina *f*; mal de
    madre *m*; náuseas del embara-
    zo; vómitos del embarazo; to-
    morrow ~ mañana por la
    mañana; ~ tongue lengua pas-
    tosa; ~-after vomiting vómito
    matutino
morose, (*gloomy*) taciturno *adj*
morphine[7], morfi[2]; morfina[2]
morphogenesis, morfogénesis *f*
morphological constitutional type,
    tipo constitucional morfológico
morphology, morfología
morsel, bocado
mortal, mortal *adj*

mortality, mortalidad *f*; **annual actual ~** mortalidad actual anual; **~ rate** índice de mortalidad *m*; tasa de mortalidad; **perinatal ~** mortalidad perinatal

mortuary, depósito de cadáveres; mortuorio *adj*

mosquito, mosquito; zancudo *Chicano*

mother, madre *f*; mamá; **nursing ~** mujer lactante *f*

motion,~ (*movement*) movimiento; **~ sickness** mareo; **~** (*gesture*) ademán *m*

motion, to, indicar con la mano

motionless, inmóvil *adj*

motor, motor *m*; **~ functions** motricidad *f*; **~ neuron** neurona motora; **~ speech area** centro del lenguaje

mottled, jaspeado *adj*; **~ areas** zonas moteadas; **~ enamel** fluorosis dental *f*; **~ teeth** dientes moteados *m*; **~** (*skin*) con manchas

mottling, moteado *adj*

mountain sickness, puna *SpAm, Med*; soroche *m, SpAm*

mounting, montaje *m*

mourn for, to, llorar la muerte de

mourning, luto; **deep ~** luto rigoroso; **to be in ~** estar de luto; **to come out of deep ~** aliviar el luto; **to be in ~ for** llevar luto por; **to come out of ~** dejar el luto; quitarse el luto; **to go into ~** ponerse de luto; vestirse (i) de luto

mouse, ratón *m*

moustache, bigote *m*; mostacho

mouth, **~** boca *Anat*; bucal *adj, Anat*; trompa *Anat, fam*; **~ cavity** cavidad bucal *f*; **~-breathing** respiración bucal *f*; **~-to mouth breathing** respiración boca a boca *f*; **~ -to-mouth resuscitation** resucitación boca a boca *f*; **roof of the ~** cielo de la boca; **through the ~** por vía bucal *prep phr*; **trench ~** boca de trinchera; **~ wash** enjuagatorio; lavado bucal;

listerina *fam*; **~** (*entrance*) entrada; **~** (*of a tube, etc.*) abertura

mouthful, **~** (*eating*) bocada; **~** (*of smoke, air, etc.*) bocanada

mouth-of-the-womb, hocico de tenca

mouthpiece, bocal *m*; boquilla; pieza bucal; portavoz *m*

move, to, mover (ue); **~ the bowels** hacer caca *vulg*; obrar

movement, movimiento; **associated ~** movimiento asociado; **automatic ~** movimiento automático; **bowel ~** defecación *f, form*; evacuación *f*; **fetal ~** movimiento fetal; **functional mandibular ~** movimiento mandibular funcional; **rapid eye ~** movimientos oculares rápidos; **reflex ~** movimiento reflejo; **spontaneous ~** movimiento espontáneo; **sudden ~** repente *m*

mucilage, mucílago

mucoid, mucoide *adj*

mucosa, mucosa

mucosity, mucosidad *f*

mucous, mucoso *adj*; **~ colitis** colitis mucosa *f*; **~ membrane** mucosa; **~ rale** estertor *m*

mucus, flema; frío *slang, Mex*; moco; mocosidad *f*; moquera *fam*

mud, barro; lodo; **~** (*thick*) fango; **~ bath** baño de fango; **~** (*in a river*) limo

muddy, limoso *adj*; fangoso *adj*; lleno de barro *adj*

muffled, **~ sound** sonido sordo; **~ voice** voz apagada *f*

muggy, (*weather*) bochornoso *adj*

muguet, (*See thrush.*)

multicare health facility, centro médico polivalente

multicellular, multicelular *adj*

multifunctional, multifuncional *adj*; polivalente *adj*

multipara, (*pl, multiparae*) multípara

multiparity, multiparidad *f*

multiparous, multíparo *adj*

multiple, múltiple *adj*; ~ **birth** alumbramiento múltiple; parto múltiple; ~ **myeloma** mieloma múltiple *m*; ~ **organ failure** fallo múltiple de órganos; ~ **personality** personalidad múltiple *f*; ~ **pregnancy** gravidez múltiple; ~ **sclerosis** esclerosis diseminada *f*; esclerosis en placa *f*; esclerosis múltiple *f*

multiplication, multiplicación *f*

mumble, to, decir entre dientes; mascullar; refunfuñar

mumbling, mascullamiento; refunfuño

mummification, momificación *f*

mummy, momia

mumps, bolas *Chicano*; buche *m*, *Mex*; chanza *Chicano*; coquetas *Mex*; farfallota *PR*; mompes *m*, *pl*, *Chicano*; paperas; parótida; parótidas *pl*; parotiditis *f*

murmur, ~ (*general term*) murmullo; ~ (*abnormal heart sound*) soplo *Med*; **aneurysmal** ~ soplo aneurismático; **aortic** ~ soplo aórtico; **arterial** ~ soplo arterial; **bellows** ~ soplo de fuelle; **cardiac** ~ soplo cardíaco; **cardiopulmonary** ~ soplo cardiopulmonar; **cardiorespiratory** ~ soplo cardiorrespiratorio; **diastolic** ~ soplo diastólico; **endocardial** ~ soplo endocardíaco; **functional** ~ soplo funcional; **heart** ~ soplo cardíaco; **mitral** ~ soplo mitral; **organic** ~ soplo orgánico; **pansystolic** ~ soplo pansistólico; **prediastolic** ~ soplo prediastólico; **presystolic** ~ soplo presistólico; **regurgitant** ~ soplo regurgitante; **stenosal** ~ soplo estenósico; **systolic** ~ soplo sistólico; **tricuspid** ~ soplo tricuspídeo; **vesicular** ~ soplo vesicular; ~ (*noise*) ruido; **mewing** ~ ruido de maullido; ~ (*of voice, etc.*) murmullo

muscle, músculo; **antagonistic** ~ músculo antagonista; ~**s of the back** músculos dorsales; **cardiac** ~ músculo cardíaco; **cutaneous** ~ músculo dérmico; **flexor** ~ músculo flexor; **hamstring** ~**s** músculos posteriores del muslo; **involuntary** ~ músculo involuntario; **pulled** ~ desgarro leve; estiramiento *form*; ~ **relaxants** relajadores musculares *m*; miorrelajantes *m*; ~ **rods** miofibrillas; **sartorius** ~ músculo sartorio; **skeletal** ~ músculo esquelético; **smooth** ~ músculo liso; ~ **spindles** husos musculares; **striated** ~ músculo estriado; ~ **tone** tono muscular; **visceral** ~ músculo visceral; **vo-luntary** ~ músculo voluntario; **not to move a** ~ permanecer impasible *fam*

muscular, muscular *adj*; ~ **contractions** contracciones musculares *f*; ~ **dystrophy** distrofia muscular; **progressive** ~ **dystrophy** distrofia muscular progresiva; ~ **fatigue** fatiga muscular; ~ **function test** prueba funcional muscular; ~ **relaxation** relajamiento muscular; ~ **twitching** sacudida muscular

musculature, musculatura

musculoskeletal, musculoesquelético *adj*

mushroom, champiñón *m*; hongo; seta; ~ **poisoning** intoxicación por hongos *f*

mushy stool, caca aguada *slang*; excremento aguado

mussel, almeja

mustard, mostaza; ~ **bath** baño de mostaza; ~ **plaster** cataplasma de mostaza; sinapismo; ~ **water** agua³ con mostaza

mutagen, mutágeno

mutant, mutante *adj*

mutation, mutación *f*

mute, calloso *adj*; mudo *adj*; silencioso *adj*

mutilate, to, mutilar

mutilation, mutilación *f*

mutter, to, cuchichear *fam*; decir entre dientes; ~ (*angrily*) refunfuñar

muzzle, hocico

myalgia, mialgia; miodinia

myasthenia gravis, miastenia grave *f*

myatrophy, miatrofia; amiotrofia

mycosis, micosis *f*

myelasthenia, mielastenia

myelin, mielina

myelinated, mielinado *adj*

myelinization, mielinización *f*

myelitis, mielitis *f*

myeloblast, mieloblasto

myelocyte, mielocito

myelogram, mielograma *m*

myeloid, mieloide *adj*

myocardia, miocardia

myocardial, miocárdico *adj*; ~ **infarction** ataque al corazón *m*; infarto de(l) miocardio; infarto miocardíaco; infarto miocardiaco

myocardiography, miocardiografía

myocardiopathy, miocardiopatía

myocarditis, miocarditis *f*

myocardium, miocardio

myoceptor, mioceptor *m*

myopia, (*nearsightedness*) cortedad de la vista *f*; miopía; **progressive** ~ miopía progresiva

myopic, (*nearsighted*) miope *m/f*, *adj*; miópico *adj*

---

[1] I have followed the spelling given in the *Diccionario de la lengua española*, RAE, 21st edition, 1990. Spanish does recognize variations using *j* and *h*.

[2] This is new vocabulary, not necessarily listed yet recognized by the Royal Academy of Spanish Grammar. It is understood that this vocabulary is primarily slang. Unless otherwise indicated, the gender of nouns is assumed to be obvious.

[3] For pronunciation purposes, the masculine definite and indefinite articles, *el* and *un*, not *la* or *una*, are used when the article immediately precedes the feminine singular noun which begins with stressed *a* or any other that begins with stressed *ha*.

[4] Current English street terminology for *marijuana* includes: a-bomb, a-stick, Acapulco gold, ace, African black, Alice B. Toklas, baby, bale, bar, bhang, black gunion, boo, brick, broccoli, buddha sticks, bush, butter flower, can, Canadian black, cannabis sativa, charge, cocktail, colombo, Colombian, Colombian red, C.S. dagga, dawamesk, doobee, dope, dry high, dube, duby, fatty, finger lid, flower tops, fuma d'Angola, funny stuff, gage, Gainesville green, ganga, gangster, ganja, giggle weed, giggles-smoke, goblet of jam, gold, gold Colombian, golden leaf, gold star, goof but, grass, grasshopper, green, grefa, greta, griefo, griefs, grifa, griffo, gunga, gungeon, gunja, haircut, has, Hawaiian, hay, hemp, herb, hooch, Indian hay, Indian hemp, intsagu, intsagu, J, Jane, jay, jay smoke, jive, jive stick, Juana, Juanita, Juanita weed, juja, kaif, Kansas grass, kauii, kee, key, ki, kick sticks, kif, killer weed, kilter, light stuff, loaf, loco, locoweed, loveweed, mach, macon, maconha, marihuana, mariguana, Mary, Mary Anne, Mary Jane, Mary Warner, Mary Werner, Mary Wearver, Mary Worner, match box, mauii, Mex, Mexican, Mexican brown, Mexican green, Mexican locoweed, M.J., mohasky, moocah, moota, mooters, mootie, mor a grifa, mota, moto, mu, muggles, muta(h), nail, nigra, number, Panama gold, Panama red, panatella, pin, pod, pot, potlikker, P.R. (Panama red), Puff the Dragon, rainy day woman, red dirt marijuana, reefer, righteous bush, roach, root, rope, Rose Maria, rough stuff, sativa, seeds, shit, sinsemilla, skinny, smoke, smoke Canada, snop, stack, stems, stick, super pot, Sweet Lucy, T, tea, Texas tea, thrupence bag, thumb, tustin, twist, weed, wheat, yesca.

[5] Current English terminology for *mescaline* includes: anhalonium, beans, big chief, blue caps, blue devils, buttons, cactus, full moon, hikori, huatari, mesc, mescal, mescal buttons, moon, plants, seni.

[6] Current English street terminology for *morning glory seeds* includes: badoh negro, blue star, flying saucers, glory seeds, heavenly blues, pearly gates, pearly whites, seeds.

[7] Current English street terminology for *morphine* includes: cobies, cube, dope, em-sel, first line, goods, hard stuff, hocus, junk, M, morf, morphie, morpho, morphy, mud, Miss Emma, mojo, sister.

[8] Part of the Drug Abuse Vocabulary.

[9] English words that have an initial *ps* now may be spelled either with or without the *p* in Spanish. In either case, the *p* is silent when the Spanish word is pronounced. This dictionary will show such words with a parenthesis around the *p*.

N

nag, to, ~ (*to bother insistently*) machacar; ~ (*the conscience*) remorder (ue)

nagging, ~ (*complaining*) quejica *adj*; ~ (*constant*) persistente *adj*; ~ (*pain*) lancinante *adj*; punzante *adj*

nail, ~ (*metal spike*) clavo; ~ (*needle for drug injection*) abuja²; aguja²; filero²; hierro²; jeringuilla²; punta²; ~ (*of a finger, toe*) uña; ~ **bed** lecho de la uña; lecho ungueal; matriz de la uña *f*; ~ **biting** onicofagia *form*; ~ **clippers** cortauñas *m, inv*, ~ **file** lima para las uñas; **finger~** uña; ~ **fold** borde de las uñas *m*; ~ **groove** surco ungueal; **ingrown** ~ uña enterrada; ~ **polish** esmalte para las uñas *m*; ~ **scissors** tijeras para las uñas; ~ **scratch** arañazo; ~ **wall** repliegue ungueal *m*; **to be as hard as** ~ tener un corazón de piedra; **to bite one's** ~ comerse las uñas

naive, ingenuo *adj*

naiveté, ingenuidad *f*

naked, ~ (*body, part of body*) desnudo *adj*; empelotado *adj, Col, Chi, Cu, Mex*; veringo *adj, Col*; viringo *adj, Col, Ec*; ~ (*feet*) descalzo *adj*; ~ (*head*) descubierto *adj*; ~ **eye examination** examen a simple vista *m*; ~ (**from the waist down**) pilucho *adj, Chi*; **to strip (oneself)** ~ desnudarse; encalatarse *Perú*

name, ~ (*Christian name*) nombre *m*; ~ (*surname*) apellido

nanism, nanismo; enanismo

nap, siesta

nap, to, dormitar; **to take a** ~ echar una siesta; tomar una siesta

napalm, napalm *m*

nape, (*of the neck*) nuca; cogote *m, fam*

naphtha, nafta

naphthol, naftol *m*

napkin, servilleta; **sanitary** ~ paño higiénico; servilleta sanitaria

narcissism, narcisismo

narcissistic, narcisista *adj*

narcoanalysis, narcoanálisis *m*

narcohypnosis, narcohipnosis *f*

narcolepsy, narcolepsia

narcoleptic, narcoléptico *adj, m*

narcosis, narcosis *f*

narcotic, droga estupefaciente; droga somnífera; estupefaciente *m*; fármaco²; narcótico *m, adj*; ~ **pill** pinguas² *pl*; **any** ~ **substitute** la otra cosa²

narrow, estrecho *adj*; **~-breasted** estrecho de pecho *adj*; **~-chested** estrecho de pecho *adj*; **~-faced** estrecho de cara *adj*; **~-minded** de miras estrechas; **~-mindedness** estrechez de miras *f*; **~-waisted** ceñido *adj*

narrowing, estrechez *f*

nasal, nasal *adj* ~ **cavity** cavidad nasal *f*; ~ **congestion** congestión nasal *f*; ~ **drip** goteo nasal; moqueadera *Chicano*; moquera *fam*; ~ **obstruction** mormación *f, Chicano*; ~ **packing** taponamiento nasal; ~ **voice** voz gangosa *f*

nasalize, to, hablar con voz gangosa

nasociliary, nasociliar *adj*

nasogastric, nasogástrico *adj*; ~ **tube** tubo nasogástrico

nasty, ~ (*accident*) grave *adj*; ~ (*dirty*) asqueroso *adj*; ~ (*temper*) vivo *adj*; ~ (*wound, cut*) feo *adj*; **to leave** ~ **taste in the mouth** dejar mal sabor de boca; **to smell** ~

oler (ue) mal; **to taste** ~ saber mal; tener mal sabor

natal, natal *adj*; de nacimiento *prep phr*

natimortality, mortinatalidad *f*

nationality, nacionalidad *f*

native, nativo *adj*; ~ **born** oriundo de; ~ **tongue** lengua materna

natural, natural *adj*; ~ **causes** causas naturales; ~ **childbirth** parto indoloro; parto natural; ~ **defenses** defensas naturales

nature, índole *f*; naturaleza; ~ **of the illness** naturaleza de la enfermedad; ~ **treatment** tratamiento naturista

naturopath, naturalista *m/f*

naughtiness, ~ (*bad behavior*) mala conducta; ~ (*disobedience*) desobediencia; ~ (*mischief*) picardía

naughty, ~ (*bad*) malo *adj*; ~ (*disobedient*) desobediente *adj*; ~ (*mischievous*) pícaro *adj*

nausea, asco; basca; náusea(s); **morning** ~ asqueo; enfermedad matutina *f*; malestares de la mañana *m*; **to have** ~ deponer el estómago; volver (ue) el estómago

nauseated, to be ~ tener náusea(s); **to feel** ~ sentir (ie) bascas; **to make** ~ dar náusea(s)

navel, ombligo; pupo *Arg, Chi, Ec, Perú*; ~ **truss** venda umbilical

near, cercano *adj*

nearsighted, corto de vista *adj*; miope *adj*

nearsightedness, cortedad de vista *f*; miopía; vista corta

nebbis[4], amarillas[2]; gorras amarillas[2]

nebula, nube *f*

nebulization, atomización *f*; nebulización *f*

nebulize, to, atomizar

nebulizer, nebulizador *m*; atomizador *m*

necessary, necesario *adj*

necessity, necesidad *f*

neck, cuello *Anat*; ~ (*back part of*) nuca; **back of the** ~ cerviz *f*; nuca; **stiff** ~ cuello tieso; tortícolis *f*; ~ **stiffness** rigidez de nuca *f*; ~ (*front part of*) cuello; ~ (*of an instrument*) mango; ~ (*of an animal*) pescuezo; ~ (*of tooth, womb*) cuello

necklace, collar *m*

necrobiosis, necrobiosis *f*; ~ **lipoidica diabetica** necrobiosis lipóidica de los diabéticos *f*

necrology, necrología

necrophilia, necrofilia

necrophobia, necrofobia

necrose, to, (*See necrotize, to.*)

necrosis, necrosis *f*; **aseptic** ~ necrosis aséptica; **avascular** ~ necrosis avascular; **coagulative** ~ necrosis de coagulación; **colliquative** ~ necrosis colicuativa; **decubital** ~ necrosis por decúbito; úlcera por decúbito; **dry** ~ necrosis seca; **embolic** ~ necrosis embólica; **fat** ~ necrosis de tejido adiposo; necrosis grasa; **moist** ~ necrosis húmeda

necrotic, necrótico *adj*

necrotize, to, necrosar; producir necrosis; hacerse necrótico

need, necesidad *f*; **caloric** ~s necesidades calóricas; **energetic** ~s necesidades energéticas

need, to, necesitar; **to be in** ~[4] andar enfermo[2]

needle, abuja[2]; aguja; filero[2]; hierro[2]; jeringuilla[2]; punta[2]; **aneurysm** ~ aguja de aneurisma; **aspirating** ~ aguja aspiradora; ~ **aspiration** punción aspiradora *f*; ~ **biopsy** punción biópsica *f*; ~ **electrode** electrodo de aguja; ~ **holder** portaagujas *m, inv*; **hypodermic** ~ aguja hipodérmica; jaipo *slang*; jeringa; ~ **tip** punta de la aguja

negative, negativo *m, adj*; ~ **ion** ion negativo *m*

negativism, negativismo
neglect, descuido; negligencia
neglect, to, desatender (ie); descuidar
negligence, negligencia
negligent, negligente *adj* descuidado *adj*
negligible, insignificante *adj*
Negro, negro; trigueño *adj*, *SpAm*, *euph*
negroid, negro *adj*
neighbor, vecino
neighborhood, vecindad *f*; barrio
nemathelminth, nematelminto
nematocide, nematocida *m*, *adj*
nematode, nematodo
neomycin, neomicina
neon, neón *m*; ~ lighting alumbrado de neón *adj*
neonatal, neonatal *adj*
neonate, neonato *m*, *adj*
neonatologist, neonatólogo
neonatology, neonatología
neophyte, neófito *m*, *adj*
neoplasm, neoplasma *m*
neoplastic, neoplástico *adj*
nephew, sobrino
nephralgia, dolor en el riñón *m*; nefralgia
nephrectomy, nefrectomía
nephritic, nefrítico *adj*
nephritis, nefritis *f*; acute interstitial ~ nefritis aguda intersticial; bacterial ~ nefritis bacteriana; chronic ~ nefritis crónica; chronic interstitial ~ nefritis intersticial crónica; riñón atrófico *m*; riñón contraído *m*; embolic ~ nefritis embólica; focal ~ nefritis focal; suppurative ~ nefritis supurada
nephrocalcinosis, nefrocalcinosis *f*
nephrocystitis, nefrocistitis *f*; inflamación de riñones y vejiga urinaria *f*
nephrogram, nefrograma *m*; radiografía del riñón

nephrolith, (*form*, *kidney stone*) nefrolito
nephrologist, nefrólogo
nephrology, nefrología
nephrolysis, nefrólisis *f*
nephroma, nefroma *m*; tumor del riñón *m*
nephropathy, nefropatía
nephrosclerosis, nefrosclerosis *f*; nefroesclerosis *f*
nephrosis, nefrosis *f*; acute ~ nefrosis aguda; chronic ~ nefrosis crónica; diabetes albuminúrica *f*
nephrotic, nefrótico *adj*
nephrotomy, incisión en el riñón *f*; nefrotomía
nerve, nervio; ~ block bloqueo del nervio; bloqueo nervioso; ~ cavity cavidad del diente *f*; cavidad pulpar *f*; ~ cell célula nerviosa; neurona; ~ center centro nervioso; ~ conduction conducción nerviosa *f*; cranial ~ nervio craneal; ~ deafness nervio acústico; ~ degeneration degeneración nerviosa *f*; ~ ending terminación del nervio *f*; entrapped ~ nervio comprimido; ~ fiber fibra nerviosa; a fit of ~s ataque de nervios *m*; motor ~ nervio motor; parasympathetic ~ nervio parasimpático; pinched ~ nervio atrapado; nervio pellizcado; ~ root raíz nerviosa; sciatic ~ nervio ciático; sensory ~ nervio sensorial; ~ supply inervación *f*; sympathetic ~ nervio simpático; ~ tissue tejido nervioso; to deaden the ~ adormecer el nervio
nervous, agitado *adj*; nervioso *adj*; autonomic ~ system aparato nervioso autónomo; sistema nervioso autónomo *m*; ~ breakdown agotamiento; choque nervioso; colapso; colapso

nervioso; crisis nerviosa *f, inv*; desarreglo nervioso; neurastenia; **central ~ system** aparato nervioso central; sistema nervioso central *m*; **~ disorder** desorden nervioso *m*; trastorno nervioso; **~ dyspepsia** dispepsia nerviosa; **~ impulse** impulso nervioso; **~ jerk** sacudida nerviosa; **~ shock** choque nervioso *m*; **~ tension** tensión nerviosa *f*; **vegetative ~ system** sistema nervioso vegetativo

nervousness, nerviosidad *f*; nerviosismo

nest, nido

net, red *f*

nettle-fever, urticaria

network, red *f*; retículo; **cell ~** red celular; **neurofibrillar ~** red neurofibrilar

neural, neural *adj*; **~ canal** canal neural *m*; **~ fold** pliegue neural *m*; **~ ridge** hendidura neural; **~ sheath** vaina neural

neuralgia, neuralgia; **cardiac ~** neuralgia cardíaca; angina de pecho; **degenerative ~** neuralgia degenerativa; **trigeminal ~** neuralgia del trigémino

neurasthenia, neurastenia

neurasthenic, neurasténico *adj*

neuritis, neuritis *f*; **alcoholic ~** neuritis alcohólica; **degenerative ~** neuritis degenerativa; **diabetic ~** neuritis diabética; **malarial ~** neuritis palúdica; **traumatic ~** neuritis traumática

neuroanatomy, neuroanatomía

neuroblast, neuroblasto

neuroblastoma, neuroblastoma *m*

neuroendocrinology, neuroendocrinología

neurofibroma, neurofibroma *m*

neuroleptic, neuroléptico *adj*

neurologic, neurológico *adj*

neurological, neurológico *adj*; **~ disorder** enfermedades nerviosas *f*

neurologist, neurólogo

neurology, neurología

neuroma, neuroma *m*; **amputation ~** neuroma de amputación; **myelinic ~** neuroma mielínico

neuromuscular, neuromuscular *adj*

neuron, neurona; **afferent ~** neurona aferente; **efferent ~** neurona eferente; **lower motor ~** neuronas motoras inferiores; **peripheral motor ~** neurona motora periférica; **peripheral sensory ~** neurona sensorial periférica; **postganglionic ~** neuronas posganglionares; **preganglionic ~** neuronas preganglionares; **upper motor ~** neuronas motoras superiores

neuro-ophthalmology, neurooftalmología

neuropathology, neuropatología

neuropathy, neuropatía

neuropharmacology, neurofarmacología

neurophysiology, neurofisiología

neuropsychiatrist, neuro(p)siquiatra[5] *m/f*

neuropsychiatry, neuro(p)siquiatría[5]

neurosis, neurosis *f*; **anxiety ~** neurosis de ansiedad; **association ~** neurosis de asociación; **compensation ~** neurosis de indemnización; **obsessive-compulsive ~** neurosis obsesivo-compulsiva

neuroskeletal, neurosquelético *adj*

neuroskeleton, neurosqueleto; endosqueleto

neurosurgeon, neurocirujano

neurosurgery, neurocirugía

neurosyphillis, neurosífilis *f*; **meningovascular ~** neurosífilis meningovascular

neurotic, neurótico *adj*

neurovascular, neurovascular *adj*

neuter, neutro *adj*

neutral, neutro *adj*; ~ **zone** zona neutra
neutralization, neutralización *f*
neutralize, to, neutralizar
neutrophil, neutrófilo; **filament-ed** ~ neutrófilo filamentoso; **rod** ~ neutrófilo en banda
never, nunca *adv*
never-ceasing, incesante *adj*
nevus, (*pl*, *nevi*) lunar *m*; nevo; ~ **anemicus** nevo anémico; ~ **cavernosus** nevo cavernoso; **junction** ~ nevo intermedio; ~ **pigmentosus** nevo pigmentario; ~ **vascularis** nevo vascular
new, nuevo *adj*
newborn, recién nacido *m*, *adj*; neonato
newlywed, recién casado
news, noticias
newspaper, diario; periódico
next, próximo *adj*; que viene; siguiente *adj*; ~ **of kin** pariente más cercano; ~ **to** al lado de *prep*
NG tube, tubo nasogástrico
niacin, niacina
nice, simpático *adj*
nick, rasguño
nickname, apodo; mote *m*
nicotine, nicotina
nicotinic acid, ácido nicotínico
niece, sobrina
night, noche *f*; **at** ~ de noche; por la noche; ~ **blindness** ceguera nocturna; nictalopía; **during the** ~ por la noche; **last** ~ anoche *adv*; ~ **nurse** enfermera de noche; ~**-screaming** terror nocturno *m*; ~ **sweats** sudor nocturno *m*; ~ **terrors** terrores nocturnos *m*; ~ **watch** guardia nocturna
nightclothes, ropa de dormir
nightgown, bata; camisa de noche; ~ (*hospital*) camisón *m*
nightmare, pesadilla; sueño malo
nightwalker, sonámbulo
nightwalking, sonambulismo

nippers, pinzas; tenacillas
nipple, ~ (*of a female breast*) chichi *f*, *Arg*, *slang*; pezón *m*; **cracked** ~ grieta del pezón; **engorged** ~ (*caked*) pezón enlechado *m*; ~ (*of a male*) tetilla; mamila; ~ (*of a baby/nursing bottle*) chupón *m*; mamadera; tetera *Cu*, *Mex*, *PR*; tetilla; tetina; teto; ~ (*pacifier*) chupeta; chupete *m*; ~ **line** línea mamilar; ~ **shield** escudo para el pezón; pezonera
nit, liendre *f*
nitrate, nitrato
nitrite, nitrito
nitric acid, ácido nítrico
nitrifying, nitrificante *adj*
nitrobenzene, nitrobenceno
nitrogen, nitrógeno
nitro(glycerin), nitro(glicerina)
nitrous, nitroso; ~ **acid** ácido nitroso; ~ **oxide** óxido nitroso
no one, nadie
nobody, nadie
nocturnal, nocturno *adj*; ~ **emission** eyaculación nocturna *f*
nod, to, afirmar con la cabeza; asentir (ie); ~ (*because of sleepiness*) cabecear; dar cabezadas
node, ~ (*general*) nodo; nudo; ~ nodo *Card*; **atrioventricular** ~ nodo atrioventricular; **auriculoventricular** ~ nodo auriculoventricular; **sinoatrial** ~ nodo sinoauricular; ~ (*lymph*) ganglio; ganglio linfático; nódulos linfáticos; ~ (*nodule*) nódulo; **singers'** ~ nódulo de los cantantes; nódulo vocal
nodular, nodular *adj*
nodule, nódulo; pequeño abultamiento
noise, ruido; ~ **abatement** campaña contra el ruido; **to make** ~ hacer ruido
noisy, ruidoso *adj*
nomenclature, nomenclatura; **binomial** ~ nomenclatura binaria
nonabsorbable, no absorbible *adj*

nonadherent, no adherente *adj*
nondisjunction, no disyunción *f*
none, ninguno *pron, adj*
nonflammable, ininflamable *adj*; no inflamable *adj*
nonfunctional, afuncional *adj*
nongonoccocal urethritis, uretritis no gonococal *f*
noninfectious, no infeccioso *adj*
noninvasive, no invasor *adj*
nonnucleated, anucleado *adj*
nonparous, nulípara *adj*
nonsense, disparates *m, pl*
nonspecific, inespecífico *adj*; ~ **urethritis** uretritis inespecífica *f*; uretritis no específica *f*
nonsteroidal antiinflammatory drug, antiinflamatorio no esteroide
nontaxable, no imponible *adj*
nontoxic, atóxico *adj*
nonviable, que no puede sobrevivir
non-weight bearing plaster, yeso de descarga
noodle, fideo
noon, mediodía *m*; **at** ~ a(l) mediodía
norepinephrine, norepinefrina; noradrenalina
norm, norma; **to deviate from the** ~ salir de lo normal
normal, normal *adj*; ~ **heartbeat** latido normal del corazón; ~ **solution** solución normal *f*; ~ **saline solution** solución normal salina
north, norte *m*
nose, nariz *f*; nayotas *pl, slang, Chicano*; ~ **bleed** hemorragia nasal; ~ **bleeding** epistaxis *f*; **bridge of the** ~ caballete de la nariz *m*; puente de nariz *m*; tabique de la nariz *m*; tabique nasal *m*; ~ **drops** gotas nasales; **stuffed** ~ nariz tapada; nariz tupida; **stuffed-up** ~ nariz tapada; **to blow one's** ~ sonarse (la nariz); soplarse la nariz *Carib*; **to hold one's** ~ taparse la nariz

nosebleed, epistaxis *f, form*; hemorragia nasal *form*; **to have a** ~ salirle sangre de la nariz
nosepiece, ~ (*of a microscope*) pieza revólver; porta objetivos *m, inv*; ~ (*of glasses*) puente *m*
nostalgia, nostalgia
nostril, fosa nasal; hoyo de la nariz *fam*; ventana de la nariz; ventana nasal; ventanilla de la nariz
notch, escotadura
notched, dentellado *adj*
noteworthy, chocante *adj*
nothing, nada; ~ **by mouth** nada por la boca
notice, atención *f*
notice, to, fijarse (en); notar; observar
noticeable, perceptible *adj*
notifiable disease, enfermedad de declaración obligatoria *f*
notify, to, notificar
not look well, to, quedar desmejorado
notoriety, notoriedad *f*
not predictable, impredecible *adj*, *CA, Mex, PR*; impredictible *adj*; imprevisible; impronosticable *adj*
nourish, to, alimentar; nutrir
nourishing, nutritivo *adj*
nourishment, alimentación *f*; alimento; nutrición *f*
novocaine, novocaína
now, ahora *adv*; **right** ~ ahora mismo
noxious, nocivo *adj*; pernicioso *adj*
NPO/nihil per os/nothing by mouth, nada por boca
NSR/normal sinus rhythm, ritmo sinusal normal
NSS/normal saline solution, solución salina normal *f*
nuclear, nuclear *adj*; ~ **stain** núcleo coloreado; colorante nuclear *m*; ~ **war** guerra nuclear
nucleated leukocytes, leucocitos nucleados; **acidophiles** acidófi-

los; **basophiles** basófilos; **blood platelet** plaqueta sanguínea; **eosinophiles** eosinófilos; **lymphocytes** linfocitos; **monocytes** monocitos; **polymorphonuclear neutrophiles** neutrófilos polimorfonucleares; **polymorphs** polimorfos; **reticulocytes** reticulocitos; **thrombocytes** trombocitos

nucleolus, nucléolo

nucleus, núcleo

nude, desnudo *adj;* veringo *adj, Col*

nudeness, desnudez *f*

nudge, to, dar un codazo (a)

null, nulo *adj*

nulligravida, nuligrávida

nulliparous, nulípara *f, adj*

numb, adormecido *adj;* aterido *adj;* dormido *adj;* entumecido *adj;* entumido *adj;* ~ (*limb*) insensible *adj, Med*

numb, to, entumecer; **to be** ~ tener adormecido; **to become** ~ adormecerse; dormirse; **to go** ~ (*limbs*) engarrotarse *SpAm*

number, número; **atomic** ~ número atómico; ~ **one** *euph* pipi *fam;* el orinar; ~ **two** *euph* caca *fam;* el defecar

numbness, adormecimiento; entorpecimiento; entumecimiento; falta de sensación; paralización *f*

nun, monja

nurse, ~ (*for the sick*) enfermera; norsa *Chicano;* **~s' aide** auxiliar de enfermeras *m/f;* auxiliar en enfermeras *m/f;* ayudante de enfermeras; enfermero asistente; enfermero auxiliar; **~anesthetist** enfermera anestesista; **charge** ~ enfermera de cargo; jefa de turno; jefe de turno *m;* **child's** ~ enfermera pediátrica; **general duty** ~ enfermera general; **graduate** ~ enfermera graduada; **head** ~ jefa de enfermeras; enfermera jefe/je-

fa; **home** ~ enfermera domiciliaria; **hospital** ~ enfermera de hospital; ~ **on duty** enfermera de guardia; **practical** ~ enfermera práctica; **private** ~ enfermera privada; **public health** ~ enfermera de salud pública; **registered** ~ enfermera graduada; enfermera titulada; **school** ~ enfermera escolar; **visiting** ~ enfermera visitadora; **ward** ~ enfermera de piso; enfermera de planta; ~ (*nursemaid*) niñera; **baby** ~ ama de cría; niñera; nodriza; **wet** ~ chichi *f, fam, Guat, Mex;* chichigua *vulg, SpAm;* nodriza

nurse, to, (*to give nourishment*) amamantar; criar a los pechos; dar de mamar; dar el pecho al niño; lactar; mamar

nursemaid, chiche *f, Mex*

nursery, cuarto de los niños; guardería; guardería infantil; **newborn** ~ sala de los recién nacidos

nurses' aide, (*See nurse.*)

nursing, (*general term*) enfermería; ~ (*suckling*) amamantamiento; crianza; de crianza *adj;* lactancia; lactante *adj;* ~ (*for the sick*) asistencia a los enfermos; ~ **bottle** biberón *m;* mamadera; tetera, tetero *Col, PR, Ven;* ~ **bra** sostén de maternidad *m;* ~ **care** cuidados auxiliares; **general duty** ~ enfermería general; ~ **home** asilo de ancianos; clínica de reposo; hogar de ancianos; hospicio para ancianos; ~ **home care** cuidado en los asilos; cuidado en un hospicio para ancianos; ~ **mother** mujer lactante *f;* ~ **pad** almohadita; ~ **profession** profesión de enfermería *f;* **special** ~ enfermería especial; ~ **staff** personal sanitario auxiliar *m;* ~ **supervisor** jefe/jefa de enfermeras *m/f*

nut, ~ (*edible*) nuez *f*; ~ (*insane*) loco *adj*; ~ (*screw*) tuerca

nutrient, nutricio; nutritivo *adj*; sustancia nutritìva; ~ **enema** enema alimenticia *f*/ *m* [*Ú.m.c.f.*]

nutriment, nutrimento; nutrición *f*

nutrition, nutrición; **total parenteral** ~ nutrición parenteral total *f*

nutritional, nutritivo *adj*; nutricional *adj*; alimenticio *adj*; ~ **diet** dieta alimenticia

nutritionist, nutriólogo

nutritious, nutritivo *adj*

nutshell, cáscara de nuez

NWB/non-weight bearing, no soporta peso

nyctalopia, nictalopía; (*See blindness, night.*)

nycturia, nicturia

nylon, nilón *m*

nymphomania, ninfomanía

nymphomaniac, ninfómana

nystagmus, nistagmo; **amblyopic** ~ nistagmo amaurótico

---

[2] This is new vocabulary, not necessarily listed nor yet recognized by the Royal Academy of Spanish Grammar. It is understood that this vocabulary is primarily slang. Unless otherwise indicated, the gender of the nouns is assumed to be obvious.

[4] Part of the Drug Abuse Vocabulary.

[5] English words that have an initial *ps* now may be spelled either with or without the *p* in Spanish. In either case, the *p* is silent when the Spanish word is pronounced. This dictionary will show such words with a parenthesis around the *p*.

oath, juramento; **Hippocratic ~** juramento hipocrático

oatmeal, avena

obduction, autopsia médico-legal

obedience, obediencia

obedient, obediente *adj*

obese, corpulento *adj*; obeso *adj*

obesity, gordura; obesidad *f*

obey, to, obedecer

obfuscation, confusión mental *f*

obituary, obituario; registro de defunciones

object, objeto; **~ blindness** ceguera de objetos

object, to, objetar; tener inconveniente; molestar

objection, objeción *f*; **~** (*difficulty*) inconveniente *m*

objective, objetivo *m*, *adj*; **~ symptoms** síntomas objetivos *m*

obligate, to, obligar

obligated, obligado *adj*

obligation, obligación *f*

obligatory, obligatorio *adj*; obligado *adj*

oblique, oblicuo *adj*

obliterate, to, destruir

obmutescence, pérdida de la voz

obnubilation, obnubilación *f*

obscure, to, enmascarar

observant, observador *adj*

observation, observación *f*; estudio; examen *m*

observe, to, notar; observar; examinar

obsession, obsesión *f*

obsessive-compulsive, obsesivo-compulsivo *adj*

obsolescence, caducidad *f*

obsolete, anticuado *adj*; sin utilidad *prep phr*

obstacle, obstáculo; traba *fam*

obstetric, obstétrico *adj*

obstetrical, obstétrico *adj*

obstetrician, obstetra *m/f*; obstétrico; tocólogo

obstetrics, obstetricia; tocología

obstruct, to, obstruir

obstruction, bloqueo; impedimento; obstrucción *f*; **intestinal ~** obstrucción intestinal; **nasal ~** mormación *f*, *Chicano*; **stomach ~** entablazón *f*, *Chicano*

obstructive, obstructivo *adj*

obtain, to, conseguir (i); adquirir (ie); obtener

obturate, to, obturar; rellenar; tapar

obturation, obturación *f*; bloqueo de un pasaje

obturator, bloqueador *m*, *adj*; obturador *m*, *adj*

obtuse, obtuso *adj*

obtusion, torpeza intelectual

obviate, to, evitar inconvenientes

obvious, obvio *adj*

occasionally, a veces

occipital, occipital *m*, *adj*; **~ bone** hueso occipital; **~ condyle** cóndilo occipital; **~ lobe** lóbulo occipital; **~ protuberance** protuberancia occipital; **~ sinus** seno occipital

occiput, cerebro; occipucio

occlude, to, ocluir; ocluirse *Dent*

occluding, oclusante *adj*

occlusal, oclusal *adj*; **~ analysis** análisis oclusal *m*, *inv*; **~ correction** corrección oclusal *f*; **~ form** forma oclusal; **~ path** vía oclusal; **~ plane** plano de oclusión; **~ rest** sostén oclusal *m*; **~ surface** superficie oclusal *f*; **~ wear** desgaste oclusal *m*

occlusion, oclusión *f*; **abnormal ~** oclusión anormal; **buccal ~** oclusión bucal; **distal ~** oclusión distal; **labial ~** oclusión labial;

lingual ~ oclusión lingual; ~ **rim** anillo de oclusión

occlusive, oclusivo *adj*; ~ **pessary** pesario oclusivo

occult, oculto *adj*; escondido *adj*; ~ **blood** sangre oculta *f*

occupation, ocupación *f*; oficio; trabajo

occupational, ocupacional *adj*; ~ **disease** enfermedad profesional *f*; ~ **neurosis** neurosis profesional *f*; ~ **therapist** terapeuta ocupacional *m/f*; ~ **therapy** terapia laboral; terapia ocupacional; terapia profesional

occupied, ocupado *adj*

occupy, to, ocupar

occur, to, ocurrir

ochronosis, ocronosis *f*

octane, octano

ocular, ocular *m*, *adj*; ~ **enucleation** oculectomía; ~ **muscles** músculos oculares; ~ **pressure** presión ocular *f*

oculist, oculista *m/f*

o.d./oculus dexter/right eye, ojo derecho

odd, ~ (*unpaired*) impar *adj*; ~ (*strange*) chocante *adj*

odontalgia, dolor de los dientes *m*

odontologist, dentista *m/f*; odontólogo

odontology, odontología

odontoscope, odontoscopio

odor, olor *m*; **underarm** ~ sajín *m*, CA; sajino *m*, CA; sobaquera CA, Mex, PR; sobaquina; sobasquera CA, Mex, PR

odorless, inodoro *adj*; sin olor *prep phr*

of, de *prep*

off, fuera de *prep*; **to be** ~ irse; **to put** ~ posponer; **to take** ~ quitarse; **to turn** ~ apagar

offense, ofensa

offensive, chocante *adj*, Arg

offend, to, ofender; insultar

offer, oferta; ofrecimiento

offer, to, ofrecer

office, oficina; **dental** ~ consultorio dental; ~ **hours** horas de consulta; horas de oficina; **medical** ~ consultorio

official, oficial *m*, *adj*; autorizado *adj*

offspring, hijos; progenitura; vástago

often, a menudo *adv*; con frecuencia *prep phr*; frecuentemente *adv*; muchas veces *adv*

oil, aceite *m*; **baby** ~ aceite para niños; **bitter almond** ~ aceite de almendras amargas; **castor** ~ aceite de ricino; aceite de castor; **clove** ~ esencia de clavos; **coconut** ~ aceite de copra; **cod liver** ~ aceite de hígado de bacalao; **cooking** ~ aceite de cocinar; **corn** ~ aceite de maíz; **cottonseed** ~ aceite de algodón; **eucalyptus** ~ esencia de eucalipto; **lavender** ~ esencia de espliego; **lemon** ~ esencia de limón; **linseed** ~ aceite de linaza; **mineral** ~ aceite mineral blanco; **olive** ~ aceite de oliva; **palm** ~ aceite de palma; **peanut** ~ aceite de cacahuete; **safflower** ~ aceite de cártamo; ~ **of Wintergreen** aceite de gaultería; esencia de Wintergreen

oily, grasiento *adj*; oleoso *adj*

ointment, crema; pomada[4]; ungüento[4]; untadura *Med*; unto; **bacitracin** ~ pomada de bacitracina; **calamine** ~ pomada de calamina; **hydrocortisone acetate** ~ pomada de acetato de hidrocortisona; **zinc oxide** ~ pomada de óxido de cinc

o.l./oculus laevus/left eye, ojo izquierdo

old, viejo *adj*; ~ **age** vejez *f*; envejecimiento; senectud *f*; ~ **man** anciano; viejo; ~ **wives' tale** cuento de viejas; ~ **woman** anciana; vieja

older, mayor *adj*

oleander, adelfa
oleic acid, ácido oleico
olfactory, olfatorio *adj*; olfativo *adj*; olfato *adj*; ~ **bundle** huso olfatorio; ~ **nerve** nervio olfatorio
olive, aceituna; oliva; ~-**skinned** trigueño *adj*
o.m./omni mane/every morning, cada mañana
omit, to, omitir
omphalocele, hernia congénita del ombligo; onfalocele *m*
o.n./omni nocte/every night, cada noche
on, en *prep*; sobre *prep*; **to be ~ drugs** drogarse; ~ **holiday** de vacaciones; ~ **one's back** boca arriba; ~ **one's stomach** boca abajo; **to be ~ pills** tomar píldoras; ~ **the left** a la izquierda; ~ **the right** a la derecha; **to be ~ the staff** estar en la plantilla
onanism, onanismo
once a week, cada ocho días; una vez por semana
oncogenic, oncógeno *adj*
oncologist, oncólogo
oncology, oncología
oncotherapy, oncoterapia
one-armed, manco *adj*; choco *adj*, *CA, Chi, Mex*; chueco *adj*, *Mex*
one-eyed, ~ (*monocular*) monóculo *adj*; ~ (*having only one eye*) tuerto *adj*; virulo *adj*, *Chicano*; choco *adj*, *CA, Chi, Mex*; ~ **person** tuerto
one-handed, manco *adj*
one-legged, choco *adj*, *CA, Chi, Mex*; chueco *adj*, *Mex*
onion, cebolla
only, único *adj*
onset, comienzo; principio; acceso *Med*; ataque *m, Med*
onychia, oniquia; oniquiasis *f*
onychosis, onicosis *f*
onychophagia, onicofagia
oogenesis, oogénesis *f*; ovogénesis *f*
oophorectomy, ooforectomía; ovariectomía

ooze, to, superar; rezumar; ~ (*blood*) destilar *Med*
opacity, opacidad *f*; ~ (*of the eye*) nube *f*
opaque, opaco *adj*; ~ **lens** cristalino opaco
open, abierto *adj*
open, to, abrir
opening, (*general term*) apertura; ~ (*aperture*) abertura
operable, operable *adj*
operate, to, operar; hacer una intervención quirúrgica; ~ **to** intervenir *Med*
operating, ~ **chair** silla de operaciones; ~ **room** quirófano; sala de cirugía; sala de operaciones; ~ **table** mesa de cirugía; mesa de operaciones
operation, operación *f*; intervención *f, Med*; intervención quirúrgica *f*; **to have an ~** operarse
operative, operativo *adj*
ophthalmia, (*inflammation of the eye*) oftalmía; inflamación de los ojos *f*
ophthalmic, oftálmico *adj*
ophthalmologist, especialista en enfermedades de los ojos *m/f*; oftalmólogo
ophthalmology, oftalmología
ophthalmoplegia, oftalmoplejía
ophthalmoscope, oftalmoscopio
ophthalmoscopy, oftalmoscopia
opiate, opiáceo *m, adj*; opiado; opiato
opinion, opinión *f*; **second ~** segunda opinión; **to be of the same ~** estar de acuerdo
opium[5], chinaloa[2] *slang*; goma[2] *slang*; material negro[2]; opio; ~ **addict** opiómano[2]; ~ **addiction** opiomanía[2]; **granulated ~** opio granulado; ~ **habit** abuso habitual del opio; **powdered ~** opio pulverizado
opotherapy, opoterapia
opportunist, oportunista *m/f, adj*

opportunistic, oportunista *adj*; ~ **infectious disease** enfermedad oportunista infecciosa *f*
opportunity, oportunidad *f*
oppose, to, oponer
opposite, lo contrario; opuesto *adj*; enfrente *adv*; enfrente de *prep*; frente a *prep*
opposition, oposición *f*
oppress, to, oprimir
oppressive, opresivo *adj*; ~ (*atmosphere*) sofocante *adj*; ~ (*mental burden*) agobiante *adj*
optic, óptico *adj*; ~ **atrophy** atrofia óptica; ~ **disc** disco óptico; punto ciego de la retina; ~ **nerve** nervio óptico
optical, óptico *adj*; ~ **activity** actividad óptica *f*
optician, óptico
optics, óptica
option, opción *f*
optometrist, especialista en lentes *m/f*; optometrista *m/f*
optometry, optometría
or, o
oral, oral *adj*; ~ **contraceptive** píldora anticonceptiva; (*See birth control.*); ~ **vaccine** (*Sabin polio*) gotas de polio; bucal *Dent adj*; ~ **diagnosis** diagnóstico bucal; ~ **hygiene** higiene bucal
orally, por vía bucal *prep phr*
orange, ~ (*fruit*) naranja; ~ **juice** jugo de naranja; ~ (*color*) anaranjado *adj*
orbit, órbita
orchidectomy, orquidectomía; orquiectomía
orchiectomy, orquiectomía; orquidectomía
orchiotomy, orquiotomía
orchis, testículo
orchitis, orquitis *f*
order, orden *f*; ~ (*authorization*) orden *f*; **written** ~ orden escrita; ~ (*harmony; series*) orden *m*
order, to, ordenar; mandar *Med*; ~ (*to prescribe*) recetar

orderly, asistente médico; asistente de enfermeras *m*; ayudante médico; camillero; mucamo; arreglado *adj*; metódico *adj*; ordenado *adj*
organ, órgano; **absorbent** ~ órgano absorbente; **sense** ~**s** órganos de los sentidos; ~ **of shock** órgano de choque; **wandering** ~ órgano errante
organic, orgánico *adj*; ~ **chemistry** química orgánica
organism, organismo
organization, organización *f*
organize, to, organizar
organizer, organizador, -ra *m/f*
orgasm, orgasmo; **to experience** ~ acabar
oriental, oriental *adj*
orientation, orientación *f*
orifice, orificio
origin, origen *m*
original, original *adj*
orphan, huérfano; guacho *Chi, Perú, Ríopl*; pepenado *CA, Mex*
orphanage, hospicio
orphaned, guacho *adj, Chi, Perú, Ríopl*
orthodontia, ortodoncia
orthodontic, ortodóntico *adj*
orthodontics, ortodoncia
orthodontist, ortodoncista *m/f, adj*; ortodontista *m/f, adj*; ortopédico dental
orthopedic, ortopédico *adj*; ~ **brace** aparato ortopédico; ~ **shoes** calzado ortopédico; ~ **surgeon** cirujano ortopédico; ~ **surgery** cirugía ortopédica
orthopedics, ortopedia
orthopedist, especialista en fracturas *m/f*; especialista en ortopedia *m/f*; ortopédico; ortopedista *m/f, adj*
orthoptic, ortóptico *adj*; ~ **training** método ortóptico; método que corrige la oblicuidad de los ejes visuales
orthoptics, ortóptica

orthoptist, ortoptista *m/f*
orthoptoscope, ortoptoscopio
orthoscope, ortoscopio
orthoscopic, ortoscópico *adj*
oscillate, to, oscilar
oscillation, oscilación *f*
oscillograph, oscilógrafo
oscillator, oscilador *m*
oscilloscope, osciloscopio
osseous, óseo *adj*
ossicle, huesecillo; huesillo; osículo
ossification, osificación *f*
ossify, to, osificar
osteitis, osteítis *f*; **fibrosa cystica ~** osteítis fibroquística
ostensive, aparente *adj*
osteoarthritis, osteoartritis *f*
osteoblast, osteoblasto
osteocope, osteócopo *form*; dolor intenso en los huesos *m*
osteocopic pain, dolor intenso en los huesos *m*
osteogenesis, osteogénesis *f*; **~ imperfecta** osteogénesis imperfecta
osteogenic, osteogénico *adj*
osteology, osteología
osteoma, osteoma *m*
osteomyelitis, osteomielitis *f*; inflamación de la médula del hueso *f*
osteonecrosis, osteonecrosis *f*
osteopath (D.O.), osteópata *m/f*
osteopathic, osteopático *adj*
osteopathy, osteopatía
osteophyte, osteofito
osteoporosis, osteoporosis *f*; **adipose ~** osteoporosis adiposa
osteosarcoma, osteosarcoma *m*
osteosclerosis, osteosclerosis *f*
osteosis, osteosis *f*
osteotomy, osteotomía
otalgia, otalgia *form*; dolor de oídos *m*
other, otro *adj*
otic, ótico *adj*
otitis, otitis *f*; **~ externa** otitis externa; **~ interna** otitis interna; **~ media** otitis media
otolaryngologist, otorrinolaringólogo

otolaryngology, otorrinolaringología
otologist, otólogo
otology, otología
otopharyngeal, otofaríngeo, *adj*; **~ tube** tubo otofaríngeo
otoplasty, cirugía plástica del oído
otorhinolaryngologist, otorrinolaringólogo
otorhinolaryngology, otorrinolaringología
otorrhea, otorrea
otosalpinx, otosalpinge *m*; trompa de Eustaquio
otosclerosis, otosclerosis *f*
otoscope, otoscopio
otoscopy, otoscopia
ought to, to, deber
ounce, onza; **fluid ~** onza líquida
out of sorts, to be, desazonarse *Med*
outbreak, **~ (*of a disease*)** epidemia; **~ (*of an epidemic*)** brote *m*; **~ (*of pimples*)** erupción *f*; **new ~** retroceso *Med*; recrudescencia; recrudecimiento
outcome, resultado
outdated, anticuado *adj*; **~ (*medication*)** caducado *adj*; vencido *adj*
outdoors, al aire libre *prep phr*
outer, exterior *adj*; externo *adj*; **~ ear** oído externo; oreja
outfit, **~ (*clothes*)** traje *m*; **~ (*gear*)** equipo
outgoing, **~ (*character*)** extrovertido *adj*; **~ (*departing*)** saliente *adj*
outgrow, to, **~ (*clothes*)** hacerse demasiado grande para; **~ (*a habit, etc.*)** perder (ie) con la edad; **~ (*an illness, etc.*)** curarse de ___ con la edad
outgrowth, **(*sth. that grows*)** excrecencia; evaginación *f*
outlet, toma *Elect*; tomacorriente *f*, *Elect*; desahogo *Psyc*; **~ (*way out*)** salida; **to be an ~** servirle (i) de desahogo a alguien
outline, to, perfilar

outlive, to, ~ (*to last longer than*) durar más (tiempo) que; ~ (*to live down*) hacer olvidar; ~ (*s.o.; a disgrace*) sobrevivir

outlook, actitud *f*; perspectiva

outnumber, to, exceder en número

outpatient, paciente ambulante *m/f*; paciente ambulatorio; paciente de consulta externa *m/f*; paciente externo; ~ **clinic** clínica de consulta externa; consultorio externo; ~ **department** servicio de consulta externa

output, total expedito *m*; total producido *m*; gasto; **energy** ~ gasto energético; **urinary** ~ gasto urinario; ~ (*of a machine*) rendimiento

outrage, ~ (*atrocity*) atrocidad *f*; ~ (*on one's rights, feelings*) agravio; ~ (*public scandal*) escándalo; ~ (*suffered by someone*) indignidad *f*

outrage, to, ~ (*to rape*) violar; ~ (*the law*) atropellar

outrageous, (*provoking disapproval*) escandaloso *adj*

outright, ~ (*complete*) entero *adj*; ~ (*forthright*) franco *adj*; ~ (*refusal*) rotundo *adj*; ~ (*at once*) en el acto *prep phr*, ~ (*openly*) francamente *adv*

outside, afuera *adv*; ~ **of** fuera de *prep*

outspoken, to be, no tener pelos en la lengua

outstanding, destacado *adj*; sobresaliente *adj*; ~ (*still to be done*) pendiente *adj*; ~ (*unpaid*) sin pagar

outweigh, to, pesar más que

oval, oval *m, adj*

ovarian, ovárico *adj*; ovario *adj*; ~ **cancer** cáncer del ovario *m*; cáncer ovárico *m*; ~ **cyst** quiste ovárico *m*; ~ **disorders** trastornos ováricos; ~ **pregnancy** embarazo ovario

ovariectomy, ovariectomía

ovariotomy, ovariotomía

ovary, ovario; **cysts on the ovaries** quistes en los ovarios *m*; **polycystic** ~ ovario poliquístico

oven, horno

over, sobre; **to bend** ~ doblar; inclinarse

overanxious, ~ (*eager*) demasiado deseoso (de) *adj*; ~ (*worried*) preocupado sin motivo *adj*

overbearing, (*domineering*) autoritario *adj*

overbite, sobremordida

overburden, to, agobiar (de)

overcareful, excesivamente cuidadoso *adj*

overcautious, demasiado cauteloso *adj*

overcharge, ~ (*extra charge*) sobreprecio; ~ (*very high price*) precio excesivo

overcharge, to, ~ (*to charge too much*) cobrar un precio excesivo (a); ~ (*to load too highly with electricity*) poner una carga excesiva (a) *Elect*

overcoat, abrigo

overcome, to, (*difficulty*) vencer; **to be** ~ **by fear** estar muerto de miedo; **to be** ~ **by pain** estar postrado de dolor

overcompensation, compensación excesiva *f*

overconfidence, exceso de confianza

overcorrection, sobrecorreción *f*

overcrowded, (*with people*) atestado *adj*

overcrowding, atestamiento

overdo, to, esforzarse (ue) demasiado; exagerar

overdose, dosis excesiva *f, inv*; sobredosis *f, inv*; sobredosis tóxica *f, inv*

overdose, to, dar una dosis excesiva (a); doblar(se); **to take an** ~ darse una dosis excesiva; tomar una dosis excesiva

overdue, ~ (*plane, etc.*) atrasado *adj*; ~ (*pregnancy*) tardío *adj*

overexert, to, agotar; ~ **oneself** hacer un esfuerzo excesivo

overextension, sobreextensión *f*

overfatigue, to, agotar

overflow, derrame *m*; rebosamiento

overhear, to, oír por casualidad

overindulge, to, ~ (*a child*) mimar con exceso; ~ (*a passion, etc.*) dar rienda suelta (a); ~ **in** abusar de

overjoyed, lleno de alegría *adj*

overload, to, sobrecargar

overnight, por una noche; **to stay** ~ pasar la noche

overpopulated, superpoblado *adj*

overpower, to, abrumar

overpowering, abrumador *adj*

overreaching, alcanzamiento

override, to, hacer caso omiso de

overrule, to, (*to rescind*) anular

oversee, to, supervisar

oversight, ~ (*neglect*) descuido; ~ (*supervision*) supervisión *f*

oversize, ~ (*too large*) demasiado grande; ~ (*unusually large*) de tamaño descomunal

oversleep, to, dormir (ue) demasiado; dormir (ue) más de lo previsto

overstrain, cansancio excesivo

over-the-counter, que no requiere receta médica *adj*

overtime, horas extraordinarias *f, pl*

overweight, exceso de peso; sobrepeso; excesivamente gordo *adj*; excesivamente grueso *adj*

overwhelm, to, ~ (*with work, etc.*) abrumar; ~ (*with grief, etc.*) postrar; ~ **with honors** colmar de honores; **to be** ~**ed with joy** rebosar de alegría

overwork, to, trabajar demasiado

overwrought, sobreexcitado *adj*; ~ (*exhausted*) con los nervios destrozados

oviduct, oviducto

ovulate, to, ovular

ovulation, ovulación *f*; **menstrual** ~ ovulación amenstrual

ovum, (*pl, ova*) huevo *fam*; óvulo

owe, to, deber

own, to, tener

oxalic acid, ácido oxálico

oxidase, oxidasa

oxidation, oxidación *f*

oxide, óxido

oxidize, to, oxidar

oxygen, oxígeno; ~ **cylinder** balón de oxígeno *m*; ~ **deficiency** falta de oxígeno; ~ **mask** máscara de oxígeno; ~ **tank** tanque de oxígeno *m*; ~ **tent** cámara de oxígeno; tienda de oxígeno; ~ **therapy** terapia de oxígeno; ~ **treatment** oxigenoterapia

oxygenate, oxigenado *adj*;

oxygenate, to, oxigenar

oxygenation, oxigenación *f*

oxygenator, oxigenador *m*

oxygenize, to, oxigenar; oxidar

oxytocia, oxitocia; parto rápido

oxytocic, oxitócico *adj*; ocitócico *adj*

oxytocin, oxitocina

oyster, ostra

ozone, ozono

---

[2]   This is new vocabulary, not necessarily listed nor yet recognized by the Royal Academy of Spanish Grammar. It is understood that this vocabulary is primarily slang. Unless otherwise indicated, the gender of nouns is assumed to be obvious.

[4]   Originally the word *pomada* was used to describe any dermatologic salve or therapeutic agent for the skin. When the ointment contained vegetable resins, however, the term *ungüento* was used. Nowadays the two words are used as synonyms.

[5]   Current English street terminology for *opium* includes: black, black stuff, gow, gum, hop, leaf, Mash Allah.

P

pabulum, pábulo

pacemaker, aparato cardiocinético; marcador de paso *m*; marcador de ritmo *m*; marcapaso(s); monitor cardíaco *m*; seno auricular

pachymeningitis, paquimeningitis *f*

pachymeninx, paquimeninge *f*

pacifier, chupeta; chupete *m*; chupón *m*; mamón *m*, *Chicano*

pack, compresa *Med*; paño (caliente) *Med*; ~ (**bundle**) lío; ~ (*packet*) paquete *m*; ~ **of cigarettes** cajetilla

pack, to, ~ (*a suitcase, etc.*) hacer; empacar *Med*; rellenar *Med*; ~ **the wound with gauze** rellenar la herida con gasa

package, paquete *m*; ~ **insert** instructivo; ~ **of heroin** gramo

pad, almohadilla; cojín *m*; cojincillo; **alcohol** ~ gasita con alcohol; **heating** ~ almohadilla eléctrica; cojín eléctrico *m*

padding, guata *Surg, Ortho*; enguatado; acolchonado

page, página

page, to, llamar por vocina; llamar por bíper

pager, bíper *m*, *Chicano*

pail, cubo

pain, dolor *m*; ~ (*ache*) dolor; **bearing-down** ~ sensación de pesantez en el perineo *f*; dolor de pujos; **boring** ~ dolor penetrante; **burning** ~ dolor quemante; dolor con ardor; ~ **in the chest** dolor de pecho; **colicky** ~ dolor cólico; **constant** ~ dolor constante; **dull** ~ dolor sordo; **expulsive** ~ dolores expulsivos; **false** ~ dolores falsos; **flank** ~ dolor del costado; dolor del ijar; **ghost** ~ dolor fantasma; **gnawing** ~ punzada; **growing** ~ dolor de crecimiento; **hunger** ~ dolores de hambre; ~ **in the side** punto de costado *Med*; **intermenstrual** ~ dolores intermenstruales; **intermittent** ~ dolor que viene y se va; **internal** ~ ijada *Med*; ~ **killer** analgésico; calmante *m*; sedante *m*; **labor** ~ dolor de parto; dolores de parto; **localized** ~ dolor localizado; **mild** ~ dolor leve; **moderate** ~ dolor moderado; **phantom limb** ~ dolor de miembro fantasma; **postoperative** ~ dolor posoperatorio; **premonitory** ~ dolores premonitorios; **pressure-like** ~ dolor opresivo; **prickling** ~ hormigueo; **punching** ~ dolor pungitivo; **radiating** ~ dolor irradiado; **referred** ~ dolor referido; **root** ~ dolor radicular; **scalding** ~ dolor urente; **severe** ~ dolor fuerte; dolor severo; **sharp** ~ dolor agudo; dolor clavado; puntada *SpAm, Med*; punzada; **sharp internal** ~ torzón *m*; **sharp rheumatic** ~ hincada *Perú, PR*; **sensation of slight** ~ dolorimiento; **shooting** ~ dolor fulgurante; punzada *Med*; **small** ~ yaya *m, Chi, Col, Cu, Perú*; **smarting** ~ escozor *m*; **steady** ~ dolor continuo; **subjective** ~ dolor subjetivo; **thoracic** ~ dolor torácico; **twinge** ~ latido; **wandering** ~ dolor errante; dolor migratorio; ~ **when urinating** dolor al orinar; **to be in** ~ tener dolor

painful, ~ (*physically*) doloroso *adj*; ~ (*result of a blow*) dolorido *adj*; ~ (*difficult*) penoso *adj*; tra-

bajoso *adj*; ~**ly** dolorosamente *adv, Med*
painless, ~ (*physically*) indoloro *adj*; sin dolor; ~ (*not difficult*) sin dificultad
paint, pintura; **lead-based** ~ pintura con plomo
paint, to, pintar; ~ dar unos toques (a) *Med*; untar
pair, par *m*
pajamas, pijamas *f, pl*; piyamas *f, pl*
palatal, palatino *adj, Anat*
palate, paladar *m*; cielo de la boca; **bony** ~ paladar duro; paladar óseo; **cleft** ~ paladar hendido; palatosquisis *f*; **hard** ~ bóveda ósea del paladar; paladar duro; **soft** ~ paladar blando; paladar membranoso; velo del paladar; velo palatino
pale, pálido *adj*; trabajoso *adj, Med*
palliative, paliativo *m, adj*
pallium, palio; manto
pallor, palidez *f*
palm, palma de la mano
palmar, palmar *adj*
palpate, to, palpar
palpation, palpación *f*
palpitate, to, latir; palpitar
palpitation, palpitación *f*; latido *Chicano*; **heart** ~ palpitación cardíaca
palsied, paralítico *adj*; perlático *adj*; paralizado *adj, Med*
palsy, parálisis *f*; paralización *f*; perlesía; **Bell's** ~ parálisis facial; **cerebral** ~ parálisis cerebral; **shaking** ~ (*Parkinson's disease*) enfermedad de Parkinson *f*; parálisis agitante
paludism, paludismo; fiebre telúrica *f*; intoxicación palúdica *f*; (*See malaria.*)
pamphlet, folleto
pancreas, páncreas *m*
pancreatic, pancreático *adj*; ~ **juices** jugos pancreáticos
pancreatin, pancreatina

pancreatitis, pancreatitis *f*
pancreozymin, pancreocimina
panniculus adiposus, subcutaneous, paniculo adiposo subcutáneo
pant, to, acezar; jadear; resollar (ue)
panting, jadeante *adj*
pants, pantalones *m*
panty/panties, bragas *f, pl*; pantaletas *Mex*; calzoncillos; ~ **hose** pantimedias
Pap smear, examen vaginal para el cáncer *m*; frotis de Papanicolaou *m*; Papanicolaou *m*; untos de Papanicolaou *m*
Pap stain, coloración de Papanicolaou *f*
paper, papel *m*; **toilet** ~ papel de baño
papilla, papila
papilloma, papiloma *m*; **human** ~ **virus/HPV** papilomavirus humano *m*; virus de papiloma humano *m*
papule, pápula
para-aminobenzoic acid, ácido para-aminobenzoico; PABA
para-aminosalicylic acid/PAS, ácido para-aminosalicílico/PAS
paracentesis, paracentesis *f*
paradentitis, paradentitis *f*
paradentium, paradentio
paradentosis, paradentosis *f*
paradigm, modelo
paraffin, parafina
parakinesia, paracinesia
parallel bars, barras paralelas *f, pl*
paralysis, parálisis *f*; paralización *f*; perlesía; **acute ascending** ~ parálisis ascendente aguda; **creeping** ~ parálisis progresiva; **Duchenne's** ~ enfermedad de Duchenne *f*; faringolaríngea; parálisis labiogloso; parálisis bulbar crónica progresiva; **familial periodic** ~ parálisis periódica familiar; **infantil** ~ parálisis infantil; (*See polio*[*myelitis*].); **obstetrical** ~ parálisis obstétrica

paralytic, paralítico *m*, *adj*; perlático *adj*; sucho *adj*, *Arg*, *Ec*

paralyze, to, paralizar

paralyzed, paralítico *adj*; **to be ~** estar paralizado *adj*

paramedic, paramédico; socorrista *m/f*

parameter, parámetro

parametrium, parametrio

paranoia, paranoia

paranoid, paranoico *m*, *adj*

paraphasia, parafasia

paraplasm, paraplasia; displasia

paraplegia, parálisis de la mitad inferior del cuerpo *f*; paraplejía; **alcoholic ~** paraplejía alcohólica; **congenital spastic ~** paraplejía espástica infantil

paraplegic, parapléjico *adj*

parapsychology, para(p)sicología[6]

parasite, parásito; **amoeba** ameba; amiba; **ascaris (*roundworm*)** ascáride *f*; ascaris *f*; lombriz grande redonda *f*; **chigger flea** garrapata; güina *Mex*; nigua; **common name** nombre común *m*; **cysticercus (*bladderworm*)** cisticerco; **distribution** distribución *f*; **form of ~ in feces** forma de los parásitos en heces; **flea** pulga; **focus of infection** foco de la infección; **giardia** giardia; **gnat** bobito *Chicano*; jején *m*, *CA*; **louse** piojo; **crab louse** ladilla; **head louse** piojo de la cabeza; **nit** liendre *f*; **metazoos** metazoos; **mite** ácaro; **parasitic cyst** ladilla; quiste *m*; **~ infestation** parasitosis *f*; **pediculosis (*infestation*)** pediculosis *f*; piojería; **protozoa** protozoarios; **flagellates** flagelados; **route of entry** vía de entrada; **schistosoma** bilharzia; esquistosoma *m*; **solium (*tapeworm*)** gusano tableado; solitaria; **sporozoa** esporozoarios; **tapeworm** lombriz solitaria *f*; solitaria; tenia; **threadworms** lombriz chiquita afilada *f*; oxiuro; **trichinosis** triquinosis *f*; **trichocephalus** lombriz de látigo *f*; tricocéfalo; **uncinaria (*hookworm*)** lombriz de gancho *f*; uncinaria; **worm** gusano; lombriz *f*; **intestinal ~** verme *m*

parasitic, parasitario *adj*; parásito *adj*

parasitism, parasitismo

parasitology, parasitología

parasympathetic, parasimpático *adj*; **~ nerve** nervio parasimpático

parathyroid, paratiroides *f*, *adj*; paratifoideo *adj*

parathyroidectomy, paratiroidectomía

paratyphoid, paratifoidea *f*; **~ fever** paratifus *f*

parched, reseco *adj*

pardon, perdón *m*; **~ me** discúlpeme; dispénseme; perdóneme

pardon, to, perdonar

paregoric, paregórico

parenchyma, parénquima *m*

parents, padres *m*, *pl*

paresis, paresia

parietal, parietal *adj*; **~ bone** hueso parietal; **~ cells** células parietales; **~ lobe** lóbulo parietal

Parkinson's disease, enfermedad de Parkinson *f*; parálisis agitante *f*

paronychia, paroniquia

parorchidium, parorquidia

parotid, parótida; parotídeo; **~ gland** glándula parótida

paroxysm, paroxismo

paroxysmal, paroxístico *adj*; **~ hypertension** hipertensión paroxística *f*; **~ tachycardia** taquicardia paroxística; **~ atrial tachycardia** taquicardia auricular paroxística; **~ auricular tachycardia** taquicardia auricular paroxística; **~ ventricular tachycardia** taquicardia ventricular paroxística

parsley, perejil *m*

part, parte *f*; **~ (*of the hair*)** raya

parthenogenesis, partenogénesis *f*

partial, parcial *adj*; ~ **denture plate** dentadura parcial; ~ **pressure** presión parcial *f*
participate, to, participar
participation, participación *f*
particular, particular *adj*
part one's hair, to, hacerse la raya
part time, de media jornada *adj*; tiempo parcial *adv*
parturition, parturición *f*
pass, to, pasar; ~ **gas** pasar gas; tirar viento *slang*; ~ **over** atravesar (ie); pasar por; ~ (*stones, parasites, etc.*) eliminar; ~ **on** (*a disease*) pegar; ~ **on** (*to die*) fallecer
passage, tubo *Anat*; ~ (*hall*) pasillo; ~ **of time** paso del tiempo
passive, pasivo *adj*; ~-**aggressive** pasivo-agresivo *adj*; ~ **congestion** congestión pasiva *f*; ~ **immunity** inmunidad pasiva *f*; ~ **movements** movimientos pasivos
pasteurization, pasteurización *f*
pasteurize, to, pasteurizar
pastime, pasatiempo
pastry, pastel *m*
patch, parche *m*; ~ (*for the eyes*) tapaojo *m*, *SpAm*; **mucous** ~ parche mucosa
patella, patela; rótula
patellar, patelar *adj*; rotuliano *adj*; ~ **reflex** reflejo rotuliano
patellectomy, patelectomía
path, senda; vía
pathetic, patético *adj*
pathogen, patógeno
pathogeny, patogenia
pathological, patológico *adj*
pathologist, patólogo
pathology, patología; **clinical** ~ patología clínica
patience, paciencia
patient, paciente *m/f*, *adj*; enfermo; doliente *m/f*, *Med*; (*See outpatient.*); paciencioso *adj*, *Chi*, *Ec*; paciente *adj*
paunch, barriga; guata *Arg, Chi, Perú*; panza
paunchy, guatón *adj*; panzudo *adj*

pay (for), to, pagar
payment, pago
PCB/polychlorinated biphenyls, BPC[8]/bifenilo policlorinado
PCP/phencyclidine[4], PCP; amiba[2]; cucuy[2] *m*; Sherm[2]; fencycladina; líquido[2]; polvo[2]
pea, chícharo; guisante *m*
peace, paz *f*
peach, durazno; melocotón *m*
peak, punto máximo
peanut, cacahuete *m*; maní *m*; ~ **butter** manteca de cacahuete; crema de cacahuete *m*; ~ **oil** aceite de cacahuete *m*
pear, pera; ~-**shaped** piriforme *adj*
pectin, pectina
pectoral, pectoral *adj*
peddler[5,9], (*drug dealer*) burro[2]; madre[2]; narcotraficante[2]; pusheador[2]; traficante[2]; vendedor de drogas
pediatric, pediátrico *adj*
pediatrician, pediatra *m/f*; pédiatra *m/f*
pediatrics, pediatría
pediculosis, pediculosis *f*
pedicure, pedicura
pedodontia, pedodoncia
pedodontist, pedodontista *m/f*; dentista especialista de niños *m/f*; dentista pediátrico
pee, pipí *m*, *fam*; pis *m*, *fam*
pee, to, hacer pipí; (*See urinate, to.*)
peel, ~ (*skin*) piel *f*; ~ (*removed skin of oranges, potatoes, etc.*) cáscara
peel, to, ~ (*to take skin off*) pelar; ~ **off** (*human skin*)/**to be peeling** depellejarse; ~ **off** (*clothes*) quitarse; ~ **off** (*paint*) descancharse; ~ **off** (*wallpaper, etc.*) despegar
peeling, peladura; **chemical** ~ peladura química
peg, clavija
pellagra, pelagra; erisipela lombarda; lepra italiana; mal de la rosa *m*; mal de sol *m*
pelvic, pelviano *adj*; pélvico *adj*;

examen ginecológico *m*; ~ **abscess** absceso pélvico; ~ **cellulitis** celulitis pélvica *f*; ~ **index** índice pélvico *m*; ~ **inflammatory disease** (*See PID.*)

pelvimeter, pelvímetro

pelvimetry, pelvimetría

pelvis, bacinete *m*; pelvis *f*; **renal** ~ bacinete renal; pelvis renal

pen, ~ (*for writing*) pluma; **ball point** ~ bolígrafo; **felt-tipped** ~ rotulador *m*; **fountain** ~ pluma estilográfica; plumafuente *SpAm*; ~ (*for farm animals*) corral *m*; ~ (*for pigs*) pocilga; **play** ~ parque de niños *m*

pencil, lápiz *m*

pending, pendiente *adj*

pendulous, penduloso *adj*

penetrate, **to**, penetrar

penetrating, penetrante *adj*

penetration, penetración *f*

penicillin, penicilina; ~ **eye ointment** pomada oftálmica de penicilina; ~ **injection** inyección de penicilina *f*; ~ **resistance** penicilinorresistencia

penis, pene *m*, *form*; balone *m*, *Chicano*; bastón *m*, *slang*, *Mex*; camote *m*, *slang*, *Mex*; chicote *m*, *slang*; chile *m*, *slang*; chorizo *vulg*; explorador *m*, *slang*, *Mex*; miembro; pija *slang*, *Arg*; pito *slang*; ~ (*cock*) cañón *m*, *vulg*; ~ (*dick*) verga *vulg*; ~ (*prick*) cuerno *slang*; hierro *slang*; palo *slang*; ~ (*lit. 3rd leg*) trespata *vulg*; **head of** ~ ñema *vulg*; porra *vulg*

penknife, cortaplumas *m*, *inv*

pennyroyal leaves, hojas de poleo

pepper, pimienta; **bell** ~ pimiento; **black** ~ pimienta negra; **hot** ~ chile *m*; **sweet** ~ pimiento morrón

pepper, **to**, sazonar con pimienta

pep pill[9], estimulante *m*

pepsin, pepsina

peptic, péptico; ~ **ulcer** úlcer péptica

peptide, péptido *adj*

peptone, peptona

per, por; ~ **anum** por el año; ~ **capita** por cabeza; ~ **diem** por día; ~ **minute** por minuto; ~ **month** por mes; al mes; ~ **week** a la semana; por la semana

perceive, **to**, percibir

percentage, porcentaje *m*

perception, percepción *f*

percussion, percusión *f*

percutaneous transluminal angioplasty/PTA angioplastia transluminal percutánea/ATP[8]

perfect, perfecto *adj*

perfectionist, perfeccionista *m/f*

perfectly, perfectamente *adv*

perforate, **to**, perforar

perforated eardrum, tímpano perforado

perforation, perforación *f*

perform, **to**, desempeñar

performance, funcionamiento

perfume, perfume *m*

perfusion, perfusión *f*

perhaps, quizá(s) *adv*; tal vez *adv*

pericardial, pericárdico *adj*

pericardiocentesis, pericardiocentesis *f*

pericarditis, pericarditis *f*; **adhesive** ~ pericarditis adhesiva; **constrictive** ~ pericarditis constrictiva; **hemorrhagic** ~ pericarditis hemorrágica; ~ **with effusion** pericarditis con derrame

pericardium, pericardio

perichondrium, pericondrio

pericystitis, pericistitis *f*

perimetrium, perimetrio

perineal, perineal *adj*

perineum, periné *m*; perineo

period, período; **child-bearing** ~ período reproductivo; **incubation** ~ período de incubación; **lag** ~ período de rezago; ~ (*menstrual*) período; período menstrual; regla; (*See menstruation.*); **to miss a** ~ no bajar la regla; **postpartum** ~ puerperio; ~ (*punctuation*) punto; **quaran-**

tine ~ período de cuarentena; **safe** ~ período de seguridad
periodical, periódico *adj*
periodontal, periodontal *adj*
periodontia, periodoncia
periodontics, periodoncia
periodontist, periodontista *m/f*
periodontitis, periodontitis *f*; **apical** ~ periodontitis apical
periodontium, periodontio
periodontology, periodontología
periodontosis, periodontosis *f*
perionychia, perioniquia
perionychium, perioniquio
periosteum, periostio
peripheral, periférico *adj*
peristalsis, peristaltismo
peristaltic, peristáltico *adj*
peritoneal, peritoneal *adj*
peritoneum, peritoneo
peritonitis, abdomen aguda *m, slang*; panza peligrosa *slang*; peritonitis *f*; **acute** ~ peritonitis aguda; **chronic adhesive** ~ peritonitis crónica adhesiva; **perforative** ~ peritonitis por perforación
permanent, permanente *f, adj*; ~ **address** domicilio
permanently, de modo definitivo *prep phr*; permanentemente *adv*
permission, permiso; **to ask** ~ pedir (i) permiso; **to give** ~ dar permiso; **to have** ~ tener permiso
permit, permiso
permit, to, permitir
pernicious, pernicioso *adj*; ~ **anemia** anemia perniciosa; ~ **malaria** malaria perniciosa; ~ **vomiting** vómito pernicioso
peroneal, peroneal *adj*; ~ **muscular atrophy** atrofia muscular del peroneo
peroneum, peroneo
peroxide, agua[3] oxigenada; peróxido; **hydrogen** ~ agua[3] oxigenada; peróxido de hidrógeno
perpetuate, to, perpetuar
perplex, to, confundir
perseveration, perseveración *f*

persist, to, persistir (en)
persistence, persistencia
person, persona; ~ **about seventy** setentón, *m, adj*; ~ **about sixty** sesentón *m, adj*; ~ **blind in one eye** tuerto; ~ **high on drugs** cócono[2]; **mentally unbalanced** ~ perturbado; **short, stocky** ~ tachuela *f, Arg, Chi, Guat, Mex*
personal, personal *adj*; ~ **hygiene** aseo personal; higiene personal *f*; ~ **stress** estrés personal *m*
personality, personalidad *f*; **antisocial** ~ personalidad antisocial; **borderline** ~ personalidad limítrofe; ~ **change** cambio de personalidad; ~ **disorder** trastorno de la personalidad; **obsessive-compulsive** ~ personalidad obsesivo-compulsiva; **paranoid** ~ personalidad paranoide; **passive-aggressive** ~ personalidad pasivo-agresiva; **psychopathic** ~ personalidad (p)sicopática[6]; **schizoid** ~ personalidad esquizoide
personnel, personal *m*
perspiration, sudor *m*; perspiración *f*; **to be bathed in** ~ estar todo sudoroso
perspire, to, sudar
perspiring, pasoso *adj, Chi*
perturb (mentally), to, perturbar
pertussis, coqueluche *f*; tos convulsiva *f*; tos ferina *f*; tosferina
perversion, perversión *f*; **sexual** ~ perversión sexual
pervert, sexual, pervertido sexual
pessary, pesario; **diaphragm** ~ pesario de diafragma
pessimism, pesimismo; **therapeutic** ~ pesimismo terapéutico
pesticide, pesticida *m*; plaguicida *m*
pestilence, pestilencia
PET/positron emission tomography, TEP/tomografía por emisión de positrones *f*; tomografía transaxial de emisión de positrones

petechia, (*pl, petechiae*) petequia
petit mal, pequeño mal *m*
petrifaction, petrificación *f*
petroleum, petróleo
peyote, peyote *m*
pH, pH^8 *m*
phalanx, falange *f*
phallic, fálico *adj*
phallus, falo
pharmaceutical, farmacéutico *adj*
pharmacist, farmacéutico; boticario
pharmacologist, farmacólogo
pharmacology, farmacología
pharmacy, botica; farmacia
pharyngitis, faringitis *f*
pharynx, faringe *f*
phase, fase *f*
phencyclidine^9, fenciclidina; (*See PCP.*)
phenobarbital, fenobarbital *m*
phenomenon, fenómeno
phenylketonuria/PKU, fenilcetonuria; fenilquetonuria; prueba del pañal *fam*
phlebitis, flebitis *f*; tromboflebitis *f*
phlebography, flebografía
phlebogram, flebograma *m*
phlebotomist, flebotomista *m/f*
phlebotomy, flebotomía; sangría *fam*; venotomía; **bloodless ~** flebotomía incruenta
phlegm, flema; mocosidad *f*; moquera *fam*; desgarro *SpAm*
phobia, fobia
phosphate, fosfato
phosphoric acid, ácido fosfórico
phosphorus, fósforo
photography, fotografía
photosensitive, fotosensible *adj*
phrenic, frénico *adj*
phthisis, consunción *f*; tisis *f*; tuberculosis *f*
physical, físico *adj*; **~ activity** actividad física *f*; **~ diagnosis** diagnóstico físico; **~ examination** reconocimiento médico; **~ exercise** ejercicio físico; **~ health** salud física *f*; **~ problems** problemas físicos *m*; **~ signs** signo

físico; **~ therapist** terapista físico; **~ therapy** fisioterapia
physically, físicamente *adv*
physician, doctor; médico; **attending ~** médico a cardo; médico adscrito; médica adscrita; médico asistente; médico de cabecera; **consulting ~** médico consultor; médica consultora; **family ~** médico de la familia; **house/resident ~** médico residente; **~ on call** médico de guardia; **referring ~** médico recomendante
physicist, fisicista *m/f*
physics, física
physiological, fisiológico *adj*
physiologist, fisiólogo
physiology, fisiología
physiotherapist, fisioterapeuta *m/f*; fisioterapista *m/f*
physiotherapy, fisioterapia
physique, (*man's*) talle *m, Anat*
pia mater, piamadre *f*
pick, to, ~ (*a scab*) rascarse; **~ one's nose** hurgarse la nariz; **~ up** recoger
pickle, pepinillo
picture, to take a, sacar fotos
PID/pelvic inflammatory disease, enfermedad inflamatoria pélvica *f*; enfermedad inflamatoria de la pelvis *f*; infección pélvica *f*
pie, pastel *m*
piece, ~ (*section*) pedazo; **~ of advice** consejo
pierce, to, perforar; penetrar
piercing, (*pain*) terebrante *adj*
pigeon, paloma; **~-toed** patizambo *adj*; chueco *adj, Arg, Perú*
pigment, pigmento
pigmentary, pigmentario *adj*
pigmentation, pigmentación *f*; **extraneous ~** pigmentación extrínseca; **malarial ~** pigmentación palúdica
piles, almorranas *f, pl*; hemorroides *f, pl*
pill, ~ (*capsule*) cápsula; ~ (*solid*)

comprimido; pastilla; píldora; tableta; **birth control** ~ pastilla para no tener niños; píldora anticonceptiva; píldora para control de(l) embarazo; ~ **freak**[9] píldoro[2]; ~ **head**[9] píldoro[2]; ~ **popper** píldoro[2]; **sleeping** ~ píldora para dormir; píldora somnífera; sedativo; somnífero; soporífera; **thyroid** ~ medicación tiroides *f*

pillbox, cajita de píldoras

pillow, almohadilla; ~ (*inflatable rubber doughnut*) almohadilla neumática en forma de anillo

pillowcase, funda de almohada

pimple, barrillo; buba; butón *m*; grano de la cara; pupa *Med*; pústula; suche *m*, *Arg*; **blackhead** ~ (*due to acne*) barro; espinilla

pin, alfiler *m*; clavo *Ortho*; ~**s and needles** hormigas *Med*

pinched nerve, nervio aplastado

pineal, pineal *adj*; ~ **gland** glándula pineal

pineapple, piña

pine oil, aceite de pino *m*

pink, rosado *adj*

pinkeye, conjuntivitis catarral aguda *f*; mal de ojo *m*; oftalmia contagiosa

pinprick, hincadura de alfiler; alfilerazo

pint, pinta

pinworm, oxiuro

pipe, ~ (*for smoking*) pipa; ~ (*tube*) tubo

piperazine, anterobius *m*; piperawitt *m/f*; piperacina; piperidol *m*

pipette, pipeta

pit, ~ (*of stomach*) boca del estómago; epigastrio; hueco epigástrico; ~ (*of fruit*) hueso; ~ (*in skin, from smallpox, etc.*) picadura; ~ (*hole in ground*) hoyo

pit, to ~ (*fruit*) deshuesar; ~ (*with smallpox*) marcar con viruelas

pitch, (*tone*) tono

pitcher, jarra

pitocin, pitocín *m*; pitocina

pituitary, pituitario *adj*; pituitaria *f*; glándula pituitaria; ~ **gland** glándula pituitaria

pity, lástima; pena

PKU/phenylketonuria, fenilcetonuria; fenilquetonuria; prueba del pañal

place, (*position*) lugar *m*; **out of** ~ fuera de lugar

place, to, (*to put*) colocar; poner

placebo, placebo

placenta, lo demás *slang*; placenta; secundinas; segundo parto *Chicano*; ~ **abruptio** desprendimiento prematuro de la placenta; ~ **previa** placenta previa

placental, placentario *adj*; ~ **insufficiency** insuficiencia placentaria

placentography, placentografía

plague, ~ (*disease*) peste *f*; **bubonic** ~ peste bubónica; tifo de Oriente; peste *f*, *Perú, PR*; ~ (*social scourge*) plaga

plain, ~ (*simple*) sencillo *adj*; (*clear*) claro *adj*; evidente *adj*; ~ (*flat, even*) plano *adj*; ~ (*unmixed*) sin mezcla *prep phr*

plane, ~ (*aircraft*) avión *m*; ~ (*carpenter's tool*) cepillo; ~ (*level*) nivel *m*

planned parenthood, natalidad dirigida *f*; procreación planeada *f*

planning, planificación *f*; **family** ~ planificación familiar

plaque, placa bacteriana *Dent*; sarro *Dent*; plaqueta *Med*; plastocito *Med*; globulino *Med*; hematoblasto *Med*; trombocito *Med*

plasma, plasma *m*; **blood** ~ plasma sanguíneo; ~ **substitute** substitutivo de plasma; ~ **thromboplastic antecedent** antecedente tromboplástico del plasma *m*; ~ **thromboplastic component** componente tromboplástico del pla ma *m*; ~ **thromboplastic factor** factor tromboplástico del plasma *m*

plasmapheresis, plasmaféresis *f*

plaster, ~ (*for a cast*) yeso; ~ **cast** apósito enyesado; vendaje enyesado *m*; ~ **of Paris** yeso mate; ~ **splint** férula de yeso; emplasto *Med*; cataplasma *f*, *Med*; **adhesive** ~ emplasto adhesivo; **mustard** ~ sinapismo; cataplasma/emplasto de mostaza; ~ (*for an injury*) escayola

plastic, plástico *m*, *adj*; ~ **surgery** cirugía plástica

plate, ~ (*dish*) plato; ~ (*x-ray*) placa *Dent*, *Med*; **denture** ~ dentadura postiza; placas

platelet, plaqueta

play, to, jugar (ue)

pleasant, agradable *adj*

please, por favor

plenty, (*enough*) bastante *adv*

pleura, pleura

pleural tap, toracentesis *f*

pleurisy, pleuresía; inflamación de los bofes *f*, *Chicano*; pleuritis *f*

plexus, plexo

pliers, pinzas

plum, ciruela

plump, ~ (*body*) petacón *adj*, *Mex*, *Perú*, *Ríopl*; rechoncho *adj*; ~ (*face*) mofletudo *adj*

pluripara, plurípara *f*, *adj*

PMS/premenstrual syndrome, síndrome premenstrual *m*

pneumatosis, neumatosis *f*

pneumaturia, neumaturia

pneumococcus, neumococo

pneumograph, neumógrafo

pneumonectomy, neumonectomía

pneumonia, neumonía; neumonitis *f*; pulmonía; **aspiration** ~ neumonía por aspiración; pulmonía por aspiración; **broncho~** bronconeumonía; pulmonía bronquial; **lipoid** ~ pulmonía por grasa; pulmonía por lípidos; **pneumococcal lobular** ~ pulmonía neumocócica lobular; **streptococcus** ~ pulmonía estreptocócica; **viral** ~ pulmonía por virus; pulmonía vírica

pneumothorax, neumotórax *m*

POA/power of attorney, poder legal *m*

pock, cacaraña *Mex*, *Guat*; postilla; viruela

pockmarked, borrado *adj*, *Perú*; picado de viruelas *adj*; picarazado *adj*, *Cu*, *PR*; picoso *adj*; sipo *adj*, *Ec*; tuso *adj*, *Col*, *Ven*

pockmarks, to have, estar cacarizo

podiatrist, podiatra *m/f*; podiatrista *m/f*; quiropodista *m/f*

podiatry, podiatría

point, punto; ~ (*sharp end*) punta

point to, to, indicar; señalar

poison, intoxicante *m*; ponzoña; veneno; ~ (*snake, etc.*) ponzoñoso *adj*; venenoso *adj*; ~ (*gas, drug, etc.*) tóxico *adj*; **common** ~ veneno común; ~ **gas** gas asfixiante *m*; gas tóxico *m*; ~ **hemlock** cicuta; **inhaled** ~ veneno aspirado; **injected** ~ veneno inyectado; ~ **ivy** chechén *m*; hiedra venenosa; yedra venenosa; zumaque venenoso *m*; **oral** ~ veneno tomado por la boca; **to take** ~ envenenarse

poison, to, emponzoñar; intoxicar; ~ (*oneself*) envenenar(se); enyerbarse *Guat*, *Mex*; **to be ~ed** envenenarse

poisoning, envenenamiento; intoxicación *f*; **botulism** ~ intoxicación botulínica; **carbon monoxide** ~ intoxicación por monóxido de carbono; **food** ~ envenenamiento por comestibles; intoxicación con alimentos; **lead** ~ envenenamiento plúmbico; envenenamiento del plomo; plumbismo; saturnismo; **salmonella** ~ intoxicación por salmonelas; **staphylococcal** ~ intoxicación por estafilococos

poisonous, ponzoñoso *adj*; venenoso *adj*

poke, ~ (*with elbow*) codazo; ~ (*shove*) empujón *m*; puntazo *SpAm*, *Cu*, *Mex*

police, (*force*) policía *f*

policeman, policía *m*

policy, (*insurance*) póliza; **dental insurance** ~ póliza de seguros de cuidado dental; **health insurance** ~ póliza de seguros de salud; **life insurance** ~ póliza de seguros de vida; póliza de seguros sobre la vida

polio(myelitis), parálisis infantil *f*; poliomielitis *f*

polish, to, ~ (*style*) limar; ~ (*floors, furniture*) sacar brillo a; ~ (*glass, metal*; *to perfect*) pulir

pollen, polen *m*

polluting agent, contaminante *m*

pollution, polución *f*; contaminación *f*; **air** ~ contaminación del aire; **water** ~ contaminación del agua

polycystic, poliquístico *adj*

polydipsia, polidipsia *form*; **to have** ~ tener mucha sed excesiva

polyp, pólipo; **bleeding** ~ pólipo hemorrágico; **fleshy** ~ pólipo carnoso; **gelatinous** ~ pólipo gelatinoso; **nasal** ~ pólipo nasal

polyphagia, polifagia *form*; **to have** ~ tener mucho apetito

polyunsaturated, poliinsaturado *adj*

polyuria, poliuria *form*; el orinar demasiado

polyvalent, polivalente *adj*

pomade, pomada

ponder, to, ponderar

pool, (*of blood*) remanso; charco

poor, pobre *adj*; **in** ~ **health** jodido *adj*

popcorn, palomitas de maíz *f*, *pl*; pororó *Ríopl*

popping, (*eyes*) saltón *adj*

poppy, amapola; adormidera

population, población *f*

porcelain, porcelana

pore, poro

pork, carne de puerco *f*; cerdo; ~ **chop** chuleta de puerco; ~ **ribs** costillas asadas

portable, portátil *adj*

portion, porción *f*; ~ (*of food*) ración *f*

position, posición *f*

positive, ~ (*not negative*) positivo *adj*; ~ (*convinced*) seguro *adj*; ~ (*definite*) auténtico *adj*; ~ **proof** prueba evidente

possible, posible *adj*

post, espiga *Dent*; pequeña claviga *Dent*

postal zone/zip code, zona postal; código postal

poster, cartel *m*

posterior, posterior *adj*

postmortem, post mortem *f*, *adj*; autopsia; examen necrópsico *m*

postnasal drip, escurrimiento posnasal

postnatal care, cuidado postnatal

post office, casa de correos; **p. o. box** apartado postal

postoperative, posoperatorio *adj*; ~ **pain** dolor posoperatorio

postpartum, posparto; puerperio; ~ **flow of milk** subida de la leche

potash, potasa

potassium, potasio; ~ **cyanide** cianuro de potasio; ~ **iodide** yoduro de potasio; ~ **nitrate** nitrato de potasio; ~ **permanganate** permanganato de potasio

potato, (*pl, potatoes*) papa *SpAm*; patata; ~ **peeler** pelapatatas *m*, *inv*

potbellied, barrigón *adj*; panzón *adj*; panzudo *adj*; guatón *adj*, *Arg, Chi, Perú*; lipón *adj*, *Ven*; petacón *adj*, *Col*; torombolo *adj*, *Cu*

potency, potencia; fuerza; eficacia

potent, ~ (*poison*) poderoso *adj*; ~ (*a remedy*) eficaz *adj*; ~ (*drink*) fuerte *adj*

potential, potencial *m*, *adj*

potion, dosis *f*, *inv*; poción *f*; pócima

poultice, cataplasma; emplasto; sinapismo

pound, ~ (*weight, money*) libra; ~(*for cars, animals*) depósito

pound, to, ~ (*to crush*) machacar; ~ (*to grind*) moler (ue); ~ (*the sea*) azotar; ~ (*to strike*) dar golpes; ~ (*heart*) latir violentamente; palpitar; ~ (*with a hammer*) martillear

powder, polvo; **talcum** ~ polvos de talco *m*, *pl*; talco
powdered, en polvo *prep phr*
powdery, empolvado *adj*; polvoriento *adj*; polvoroso *adj*
power, ~ (*in general*) poder *m*; ~ (*Math*; *Mech*) potencia; ~ **of attorney/POA** carta de personería; poder (legal) *m*; ~ (*mental*) facultad *f*; **mental ~s** facultades mentales
powerful, potente *adj*
PPO/preferred provider organization, OPP[8]/organización de proveedor preferido *f*
practice ~ (*of profession, etc.*) práctica; ~ (*habit*) costumbre *f*; ~ (*Med: number of patients*) clientela
practice, to, practicar
practitioner, general/GP, médico general
precarious, precario *adj*
precaution, precaución *f*
precautionary, preventivo *adj*; ~ **measures** medidas preventivas
precautious, cauteloso *adj*
precedence, precedencia; prioridad *f*; **to take ~ over s.o.** preceder a uno
precedent, precedente *m*
preceding, precedente *adj*
precept, precepto
precipitate, precipitado *Chem*; ~ (*hasty*) precipitado *adj*; apresurado *adj*
precipitate, to, precipitar *Chem*; ~ (*to cause*) producir; ~ (*to hasten*) acelerar; apresurar; precipitar
precise, preciso *adj*
precision, precisión *f*
precocious, precoz *adj*
precursor, precursor, -ra *m/f*
predict, to, predecir; pronosticar
predispose, to, predisponer
predisposition (to), predisposición (a) *f*
prednisone, prednisona
predominant, predominante *adj*
predominate, to, predominar
preeclampsia, preeclampsia

preexist, to, preexistir
preexistence, preexistencia
preexistent, preexistente *adj*
prefer, to, preferir (ie)
preferable, preferible *adj*
preference, preferencia; **What is your ~**? ¿cuál le gusta más?
preferential, preferencial *adj*; preferente *adj*; ~ **treatment** trato preferente
pregnancy, embarazo; estado interesante *euph*, *Chicano*; gravidez *f*; preñez *f*; **ectopic ~** embarazo ectópico; embarazo fuera de la matriz; **false ~** embarazo falso; **hysteria ~** embarazo histérico; **incomplete ~** embarazo incompleto; ~ **toxemia** toxemia gravídica; **tubal ~** embarazo en los tubos; embarazo tubárico
pregnant, embarazada *adj*; en estado *prep phr*, *fam*; encinta *adj*; grávida *adj*; gruesa *adj*, *fam*; panzona *vulg*; preñada *adj*; **to be ~** estar embarazada; estar en estado; estar encinta; estar de encargo *Arg*, *RD*, *Ur*; estar ocupada (*for women*); **to be ____ months ~** estar embarazada de ____ meses; **to become ~** embarazarse; **to get ~** preñar *fam*
preheat, to, precalentar (ie)
prejudice, ~ (*biassed view*; *detriment*) prejuicio; ~ (*hostility*) mala voluntad *f*
prejudiced, predispuesto *adj*; **to be ~ against** estar predispuesto contra; **to be ~ in favor of** estar predispuesto a favor de
preliminary, preliminar *m*, *adj*
premature, prematuro *adj*: ~ **atrial contraction/PAC** contracción auricular prematura *f*; ~ **ventricular contraction/PVC** contracción ventricular prematura *f*; ~ **beat** (*extrasystole*) extrasístole *f*, ~ (*birth*) chaucha *adj*, *Chi*, *Ec*; ~ (*lit. seven months*) sietemesino *adj*, *m/f*; ~ (*baldness, etc.*) precoz *adj*
prematurity, premadurez *f*

premedication, premedicación *f*
premenstrual syndrome/PMS, síndrome premenstrual *m*
premium, (*in commerce, insurance*) prima; **insurance** ~ prima de seguros
premonition, presentimiento; **to have a** ~ presentir (ie)
prenatal, prenatal *adj*; ~ **care** cuidado prenatal
preoperative, preoperatorio *adj*
prepaid, pagado con anticipación *adj*
preparation, preparación *f*; preparado *Pharm*
preparatory, preparatorio *adj*
prepare, to, preparar
prepuce, prepucio, *Anat*
presbyopia, (*farsightedness*) hipermetropía; presbicia; presbiopía; vista cansada
prescribe, to, prescribir; prescribir un remedio; recetar; ~ **for oneself** autorecetarse
prescribed, recetado *adj*; prescrito *adj*
prescription, prescripción *f*; receta; **medical** ~ prescripción facultativa; receta médica
presence, presencia
present, presente *adj*; ~ (*gift*) regalo
presentation, presentación *f*; **breech** ~ presentación de nalgas *Obst*; **frank breech** ~ presentación franca de nalgas *Obst*; **brow** ~ presentación de frente *Obst*; **cephalic** ~ presentación cefálica *Obst*; **face** ~ presentación de cara *Obst*; **footling** ~ presentación de pies *Obst*; **placental** ~ presentación placentaria *Obst*; ~ **shoulder** ~ presentación de hombro *Obst*; **transverse** ~ presentación transversa *Obst*
press, ~ (*pressure*) presión *f*; ~ (*of hand*) apretón *m*
press, to, ~ (*to iron*) planchar; ~ (*to push*) apretar (ie)
pressure, presión *f*; tensión *f, Med*;

blood ~ presión arterial; presión de sangre; presión sanguínea; tensión arterial; (*See blood pressure.*); **diastolic** ~ presión diastólica; ~ **sore** úlcera por presión; **systolic** ~ presión sistólica; ~ **sensations** sensaciones de ser apretado *adj*; **to exert** ~ **on** ejercer presión sobre; **to take the blood** ~ tomar la presión
presume, to, suponer
presumption, presunción *f*
presurgical, prequirúrgico *adj*
presystole, presístole *f*
pretence, (*See pretense.*)
pretend, to, ~ (*to claim*) pretender; ~ (*to feign*) fingir; ~ **to be** fingirse
pretense, ~ (*claim*) pretensión *f*; ~ (*display*) afectación *f*; ~ (*pretext*) pretexto; ~ (*make-believe*) fingimiento
prevent, to, impedir (i); prevenir
preventable/preventible, prevenible *adj*; evitable *adj*
prevention, prevención *f*
preventive, preventivo *adj*; ~ **measure** medida preventiva; ~ medicamento profiláctico *Med*; profiláctico
previous, previo *adj*; anterior *adj*
prick, ~ (*of a needle*) pinchazo; puntura; punzada; estacada *SpAm*; piquete *m, Mex*; puyón *m, Col, Guat, PR* ; polla *Anat*; (*See penis.*); ~ (*of an insect*) picadura
prick, to, pinchar; estacar *Ven*; puyar *SpAm*
prickly heat, erupción debida al calor *f*; picazón *f*; sarpullido causado por exceso de calor
pride, orgullo
priest, cura *m*; sacerdote *m*; **parish** ~ párroco
primary, primario *adj*; ~ **care** cuidado básico; cuidado general; ~ **care physician** médico de cuidado general; ~ **disease** enfermedad primaria *f*

prime, ~ (*chief*) primero *adj*; ~ (*of life*) flor de la vida *f*
primigravida, primigrávida
primipara, primípara *f, adj*
primitive, primitivo *adj*
principal, principal *adj*; ~ (*of a school, etc.*) director, -ra *m/f*
principle, principio
print, (*of finger, foot, etc.*) huella
priority, prioridad *f*
privacy, soledad *f*
private, privado *adj*; confidencial *adj*; particular *adj*; ~ **clinic** clínica privada; ~ **hospital** clínica; ~ **parts** partes *f, pl*; partes privadas *f, pl*; genitales *m, pl*; partes pudendas *f, pl*; ~ **practice** consulta particular
privileged, privilegiado *adj*; confidencial *adj*; ~ **information** información confidencial *f*
p.r.n./pro re nata, según las necesidades *prep phr*; según las circunstancias *prep phr*
probe, cánula; estilete *m*; sonda; tienta
probe, to, ~ (*to investigate*) indagar; ~ (*with a medical probe*) explorar *Med*; sondar *Med*; sondear *Med*; tentar (ie) *Med*
probing, sondeo
problem, problema *m*; trastorno
procaine, procaína
procedure, procedimiento; **clinical** ~ procedimiento clínico; **rules of** ~ reglamento interno; **surgical** ~ procedimiento quirúrgico
proceed, to, proceder; proseguir (i)
process, apófisis *f, Med*; proceso
procreate, to, procrear
proctitis, proctitis *f*
proctologist, proctólogo
proctology, proctología
proctoscope, proctoscopio
produce, to, producir
product, producto; ~ **IV**[9] combinación de PCP y LSD; **milk** ~**s** productos lácteos *m, pl*; **waste** ~**s** desperdicios *m, pl*

profession, profesión *f*
professional, profesional *adj*; ~ **services** servicios profesionales; ~ **training** formación profesional *f*
profile, (*of face*) perfil *m*; ~ (*of body*) silueta
profound, hondo *adj*
profoundly, profundamente *adv*
profuse, profuso *adj*
progeny, progenie *f*; prole *f*
progesterone, progesterona
prognose, to, pronosticar
prognosis, (*pl, prognoses*) pronóstico
prognosticate, to, pronosticar
program, programa *m*
progress, progreso; ~ (*of a disease*) curso; **in** ~ en curso
progress, to, progresar *Med*; mejorar, *Med*
progression, progresión *f*
progressive, progresivo *adj*; ~ **illness** enfermedad progresiva *f*
prohibit, to, ~ (*to forbid*) prohibir; **smoking is** ~**ed** se prohibe fumar; ~ (*to prevent*) impedir (i)
project, (*plan*) proyecto
project, to, proyectar
projection, proyección *f*
prolapse, prolapso; ~ **of the uterus** caída de la matriz; descenso del útero *Med*; **mitral valve** ~ prolapso valvular mitral; ~**d umbilical cord** prolapso del cordón umbilical; ~ **of the rectum** prolapso del recto
prolific, prolífico *adj*
prolong, to, ~ (*in space*) prolongar; ~ (*in time*) extender (ie)
prolongation, prolongación *f*
prolonged, prolongado *adj*
prominent, ~ (*cheekbone, tooth, etc.*) saliente *adj*; ~ (*eye*) saltón *adj*; ~ (*jutting out*) prominente *adj*; ~ (*outstanding*) destacado *adj*
promiscuous, (*sexually*) libre *adj*; promiscuo *adj*
promise, promesa
prompt, inmediato *adj*; en punto *prep phr*

prone, ~ (*person*) acostado boca abajo *adj*; ~ (*inclined*) propenso *adj*
proof, prueba
propagation, propagación *f*
property, propiedad *f*
prophylactic, profiláctico *m*, *adj*; condón *m*; (*See birth control.*)
prophylaxis, profilaxis *f*, *Med*; profilaxia *Med*
proportion, proporción *f*
prostaglandins, prostaglandinas
prostate, próstata; prostático *adj*; ~ gland próstata
prostatic, prostático *adj*
prostatitis, prostatitis *f*; tapado de orín
prosthesis, miembro artificial; parte artificial *f*; prótesis *f*; dental ~ prótesis dental; maxillofacial ~ prótesis maxilofacial; postsurgical ~ prótesis posquirúrgica
prosthetic, prostético *adj*; ~ dentistry odontología prostética
prosthetics, protética
prosthodontia, prostodoncia
prosthodontics, prostodoncia
prostitute, prostituta; puta *vulg*
prostitution, prostitución *f*
prostrate, postrado *adj*; to be ~d by grief ser postrado por el dolor
prostrate, to, postrar *Med*; ~ oneself postrarse
prostration, postración *f*; heat ~ postración por el calor
protect, to, proteger
protection, protección *f*
protective, proteccionista *adj*; protector *adj*; ~ custody detención preventiva *f*
protein, proteína
prothrombin, protrombina; trombógeno; ~ consumption test test del consumo de protrombina *m*; ~ time tiempo de protrombina
protoplasm, protoplasma *m*
protruding, ~ (*eyes*) saltón *adj*; ~ (*bowel*) herniado *adj*, *Med*; ~ (*jaw, forehead*) saliente *adj*
protrusion, protuberancia, saliente *m*

protuberance, protuberancia
proud, orgulloso *adj*
prove, to, ~ (*to test*; *to try out*) probar (ue); ~ (*to result*) resultar
provide, to, ~ (*to supply*) proveer; ~ (*to give*; *to furnish*) proporcionar; ~ an addict with a fix curar²
provision, provisión *f*; ~s (*food*) provisiones *f*, *pl*; suministro; comestibles *m,pl*; víveres *m*, *pl*
provoke, to, provocar
prune, ciruela pasa
pruritus, (*severe itching*) prurito; comezón intensa *f*; bath ~ prurito del baño; ~ vulvae prurito vulvar
pseudocyesis, (p)seudociesis⁶ *f*; embarazo falso; embarazo imaginario
psilocybin⁷,⁹, hongos²; mujercitas²; niños²
psoriasis, mal de pintas *m*; (p)soríasis⁶ *f*
psyche, (p)sique⁶ *f*
psychedelic⁹, droga (p)sicodélica⁶; (p)sicodélico⁶ *m*, *adj*
psychiatric, (p)siquiátrico⁶ *adj*; ~ intervention intervención (p)siquiátrica⁶ *f*
psychiatrist, (p)siquiatra⁶ *m/f*
psychiatry, (p)siquiatría⁶
psychic, (p)síquico⁶ *adj*
psycho, (p)sicópata⁶ *m/f*; persona anormal *f*
psychoanalysis, (p)sicoanálisis⁶ *f*
psychoanalyst, (p)sicoanalista⁶ *m/f*
psychoanalyze, to, (p)sicoanalizar⁶
psychodrama, (p)sicodrama⁶ *m*
psychologic(al), (p)sicológico⁶ *adj*
psychologically, (p)sicológicamente⁶ *adv*
psychologist, (p)sicólogo⁶
psychology, (p)sicología⁶
psychometry, (p)sicometría⁶
psychomotor, (p)sicomotor⁶ *adj*
psychoneuroimmunology, (p)siconeuroinmunología⁶
psychoneurosis, (p)siconeurosis⁶ *f*
psychopath, (p)sicópata⁶ *m/f*

psychopathic, (p)sicopático[6] *adj*
psychopathology, (p)sicopatología[6]
psychopathy, (p)sicopatía[6]
psychosis, (p)sicosis[6] *f*; **manic-depressive ~** (p)sicosis[6] maníaco-depresiva; **situational ~** (p)sicosis[6] situacional; (p)sicosis[6] de situación
psychosocial, (p)sicosocial[6] *adj*
psychosomatic, (p)sicosomático[6] *adj*
psychotechnics, (p)sicotecnia[6]
psychotherapeutics, (p)sicoterapia[6]
psychotherapy, (p)sicoterapia[6]
psychotic, (p)sicótico[6] *m, adj*
PTA/Plasma Thromboplastic Antecedent, antecedente tromboplástico del plasma *m*
pterygium, carnosidad *f, fam*; pterigión *m*
ptomaine, ptomaína; ptomaínico *adj*; tomaína; **~ poisoning** envenenamiento ptomaínico
ptosis, ptosis *f*
puberty, pubertad *f*
pubescence, pubescencia
pubic, púbico *adj*; **~ hair** pelitos *m, pl, Chicano*; pelo púbico; pendejos *fam, slang, Arg*; vello púbico; **~ region** partes ocultas *f*; pubis *m*; verijas *pl*
public, público *m, adj*; **~ funds** fondos públicos; **~ health** salud pública *f*; salubridad pública *f*; **~ health agency** agencia de salud pública; **~ health services** servicios de salud pública
pudendal, pudendo *adj*
puerile, pueril *adj*
puerperal, puerperal *adj*
puerperium, puerperio
puff to, **~** (*to blow*) soplar; **~** at (*cigar, cigarette*) dar chupadas a; **~ and pant** jadear; **~ out** inflar (se)
pull, to, jalar; **~** (*to tug at*) tirar (de); **~** (*to extract*) sacar; **~** (*back foreskin of penis*) pelársela; **~ a muscle** desgarrarse un músculo; sufrir un tirón; **~ out** extraer; **~ up (one's) knees** encoger las rodillas; **~ through** recobrar la salud; **to have a ~ed muscle** tener un tirón en un músculo

pulmonary, pulmonar *adj*; **~ artery wedge pressure** presión diferencial de la arteria pulmonar; **~ disease** (*lung*) enfermedad pulmonar *f*; **~ edema** edema pulmonar *m*; **~ embolism** embolia pulmonar; **~ emphysema** enfisema pulmonar *m*; **~ insufficiency** insuficiencia pulmonar; **~ stenosis** estenosis pulmonar *f*
pulmonologist, neumólogo
pulp, pulpa; **dental ~** pulpa dentaria; pulpa dental; **devitalized ~** pulpa desvitalizada; pulpa muerta
pulpotomy, pulpotomía
pulsation, pulsación *f*
pulse, pulso; **abdominal ~** pulso abdominal; **arterial ~** pulso arterial; **capillary ~** pulso capilar; **high-tension ~** pulso hipertenso; **intermittent ~** pulso intermitente; **irregular ~** pulso arrítmico; pulso irregular; **jerky ~** pulso espasmódico; **jugular ~** pulso yugular; **low-tension ~** pulso hipotenso; **quick ~** pulso rápido; **slow ~** pulso lento; **strong ~** pulso fuerte; **venous ~** pulso venoso; **to feel s.o.'s ~** pulsar a uno; **to take the ~** registrar el pulso; **to take s.o.'s ~** pulsar a uno; tomar el pulso a uno
pumice stone, piedra pómez
pump, bomba; **injection ~** bomba de inyección; **stomach ~** bomba gástrica; **suction ~** bomba aspirante; **~** (*gasoline*) surtidor *m*; **gas ~** surtidor de gasolina; **~** (*shoe*) escarpín *m*
pump, to, **~** (*blood*) impulsar; **~** (*milk*) sacar (leche) por medio de una bomba
punch, **~** (*blow with fists*) puñetazo; **~** (*for making holes in paper*) perforadora; **~** (*a drink*) ponche *m*

punch, to, dar un puñetazo (a); pegar con los puños; ~ (*in paper*) perforar

puncture, punción *f, Med*; puntura *Med*; piquete *f, Med, Mex*; **lumbar** ~ punción lumbar

pupil, pupila *Anat*; **to dilate the ~s** dilatar las pupilas

purgation, purgación *f*

purgative, catártico *adj*; purgativo *adj*; purga *Med*; purgante *m, adj*

purge, lavado; lavativo; purga; purgante *m*

purge, to, ~ (*bowels*) purgar *Med*; **to take a** ~ purgarse *Med*; ~ (*blood*) purificar

purification, purificación *f*; depuración *f*

purify, to, purificar

purple, ~ (*bruise*) morado *adj*; ~ (*color*) purpúreo *adj*; púrpura

purse, bolsa; cartera; bolso

pursue, to, perseguir (i)

purulent, purulento *adj*

pus, pus *m*; flujo purulento; postema *Med, Mex*

push, (*shove*) empujón *m*

push, to, ~ (*to press or shove*) empujar; ~ (*to strain*) pujar *Obst*; ~ **out** hacer salir; ~ (*drugs*)[9] pushar[2, 5]

pustule, bubón *m*; grano; pústula

put, to, poner; ~ **heroin in capsules**[9] capear[2]; capiar[2]; ~ **in a plaster cast** enyesar; ~ **ointment on** ungir *Med*; ~ **on** (*clothing*) ponerse (+ *noun*); ~ **on the defensive** poner a la defensiva; ~ **to sleep** adormecer por anestesia

putrefaction, putrefacción *f*

putrescine, putrescina

putrid, podrido *adj*; gangrenoso *adj, Med*

PVS/persistent vegetative state, estado vegetativo persistente

pyelitis, pielitis *f*

pyelocystitis, pielocistitis *f*

pyelogram, pielograma *m*; **intravenous** ~/**IVP** pielograma intravenoso

pyelography, pielografía

pyelonephritis, pielonefritis *f*

pyloric, pilórico *adj*

pylorus, (*pl, pylori*) píloro *Anat*

pyorrhea, mal de las encías *m*; piorrea

pyromania, obsesión con el fuego *f*

pyuria, piuria

---

[2] This is new vocabulary, not necessarily listed nor yet recognized by the Royal Academy of Spanish Grammar. It is understood that this vocabulary is primarily slang. Unless otherwise indicated, the gender of nouns is assumed to be obvious.

[3] For pronunciation purposes, the masculine definite and indefinite articles, *el* and *un*, not *la* or *una*, are used when the article immediately precedes the feminine singular noun which begins with stressed *a* or any other that begins with stressed *ha*.

[4] The current English street terminology for *PCP* includes: amoeba, angel dust, angel hair, animal tranquilizer, cadillac, C.J., crystal, crystal joints, cyclones, dead on arrival, D.O.A., dust, elephant tranquilizer, goon, hog, horse tranquilizer, killer weed, K. J., mist, peace pill, pig tranquilizer, rocket fuel, scuffle, sheets, snorts, soma.

[5] Other slang terms include: dealer, mother, pusher.

[6] English words that have an initial *ps* now may be spelled either with or without the *p* in Spanish. In either case, the *p* is silent when the Spanish word is pronounced. This dictionary will show such words with a parenthesis around the *p*.

[7] Current English terminology for *psilocybin* includes: hombrecitos, little children, little men, little women, magic mushroom, las mujercitas, mushrooms, los niños, noble princess of the waters.

[8] Use the Spanish pronunciation of these letters.

[9] Part of the Drug Abuse Vocabulary.

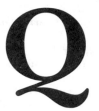

q.d./quaque die/every day, cada día

q.h./quaque hora/every hour, cada hora

q. 2h./quaque secunda hora/every two hours, cada dos horas

q. 3h./quaque tertia hora/every three hours, cada tres horas

q.i.d./quater in die/4 times a day, cuatro veces al día

q.l./quantum libet / at will, a voluntad

q.m./quaque matin/every morning, cada mañana

q.n./quaque nox/every night, cada noche

q.q.h./quater quarta hora/every 4 hours, cada cuatro horas

q.s./quantum satis/as much as necessary, cantidad suficiente *f*

quack, matasanos *m*, *inv*; charlatán, -na *m/f*, *fam*; sobador, -ra *m/f*, *Col*, *Mex*; sobandero *Col*, *Ven*; ~ **doctor** chamarrero *Ven*; lupia *m/f*, *Hond*; piache *m*, *Ven*; ~ **remedy** ensalmo *Med*; ~ **treatment** ensalmo *Med*

quackery, charlatanería; charlatanismo

quadrangle, cuadrángulo

quadrant, cuadrante *m*

quadriceps, cuadríceps *m*, *adj*

quadricuspid, cuadricúspide *adj*

quadrigeminal, cuadrigémino *adj*

quadrigeminum, (*pl*, *quadrigemina*) cuadrigémino

quadripara, cuadrípara

quadriparous, cuadrípara *adj*

quadriplegia, cuadriplejía; tetraplejía

quadriplegic, cuadripléjico *m*, *adj*; tetrapléjico *m*, *adj*

quadripolar, cuadripolar *adj*

quadrisect, cuadrisección *f*

quadruplet, cuádruple *m/f*; cuadrúpleto *adj*; cuadrillizo; cuatrillizo

quadruplicate, to, sacar cuatro copias de

quaint, (*odd*) extraño *adj*

quake, temblor *m*

quake, to, ~ (*to shake inwardly*) estremecerse; ~ (*to shake violently*) temblar; ~ **with fear** temblar de miedo; ~ **at the knees** flaquearle las piernas a alguien; temblarle a uno las rodillas

Quaker, cuáquero *m*, *adj*

qualification, ~ (*skilled*) calificación *f*; ~ (*competence*) capacidad *f*; competencia; ~ (*degree*) título

qualified, ~ (*trained*) calificado *adj*; ~ (*fit*) competente *adj*; ~ (*professionally*) titulado *adj*

qualitative, cualitativo *adj*; ~ **analysis** análisis cualitativo *m*; ~ **test** prueba cualitativa

quality, ~ (*nature*, *kind*) calidad *f*; ~ **control** control de la calidad *m*; ~ **of life** calidad de la vida; ~ (*characteristic*) cualidad *f*

qualm, ~ (*feeling of nausea*) bascas *f*, *pl*; náusea; ~ (*scruple*) escrúpulo; ~ (*worry*) aprensión *f*

quandary, dilema *m*; **to be in a** ~ estar en un dilema

quantify, to, cuantificar

quantimeter, cuantímetro

quantitative, cuantitativo *adj*; ~ **analysis** análisis cuantitativo *m*; ~ **test** prueba cuantitativa

quantity, cantidad *f*

quarantine, cuarentena; **to put in** ~ poner en cuarentena

quarrel, riña

quarrel, to, (*to argue*) reñir (i)
quarrelsome, (*inclined to quarrel*) pendenciero *adj*
quart, cuarto
quarter, ~ (*fourth part*) cuarto; ~ **of an hour** un cuarto de hora; ~ (*trimester*) trimestre *m*; ~ (*of town*) barrio
quarterly, trimestral *adj*; cada tres meses *adv*
quarters, alojamiento; **to take up** ~ alojarse (en)
quartz, cuarzo
quaver, to, (*voice*) temblar; decir con voz trémula
quavering voice, voz temblorosa *f*
queasiness, (*feeling sick*) náuseas *f, pl*; bascas *f, pl*
queasy, con náuseas; bascoso *adj*, *Med*; nauseabundo; **to have a** ~ **stomach** tener náuseas
queer, ~ (*homosexual*) *slang* homosexual *m, adj*; maricón *m, adj, slang*; ~ (*odd*) extraño *adj*; ~ (*unwell*) enfermo *Med, adj*
quell, to, calmar
quench, to, ~ (*thirst*) apagar; ~ (*emotions*) reprimir
question, ~ (*matter*) cuestión *f*; ~ (*interrogative*) pregunta
question, to, hacer una pregunta; preguntar
questionable, discutible *adj*; sospechoso *adj*
questionnaire, cuestionario
queue, cola
queue up, to, hacer cola
quick, rápido *adj, adv*; ~-**acting** extrarrápido *adj*
quickly, rápidamente *adv*
quicken, to, acelerar
quickening, *Obst*, desencogimiento; primer movimiento del feto; primera señal de vida que da el feto *f*
quicklime, cal viva *f*
quicksilver, azogue *m*

quick-tempered, de genio vivo *prep phr*
quiet, ~ (*person's nature*) callado *adj*; ~ (*silent*) silencioso *adj*; ~ (*calm*; *unworried*) tranquilo *adj*
quiet down, to, calmarse
quilt, colcha
quilt, to, acolchar
quinic, quínico *adj*
quinidamine, quinidamina
quinidine, quinidina
quinine, quinina; ~ **and urea hydrochloride** clorhidrato de quinina y urea; ~ **bisulfate** bisulfato de quinina; ~ **dihydrochloride** diclorhidrato de quinina; ~ **sulfate** sulfato de quinina
quinsy, (*sore throat*) absceso periamigdalino; absceso retrofaríngeo; amígdalitis supurativa *f*; angina; esquinancia
quint, quintillizo
quintipara, quintípara *f, adj*
quintuplet, quintillizo; quíntuple *m/f*
quirk, ~ (*oddity*) peculiaridad *f*; ~ (*in writing*) rasgo
quit, abandonar
quitclaim, renuncia
quite, bastante *adv*
quiver, temblor *m*
quizzical, curioso *adj*
quota, cuota
quotation, (*words*) cita
quotient, cociente *m*; **achievement** ~ cociente de realización; **blood** ~ cociente sanguíneo; **caloric** ~ cociente calórico; **growth** ~ cociente de crecimiento; **intelligence** ~ cociente de inteligencia; cociente intelectual; **protein** ~ cociente proteínico; **rachidian** ~ cociente raquídeo; **respiratory** ~ cociente respiratorio; **spinal** ~ cociente espinal

R

rabbit, conejo; ~ **fever** tularemia; ~ **test** examen de conejo *m*

rabid, rabioso *adj*

rabies, hidrofobia; rabia; ~ **virus** virus de la rabia *m*; **to have** ~ rabiar *Med*

raccoon, mapache *m*

race, raza

race, to, (*heart, pulse, etc.*) latir a ritmo acelerado

rachialgia, raquialgia; dolor en la columna vertebral *m*

rachiotomy, raquiotomía; laminectomía

rachischisis, raquisquisis *f, form*; espina bífida

rachitic, raquítico *adj*

rachitis, raquitis *f*; raquitismo; enfermedad inflamatoria de la columna vertebral *f*

racked with pain, transido de dolor *adj*

radial cracks, grietas radiales

radiant, radiante *adj*

radiate, to, radiar

radiating, radiante *adj*; radiado *adj*; ~ **pain** dolor irradiado *m*; ~ **scars** cicatrices radiadas *f*

radiation, radiación *f*; ~ **biologist** radiobiólogo, ~ **energy** energía radiante; ~ **shield** blindaje contra la radiación *m*; ~ **therapy** radioterapia; ~ **treatment** radiaciones *f*

radical, radical *adj*; ~ **mastectomy** mastectomía radical

radicotomy, radicotomía *f*

radioactive, radiactivo *adj*; radioactivo *adj*; ~ **material** materia radioactiva; ~ **substance** substancia radioactiva

radioactivity, radiactividad *f*; radioactividad *f*

radiodiagnosis, radiodiagnóstico

radiography, radiografía

radioisotope, isótopo radioactivo; radioisótopo

radiologist, radiólogo

radiology, radiología

radiolucency, radiotrasparencia

radiolucent, radiolúcido *adj*; radiotransparente *adj*

radiosensibility, radiosensibilidad *f*

radiotherapy, radioterapia

radiothermy, radiotermia

radiowaves, radioondas

radish, rábano

radium, radio; ~ **therapy** radioterapia; radiumterapia

radius, radio

radon, radón *m*

rag, trapo; chira *Col*

rage, furor *m*

RAI/radioactive iodine, yodo radiactiva

rain water, agua³ de lluvia *f*

raise, to, ~ (*children*) criar; ~ (*to elevate*) elevar; ~ (*a family*) mantener; ~ (*to lift*) levantar; ~ **one's head** levantar la cabeza hacia arriba; ~ **oneself** (*to get up*) levantarse; ~ (*blisters, etc.*) producir *Med*

raisin, pasa

rale, estertor *m*; **bubbling** ~ estertor de burbujas; **clicking** ~ estertor de chasquido; **dry** ~ estertor seco; **moist** ~ estertor húmedo; **rackling** ~ estertor crujiente; **redux** ~ estertor de retorno; **sibilant** ~ estertor sibilante

ramify, to, ramificar(se)

rancid, rancio *adj*

random, al azar; ~ **sample/sampling** muestreo al azar; ~ **test** prueba al azar

range, amplitud *f*; campo; límites *m*; margen *f*; rango; variación *f*; ~

(*of knowledge*, *voice*) extensión *f*; ~ (*of frequencies*, *colors*, *etc*.) gama; ~ **of error** margen de error; ~ **of motion** límite(s) de movimiento; rango de movimiento; ~ **of vision** campo visual

rape, violación *f*; estupro; rapo *Chicano*; **attempted** ~ intento de violación

rape, to, violar; atacar

rapid, rápido *adj*; **~-developing film** placa de revelado rápido

rapist, violador *m*

rash, ~ (*action*) precipitado *adj*; ~ (*person*) impetuoso *adj*; ~ (*skin eruption*) alfombra *PR*, *Chicano*; alfombrilla *Cu*; erupción (cutánea) *f*; exantema *m*, *form*; salpullido; sarpullido; pitra *Chi*; **diaper** ~ pañalitis *f*; chincual *m*, *Mex*; **drug** ~ exantema medicamentoso; **heat** ~ exantema por calor; **wheals** (*hives*) ronchas

raspberry, frambuesa; ~ **mark** angioma elevado *m*

rasping sound, ruido áspero; ruido chirrido

rat bite, mordedura de ratas; ~ **fever** fiebre por mordedura de ratas *f*; sodoku *m*

rate, frecuencia; ritmo; índice *m*; intensidad *f*; tasa; velocidad *f*; **basal metabolic** ~ intensidad del metabolismo basal; **birth** ~ índice de natalidad; **death** ~ índice de mortalidad; **erythrocite sedimentation** ~ velocidad de eritrosedimentación; **growth** ~ intensidad de crecimiento; **heart** ~ frecuencia cardíaca; **morbidity** ~ índice de morbilidad; **pulse** ~ frecuencia del pulso; **respiratory** ~ frecuencia respiratoria; **sickness** ~ índice de enfermedad; **stillbirth** ~ índice de mortinatalidad

ratio, proporción *f*; relación *f*; **body-weight** ~ relación peso-

talla ; **cardiothoracic** ~ relación cardiotorácica; **urea excretion** ~ proporción de excreción de urea

rational, racional *adj*

rationalization, racionalización *f*

rattlesnake, crótalo; serpiente de cascabel *f*

rattling, estertor *m*

ravage, to, destrozar

ravaged by disease, face, cara desfigurada por la enfermedad

rave, to, delirar; desvariar; ~ **in one's delirium** desvariar en su delirio; ~ **about** entusiasmarse por

ravenous, hambriento *adj*; **to be** ~ tener un hambre[3] canina

raving, delirante *adj*; desvariado *adj*; delirio; desvarío; ~ **mad** loco de atar *adj*

raw, ~ (*food*) crudo *adj*; ~ **meat** carne cruda; ~ (*flesh*) vivo *adj*; ~ (*wound*) en carne viva; ~ (*nerves*) aflor de piel

ray, rayo; **cathode ~s** rayos catódicos; **infrared ~s** rayos infrarrojos; **ultraviolet** ~s rayos ultravioletas; **x-~s** rayos equis; rayos x; radiografías; retrato del x-ray *Chicano*

razor, navaja de afeitar; cuchilla de afeitar; **safety** ~ máquina de afeitar; maquinilla de afeitar; maquinilla de seguridad; ~ **blade** hoja de afeitar; navajita; gillette *m*, *CA*

RBC/red blood count, NGR[5]/numeración de glóbulos rojos *f*; recuento de glóbulos rojos

reach, alcance *m*; **out of** ~ **of children** fuera del alcance de niños

reach, to, alcanzar

reactant, reactivo *adj*

reaction, reacción *f*; **accelerated** ~ reacción acelerada; **acid** ~ reacción ácida; **adverse** ~ reacción adversa; **alkaline** ~ reacción alcalina; **allergic** ~ reacción alérgica; **anaphylactic** ~ reacción anafiláctica; **chain** ~ reacción en cadena; **delayed** ~ reacción tardía; **false positive** ~ reacción falsa positiva; **skin** ~ reacción de la piel; **~-formation** reacción-formación *f*; ~ **time** tiempo de reacción

reactivate, to, reactivar

reactive psychosis, (p)sicosis[6] reactiva *f*

reactor, nuclear, reactor nuclear *m*

read, to, leer

reading, lectura

ready, listo *adj*; **to get** ~ prepararse

reagent, reactivo

reality, realidad *f*; **in** ~ en realidad

realize, to, darse cuenta (de)

really, de veras *adv*; realmente *adv*

reamer, ensanchador *m*

reappear, to, reaparecer

rear, trasero *m, adj*

reason, razón *f*

reassure, to, dar seguridades; tranquilizar

reattach, to, reatar; religar

rebase, rebase *f, Dent*

rebound, rebote *m*

receding, *(forehead)* huyente *adj*

receipt, recibo

receive, to, recibir

receiver, receptor *m*

recent, reciente *adj*

receptacle, vasija

reception, recepción *f*; ~ **clerk** recepcionista *m/f*; ~ **desk** recepción; ~ **room** sala de espera

receptionist, recepcionista *m/f*

receptivity, receptividad *f*

receptor, receptor *m*

recess, ~ *(rest)* descanso; ~ *(small cavity)* nicho; ~ *(fossa, sinus, cleft, etc.)* fosa *Anat*

recessive, recesivo *adj*; ~ **character** carácter recesivo *m*

recidivation, recidiva

recognize, to, identificar; reconocer

recommend, to, recomendar (ie)

recommended dietary allowance/RDA, dosis diaria recomendada *f, inv*

reconstructive surgery, cirugía reparadora

record, ~ *(of medication, etc.)* registro; ~ *(patient's chart)* historial médico *m*; historia clínica *f*; expediente *m*

record, to, ~ *(to make note of)* apuntar; ~ *(to register)* registrar; ~ *(a thermometer, etc.)* marcar; ~ *(a birth or death)* declarar; ~ *(on tape)* grabar

recover, to, ~ *(from an illness)* aliviarse; curarse; recuperarse; rehacerse *Med*; restablecerse; resurgir *Med*; sanar; ~ *(voice, senses, etc.)* recobrar; recuperar; ~ *(a fainting person)* hacer volver en sí; ~ **one's legs** ponerse de pie

recovery, recuperación *f*; reposición *f, Med*; restablecimiento; **past** ~ en estado desesperado *Med*; desahuciado *adj, Med*; sin cura; ~ **room** sala de recuperación; sala de restablecimiento

recreation, recreo

rectal, rectal *adj*; ~ **examination** examen tacto rectal *m*

rectify, to, rectificar

rectocele, rectocele *m*

rectoscope, rectoscopio

rectoscopy, rectoscopia

rectum, recto

recuperate, to, ~ *(one's health)* recobrar; ~ *(to recover health)* recuperar; ~ *(from an illness)* recuperarse; reponerse de una enfermedad

recuperation, recuperación *f*; restablecimiento

recur, to, repetirse (i); volver (ue) a ocurrir; reproducirse *Med*

recurrence, reaparición *f, Med*; recidiva *Med*; reproducción *f, Med*

recurrent, recurrente *adj, Anat, Med*

recurring, recurrente *adj*

red, rojo *adj*; colorado *adj*; ~ **blood cell** eritrocito; glóbulo rojo; hematíe *m*, *Med*; ~ **cell mass** hematócrito; ~ **Cross** Cruz Roja *f*; ~ **fever** erisipela; **~-green blindness** daltonismo; (*See blindness.*)

redden, to, enrojecer

reddish, rojizo *adj*; ~ (*hair*) bermejizo *adj*

red-haired, pelirrojo *adj*

redness, enrojecimiento; rojez *f*; rubor *m*

reduce, to, reducir; ~ (*inflammation*) desenconar; ~ (*weight*) hacer adelgazar; ~ **a fracture** enderezar; ~ **anxiety** reducir la ansiedad

reducing, reductor *adj*; ~ **exercises** ejercicios físicos para adelgazar; ejercicios físicos para reducir peso; ~ **valve** válvula reductora

reduction, reducción *f*

reeducation, reeducación *f*

reestablish, to, restablecer; ~ **one's health** restablecerse; recuperarse

refer, to, referir (ie); ~ (*a patient*) enviar

refill, (*of a prescription*) repuesto; relleno

refill, to, (*a prescription*) rehacer (la receta); reponer; rellenar

refined, refinado *adj*

reflect, to, reflejar

reflex, reflejo; **Achilles tendon ~** reflejo del tendón de Aquiles; reflejo aquíleo; **conditioned ~** reflejo condicionado; **cremasteric ~** reflejo cremastérico; **delayed ~** reflejo retardado; **flexion ~ of the leg** reflejo de flexión de la pierna; **gag ~** reflejo nauseoso; **inborn ~** reflejo innato; **instinctive ~** reflejo instintivo; **knee jerk ~** reflejo patelar; reflejo rotuliano; **rooting ~** reflejo del hociqueo

reflux, reflujo; flujo retrógrado

refract, to, refractar

refraction, refracción *f*

refractive, refringente *adj*; refractivo *adj*

refresh, to, refrescar

refrigeration, refrigeración *f*

refrigerator, refrigerador *m*; nevera

regain, to, recobrar; ~ **one's breath** recobrar el aliento; ~ **consciousness** recobrar el conocimiento; recobrar el espíritu; recobrar el sentido; recobrarse; volver (ue) en sí; ~ **one's composure** serenarse; ~ **one's strength, to** rehacerse *Med*

regenerate, to, regenerar

regeneration, regeneración *f*

region, región *f*

regional, regional *adj*

register, to, registrar; ~ (*deaths, births, etc.*) declarar; ~ (*emotions*) acusar

registered nurse, enfermera registrada; enfermero registrado; enfermera con título; enfermera diplomada; enfermero diplomado; enfermera titulada; enfermero titulado

regress, to, retroceder

regret, with deep, con hondo pesar

regular, regular *adj*; normal *adj*

regularly, con regularidad *adv*

regulate, to, ~ (*a flow, etc.*) regular; ~ (*to make rules for*) reglamentar

regulations, reglamentos; regulaciones *f*; órdenes *f*

regurgitation, regurgitación *f*

rehabilitate, to, rehabilitar

rehabilitation, rehabilitación *f*; **mouth ~** rehabilitación bucal; ~ **of the handicapped** rehabilitación de incapacitados

rehydrate, to, rehidratar

reimplantation, reimplantación *f*; reinjertación *f*

reinfection, reinfección *f*

reinnervation, reinervación *f*

reinoculation, reinoculación *f*
reintegrate, to, reintegrar
rejection, ~ (*of a transplant, etc.*) rechazamiento; rechazo
rejuvenation, rejuvenecimiento
relapse, atrasado *adj*; reventón *m*, *Chi, Med*; ~ (*into poor health*) recaída; recidiva; **to cause to suffer a** ~ atrasar; **to have a** ~ atrasarse; tener una recaída; **to suffer a** ~ recaer *Med*
relapsing, recidivante *adj*
relate (to), to, relacionarse (con)
related, vinculado *adj*; relacionado *adj*
relation, ~ (*kinship*) parentesco; ~ (*connection*) relación *f*; **buccolingual** ~ relación bucolingual *Dent*; **jaw** ~ relación maxilar; **occlusal jaw** ~ relación oclusal de los maxilares; **rest jaw** ~ relación de reposo del maxilar inferior; **sexual** ~**s** relaciones sexuales; **to have sexual** ~**s** conocer; dormir (ue) con alguien; tener relaciones sexuales; chingar *f, vulg*; ~ (*relative*) pariente, ta *m/f*
relationship, parentesco; relación *f*
relative, familiar *m*; pariente, -ta *m/f*
relatively, relativamente *adv*
relax, to, aflojarse; calmarse; descansar; relajar el cuerpo; relajarse; soltar (ue) *Med*; ~ (*pain*) mitigar
relaxant, relajante *m, adj*; **muscle** ~ miorrelajante *m*; relajante muscular
relaxation, descanso; relajación *f*; ~ **of tension** disminución de la tirantez *f*
release, ~ (*from obligation, duty, etc.*) descargo; ~ (*of gas, steam*) escape *m*; ~ (*of medication, light, etc.*) difusión *f*; **extended** ~ difusión prolongada *Pharm*; **slow** ~ difusión lenta *Pharm*; **sustained** ~ difusión regulada

Pharm; **timed** ~ difusión periódica *Pharm*
release, to, desencadenar; soltar (ue); ~ (*gas, etc.*) desprender
relief, alivio
relieve, to, aliviar; ayudar; socorrer
rely (on/upon), to, confiar (en)
REM/rapid eye movement, movimiento ocular rápido
remain, to, quedar(se)
remaining, persistente *adj*; sobrante *adj*
remedy, medicamento; medicina; remedio; reparo *Med*; **home** ~ remedio casero
remember, to, acordarse (ue) de; recordar (ue)
reminisce, to, recordar (ue) el pasado
remission, remisión *f*
remit, to, remitir
remittance, remitencia
remittent, remitente *adj*; ~ **fever** fiebre remitente *f*
remnant, residuo; resto
removal, ablación *f*; excisión *f*; extirpación *f, Med*; ~ (*of a suffering*) alivio
remove, to, extirpar; extraer; quitar; resecar *Med*; sacar; ~ **the nerve** matarle el nervio a alguien *Dent*; sacarle el nervio a alguien *Dent*
renal, renal *adj*; ~ **blockade** anuria; ~ **failure** insuficiencia renal; ~ **shutdown** cierre renal *m*; colapso renal
renin, renina
repair, to, restaurar; reparar
repeat, to, repetir (i)
repellent, repelente *m, adj*; **insect** ~ repelente contra insectos
repent, to, arrepentir(se) (ie)
replace, to, ~ (*to take the place of*) reemplazar; sustituir; ~ (*to put back*) reponer
replacement, ~ (*something that replaces*) reemplazo; **partial knee** ~ reemplazo parcial de la rodi-

lla; **total hip** ~ reemplazo total de la cadera; **total knee** ~ reemplazo total de la rodilla; ~ (*spare part*) repuesto; ~ (*someone who replaces*) sustituto

replicate, to, reduplicar; repetir(i)

replication, repliegue *m*

report, ~ (*official*) dictamen *m*; informe *m*; ~ (*spoken account*) relato

represent, to, representar

repress, to, reprimir

repression, represión *f*

reproduction, reproducción *f*

reproductive, reproductivo *adj*; reproductor *adj*

reputation, fama; reputación *f*

request, petición *f*; solicitud *f*

request, to, requerir(ie); solicitar; pedir(i)

require, to, requerir (ie); exigir

rescue, rescate *m*; salvamento; **to go to the** ~ **of** ir en auxilio de

rescue, to, rescatar; salvar

research, investigación *f*

researcher, investigador, -ra *m/f*

resect, to, resecar *Med*

resection, resección *f*; **gastric** ~ resección gástrica; **transurethral** ~ resección transuretral

reserpine, reserpina

reserve, cardiac, reserva cardíaca

residence, residencia

resident, residente *m/f*; ~ **physician** interno; médico de hospital; **surgical** ~ residente en cirujía

residue, residuo

resin, resina

resist, to, resistir

resistance, resistencia; **bacterial** ~ resistencia bacteriana; **globular** ~ resistencia globular; **to build up a** ~ (**to**) hacerse resistente (a) *Med*

resistant, resistente *adj*

resolution, resolución *f*

resolve, to, resolver(se) (ue)

resonance, resonancia

resonant, resonante *adj*

resonator, resonador *m*

resorption, resorción *f*

resort to, (**to**), recurrir (a)

resource, recurso

respiration, respiración *f*; **abdominal** ~ respiración abdominal; **artificial** ~ respiración artificial; **fetal** ~ respiración fetal; **stertorous** ~ respiración estertorosa

respirator, respirador *m*

respiratory, respiratorio *adj*; ~ **ailment** enfermedad respiratoria *f*; ~ **distress** disnea; ~ **exchange** intercambio respiratorio; ~ **function tests** pruebas de función respiratoria; ~ **quotient** cociente respiratorio *m*; ~ **rate** ritmo respiratorio; ~ **system** aparato respiratorio; sistema respiratorio *m*; ~ **tract infection** infección de las vías respiratorias *f*

respirometer, respirómetro

respond, to, responder

response, reflejo; respuesta

responsibility, responsabilidad *f*

responsible, responsable *adj*; sensible *adj*

rest, descanso; reposo; **complete** ~ reposo absoluto *Med*; ~ (*remainder*) resto *Dent*

rest, to, descansar; ~ (*to stop*) pararse; ~ (*to lean against*) apoyar *m*

resting, ~ **metabolism** metabolismo en reposo; ~ **potential** potencial de reposo; ~ **rigidity** rigidez estática *f*; ~ **tremor** temblor estático *m*

restless, inquieto *adj*

restlessness, ~ (*worry*) inquietud *f*; intranquilidad *f*; ~ (*impatience*) impaciencia; ~ (*sleeplessness*) insomnio; ~ (*agitation*) agitación *f*

restoration, restauración *f*; **buccal** ~ restauración bucal

restorative, restaurativo *m*, *adj*; reconstituyente *m*, *adj*

restore, to, restituir; reintegrar; ~ **s.o. to health** devolver (ue) la salud a alguien; ~ **s.o.'s sight**

devolver (ue) la vista a alguien; ~ **s.o.'s strength** restaurar las fuerzas a alguien

restrain, to, ~ (*to repress*) reprimir; ~ **s.o. from** (+ *gerund*) disuadir a alguien de (+ *infinitive*); ~ (*to hold down*) sujetar

restraining device, coercitivo; medio de restricción

restraint, restricción *f*; ~ (*physical*) atadura; **chemical** ~ restricción química

restrict, to, restringir

restrictive, restringido *adj*

restroom, aseos *m, pl*; baño; comodidades *f, pl*; cuarto de baño; excusado; servicios *m, pl*; tocador *m*; WC[5] *m*

result, resultado

resurgence, recrudecimiento; resurgimiento

resuscitate, to, resucitar

resuscitation, resucitación *f*; reanimación *f*; **cardiopulmonary** ~/**CPR** resucitación cardiopulmonar/RCP[5]; **mouth-to-mouth** ~ resucitación boca a boca

resuscitator, resucitador *m*

retain, to, retener

retainer, retenedor *m, Dent*; **continuous bar** ~ retenedor por barra continua *Dent*

retardation, retardo; retardación *f*; **mental** ~ retardo mental; **psychomotor** ~ retardo psicomotor

retarded, atrasado *m, adj*; retardado *m, adj*; **mentally** ~ atrasado mentalmente *adj*; **mentally** ~ **person** retardado mental; atrasado mental

retch, to, nausear; arquear; ~ **violently** echar las tripas *fam*

retching, arcada; basca; vómito seco; vomitera *Cu, PR*

retention, retención *f*; ~ **arm** brazo de retención *Dent*; **fecal** ~ retención fecal; ~ **of urine** retención de (la) orina; retención urinaria

reticulocyte, reticulocito

reticulum, retículo

retina, retina; **detachment of the** ~ desprendimiento de la retina

retinitis, retinitis *f*

retinochoroiditis, retinocoroiditis *f*

retinopathy, retinopatía

retinoscope, retinoscopio

retinoscopy, retinoscopia; oftalmoscopia

retired, (*not working*) jubilado *adj*

retraction, retracción *f*; **gingival** ~ retracción gingival; **mandibular** ~ retracción mandibular; ~ (*of claim, etc.*) retractación *f*

retractor, retractor *m*; separador *m*

retroflexion, retroflexión *f*

retrograde, retrógrado *adj*

return, (*coming back*), regreso; retorno; vuelta; ~ (*giving back*) devolución

return, to, ~ (*to come back*) volver (ue); ~ (*to give back*) devolver (ue)

reusable, utilizable de nuevo *adj*

reuse, to, volver (ue) a emplear

revealing, revelador *adj*

reversal, inversión *f*; **sex** ~ inversión del sexo

reversible, reversible *adj*

reversion, reversión *f*

review of systems, revisión sistémica *f*

review, to, revisar

Rh factor, factor Rh *m*; factor Rhesus *m*; **Rh negative** Rh-negativo *adj*; **Rh positive** Rh-positivo *adj*

rheostat, reóstato

rheum, ~ (*discharge from mucous membranes*) reuma *m/f* [*Ú.m.c.m.*]; reúma *m/f* [*Ú.m.c.m.*]; ~ (*in the eyes*) legaña; ~ (*in the nose*) mucosidades *f, pl, Med*

rheumatic, reumático *adj*; ~ **fever,** fiebre reumática *f*

rheumatism, reuma(s) *m/f* [*Ú.m.c.m.*]; reúma *m/f* [*Ú.m.c.m.*]; reumatismo; **acute articular** ~

reumatismo articular agudo; fiebre reumática (aguda); **chronic articular** ~ reumatismo articular crónico; gota asténica; ósteoartritis *f*; **subacute** ~ reumatismo subagudo

rheumatoid, reumatoide *adj*; reumatoideo *adj*; ~ **arthritis** artritis reumatoide *f*; artritis reumatoidea *f*

rheumatologist, reumatólogo

rheumatology, reumatología

rhinitis, coriza; escurrimiento de la nariz; rinitis *f*; **acute catarrhal** ~ rinitis catarral aguda; oriza; **allergic** ~ (*See fever, hay.*)

rhinoplasty, rinoplastia

rhinorrhagia, rinorragia

rhinoscopy, rinoscopia

rhodium, rodio

rhogam, rogam *m*

rhubarb, ruibarbo

rhythm, ritmo; **alpha** ~ ritmo alfa; **beta** ~ ritmo beta; **circadian** ~ ritmo circadiano; **gallop** ~ ritmo de galope; ~ **method** método del ritmo; ritmo; **sinus** ~ ritmo sinusal

rib, costilla; ~ **cage** caja costal; caja torácica; caja de las costillas; **cervical** ~ costilla cervical; **false** ~ costilla falsa; **floating** ~ costilla flotante; **true** ~ costilla verdadera

ribbon, cinta

riboflavin, riboflavina

rice, arroz *m*; ~**-water stools** deposición colérica *f*

rich, ~ (*color*) vivo *adj*; ~ (*food*) sabroso *adj*; ~ (*wealth*) rico *adj*; ~ (*wine*) generoso *adj*

rickets, raquitis *f*; raquitismo

ridge, elevación *f*; reborde *m*, *Dent*; **alveolar** ~ reborde alveolar; **buccocervical** ~ reborde bucocervical; **dental** ~s rebordes dentales; **linguocervical** ~ reborde linguocervical; **marginal** ~s rebordes marginales

right, derecho *m*, *adj*; ~ **away** aho-

ra mismo *adv*; en seguida *prep phr*; ~**-handed** manidiestro *adj*; ~ **now** ahorita *fam*; **to be** ~ tener razón; **to the** ~ a la derecha; **patient's** ~**s** derechos del/de la paciente; **everything will be all** ~ todo saldrá bien

rigid, rígido *adj*; tieso *adj*

rigidity, rigidez *f*

rigor mortis, rigidez cadavérica; rigor mortis *m*

rind (*of fruits*), cáscara

ring, anillo; argolla *parts of SpAm*; ~ (*IUD*) anillo; ~ (*jeweled*) sortija; **engagement** ~ anillo de prometida; anillo de compromiso *Mex*; **wedding** ~ alianza; anillo/sortija de matrimonio; anillo/sortija de boda; anillo/sortija de casamiento; ~ (*sound*) sonido; ~ (*of the voice*) timbre *m*; ~ (*of people*) grupo

ring, to, tocar; sonar (ue); ~ (*ears*) zumbar

Ringer's solution, solución de Ringer *f*; solución salina normal *f*

ringing, (*in ears*) zumbido; pitido

ringworm, culebrilla *fam*; empeine *m*; serpigo; tiña *form*; ~ **of the beard** tiña de la barba; ~ **of the body** tiña del cuerpo; ~ **of the groin** tiña crural; ~ **of the scalp** porrigo

rinse, ~ (*mouthwash*) enjuague *m*; enjuagadientes *m, inv*; ~ (*of clothes, hair*) aclarado

rinse, to, ~ (*clothes*) aclarar; ~ (*dishes, etc.*) enjuagar; ~ **out** (*one's mouth*) enjuagarse

ripe, (*fruit; abscess*) maduro

rise, ~ (*in rate, pressure, etc.*) aumento; ~ (*in temperature, etc.*) subida; recargo *Med*

rise, to, subir

risk, peligro; riesgo; ~ **factor** factor de riesgo *m*; **high** ~ alto riesgo; ~ **of contamination** peligro de contaminación; ~ **of infection** riesgo de infección

RN/registered nurse, enfermera titulada; (*See registered nurse.*)

roach, ~[4] (*butt of marijuana cigarette*) bacha[2]; bachilla[2]; colilla[2]; cucaracha[2]; tecla[2]; tecolota[2]; tocola[2]; ~ (*cockroach*) cucaracha

roast, asado *adj*; ~ **beef** carne asada *f*; rosbif *m*

roast, to, asar

robe, bata

robust, válido *adj*, *Med*

rod, ~ (*bacteria*) bacilo; ~ (*bar*) varilla; **metal** ~ varilla de metal; ~ (*eye*) bastoncillo; bastoncito; ~ **cells** bastoncillos de la retina; ~ **epithelium** bastoncillos; ~**s and cones** conos y bastones

roentgen, roentgen *m*

roentgenography, radiografía; **body section** ~ tomografía

roll, rollo; ~ **of fat** rosca *Anat*

roll, to, enrollar; envolver (ue); ~ **one's eyes back** poner los ojos en blanco; ~ **over** voltearse; ~ **up one's sleeve** arremangarse; subirse la manga

roller, (*hair curler*) rollo

roof, techo; ~ **of mouth** cielo de la boca; paladar *m*

room, cuarto; sala; ~ **air** aire ambiente *m*; **delivery** ~ sala de partos; **double** ~ cuarto doble; **emergency** ~ sala de emergencia; sala de urgencia; **intensive therapy** ~ sala de terapéutica intensiva; **labor** ~ sala prenatal; **postdelivery** ~ sala para puérperas; **private** ~ cuarto privado; **recovery** ~ sala de recuperación; sala de restablecimiento; ~ **temperature** temperatura ambiente; **waiting** ~ sala de recepción; sala de estar

root, raíz *f*; ~ **abscess** absceso radicular; ~ **amputation** resección de una raíz dental *f*; ~ **canal** canal de la raíz *m*; canal radicular *m*; ~ **canal work** curación del nervio *f*, *fam*; endodoncia *form*; extracción del nervio *f*

rosemary, romero

roseola, roséola; rubéola

rot, descomposición *f*

rotation, rotación *f*

rotator cuff of the shoulder, manguito rotador del hombro *m*

rotatory joint, articulación trocoide *f*

rotten, podrido *adj*

rouge, colorete *m*

rough, ~ (*skin, surface*) áspero *adj*; ~ (*hands*) calloso *adj*; ~ (*voice*) bronco *adj*; ~ (*character, language*) grosero *adj*; ~ (*weather*) tempestuoso *adj*

roughage, alimento poco digerible; material áspero inabsorbible; **low residue** ~ residuo bajo

round head of a bone, chueca *Anat*

rounds, (*of doctor*) visitas; **to make** ~ hacer visitas

roundworm, ascáride *f*, *form*; áscaris *f*; nematelminto *m*; verme cilíndrico *m*

route, parenteral, vía parenteral

routine, rutina; rutinario *adj*; ~ **test** prueba rutinaria

rub, roce *m*; fricción *f*; frotación *f*; **pericardial** ~ roce pericárdico

rub, to, frotar(se); pasar la mano sobre la superficie de; restregar; ~ **one's eyes** restregarse los párpados

rubber, caucho; goma; de caucho *adj*; de goma *adj*; ~ **bulb** pera de goma; ~ **suction ball** pera de goma; ~ **gloves** guantes de goma *m*, *pl*; ~**-dam** dispositivo de caucho; ~ (*condom*) condón *m*; bomba *slang*; caperucita en carnada *slang*; desafinador *m*, *slang*; diablito *slang*; Doña Prudencia *slang*; globito *slang*; goma; hule *m*; impermeable *m*, *slang*; paraguas *m, inv, slang*; preservativo

rubbing alcohol, alcohol para fricciones *m*

rubella, alfombría *Chicano*; alfombrilla *Chicano*; fiebre de tres días *f*; peluza *Mex*; roséola epidémica; rubéola; sarampión alemán *m*; sarampión bastardo *m*

rue, ruda

rule, regla

rule, to, ~ (*to decide*) decidir; ~ (*to dominate*) dominar; ~ **in** incluir; ~ **out** descartar

rum, ron *m*; aguardiente de caña *m*

rumble, to (*stomach*) hacer ruidos

run, to, correr; ~ (*a liquid*) hacer correr líquido

runner,[4] (*carrier of drugs*) caballo[2]; mula[2]

running, ~ **pulse** pulso trémulo; ~ **suture** sutura continua; ~ **water** agua[3] corriente; ~ **wound** herida supurante

runny nose, to have a, moquear

rupture, ~ (*abscess*) explotación *f*; ~ (*bone*) fractura; rotura; ~ (*hernia*) hernia; potra *Med*; quebradura; relajación *f*; relajadura *Mex*; reventón *m*; rotadura *Chicano*; ruptura; ~ (*womb*) descenso *Med*; **fallen womb** descenso del útero; **to have a** ~ quebrarse

rupture, to, ~ (*to burst*) romper; ~ (*an abscess*: *to burst*) explotarse; ~ **an organ** relajarse un órgano *Med*

ruptured, perforado *adj*; roto *adj*; relajado *adj, Med*

rust, ~ (*action*) corrosión *f*; ~ (*on metal*) orín *m*; herrumbre *f*; moho *m*

rust, to, enmohecer(se); oxidar(se)

rye, centeno

---

[2] This is new vocabulary, not necessarily listed nor yet recognized by the Royal Academy of Spanish Grammar. It is understood that this vocabulary is primarily slang. Unless otherwise indicated, the gender of nouns is assumed to be obvious.

[3] For pronunciation purposes, the masculine definite and indefinite articles, *el* and *un*, not *la* or *una*, are used when the article immediately precedes the feminine singular noun which begins with stressed *a* or any other that begins with stressed *ha*.

[4] Part of the Drug Abuse Vocabulary.

[5] Use the Spanish pronunciation of these letters.

[6] English words that have an initial *ps* now may be spelled either with or without the *p* in Spanish. In either case, the *p* is silent when the Spanish word is pronounced. This dictionary will show such words with a parenthesis around the *p*.

S

S/signa/mark, indique

s/sans/without, sin

sac, bolsa; saco

saccharine, sacarina; **~ diabetes** diabetes sacarina *f*; (*See diabetes mellitus.*)

saccharose, (*cane sugar*) sacarosa; azúcar de caña *m*

sacral, sacro *adj*; **~ bone** hueso sacro

sacroiliac, sacroilíaco *adj*

sacrum, sacro

sad, triste *adj*

saddleblock anesthesia, anestesia en silla de montar

sadism, sadismo

sadist, sadista *m/f*; sádico

sadistic, sádico *adj*

safe, **~** (*container for valuables*) caja fuerte; **~** (*secure*) seguro *adj*; salvo *adj*; **~** (*trustworthy*) digno de confianza *adj*; **~** (*uninjured*) indemne *adj*; **~** (*cautious*) prudente *adj*

safely, con (toda) seguridad *prep phr*; sin peligro *prep phr*

safety, seguridad *f*; **~ belt** cinturón de seguridad *m*; **~ catch** (*on gun*) seguro; **~ catch** (*on jewelry*) cadena de seguridad; retenedor *m*; **~ glass** vidrio inastillable; vidrio de seguridad; **~ lamp** lámpara de seguridad; **~ measures** medidas de seguridad; prevención *f*; **~ pin** alfiler de seguridad *m*; imperdible *m*; seguro *Mex*; **public ~** seguridad pública; **~ razor** maquinilla de afeitar

safflower, alazor *m*; cártamo; **~ oil** aceite de cártamo

saffron, azafrán *m*

sag, **to**, **~** (*flesh*) colgar (ue); **~** (*spirit*) decaer; flaquear; **~** (*shoulders*) caer

sagging, **~** (*sunken*) hundido *adj*; **~** (*spirits*) decaído *adj*; **~ abdomen** abdomen péndulo *m*; **~ breast** ptosis mamaria *f*

sagittal, sagital *adj*

Saint Anthony's fire, fuego de San Antonio

saint's day, santo

Saint Vitus's dance, (*See chorea.*)

salad, ensalada; **~ dressing** salsa para ensalada

salary, salario; sueldo; **to be on a ~** estar a sueldo

salicylate, salicilato

salicylic acid, ácido salicílico

saline, **~** (*containing salt*) salino *adj*; **~ solution** agua^3 con sal; agua^3 salina; solución salina *f*; **~** (*tasting of salt*) salado *adj*

saliva, saliva; esputo

salivary, salival *adj*; **~ gland** glándula salival; **~ juice** jugo salival

salivation, salivación *f*

salmon, salmón *m*

salmonella, salmonela

salpingectomy, salpingectomía

salpingitis, salpingitis *f*

salpingo-ovariectomy, salpingo-ovariectomía

salpingotomy, salpingotomía

salt, sal *f*; **~-free diet** dieta sin sal; **iodized ~** sal yodada; **non-iodized ~** sal corriente; **smelling ~s** sales aromáticas; sales perfumadas; **~ substitute** su(b)stituto de sal; **~ water** agua^3 salada; **to ~** (*to season/flavor*) echar sal a; **to ~** (*to treat with salt*) salar

salty, salado *adj*

salve, pomada; ungüento; bálsamo

same as, así como

same thing, lo mismo
sample, muestra; **random** ~ muestra al azar
sand, arena
sandflea, pulga de mar; pulga penetrante; nigua
sandfly, jején *m*; jijene *m*
sane, ~ (*person: sensible*) cuerdo *adj*; sensato *adj*; ~ (*person: mind*) sano *adj*; ~ (*policy*) prudente *adj*
sanguineous, sanguíneo *adj*; ~ **circulation**, circulación sanguínea *f*
sanitarium, (*place for treatments*) sanatorio
sanitary, sanitario *adj*; higiénico *adj*; ~ **napkin** absorbente higiénico *m*; almohadilla higiénica; apósito femenino; kótex *m*; servilleta sanitaria; toalla femenina *Mex*; ~ **pad** kótex *m*; servilleta sanitaria
sanity, (*soundness of mind*) juicio; cordura; lucidez *f*; **to lose one's** ~ perder (ie) el juicio; perder (ie) la razón; **to regain one's** ~ recobrar el juicio
saphenous vein, vena safena
sarcoma, sarcoma *m*; **Kaposi's** ~ sarcoma de Kaposi
sardine, sardina
sartorius muscle, músculo sartorio
satellite, satélite *m*; ~ **DNA** ADN[8] satélite
satisfy, to, satisfacer
saturated fats, grasas saturadas
saturation, saturación *f*; ~ **point** punto de saturación
sauce, salsa
saucer, platillo
sauna, sauna
saunter, (*gait*) paso lento
saunter, to, deambular
sausage, chorizo; salchicha
save, to, ~ (*to collect*) coleccionar; ~ (*electricity, money, etc.*) ahorrar; ~ (*to keep for later*) guardar; ~ (*to prevent*) evitar; ~

(*to rescue*) salvar; rescatar; ~ **one's eyes** cuidarse la vista; ~ **one's strength** escatimar sus fuerzas
say, to, decir; ~ **goodbye** (**to**) despedirse (i) (de)
saw, sierra
scab, costra; cuerín *m*, *Chicano*; cuerito *Chicano*; postilla; ~ (*mange*) roña *Vet*
scab, to, formar costra
scabby, costroso *adj*; lleno de costras *adj*; tiñoso *adj*, *Med*
scabies, escabiosis *f*; guaguana *slang*; gusto *slang*; sarna
scald, escaldadura
scald, to, (*to burn skin*) escaldar; ~ **one's hand** escaldarse la mano; ~ (*milk*) calentar (ie)
scalding, hirviendo *adj*; hirviente *adj*; urente *adj*, *Med*; escaldado *m*
scale, ~ (*instrument for measuring*) escala; **centigrade** ~ escala centígrada; escala de Celsius; **Fahrenheit** ~ escala de Fahrenheit; **sliding** ~ escala móvil; ~ (*instrument for weighing*) balanza; báscula; **bathroom** ~ peso de baño; ~ (*of disaster, etc.*) extensión *f*; ~ (*on skin*) escama *Med*; costra; ~ (*flakes*) hojuela; ~ (*on fish*) escama; ~ (*on teeth*) sarro
scale, to, quitar el sarro a *Dent*; ~ (*fish*) escamar
scalp, casco; cuero cabelludo; piel de la cabeza *f*; pericráneo *Anat*
scalpel, bisturí *m*; escalpelo
scan, escán *m*, *Chicano*; estratigrafía; gammagrafía; laminografía; planigrafía; radiografía seccional; tomografía; ~ (*nuclear*) exploración nuclear *f*; gammagrama *m*; **CAT/computerized axial tomography** TAC/tomografía axial computarizada; tomodesintometría; **CT/computed tomography** TC/tomografía computada

scanty, escaso *adj*
scapula, escápula; omóplato; omoplato
scar, cicatriz *f*; escara *Chicano*; yaya *m*, *Chi*, *Col*, *Cu*, *Perú*; ~ (*mark left by illness*) lacra *Med*; ~**-faced** caricortao *adj*, *PR*; **long** ~ tajeadura *Chi*, *Ríopl*
scar, to, cicatrizarse
scarce, escaso *adj*
scare, susto; sobresalto; **to be ~d** tener miedo; encandilarse *Col*, *Perú*, *PR*; **to get ~d** epicharse *Guat*
scare, to, asustar
scarf, bufanda
scarlet fever, fiebre escarlatina *f*
scarred, cicatrizado *adj*
schedule, programa *m*; ~ (*legal document*) inventario; ~ (*timetable*) horario; **work ~** plan de trabajo *m*; **pediatric immunization** ~ plan de inmunización pediátrica *m*
schedule, to, ~ (*appointments, etc.*) fijar la hora de; ~ (*to list*) inventariar; ~ (*plan*) programar
schistasis, esquistasis *f*
schizoid, esquizoide *adj*
schizoidism, esquizoidia; esquizoidismo
schizophrenia, esquizofrénica; (p)sicosis[7] esquizofrénica *f*; demencia precoz
schizophrenic, esquizofrénico *m/f*, *adj*
school, escuela; ~ (*of a university*) facultad *f*; **medical ~** facultad de medicina; **nursing ~** facultad de enfermería
sciatic, ciático *adj*
sciatica, ciática
science, ciencia
scientific, científico *adj*
scientist, científico
scissors, tijeras *f*, *pl*; **a pair of ~** unas tijeras
sclera, esclerótica; esclera; córnea opaca

sclerosis, esclerosis *f*
scoff[6]**, to**, *slang* ingerir (ie) narcóticos; injerir (ie) narcóticos
scoliosis, escoliosis *f*; **habit ~** escoliosis postural
scoop[6]**, to**, *slang* aspirar narcóticos
scope, ~ (*field of action*) esfera de acción; ~ (*person's responsibilities*) incumbencia; ~ (*reach*) alcance *m*; ~ (*ability*) competencia
scopolamine, escopolamina
score, (*result*) resultado; **Apgar ~** valoración de Apgar *f*
score[6]**, to**, (*See inject oneself with drugs, to.*)
scorpion bite, mordedura de escorpión
scotoma, (*spots before the eyes*) escotoma *m*, *form*; manchas frente a los ojos
scratch, ~ (*on the skin*) arañazo; rascado; rasguño; rasmillón *m*, *Chi*; raspón *m*, *SpAm*; ~ (*action to relieve itching*) rascadura; ~ (*on a surface*) raya; ~ (*makeshift*) improvisado *adj*; ~ **pad** cuadernillo de apuntes; bloc para apuntes *m*; ~ **test** cutirreacción *f*; **to feel up to ~** sentirse (ie) en forma; **to start from ~** empezar (ie) desde el principio
scratch, to, ~ (*to relieve itch*) rascar(se); rasmillar *Chi*; ~ (*to hurt*) rasguñar; arañar; chimar *CA*; rajuñar *Arg*; ~ (*hard surface*) rayar; ~ (*a chicken, etc.*) escarbar; ~ **oneself** guayarse *slang*, *PR*; ; ~ **out** tachar
scratchy, ~ (*tone*) áspero *adj*; ~ (*itchy or irritated*) que pica *adj*
scream, grito; chillido
scream, to, gritar; chillar; ~ **oneself to sleep** berrear hasta dormirse; ~ **with laughter** reír (i) a carcajadas; ~ **with pain** gritar de dolor; lanzar gritos de dolor
screen, pantalla
screen for (+ *illness*)**, to**, escrutar para detectar (+ *enfermedad*); se-

leccionar para detectar (+ *enfermedad*)

screening, escrutinio; selección *f*; **multiphasic** ~ escrutinio multifásico; selección multifásica *f*

screw, to, *slang* (*to have intercourse*); chicar *vulg*, *PR*; chingar *vulg*, *Mex*, *PR*; fregar *vulg*, *Mex*

scrofula, escrófula; escrofulismo; lamparón *m*, *Med*; linfatismo *vulg*; tifus de los nudos linfáticos *m*

scrotum, bolsa de los testículos; escroto

scrub, to, ~ (*surgically*) fregar; lavar; refregar; ~ (*clothes*) restregar; ~ (*with brush/abrasive*) estregar

scruff, (*of neck*) cogote *m*

scruffy, (*neglected looking*) desaliñado *adj*; piojoso *adj*

scruple, escrúpulo

scurvy, escorbuto

sea, mar *m*; ~ **bath** baño de mar; ~ **climate** clima de mar *m*

seal, ~ (*stamp*; *mark*) sello; ~ (*paper sticker*) precinto; **broken** ~ precinto roto; ~ (*guarantee*) garantía

seal, to, sellar

seam, sutura *Anat*

sear, to, ~ (*to cauterize*) cauterizar *Med*; ~ (*of pain, etc.*) punzar

seasick, mareado *adj*

seasickness, mal de mar *m*; mareo (marino)

season, ~ (*of year*) estación *f*; ~ (*indefinite period*) época; temporada; **cold** ~ temporada de los catarros; **flu** ~ temporada de la gripe

seasonal disease, enfermedad estacional *f*

seasoning, condimento

seat, asiento; ~ **belt** cinturón de seguridad *m*

sebaceous, sebáceo *adj*; ~ **cyst** quiste sebáceo *m*; ~ **gland** glándula sebácea

seborrhea, seborrea

seconal[4], seconal *m*; colorada[2]; diablo[2]; roja[2]; ~ **capsule** colorada[2]

second, segundo *m*, *adj*

secondary, secundario *adj*; ~ **infection** infección secundaria *f*; ~ **stage** estado secundario

secrete, to, secretar; segregar *Anat*

secretin, secretina

secretion, secreción *f*; segregación *f*, *Anat*; segregado *Anat*

section, sección *f*; corte *m*; **caesarean** ~ sección cesárea; (*See Caesarean.*); **cross** ~ sección transversal; **frontal** ~ corte frontal; **frozen** ~ corte por congelación; **paraffin** ~ corte de parafina; **sagittal** ~ corte sagital; **serial** ~ cortes en serie

security, seguridad *f*; seguro; **Social** ~ seguro social

sedate, to, dar un sedante, calmante, sedativo o soporífero

sedative, calmante *m*; sedante *m*; sedativo; soporífero

sedentary, sedentario *adj*

sediment, sedimento; hipostasis *f*; **urinary** ~ sedimento urinario

sedimentation, sedimentación *f*; **erythrocyte** ~ eritrosedimentación *f*; sedimentación de eritrocitos; ~ **rate** índice de sedimentación *m*; velocidad de sedimentación *f*

see, to, ver

seed, semilla

seek, to, buscar; ~ **a sexual partner** crusiar *Chicano*

seem, to, parecer

segment, segmento

seizure, acceso; ataque *m*; convulsión *f*; crisis *f*, *inv*; **absence** ~ crisis de ausencia; **asthmatic** ~ crisis asmática; choque asmático *m*; **grand mal** ~ crisis del haut mal; **petit mal** ~ crisis del pequeño mal

seldom, pocas veces *adv*

select, to, seleccionar; escoger; elegir (i)

selection, selección *f*
self-centered, egocéntrico *adj*
self-confidence, confianza en sí mismo *f*; seguridad en sí mismo *f*
self-confident, seguro de sí mismo *adj*; lleno de confianza en sí mismo *adj*
self-conscious, cohibido *adj*
self-control, autocontrol *m*; dominio de sí mismo
self-criticism, autocrítica
self-defense, autodefensa
self-denial, abnegación *f*
self-discipline, autodisciplina
self-esteem, amor propio *m*
self-explanatory, que se explica por sí mismo
self-help, esfuerzo personal
self-importance, presunción *f*
self-indulgent, inmoderado *adj*
self-reliant, independiente *adj*
self-respect, dignidad *f*
self-sacrificing, abnegado *adj*
self-sufficient, autosuficiente *adj*
self-supporting, económicamente independiente *adj*
self-taught, autodidacta *adj, inv*; [*Ú.c.m.y.f.*] autodidacto *adj*
sell, to, vender
semen, esperma *m*; leche *f, vulg*; mecos *m, pl, vulg*; semen *m*
semicircular duct, conducto semicircular
semicomatose, semicomatoso *adj*
semi-erection, zarasa
semilunar, semilunar *adj*
seminal, seminal *adj*; ~ **fluid** líquido seminal; ~ **vesicle** vesículo seminal
seminiferous, seminífero *adj*
seminoma, seminoma *m*
send, to, mandar; ~ **for** despachar; ~ **for the doctor** llamar al médico
sender, emisor *m*; remitente *m/f*
senile, senil *adj*; **to get** ~ padecer debilidad senil
senilism, senilismo
senility, caduquez *f*; chochez *f*, vulg*; senectud *f*; senilidad *f*; debilidad senil *f, Med*
senior citizen, jubilado
sensation, sensación *f*; sentido; **burning** ~ ardor *m*; ~ **of dizziness** sensación de mareo; ~ **slight pain** dolorimiento
sense, ~ (*bodily; insight, instinct*) sentido; ~ **of feeling** (*tactile*) sentido del tacto; ~ **of hearing** (*auditory*) sentido del oído; ~ **of humor** sentido del humor; ~ **of sight** (*visual*) sentido de la vista; ~ **of smell** (*olfactory*) sentido del olfato; ~ **of taste** (*gustatory*) sentido del gusto; ~ **organ** órgano sensorio; ~ (*meaning*) significado; ~ (*sensation*) sensación *f*; ~ **of pain** sensación de dolor; ~ **of pleasure** sensación de placer; ~**s** (*right mind*) juicio *Med*
senseless, sin sentido *prep phr*; sin conocimiento *prep phr*
sensibilization, sensibilización *f*
sensitive, sensible *adj*; enconoso *adj, Med*; **to be** ~ **to** ser sensible a
sensitivity, dolor *m*; sensibilidad *f*
sensitization, sensibilización *f*; **protein** ~ sensibilización a proteínas; **Rh** ~ sensibilización al factor Rh
sensitize, to, sensibilizar
sensitized, sensibilizado *adj*
sensorial, sensorial *adj*
separated, separado *adj*
separate from, to, desprenderse de
separation, separación *f*
sepsis, sepsis *f*; septicemia; infección *f, fam*
septic, séptico *adj*
septicemia, bacteremia; infección en la sangre *f, fam*; piemia; septicemia; toxemia
septum, tabique *m*; **atrioventricular** ~ **of heart** tabique auriculoventricular; **bronchial** ~ tabique bronquial; **deviated** ~ tabique desviado; **gingival** ~

tabique gingival; papila inter-dentaria; **interatrial ~ of heart** tabique interauricular del corazón; **intermediate cervical** ~ tabique cervical intermedio; **interventricular** ~ tabique interventricular; **nasal** ~ tabique nasal; **orbital** ~ tabique orbitario; ligamentos anchos de los párpados

sequela, secuela

sequestrum, secuestro; **bone** ~ secuestro óseo

serene, sereno *adj*

series, serie *f*

serious, serio *adj*; ~ (*illness, wound, situation*) grave *adj*; **not** ~ de pronóstico leve *prep phr*; **possibly** ~ de pronóstico reservado *prep phr*

seroagglutination, seroaglutinación *f*

seroalbumin, seroalbúmina

serodiagnosis, serodiagnóstico

serology, serología

serosa, serosa

serotherapy, seroterapia; sueroterapia

serous, seroso *adj*; ~ **membrane** membrana serosa

serum, suero; **antivenin** ~ suero antiviperino; **black widow spider antivenin** ~ suero antialacrán; **blood** ~ suero de sangre; suero sanguíneo; ~ **sickness** enfermedad de suero *f*; ~**-fast** serorresistente *adj*

serve, to, servir (i)

service, servicio

sesame, sésamo

sesamoid, sesamoideo *adj*; ~ **bone** hueso sesamoideo; ~ **cartilage** cartílago sesamoideo

session, sesión *f*

set, (*of diverse things*) conjunto

set, to, ~ (*a bone*) encajar; encasar; reducir; sobar *SpAm*; ~ **bones** ensalmar huesos; ~ **a fracture** componer una fractura; re-ducir una fractura; ~ (*to coagulate*) coagular(se)

setback, recaída *Med*; ~ (*misfortune*) revés *m*

seven-month fetus, sietemesino

seventyish, setentón *adj*

several, varios *adj*

severe, agudo *adj*; fuerte *adj*; severo *adj*

severity, severidad *f*

sewing, costura

sex, sexo; ~ **characteristics** características sexuales; ~ **chromosome** cromosoma sexual *m*; ~ **life** vida sexual; ~**-linked inheritance** herencia ligada al sexo; **oral** ~ sexo oral; **oral** ~ (*cunnilingus*) cunilinción *f*; **oral** ~ (*fellatio*) felación *f*; felatorismo; irrumación *f*

sexual, sexual *adj*; ~ **activity** actividad sexual *f*; ~ **appetite** apetito sexual; ~ **cohabitation** cohabitación sexual *f*; ~ **contact** contacto sexual; ~ **climax** orgasmo sexual; ~ **perversion** perversión sexual *f*; aberración sexual *f*; ~ **relations** relaciones sexuales *f*; coito; **to reach** ~ **climax** es-lecharse *vulg*; dar(se) leche *vulg*; venirse *vulg*

shade, sombra; ~ (*lampshade*) pantalla; ~ (*window blind*) persiana

shaft, ~ (*of a bone*) caña; ~ (*handle*) mango

shake, to, ~ (*to agitate*) sacudir; ~ (*liquid*) agitar; **shake well before using** agítese bien antes de usar; ~ (*to impair*) afectar; ~ (*to upset composure of*) desconcertar (ie); ~ **hands** darse la mano; ~ **one's head** negar (ie) con la cabeza; ~ **with cold** temblar de frío; ~ **with fear** estremecerse

shaky, ~ (*situation, etc.*) inestable *adj*; ~ (*voice, hand*) tembloroso *adj*; ~ (*voice*) trémulo *adj*; ~ (*handwriting*) temblón *adj*; **to be** ~ **on one's legs** tener las piernas poco firmes; andar con paso vacilante

shame, ~ (*feeling*) vergüenza; ~ (*dishonor*) deshonra; ~ (*pity*) lástima

shame, to, ~ (*to bring shame upon*) deshonrar; ~ (*to cause to feel shame*) avergonzar

shampoo, champú *m*

shape, ~ (*form*) forma; ~ (*condition*) estado; condición *f*; **to be in perfect** ~ no doler ni una uña *PR*

sharp, afilado *adj*; cortante *adj*; puntudo *adj*, *SpAm*; ~ (*acute*) agudo *adj*; ~ (*biting*) picante *adj*; ~ (*pain*) terebrante *adj*, ~ (*sudden*) repentino *adj*

shave, to, afeitar(se); rasurar(se)

shears, tijeras (grandes)

sheath, vaina; cubierta

shed tears, to (*a person*), lagrimear

sheepskin, piel de oveja *f*

sheet, ~ (*bed*) sábana; ~ (*shroud*) mortaja; ~ (*of paper*) hoja

shelf, estante *m*

shellfish, mariscos *m, pl*

shelter, ~ (*place of safety*) refugio; ~ (*for homeless, old*) asilo

shelter, to, proteger; ~ (*poor, etc.*) acoger

sheltered, protegido *adj*

sherbet, nieve *f*; sorbete *m*

shield, (*IUD*) escudo

shift, ~ (*at work*) turno; **day** ~ turno de día; **night** ~ turno de noche; **to work in** ~s trabajar por turnos; ~ (*change*) cambio; **to** ~ cambiar

shin, canilla; espinilla

shinbone, tibia

shine, to, ~ (*by polishing*) sacar brillo; ~ (*with health*) rebosar de; ~ (*a light*) dirigir; proyectar

shingles, herpes[5] *m/f, pl*; zona; zoster *f*

ship, to, (*to transport*) enviar

shirt, ~ (*man's*) camisa; ~ (*woman's*) blusa; ~ (*infant's*) cotita *PR*

shit, mierda; caca

shit, to, cagar(se) *vulg*

shiver, ~ (*with cold*) escalofrío; ~ (*with fear*) estremecimiento

shiver, to, ~ (*with fear*) estremecerse; temblar; ~ (*with cold*) tiritar

shock, choque *m*; conmoción nerviosa *f*; shock *m*; sobresalto; susto; **anaphylactic** ~ choque alérgico *fam*; choque anafiláctico; **emotional** ~ choque emocional; ~ **of hair** greña; ~ **therapy** shockterapia; ~ **treatment** tratamiento de choque eléctrico; descarga *Elect*; **to be suffering from** ~ padecer una postración nerviosa

shock, to ~ (*to startle*) sobresaltar; ~ (*to affect emotionally or physically*) dar un disgusto; ~ (*to give offence*) escandalizar

shoe, zapato; **tennis** ~ chambón *m*; teni *m, Chicano*

shoelace, cabetes *m, pl, Mex*; cordón *m*

shoot (up)[6], **to**, (*See inject oneself with drugs, to.*)

shoot oneself[6], **to**, (*See inject oneself with drugs, to.*)

short, ~ (*person*) bajo *adj*; chaparro *adj, Mex, CA*; petacón *adj, Mex, Perú, Ríopl*; ~ (*in length, distance*) corto *adj*; ~ (*in time*) breve *adj*; ~ (*reply*) brusco *adj*

shortage, escasez *f*

shorten, to, ~ (*to make shorter*) acortar; ~ (*to abbreviate*) abreviar

shortness of breath, ahoguijo; ahoguío *fam*; falta de aire; falta de aliento

shorts, ~ (*men's underwear*) calzoncillos; pantaloncillos; ~ (*men's bathing trunks*) trusas *PR*

shortsighted, cegato *adj, fam*; miope *adj*

short-term, a plazo corto *prep phr*

shot, ~ (*causing wound*) balazo; ~ (*injection*) inyección *f*; chot *m*,

Chicano; **to give a ~** inyectar; **~** (*dose*) dosis *f, inv*; **~** (*of drinks*) trago; **~ of rum** trago de ron; **to take a ~ of straight liquor** dar(se) un juanetazo

shoulder, **~** (*person*) hombro; **~** (*animal*) lomo; **~ blade** (*scapula*) escápula; espaldilla; omóplato; paleta *Anat*; paletilla *Anat*; **~ joint** articulación del hombro *f*

show, to, demostrar (ue); mostrar (ue); **~ one's teeth** enseñar los dientes *fam*; mostrar (ue) los dientes

shower, ducha; regadera *Mex*

shower, to, (*to take a shower*) ducharse

shown, manifiesto *adj*

shrimp, camarones *m, pl*; **freshwater ~** guábara *PR*

shrink, *slang* (p)siquiatra[7] *m/f*

shrink, to, **~** (*clothes, etc.*) encoger; **~** (*quality*) reducir(se)

shuffle, to walk with a, caminar arrastrando los pies

shunt, corto circuito; derivación *f*; desviación *f*; shunt *m*

shy, tímido *adj*; ranchero *adj, slang, Mex*

sibling, hermano

sick, enfermo *adj*; malo *adj*; **~ benefit** subsidio de enfermedad; **~ leave** baja por enfermedad; permiso de convalencia; **~ person** doliente *m/f, Med*; **to become ~** enfermarse; **to get ~ from overeating** empachar(se)

sickening, nauseabundo *adj*

sickle cell, célula falciforme; **~ anemia** drepanocitosis *f*; anemia drepanocítica; (*See anemia, sickle cell.*)

sickliness, achaque *m*; mala salud *f*

sickly, cholenco *adj, Chicano*; **~** (*appearance*) pálido *adj*; papujo *adj, Mex*; trabajoso *adj, Med*; **~** (*emaciated*) demacrado *adj*; enteco *adj*; **~** (*person*) achacoso

adj; enfermizo *adj*; **~ person** enclenque *m/f*; **~** (*smell*) nauseabundo *adj*; **~** (*smile*) forzado *adj*; **~** (*taste*) empalagoso *adj*; **~** (*weak*) enclenque *adj*; chipe *adj, CA*; enclenco *adj, Col, PR*; engerido *adj, Col, Ven*; farruto *adj, Arg. Bol, Chi*; tere *adj, Col*

sickness, dolencia; enfermedad *f*; mal *m*; padecimiento; **morning ~** vómitos del embarazo; enfermedad matutina; mal de madre; náuseas del embarazo *f*; ansias matutinas; **mountain ~** soroche *m, SpAm*; **to get mountain ~** asorocharse *Bol, Chi, Ec, Perú*; sorocharse *Bol, Chi, Ec, Perú*

side, costado; lado; **left lower ~** lado izquierdo inferior; **left upper ~** lado izquierdo superior; **right lower ~** lado derecho inferior; **right upper ~** lado derecho superior; **~ effect** efecto secundario

siderail, barandal *m*

sidewalk, acera; banqueta *Mex*; andén *m, Ven, Col, CA*; vereda *Ec, Perú, Bol, Chi*

SIDS/sudden infant death syndrome, síndrome de muerte infantil repentina *m*

Sig/signetur/directions, método

sigh, suspiro

sigh, to, suspirar

sight, **~** (*view*) visión *f*; **~** (*sense*) vista

sigmoid, sigmoide *adj*; sigmoideo *adj*; **~ colon** sigma cólico *m*; colon sigmoide *m*; colon sigmoideo

sigmoidoscope, sigmoidoscopio

sigmoidoscopy, sigmoidoscopia

sign, indicio; seña; señal *f*; signo; **vital ~s** signos vitales; **warning ~** aviso; **~** (*symptom*) síntoma *m*

sign, to, firmar; **~** (*for the deaf*) hablar por señas

signal, señal *f*; **to pick up the ~** registrar la señal

signature, firma

silica, silice *f*

silicon, silicio
silicone, silicona
silver, plata; ~ **nitrate** nitrato de plata; piedra infernal
similar, semejante *adj*
similarity, semejanza
simmer, to, hervir(ie) a fuego lento
simple, sencillo *adj*
simulation, fingimiento; simulación *f*
sinapism, sinapismo
singe, to, chamuscar; socarrar; ~ (*hair*) quemar las puntas de
single, (*not married*) soltero *adj*
single out, to, separar
sinoatrial, sinoatrial *adj*
sinoauricular, sinoauricular *adj*
sinoventricular, sinoventricular *adj*
sinus, seno; ~ **congestion** congestión nasal *f*; sinusitis *f*
sinusitis, sinusitis *f*
sip, sorbo
sip, to, sorber
sister, hermana
sister-in-law, cuñada
sit to, sentar (ie); ~ **back in one's chair** recostarse (ue) en la silla; ~ **down** sentarse (ie); ~ **up** (*in bed*) incorporarse (en la cama)
sitting with the legs apart, espatarrao *adj*
sitz bath, baño de asiento; semicupio
sixth sense, sentido sexto
sixtyish, sesentón *adj*
size, tamaño; **assorted** ~ tamaño surtido; **large** ~ tamaño grande; **small** ~ tamaño pequeño; ~ (*of shoes*, *gloves*) número; ~ (*of clothes*) talla
skeletal, esquelético *adj*; ~ **muscles** músculos esqueléticos
skeleton, armazón *m*; esqueleto
skill, destreza
skim, to, ~ (*milk*) descremar; desnatar; ~ (*a liquid*) espumar; ~ **through** hojear
skim(med) milk, leche descremada *f*

skin, cuero *fam*; piel *f*; dérmico *adj*; ~ **blemish** placa *SpAm*; ~ **cancer** cáncer de la piel *m*; cáncer cutáneo *m*; ~ **disease** enfermedad dérmica *f*; **flap of the** ~ pellejo; ~ **of the face** cutis *m*; ~ **reaction** cutirreacción *f*; ~ **test** prueba cutánea
skin, to[6], *slang* inyectar narcóticos
skinned, ~ (*injured*) arañado *adj*; raspado *adj*; **light-**~ (*light-complexioned*) despercudido *adj*; **olive-**~ (*olive-complexioned*) trigueño *adj*; **very dark-**~, **lacking negroid features** pinto *adj*; retinto *adj*
skinny, delgado *adj*; flaco *adj*; ~ **person** bacalao *PR*
skirt, falda; pollera *Ríopl*
skull, calavera *Chicano*; cráneo; caja del cráneo; caja encefálica; ~ **fracture** fractura del cráneo; **top of** ~ tapa de los sesos *fam*
slacks, pantalones *m*, *pl*
slap, ~ (*blow on face*) bofetada; ~ (*on a child's bottom*) azote *m*; ~ (*on the back*) espaldarazo; ~ (*on thigh*, *back*, *etc.*) palmada; ~ (*with the hand*) manazo *Ríopl*; guantón *m*, *SpAm*
slap, to, (*to hit*) abofetear; golpear; ~ **s.o. on the face** dar una bofetada a uno; pegar un tortazo a uno; ~ **one's knees** palmotearse las rodillas
slash, ~ (*with a knife*) cuchillada; tajo; ~ (*wound*) tajarrazo *CA*, *Mex*; ~ (*on the face*) chirlo
sleep, sueño; ~ **apnea** narcolepsia; sueño paroxístico; ~ **disorders** trastornos del sueño; **twilight** ~ sueño crepuscular; ~ **walker**[6] (*a heroin addict*) tecato[2]; adicto a heroína
sleep, to, dormir (ue); ~ **it off** dormir (ue) la mona *fam*; ~ **like a log** dormir (ue) como un lirón; ~ **on something** consultar algo con la almohada; **to cry**

oneself ~ llorar hasta dormirse; **to drop off into** ~ quedarse dormido *adj*; **to fall asleep** dormirse (ue); **to fall into a deep** ~ caer en un sueño profundo; **to go** ~ (*limb*) dormirse (ue); **to put someone** ~ dormir (ue) a alguien; **to not have a wink of** ~ **all night** no pegar ojo en toda la noche

sleepiness, somnolencia; sueñera *SpAm*

sleeping, durmiente *adj*; dormido *adj*; ~ **pill** somnífero; píldora para dormir; píldora somnífera; sedativo; soporífera; ~ **sickness** enfermedad del sueño *f*

sleepy, soñoliento *adj*; **to be** ~ tener sueño

sleeve, manga

slender, delgado *adj*; flaco *adj*

slice, ~ (*of cheese, fish, melon, etc.*) raja; ~ (*of bread*) rebanada; ~ (*of meat*) tajada

slice, to, partir en rajas (rebanadas, etc.)

slicer, máquina de cortar

slide, ~ (*photo*) diapositiva; transparencia; **color** ~ diapositiva en color; ~ (*of a microscope*) portaobjetos *m*, *inv*; platina; ~ (*in playground*) tobogán *m*

slide, to, ~ (*to slip*) resbalar; ~ (*to glide*) deslizarse; ~ (*an object*) correr

sliding, ~ (*scale*) móvil *adj*; ~ (*part*) corredizo *adj*

slight, leve *adj*

slim, ~ (*thin*) delgado *adj*; ~ (*slender*) esbelto *adj*; **to get** ~ perfilarse *SpAm*

sling, cabestrillo; **to put in a** ~ poner en cabestrillo

slip, ~ (*sliding*) resbalón *m*; ~ (*a trip*) traspié *m*; ~ (*of paper*) trozo; ~ (*mistake*) error *m*; ~ (*lingerie*) combinación *f*

slip, to, ~ (*to slide*) deslizar; ~ (*to*

stumble) resbalar; ~ **a bone** dislocarse un hueso; zafarse (un hueso) *SpAm*; ~ **unexpectedly** esgolizarse *PR*

slipped disc, disco desplazado; disco intervertebral luxado

slipper, pantufla; zapatilla

slit, raja; corte *m*

sliver, astilla

slot, (*groove for coins*) ranura

slouch, to, (*bad posture*) andar desgarbado; andar con los hombros caídos y la cabeza inclinada; ~ **in a chair** estar repantigado en un sillón

slow, lento *adj*; ~ (*stupid*) torpe *adj*; ~ **walk** paso de tortuga; **to be** ~ (*a timepiece*) atrasarse; ~ **down** (*in walking, etc.*) ir más despacio; ~ **down** (*car, etc.*) moderar la marcha

slowing, lentitude *f*

slowly, despacio *adv*; **more** ~ más despacio

slowing, lentitud *f*

slur, to, (*words*) pronunciar mal; comerse las palabras *fam*

slurred speech, lenguaje cercenado *m*

small, ~ (*size*) pequeño *adj*; ~ (*stature*) bajo *adj*; ~ (*amount*) poco; ~ **intestine** intestino delgado; ~ **of the back** región lumbar *f*

smallpox, viruelas; alfombrilla *Mex*; peste *f*, *Chi*

smart, ~ (*intelligent*) listo *adj*; inteligente *adj*; ~ (*stylish*) elegante *adj*

smarting, (*sensation*) escozor *m*; ardor *m*, *Mex, CA, Ríopl*

smart, to, escocer; arder *Mex, CA, Ríopl*; picar *Med*

smash, to, aplastar

smear, cultivo; frotis *m*; unto

smear, to, untar (de)

smegma, esmegma *m*; queso *slang*

smell, olfato; olor *m*

smell, to, oler (ue); ~ **bad** abombar(se) *PR*

smile, sonrisa

smile, to, sonreír (i)

smiling, sonriente *adj*

smoke, humo; ~ **inhalation** inhalación de humo *f*

smoke, to, fumar; ~ **marijuana** dorar[2]; enamoriscar[2]; enyerbar[2]; grifear[2]; motear[2]; motiar[2]; motorizar[2]; quemar[2]; tostar[2]; tronar(se)[2]

smooth, ~ (*surface*) liso *adj*; ~ **muscles** músculos lisos; ~ (*silky*) blondo *adj*, *SpAm*; ~ (*wine, voice, skin*) suave *adj*; ~ (*brow*) sin arrugas *prep phr*; ~ (*beardless*) lampiño *adj*; imberbe *adj*

smooth, to, ~ (*to file down*) limar; ~ (*hair*) alisar; ~ (*to polish*) pulir

snack, bocadillo; merienda; piscolabis *m, inv*; tiento *Arg. PR*

snack shop, tienda de refrescos

snake, culebra; serpiente *f*; vípora; ~ **bite** mordedura de culebra

sneeze, estornudo

sneeze, to, estornudar

sniff, to, (*snuff, smelling salts, etc.*) aspirar; ~ (*in/up*)[6] sorber por las narices[2]; ~ **glue**[6] aspirar cola[2]; hacer(se) a la glu(fa)[2]; inhalar cola[2]; respirar cola[2]; sesonar[2]; ~ **residue of powdered narcotics**[6] estufear[2]; estufiar[2]

sniffle, to, moquear

snore, ronquido

snore, to, roncar

snort[6], **to**, (*sniff residue of powdered narcotics*) aspirar narcóticos por la nariz; estufear[2]; estufiar[2]

snow, nieve *f*; ~ **bird**[6] *slang* adicto a cocaína

snow, to, nevar (ie)

soak, to, remojar; entripar *Mex*; ~ **gauze in antiseptic** empapar la gasa en un antiséptico; ~ **through** calar

soap, jabón *m*; **germicidal** ~ jabón germicida; **green** ~ jabón verde; jabón blando; **a piece of** ~ jaba *PR*; **soft** ~ jabón blando

soapy water, agua[3] jabonosa

soaring, to be, (*See blasted, to be.*)

S.O.B., *slang* cabrón *m*, *slang, Mex*

sober, sobrio *adj*

sober up, to, espabilar la borrachera

social, social *adj*; ~ **class** clase social *f*; ~ **Security** seguro social; ~ **service** servicio social; ~ **stratum** capa social; ~ **worker** trabajador social

societal values, valores de la sociedad *m*

society, sociedad *f*

socioeconomic, socioeconómico *adj*

sociotherapy, socioterapia

sock, ~ (*stocking*) calcetín *m*; ~ (*blow*) golpe *m*; porrazo; puñetazo

socket, ~ (*of an eye*) cuenca; órbita; ~ (*of a joint*) fosa; ~ (*of a tooth*) alvéolo

soda cracker, galleta blanca

sodium, sodio; ~ **carbonate** carbonato de sodio; ~ **hydroxide** hidróxido de sodio; ~ **hypochlorite** (*bleach*) blanqueador de ropa *m*; hipoclorito de sodio; ~ **pentothal** pentotal sódico *m*; pentotal de sodio *m*; ~ **peroxide** agua[3] oxigenada; peróxido de sodio; ~ **sulfate** (*in toilet cleaners*) sulfato de sodio (en limpiadores de inodoros)

sodoku, (*rat-bite fever*) sodoku *m*; fiebre por mordedura de ratas *f*

sodomy, sodomía

soft, ~ (*bland; of material, etc.*) blando *adj*; suave *adj*; ~ **lenses** lentes suaves; (*See contact lens.*); ~ (*drink*) no alcohólico *adj*; analcohólico *adj*; ~ (*flabby*) flojo *adj*; ~ (*gentle; smooth*) suave *adj*; blondo *SpAm*; ~ (*job*) fácil *adj*; ~ (*lenient*) indulgente *adj*; ~

(*low*) bajo *adj*; ~ **voice** voz baja *f*; ~ (*pliant*) blando *adj*; ~ **chancre** chancro blando; ~ **palate** velo del paladar; paladar blando *m*; (*See palate, soft.*)

soiled, ~ (*stained*) manchado *adj*; ~ (*dirty*) sucio *adj*

solar, solar *adj*; ~ **rays** rayos solares

sole, ~ (*a fish*) lenguado; ~ **of the foot** planta del pie *Anat*; ~ **of the shoe** suela

soleus (*muscle*), sóleo

solid, sólido *m*, *adj*

solidity, solidez *f*

solution, solución *f*; **physiological saline** ~ suero fisiológico; **physiological** ~ solución fisiológica *f*

solvent, solvente *m*

somatic, somático *adj*

somnambulism, sonambulismo

somniferous, somnífero *adj*

son, hijo

sonde, sonda

son-in-law, yerno

sonogram, sonograma *m*

soon, pronto *adv*; **as ~ as possible** lo más pronto posible

soporific, narcótico *m*, *adj*; somnífero *m*, *adj*; soporífero *m*, *adj*; soporífico *m*, *adj*

sore, aflicción *f*; dolor *m*; enconado; lamprea; lesión *f*; lastimadura; pena; chácara *CA, Col, Chi*; chira *CA*; cholla *CA*; lacra *Med, SpAm*; lascadura *Mex*; ñacara *CA*; ñola *Guat, Hond*; **cold** ~ pupa *Med*; ~ **ears** dolor de oídos; mal de oídos *m*; ~ **eyes** dolor de ojos; ~ **throat** garganta inflamada; dolor de garganta; mal de garganta *m*; ~ (*wound*) grano; llaga; úlcera; **bed** ~ llaga por decúbito; úlcera por decúbito; gangrena por decúbito; úlcera trófica; ~ (*painful*) (a)dolorido *adj*; ~ (*inflamed*) inflamado *adj*; ~ (*in-*

jured) lastimado *adj*; ~ (*sensitive*) sensitivo *adj*; **to be** ~ dolerle (ue) a uno (+ *noun*); tener dolor de (+ *noun*)

soreness, dolor *m*; inflamación *f*

sorrow, pesar *m*; pena; tristeza; **with heartfelt** ~ con hondo pesar *prep phr*

sorry, ~ (*regretful*) arrepentido *adj*; ~ (*sad*) triste *adj*; afligido *adj*; apenado *adj*; ~ (*condition*) lastimoso *adj*; ~ (*figure*) ridículo *adj*; **to be** ~ (*to regret*) sentirlo (ie); **to be ~ for someone** tener lástima a uno

s.o.s./**si opus sit**/**if necessary**, si es necesario

souffle, pillido *Mex*; silbido; soplo

soul, alma³

sound, ~ (*sonorous*) sonoro *adj*; ~ **effects** efectos sonoros; ~ **track** banda sonora; ~ **waves** ondas sonoras; ~ (*healthy*) sano *adj*; ~ (*health, advice, character, etc.*) bueno *adj*; ~ **character** buen carácter *m*; ~ **health** buena salud *f*; ~ (*sleep*) profundo *adj*; **to be ~ asleep** estar profundamente dormido *adj*; ~ (*hoarse, raucous*) ronquido; ~ (*noise*) ruido; sonido; **auscultatory** ~ sonido auscultatorio; **flapping** ~ sonido valvular; **friction** ~ ruido de frotación; **heart ~s** ruidos cardíacos; ~ (*probe*) sonda *Med*; **urethral** ~ sonda uretral

sound, to, sonar (ue); ~ (*with a stethoscope*) auscultar; ~ (*with a sound*) sondar; sondear

sour, agrio *adj*

source, fuente *f*; ~ **of energy** fuente de energía

space, espacio; **epidural** ~ espacio epidural

spaced (**out**)⁶, **to be**, (*See blasted, to be.*)

Spanish, español *m*, *adj*

spank, to, dar una zurra a

spanking, azotaina; zurra

spasm, contracción muscular *f*; espasmo; latido *Chicano*; punzada *Med*; **bronchial** ~ espasmo bronquial; **facial** ~ espasmo facial; **pharyngeal** ~ espasmo faríngeo

spasmodic, espasmódico *adj*; espástico *adj*; intermitente *adj*; irregular *adj*

spastic, espasmódico *adj*; espástico *adj*

speak, to, hablar

speaker, interlocutor

special, especial *adj*

specialist, especialista *m/f*

specialization, especialización *f*

specialize, to, especializarse

specialized, especializado *adj*

specific, específico *adj*; ~ **gravity** peso específico

specimen, espécimen *m*; muestra; **urine** ~ muestra de la orina

speck, (*small portion*) pizca

spectacles, anteojos (*general term*); espejuelos *Cu*; gafas; lentes *m*, *pl*, *Mex*; ~ (*wire-rimmed*) quevedos

speculum, espéculo; espejo vaginal

speech, del habla *prep phr*; lenguaje *m*; ~ **defect** defecto de dicción; **faculty of** ~ palabra; habla³; **incoherent** ~ lenguaje incoherente; **jumbled** ~ lenguaje confuso; ~ **pathologist** logopatólogo; especialista en logopedia; **power of** ~ palabra; habla³; **slurred** ~ lenguaje cercenado; ~ **therapy** logoterapia; foniatría; **to lose one's power of** ~ perder (ie) palabra; perder (ie) el habla; **to recover one's** ~ recobrar el habla

spell, ~ (*charm*) encanto; ~ (*evil spell*) maleficio; ~ (*of a disease*) ataque *m*; ~ (*period of time*) temporada; ~ (*shift/turn*) turno

spell, to, (*letter by letter*) deletrear

sperm, esperma *m*; espermatozoide *m*; mecos *m*, *slang*; semen *m*; semilla *slang*, *Mex*

spermatic cord, cordón espermático *m*

spermatocele, espermatocele *m*

spermatocyte, espermatocito

spermatogenesis, espermatogénesis *f*

spermatorrhea, pérdidas seminales

spermatozoid, espermatozoide *m*

spermicide, espermaticida *m*; **vaginal** ~ espermaticida vaginal

spermiogram, espermiograma *m*

sphere, esfera

sphincter, esfínter *m*; **pylori(c)** ~ esfínter pilórico

sphygmomanometer, *form*, esfigmomanómetro

sphygmomanometry, esfigmomanometría

spice, especia

spicy, picante *adj*

spike⁶, (*a hypodermic needle*) abuja²; aguja²; filero²; hierro²; jeringuilla; punta²

spina bifida, espina bífida

spinach, espinaca

spinal, espinal *adj*; ~ **anesthesia** anestesia espinal; anestesia raquídea; ~ **column** columna vertebral; espina dorsal; ~ **cord** médula espinal; ~ **curvature** desviación de la columna vertebral *f*; escoliosis *f*; ~ **fusion** fusión espinal *f*; ~ **medulla** médula espinal; ~ **tap** punción lumbar *f*; ~ **tuberculosis** tuberculosis de la columna vertebral *f*

spindle, huso

spine, columna vertebral

spinster, soltera; jamona *PR*

spiral, (*IUD*) espiral *m*

spirit, espíritu *m*; ánimo; **evil** ~ cuco

spiritism, espiritismo

spiritist, espiritista *m/f*; ~ **store** botánica

spirogram, espirograma *m*
spirograph, espirógrafo
spirometer, espirómetro
spirometry, espirometría; pulmometría; **bronchoscopic ~** espirometría broncoscópica; broncoespirometría
spiroscope, espiroscopio
spit, ~ (*in the mouth*) saliva; ~ esputo *Med*; ~ **of blood** esputo de sangre; ~ (*out of/expelled from mouth*) salivazo
spit, to, arrojar; escupir; ~ **blood** escupir sangre; ~ **in the bowl** escupir en la taza
spleen, bazo; espleno *fam*; esplín *Chicano*
splenectomy, esplenectomía
splenorrhagia, esplenorragia
splint, férula; tablilla; **in a ~** entablillado *adj*; **to put in ~s** entablillar
splinter, ~ (*of wood*) astilla; ~ (*of bone*) esquirla
split, partido *adj*; ~ (*in skin*) grieta; ~ **personality** desdoblamiento de la personalidad; desdoblamiento del yo
split, to, ~ (*to divide*) partir; ~ (*skin*) agrietar
spoil, to, estropear *Med*; **to begin ~** abombar(se)
spoiled, ~ (*indulged*) mimado *adj*; añiao *adj*, *PR*; ~ (*rotten*) podrido *adj*
spondyloarthrosis, espondiloartrosis *f*
spondylolysis, espondilólisis *f*
sponge, esponja
spontaneous, espontáneo *adj*; ~ **delivery** parto espontáneo
spoon, cuchara
spoonful, cucharada
sporadic, esporádico *adj*
spore, espora
sporoblast, esporoblasto
sports medicine, medicina deportiva

spot, ~ (*place*) lugar *m*; ~ (*blemish*) mancha; **black ~s** puntos negros
spotted sickness, mal de pinto *m*; pinta
spotting, manchado; manchas de sangre; **vaginal ~** manchas de flujo vaginal sanguinolento
spotty, ~ (*from infection*) con manchas *Med* ; ~ (*with pimples*) con granos *Med*
sprain, dislocación *f*; esguince *f*; falseo *Chicano*; lastimadura; torcedura; torcimiento
sprain, to, desconcertar (ie); falsear; torcer (ue); ~ **one's ankle** torcerse (ue) el tobillo
spray, pulverización *f*; pulverizador *m*; rociador *m*; espray *m*, *Chicano*
spray, to, ~ (*to propel a liquid*) pulverizar; ~ (*to sprinkle*) rociar
spread, to, propagar(se); ~ **apart** separar; ~ **out** (*to scatter*) esparcir; ~ (**out**) (*to lay out*) tender (ie); ~ **limbs** extender (ie)
spur, espolón *m*; **calcaneal ~** espolón calcáneo
sputum, esputo; flema; desgarro *SpAm*; gargao; pollo *Chicano*; saliva; **bloody ~** esputo hemático; **mucoid ~** esputo mucoso; **mucopurulent ~** esputo mucopurulento; **nummular ~** esputo numular; **purulent ~** esputo purulento; **prune juice ~** esputo de zumo de ciruelas; **red currant jelly ~** esputo de jalea de grosellas; **rusty ~** esputo herrumbroso
squash, calabaza
squat, ~ (*person*) rechoncho *adj*; chaparro *adj*, *Mex*, *CA*, *Ec*, *Perú*, *Bol*; ~ (*crouching*) en cuclillas *prep phr*
squat, to, acuclillarse; ponerse de cuclillas
squatting, eñangotao *adj*, *PR*
squeeze, to, apretar (ie)
squint, ~ (*strabismus*) bizca; biz-

quera *Col, PR*; ~ (*sidelong glance*) vistazo

squint-eyed, bisojo *adj*; bizco *adj*; bizcorneado *SD*; bizcorneto *Col, Mex*; ojituerto *adj*

squint, to, ~ (*to be cross-eyed*) bizquear; mirar bizco; ponerse bizco; bizcornear *Cu, PR*; ~ (*to keep eyes half closed*) entrecerrar (ie) los ojos

stab, ~ (*with a dagger*) puñalada; ~ (*with a knife*) navajazo; ~ (*of pain*) punzada

stab, to, ~ (*with a dagger*) apuñalar; ~ (*with a knife*) dar un navajazo; ~ **s.o. to death** matar a alguien a puñaladas; **to be stabbed to death** morir (ue) apuñalado *adj*

stabbing, punzada; ~ (*pain*) punzante *adj*

stabilize, to, estabilizar

stable, estable *adj*

staff, personal *m*; del personal *adj*

stage, etapa; fase *f*; **expulsive** ~ fase expulsiva; **placental** ~ fase placentaria; ~ **of pregnancy** fase del parto; período del parto; **first** ~ **of pregnancy** primera fase del parto; primer período del parto; **second** ~ **of pregnancy** segunda fase del parto; segundo período del parto; **third** ~ **of pregnancy** tercera fase del parto; tercer período del parto

stagger, to, tambalearse

stain, ~ (*staining*) coloración *f*; **acid-fast** ~ coloración acidorresistente; **Giemsa's** ~ coloración de Giemsa; **Gram's** ~ coloración de Gram; **methylene blue** ~ coloración de azul de metileno; **Wright's** ~ coloración de Wright; ~(**ing**) (*for microscopic study*) colorante *m*; **selective** ~ colorante selectivo; **Ziehl-Neelsen** ~ colorante de Ziehl-Neelsen; ~/**staining** tinción *f*; ~**s and staining methods** co-

loración y métodos de coloración; ~ (*mark*) mancha

stain, to, manchar

stained, manchado *adj*

stainless steel, acero inoxidable; ~ **wire** alambre de acero inoxidable *m*

stair, escalera(s); ~ (*a single step*) peldaño; **flight of** ~**s** tramo de escalera; **to go down the** ~**s** bajar la escalera; **to go up the** ~**s** subir la escalera

staircase, moving, (*escalator*) escalera mecánica

stairway, escalera

stairwell, caja de la escalera

stale, rancio *adj*

stammer, tartamudeo; balbuceo

stammer, to, tartamudear; balbucear; cancanear *CA, Col, Mex*

stammering, cancaneo *CA, Col, Mex*

stamp, estampilla *SpAm*; sello

stamp, to, ~ (*to affix*) sellar; estampar; ~ (*to mark*) imprimir; ~ **out** extirpar; ~ **one's foot** dar patadas en el suelo

stand, estante *m*

stand, to, estar de pie; ~ **out** destacar; ~ **up** levantarse; parar(se); ponerse de pie

standard, estándar *m, adj*; ~ **of living** nivel de vida *m*; **to be below** ~ estar por debajo del nivel correcto; **to be up to** ~ estar conforme con el debido nivel

standardization, estandarización *f*

standardize, to, estandarizar

standing, de pie *prep phr*; **to be** ~(**up**) estar de pie; estar parado *adj, SpAm*

stapes, estribo

staphylococcal, estafilocócico *adj*; ~ **infection** infección estafilocócica *f*

staphylococcus, (*pl, staphylococci*) estafilococo

staple, grapa

stapler, grapadora

starch, almidón *m*

starchy, almidonado *adj*; amiláceo *adj*

stare, to, fijar la mirada

start, ~ (*fright*) susto; ~ (*nervous jump*) sobresalto

start, to, empezar (ie); comenzar (ie); iniciar; precipitarse; ~ (*a machine*) poner(se) en marcha; ~ out arrancar

starvation, inanición *f*

starving, esmayao *adj*, *PR*

stash⁶, to, (*to hide a supply of drugs*) clavar²; plantar²

stasis, estasis *f*

stat/statim/immediately, inmediatamente

state, estado; ~ of anxiety estado de ansiedad; ~ of depression estado de depresión; ~ of health *s*alud *f*; estado físico; ~ of mind estado de ánimo; ~ of shock estado de choque; persistent vegetative ~ estado vegetativo persistente; resting ~ estado de reposo; in a commatose ~ en estado comatoso

static, estático *adj*

station, estación *f*; posición *f*; aid ~ estación de ayuda; puesto de socorro; nursing ~ puesto de enfermeras; test ~ prueba de posición

statistics, estadística; medical ~ estadísticas médicas; vital ~ estadísticas vitales; bioestadística

stature, estatura

status, ~ (*state*) estado; marital ~ estado civil; ~ (*position*) posición *f*; ~ symbol símbolo de prestigio

statute, ley *f*; estatuto; by ~ de acuerdo con la ley

stay, estancia

stay, to, quedarse; ~ at home quedarse en casa; ~ awake desvelarse; ~ in bed guardar cama

STD/sexually transmitted dis-ease, enfermedad pasada sexualmente *f*

steady, (*constant*) constante *adj*; ~ hand mano segura *f*; ~ job trabajo fijo; ~ pace paso regular

steam, vapor *m*

stenosis, estenosis *f*; esophageal ~ estenosis esofágica

step, paso; pisada

stepbrother, hermanastro

stepchild, hijastro

stepfather, padrastro

stepmother, madrastra

stepsister, hermanastra

stepson, hijastro

stereoscopic radiograph, cinerradiograma *m*, *Dent*

sterile, estéril *adj*; esterilizado *adj*; infecundo *adj*; aséptico *adj*; ~ syringe jeringa esterilizada

sterility, esterilidad *f*; infecundidad *f*; female ~ frío de la matriz; permanent ~ esterilidad permanente

sterilization, esterilización *f*

sterilize, to, castrar; esterilizar; ~ the bottles esterilizar las botellas

sterilized, esterilizado *adj*

sterilizer, esterilizador *m*

sternum, esternón *m*

steroid, esteroide *m*

stertor, estertor *m*; tracheal ~ estertor traqueal

stertorous, estertoroso *adj*

stethoscope, estetoscopio; fonendoscopio

stew, guisado

stick, ~ (*bar, mop, etc.*) palo; ~ (*for walking*) bastón *m*; ~ (*of chewing gum, wax, etc.*) barra; ~ (*of a needle*) pinchazo; piquete *m*, *Mex*; ~ (*of an insect; a needle*) picadura; ~ (*of celery*) rama

stick, to, ~ (*to thrust*) clavar; ~ (*with knife, dagger, etc.*) herir (ie); ~ (*to adhere*) pegar; ~ (*to sting*) picar; ~ (*to penetrate*) pinchar; ~ **out** sacar; ~ **out one's tongue** sacar la lengua

sticking plaster, pegoste *m*, CA, Col, Mex, Ven

sticky, ~ (*viscous*) amogollao *adj*, PR; pegajoso *adj*; ~ (*situation*, *person*) difícil *adj*; ~ (*weather*) húmedo y con mucho calor *adj*

stiff, ~ (*joint*) anquilosado *adj*, Med; ~ (*leg*) tieso *adj*, Med; ~ (*numb*) embotado *adj*, Med; entumecido *adj*, Med; ~ (*after exercise*) con agujetas *adj*, Med; ~ (*starched*) almidonado *adj*; ~ (*hard to move*) duro *adj*; ~ (*unbending*) rígido *adj*; ~ (*taut*) tieso *adj*; ~ **neck** nuca tiesa *fam*; tortícolis *m*; torticolis *m*; ~ (*frozen*) joint articulación envarada *f*; articulación trabada *f*; ~ **with cold** yerto de frío *adj*; **to be ~ all over** estar lleno de agujetas; **to be ~ in the legs** tener las piernas entumecidas; **to become ~** envararse Mex; **to get ~** engarrotarse SpAm

stiffen, to, ~ (*a joint*) anquilosar(se); ~ (*limbs*) embotar(se); entumecer(se); ~ (*muscles*) agarrotar(se); ~ (*to tighten up*) atiesar

stiffness, ~ (*of a joint*) anquilosamiento; ~ (*of limbs*) embotamiento; ~ (*of muscles*) agarrotamiento; ~ **of legs** (*after exercise*) agujetas en las piernas *f, pl*; ~ (*numbness*) envaramiento Mex; ~ (*rigidity*) tiesura

stigma, estigma *m*

still, todavía *adv*; ~ (*motionless*) inmóvil *adj*; quieto *adj*; ~ (*calm*) tranquilo *adj*; ~ (*noise*) sordo *adj*; ~ (*silent*) silencioso *adj*

stillbirth, mortinato; natimuerto; parto muerto; ~ **rate** tasa de natimortalidad

stillborn, mortinato *adj*; nacido muerto *adj*

stimulant, estimulante *m*; exitante[2] *m*

stimulate, to, estimular

stimulating, excitante *adj*, Med

stimulus, estímulo

sting, (*of an insect*) picadura; picotada; picotazo; piquete *m*; punzada; **ant** ~ picadura de hormiga; **bee** ~ picadura de abeja; **black widow spider** ~ picadura de ubar *fam*; picadura de viuda negra; **botfly** ~ picadura de moscardón; **chigoe/jigger/sandflea** ~ picadura de nigua; **flea** ~ picadura de pulga; **hornet** ~ picadura de avispón; **mosquito** ~ picadura de mosquito; **scorpion** ~ picadura de alacrán; **spider** ~ picadura de araña; **tick** ~ picadura de garrapata; **wasp** ~ picadura de avispa

sting, to, picar

stinger, (*of bees, wasps, etc.*) aguijón *m*

stinging, urente *adj*, Med

stingy, tacañoso *adj*; guillao *adj*, PR

stink, hedor *m*

stink, to, abombar(se)

stir, to, mezclar; revolver (ue)

stirrup bone, estribo

stitch, puntada; punto (de costado) Med; sutura; jada Med

stocking, media; ~ (*sock*) calcetín *m*; ~ (*knee-length*) calceta; **elastic** ~ calceta elástica; media elástica; **surgical** ~ calceta compresiva; media compresiva; **a pair of ~s** un par de medias; **in one's ~ feet** descalzo *adj*

stomach, estómago; barriga; panza Chicano; vientre *m*; guata Arg, Chi, Perú; estomacal *adj*; ~ **ache** dolor de estómago *m*; **to have a ~ ache** dolerle (ue) las tripas; **on an empty ~** en ayunas; **pit of ~** boca del estómago; epigastrio; hueco epigástrico; ~ **pump**

bomba estomacal; bomba gástrica; ~ **tube** sonda gástrica; ~ **ulcer** úlcera del estómago; ~ **upset** trastorno gástrico; trastorno estomacal; jaleo *PR*
stomatitis, estomatitis *f*
stomatologist, estomatólogo *m, adj*
stomatology, estomatología
stone, cálculo; piedra; **gall ~s** cálculos biliares; **kidney ~s** cálculos renales; **pumice ~** piedra pómez
stoned on marijuana, arrebatao[2] *adj*; bombiao[2] *adj*; curao[2] *adj*; espaseao[2] *adj, Chicano*; (*See marijuana.*)
stoned[6], **to be**, estar a millón[2]
stool, ~ (*feces*) defecación *f*; deposición *f*; deyecciones *f, pl*; excremento; evacuación *f*; heces *f, pl*; pupú *m, fam*; (*See feces.*); ~ **character** consistencia de las heces; ~ **culture** coprocultivo; **mucous ~** deposición mucosa; **rice water ~** deposición de agua de arroz; defecación colérica; **soapy ~** heces jabonosas; **spinach ~** heces biliosas; **spluttery ~** heces espumosas; ~ **softener** cápsula para ablandar evacuaciones; ~ **specimen** muestra de excremento; muestra de heces fecales; ~ (*seat with no back, sides, or arms*) taburete *m*
stop, to, dejar de; pararse; suprimir; ~ **up one's ears** taponar los oídos
stopped-up nose, constipación nasal *f*; nariz tapada *f*
stopper, tapón *m*
storage, almacenaje *m*
store, tienda
store, to, almacenar; guardar
story, ~ (*tale*) cuento; ~ (*floor*) piso
strabismal/strabismic, estrábico *adj*
strabismus, bizco *CA*; estrabismo *form*; desviación manifiesta *f*; **external ~** estrabismo externo;

estrabismo divergente; exotropía; **internal ~** estrabismo interno; estrabismo convergente; esoforia; esotropía; rinopsia
strabometer, estrabometro
straight, derecho *m, adj*; recto *adj*; directo *adj*; ~ (*hair*) pajón *adj, Mex*
straighten the teeth, to, enderezar los dientes
strain, ~ (*stock*) cepa *Med*; ~ (*nervous, mental*) tensión *f*; **neck ~** tensión del cuello *f*; ~ (*exhaustion*) agotamiento; torcedura *Med*
strain, to, ~ (*a muscle*) distender (ie); sufrir un tirón; ~ (*expelling fetus, B.M.*) pujar; ~ (*heart, eyes*) cansar; ~ (*laughter, voice*) forzar (ue); ~ (*nerves*) agotar los nervios; ~ (*shoulder*) dislocar; ~ (*to overtax*) dañar por esfuerzo excesivo *Med* ; ~ (*to twist back, muscles*) torcer(se) (ue); ~ (*vegetables, noodles, etc.*) colar (ue); ~ **one's back** derrengarse; ~ **one's ears** aguzar el oído; ~ **one's eyes** cansar; ~ **one's wrist** torcerse (ue) la muñeca
strained, ~ (*ankle, wrist, back*) torcido *adj*; ~ (*eyes, heart*) cansado *adj*; ~ (*joint*) dislocado *adj*; ~ (*laughter, voice*) forzado *adj*; ~ (*nerves*) tenso *adj*; ~ (*noodles, etc.*) colado *adj*
straining, (*tenesmus*) pujos
strait jacket, camisa de fuerza
strand, filamento; cabo; fibra
strange, extraño *adj*
strangulation, estrangulación *f*; **hernial ~** estrangulación herniaria
strap, correa; tira; ~ (*leather*) tira de cuero; **metal ~** banda de metal; **shoulder ~** tirante *m*; hombrera
strap, to, (*to tie up*) atar con correa; ~ **down** sujetar con correa
stratum, (*pl, strata*) capa

straw, paja; **drinking** ~ sorbeto *slang*

strawberry, fresa; ~ **mark** angioma elevado *m*; ~ **nevus** nevo cavernoso

streak, raya; **primitive** ~ línea primitiva

stream, ~ (*of water, blood*) chorro (*common*); corriente *f*; ~ (*of tears*) torrente *m*

stream, to, ~ (*liquid*) correr; fluir; ~ (*blood*) chorrear; manar

street, calle *f*

strength, fuerza; **extra** ~ fuerza extra; **inner** ~ fuerza interior; **muscular** ~ potencia muscular

strengthen, to, reconfortar *Med*

strenuous, estrenuo *adj*

strep throat, estreptococia *form*; angina estreptocócica; dolor de garganta por estreptococo *m*; mal de garganta por estreptococo *m*

streptococcus, estreptococo

streptomycin, estreptomicina

stress, estrés *m*; **emotional** ~ tensión emocional *f*; ~ **incontinence** incontinencia de esfuerzo; ~ **test** electrocardiograma de esfuerzo *m*; prueba de ejercicio; prueba de esfuerzo graduado; prueba ergométrica; **dipyridamole** ~ **test** electrocardiograma de esfuerzo con dipiridamol; **thallium** ~ **test** electrocardiograma de esfuerzo con talio

stress, to, enfatizar

stretch marks, (*stria*) estrias

stretch, to, estirar; ~ (*to unfold*) tender (ie)

stretcher, camilla; **to carry on** ~ llevar en camilla; ~ **bearer** camillero

stria, (*pl, striae*) estria; estriación *f*; **skin** ~ estriaciones cutáneas

striated, estriado *adj*; ~ **muscles** músculos estriados

strict, estricto *adj*

stricture, constricción *f*; estenosis *f*; estrechez *f, fam*; estrictura

strike, to (*with a disaster*), lacrar *Med*

string, cuerda

strip (**naked**), **to**, encuerar *Chi, Cu, Mex*; encalatarse *Perú*

stripping, safenectomía

stroke, ~ (*cerebrovascular*) accidente cerebral *m*; apoplejía; ataque cerebral *m*; ataque fulminante *m*; derrame cerebral *m*; embolia cerebral; emolio *Chicano*; estroc *m, Chicano*; hemorragia vascular; parálisis *f*; ~ (*heartbeat*) latido; ~ (*blow*) golpe *m*; **heat** ~ golpe de calor; fiebre térmica *f*; **sun** ~ golpe de sol; insolación *f*; siriasis *f*

strong, fuerte *adj*; válido *adj, Med*; ~ **tea** té cargado *m*; té fuerte *m*

strontium, estroncio

structure, estructura

strung out, to be, (*See blasted, to be.*)

strychnine, estricnina; ~ **poisoning** envenenamiento por estricnina

stub one's foot, to, dar(se) un tropezón

stubble, (*of beard*) cañones *m*

stubborn, tenaz *adj*; rebencudo *adj, Cu*

stuck, to become, pegarse

stud, *slang* garañón *m, Mex, slang*

student, estudiante *m/f*

studious, estudioso *adj*

study, estudio

stuff, (*medicine*) medicina; menjurje *m*; mejunje *m*

stuffed, relleno *adj*; ~**-up nose** nariz tapada *f*; nariz tupida *f*

stuffy, ~ (*ventilation*) mal ventilado *adj*; ~ (*congested*) congestionado *adj*; taponado *adj*

stump, ~ (*of pencil, candle, etc.*) cabo; ~ (*of cigarette*) colilla; ~ (*of an amputation*) muñón *m*; tu-

co *SpAm*; ~ (*of a tooth*; *large root*) raigón *m*; ~ (*of tree*) tocón *m*
stun, to, pasmar
stupefacient, estupefaciente *adj*
stupendous, estupendo *adj*
stupid, estúpido *adj*; ñango *adj*, *slang*
stupidity, estupidez *f*; ñanguería *slang*
stupor, estupor *m*
stutter, to, tartamudear
stutterer, tartamudo
stuttering, balbucencia; tartamudez *f*; disartria espasmódica; disfemia espasmódica
sty, orzuelo; perilla *fam, Mex*; chiquero *Ríopl*
stylet, estilete *m*
subacute, subagudo *adj*
subclass, subclase *f*
subconscious, subconsciente *m*, *adj*
subconsciousness, subconsciencia
subcutaneous, subcutáneo *adj*; ~ **implantation** implantación subcutánea *f*
subdue, to, (*pain*) aliviar
sublingual gland, glándula sublingual
submaxillary gland, glándula submaxilar
submissive, ñangotao *adj, slang*
submit, to, someter
subscribe, to, su(b)scribir
subside, to, calmarse
subsidize, to, ~ (*an enterprise*) subvencionar; ~ (*people*) dar subsidios a
subsidized, (*an enterprise*) subvencionado *adj*; ~ **transport** transporte subvencionado
subsidy, ~ (*to an enterprise*) subvención *f*; ~ (*to a person*) subsidio
subspecialty, subespecialidad *f*
substance, substancia; **radioactive** ~ substancia radioactiva; **residue** ~ substancia de desecho
substitute, su(b)stituto; ~ (*thing*)

su(b)stitutivo *m, adj*; **plasma** ~ su(b)stitutivo de plasma
substitute, to, sustituir
subtract, to, deducir; restar; sustraer
success, éxito
successive, sucesivo *adj*
succinylcholine, succinilcolina
suck, to, chupar; mamar
suckle, mamada; tetada
suckle, to, amamantar
suckling, lactante *m/f*
suction, succión *f*; aspiración *f*; ~ **biopsy** biopsia aspirativa; biopsia por succión; ~ **cup method** método de succión con ventosa; ~ **drainage** drenaje por succión *m*; drenaje por aspiración *m*
sudden, súbito *adj*; repentino *adj*; ~ **infant death syndrome/SIDS** síndrome de muerte infantil repentina *m*; síndrome de muerte en la cuna *m*
suddenly, de repente
sue, to, poner pleito
suffer (from), to, padecer (de); sufrir (de)
sufferer, AIDS, sidoso *fam*
suffering, padecimiento; sufrimiento
sufficient, bastante *adv*; suficiente *adv*
suffocate, to, ahogar(se); sofocar(se)
suffocation, asfixia; ahogo; sofocación *f*
suffusion, hemorrhagic, sufusión hemorrágica *f*
sugar, azúcar *m/f*; **beet** ~ azúcar de remolacha; **blood** ~ azúcar sanguínea; **brown** ~ azúcar morena; azúcar negro; **cane** ~ azúcar de caña; **grape** ~ glucosa; azúcar de uva; **lump** ~ azúcar en terrones; **refined** ~ azúcar refinada; **starch** ~ azúcar de almidón; dextrina; ~**coated pill** gragea

sugarless, sin azúcar *prep phr*
sugary, azucarado *adj*
suggest, to, sugerir (ie)
suggestion, sugerencia; ~ (*psychiatric*) sugestión *f*; **hypnotic** ~ sugestión hipnótica; **posthypnotic** ~ sugestión poshipnótica
suicide, suicidio; **to attempt** ~ atentar (ie) el suicidio; **to commit** ~ suicidarse
suit, ~ (*legal*) pleito; ~ (*of clothing*) traje *m*; flux *m*, *Ven, Carib*
suitcase, maleta
sulfa drug, sulfamida
sulfate, sulfato
sulfathiazole, sulfatiazol *m*
sulfide, sulfuro; **carbon** ~ sulfuro de carbono
sulfonamide, sulfamida
sulfonyluria, sulfoniluria
sulfur, azufre *m*; ~ **powder** polvo de azufre; **total** ~ azufre total
sulfuric acid, ácido sulfúrico
sulph-, *For words that begin with these letters, see those that have "sulf." (Para las palabras que comienzan con este prefijo, ver tambien las que comienzan con "sulf.")*
sum, suma
summary, resumen *m*
summer, estival *adj*
sun, sol *m*; ~ **cure** cura por el sol; ~ **therapy** cura de sol
sunbathe, to, tomar el sol
sunbathing, baños de sol *m, pl*
sunburn, ~ (*burn*) quemadura de sol; eritema solar *m*; ~ (*tan*) bronceado *m*
sunburn, to, ~ (*to burn*) quemar al sol; sufrir quemaduras de sol; ~ (*to tan*) broncear(se)
sunburned/sunburnt, ~ (*burn*) quemado del sol *adj*; ~ (*tanned*) bronceado *adj*; tostado por el sol *adj*; **to get** ~ asolearse; broncearse; sufrir quemaduras del sol
sunglasses, anteojos oscuros; gafas de sol

sunlamp, lámpara solar
sunlight, luz del sol *f*; luz solar *f*
sunscreen, filtro solar; protector del sol *m*
sunstroke, insolación *f*; solanera; asoleada *Chi, Col, Guat*; asoleo *Mex*; chavalongo *Arg, Chi*; soleada *SpAm*; **to get** ~ asolearse *Arg, Mex*
suntan, bronceado; ~ **lotion** loción bronceadora *f*; loción para el sol *f*
suntanned, bronceado *adj*; tostado *adj*
superficial, superficial *adj*
superimposed, sobreañadido *adj*
superior, superior *adj*
supermarket, supermercado
supernatural, sobrenatural *adj*
supervise, to, supervisar
supervision, supervisión *f*
supine, supino *adj*
supper, cena
supplement, suplemento
supplementary, suplementario *adj*; ~ **feeding** alimentación suplementaria *f*
supply, suministro
supplies, (*food*) provisiones *f, pl*; víveres *m, pl*
support, apoyo; soporte *m*; sostén *m*; **financial** ~ ayuda económica; **moral** ~ apoyo moral
support, to, ~ (*to keep from falling*) apoyar; sostener; ~ (*to bear*) soportar; ~ (*to provide for*) mantener; sustener
supported, mantenido *adj*
supporter, faja médica; **athletic** ~ suspensorio
suppository, cala; calilla; supositorio; **vaginal** ~ óvulos *m, pl*
suppress, to, suprimir
suppuration, supuración *f*
suprarenal, suprarrenal *adj*
sure, seguro *adj*; **to be** ~ estar seguro; **to make** ~ asegurarse
surface, superficie *f*; **body** ~ su-

perficie corporal; **corporal** ~ superficie corporal; **working occlusal** ~ superficie oclusal funcional

surgeon, cirujano; quirurgo; **dental** ~ dentista *m/f*; odontólogo; **veterinary** ~ veterinario

surgery, ~ (*surgeon's work*) cirugía; **arthroscopic** ~ cirugía artroscópica; **cardiac** ~ cirugía cardíaca; **clinical** ~ cirugía clínica; **conservative** ~ cirugía conservadora; **cosmetic** ~ cirugía cosmética; cirugía estética; **dental** ~ odontología quirúrgica; **elective** ~ cirugía electiva; **general** ~ cirugía general; **major** ~ cirugía mayor; **minor** ~ cirugía menor; **open-heart** ~ cirugía de corazón abierto; **orthopedic** ~ cirugía ortopédica; **plastic** ~ cirugía estética; cirugía plástica; **radical** ~ cirugía radical; **reconstructive** ~ cirugía reconstructiva; ~ (*clinic*) clínica; ~ (*dispensary*) dispensario

surgical, quirúrgico *adj*; ~ **assistant** asistente en cirugía *m/f*; ~ **bed** cama quirúrgica; ~ **dressing** vendaje quirúrgico *m*; ~ **forceps** pinzas quirúrgicas; ~ **intervention** intervención quirúrgica *f*

surname, apellido

surrogate, subrogado *adj*

surrogate, to, subrogar

surround, to, circundar; rodear

surrounded, rodeado *adj*

surveillance, vigilancia; **to be under** ~ estar fichao *slang*

survival, supervivencia

survive, to, sobrevivir

survivor, sobreviviente *m/f*

susceptible, susceptible *adj*

suspect, to, sospechar

suspension, suspensión *f*

suspensory, suspensorio *adj*

sustain, to, ~ (*bear weight of; effort*)

sostener; ~ (*effort, talk; to feed*) mantener; ~ (*to endure*) aguantar; ~ (*injury, attack, loss, etc.*) sufrir; ~ (*life*) sustener; ~ (*to support a theory, etc.*) apoyar

sustained-release, de difusión prolongada *Pharm*, *prep phr*; de liberación prolongada *prep phr*; de difusión sostenida *adj*; (*See release, sustained.*)

suture, comisura; puntada; sutura; **absorbable** ~ sutura absorbible; **buried** ~ sutura incluida; **chain** ~ sutura en cadena; **circular** ~ sutura circular; **continuous** ~ sutura continua; **dental** ~ sutura dentada; **dissolving** ~ sutura absorbible; **hemostatic** ~s puntos de sutura hemostáticos; **lockstitch** ~ sutura en punto de ojal; **horizontal mattress** ~ sutura horizontal de colchonero; **right angle mattress** ~ sutura en ángulo recto de colchonero; **over-and-over** ~ sutura de punto sobre punto; **purse-string** ~ sutura en bolsa de tabaco; **quilled** ~ sutura emplumada; ~ **thread** hilos de sutura

suture, to, suturar; coser

swab, escobillón *m*

swallow, trago

swallow, to, tragar; deglutir

swallowing, deglución *f*

swarthy, atezado *adj*; moreno *adj*; choco *adj*, *Bol*, *Col*, *Ec*, *Ríopl*; trigueño *adj*, *PR*

sweat, sudor *m*

sweat, to, sudar; ~ **a little** resudar

sweater, (*sudorific*) sudorífico *m*, *adj*, *Med*

sweating, sudación *f*

sweaty, pasoso *adj*, *Chi*; sudón *adj*, *SpAm*

sweet, dulce *m*, *adj*; ~**-and-sour** agridulce *adj*

sweetener, dulcificante *m*

sweets, dulces *m*, *pl*; golosinas *f*, *pl*

swell, to, hinchar; inflar(se); **~ up** (*a part of the body*) hincharse

swelling, hinchado *adj*; hinchazón *f*; tumefacción *f*; tumor *m*, *fam*; chibola *CA*; chibolo *Col, Ec, Hond, Perú*; pectora *Chi, Anat*; poporo *Col, Ven*; porcino *Med*; tolondro *Med*; **~** (*bruise*) bulto; chichón *m*; **~** (*from a bite*) roncha; salpullido

swelter, to, sofocarse de calor

sweltering, ~ (*day, office, etc.*) sofocante *adj*; **~** (*person*) chorreando sudor *adj*

swill, bazofia *fam*

swim, to, nadar

switch, interruptor *m*, *Elect*

swollen, hinchado *adj*; papujo *adj*, *Mex*

symbiosis, simbiosis *f*, *inv*

symbol, símbolo

symmetrical, simétrico *adj*

symmetry, simetría

sympathetic, ~ (*kind*) amable *adj*; **~** (*showing pity*) compasivo *adj*; **~** (*understanding*) comprensivo *adj*; **~** (*nerve, pain*) simpático *adj*; **~ nervous system** sistema nervioso simpático *m*

sympathize (with), to, compadecerse (de); **~ s.o. in his/her bereavement** dar el pésame a alguien por la muerte de ...

sympathy, simpatía

symphysis, sínfisis *f*

symptom, síntoma *m*; retoque *m*, *Med*; **characteristic ~** síntoma característico; **delayed ~** síntoma demorado; **equivocal ~** síntoma equívoco; **general ~** síntoma general; **presenting ~** síntoma presente; **sympathetic ~** síntoma por simpatía; **withdrawal ~** síntomas de supresión

symptomatic, sintomático *adj*

symptomless, asintomático *adj*

synapsis, sinapsis *f*

syncope, síncope *m*

syndrome, síndrome *m*; complejo sintomático; **acquired immunodeficiency ~/AIDS** síndrome de inmuno-deficiencia adquirida/SIDA; **acute radiation ~** síndrome agudo por radiación; **adult respiratory distress ~/ARDS** síndrome de insuficiencia respiratoria del adulto; síndrome de dificultad respiratoria del adulto; **anxiety ~** síndrome de ansiedad; **asthmatic ~** síndrome asmático; **battered child ~** síndrome del niño golpeado; **carotid sinus ~** síndrome del seno carotídeo; síndrome carotídeo; **carpal tunnel ~** síndrome del túnel del carpo; síndrome del túnel carpiano; síndrome del canal del carpo; **compression ~** síndrome por aplastamiento; síndrome por compresión; **~ deficiency** síndrome de deficiencia de __; **Down's ~** síndrome de Down; mongolismo; idiocia mongólica; **Dressler's ~** síndrome de Dressler; síndrome posinfarto de miocardio; **dumping stomach ~** síndrome de estómago de vaciamiento rápido; **fetal alcohol ~** síndrome alcohólico fetal; síndrome fetal alcohólico; **hyaline membrane ~** síndrome de insuficiencia respiratoria del recién nacido; síndrome de la membrana hialina; síndrome de dificultad respiratoria del recién nacido; **irritable bowel ~** síndrome del colon irritable; **menopausal ~** síndrome del climaterio femenino; síndrome menopáusico; **myofacial pain disfunction ~** síndrome funcional doloroso miofacial; **premenstrual ~/PMS** síndrome premenstrual; **restless legs ~**

síndrome de las piernas inquietas; **scalded skin** ~ síndrome de la piel escaldada; necrólisis epidérmica tóxica *f*; **sudden infant death** ~/**SIDS** síndrome de la muerte súbita del lactante; **toxic shock** ~ síndrome de choque tóxico

synechia, sinequia; adherencia anormal

synergism, sinergismo

synergy, sinergía

synovial, sinovial *adj*; ~ **fluid** líquido sinovial; ~ **membrane** membrana sinovial; ~ **sheath** vaina sinovial

synthesize, to, sintetizar

synthetic, sintético *adj*

syphilis, sífilis *f*; avariosis *f*, *SpAm*; infección de la sangre *f, euph*; lúes *f*; mal de bubas *m, slang*; mal francés *m, slang*; mal napolítano *m, slang*; sangre mala *f, slang*; **congenital** ~ sífilis congénita; **tertiary** ~ sífilis terciaria

syphilitic, sifilítico *m, adj*; ~ **chancre** chancro sifilítico

syringe, jeringa; jeringuilla visitadora *SpAm*; (*See spike.*); **disposable** ~ jeringa desechable; jeringuilla descartable; **glass cylinder** ~ jeringa con cilindro de cristal; **hollow needle** ~ jeringa con aguja hueca; **hypodermic** ~ jeringuilla hipodérmica; ~ **piston**/~ **plunger** émbolo

syrup, ~ (*culinary*) almibar *m*; ~ (*medication*) jarabe *m*; **cherry** ~ jarabe de cereza; **cough** ~ jarabe para la tos; ~ **of ipecac** jarabe de ipeca; jarabe de ipecacuana; **licorice** ~ jarabe de regaliz

system, constitución *f*; organismo; sistema *m*; **alimentary** ~ sistema alimenticio; **autonomic nervous**

~ aparato nervioso autónomo; sistema nervioso autónomo; sistema neurovegetativo; sistema nervioso involuntario; sistema nervioso vegetativo; sistema nervioso de la vida orgánica; sistema nervioso de los ganglios; sistema nervioso idiotropo; **biological** ~ sistema biológico; **blood-vascular** ~ sistema vascular sanguíneo; sistema hematicovascular; **bulbospiral** ~ sistema bulboespiral; **cardiovascular** ~ sistema cardiovascular; **centimeter-gram-second** ~ sistema cegesimal; sistema C.G.S.; **central nervous** ~ aparato nervioso central; sistema nervioso central; sistema cerebroespinal; **circulatory** ~ sistema cardiovascular; sistema circulatorio; **digestive** ~ sistema alimentario; sistema digestivo; **ecological** ~/**ecosystem** ~ sistema ecológico; **endocrine** ~ sistema endocrino; glándulas de secreción interna; **genitourinary** ~ sistema genitourinario; **hematopoietic** ~ sistema hematopoyético; **immune** ~ sistema de inmunidad; **integumentary** ~ sistema integumentario; **kinesodic** ~ sistema cinesódico; sistema quinesódico; **lymphatic** ~ sistema linfático; **masticatory** ~ sistema masticatorio; **metric** ~ sistema métrico; **muscular** ~ sistema muscular; **musculoskeletal** ~ sistema musculoesquelético; **nervous** ~ sistema nervioso; **oxidation-reduction** ~ sistema de oxidación-reducción; **parasympathetic nervous** ~ sistema nervioso parasimpático; sistema nervioso craneosacral; **peripheral nervous** ~ sistema nervioso periférico; **reproductive** ~ sistema reproductivo; **respiratory** ~ sistema respiratorio; aparato respiratorio; **reticuloendothelial** ~ sistema reticuloendotelial; **review of** ~**s** repaso de sistemas; **skeletal** ~ sistema esquelético; **static** ~ sistema estático; sistema postural; **sympathetic nervous** ~ gran simpático *m*; sistema nervioso simpático; **urogenital** ~ sistema urogenital; **vascular** ~ sistema vascular; **vasomotor** ~ sistema vasomotor; **vestibular** ~ sistema vestibular; sistema laberíntico

systemic, sistemático *adj*; general *adj*; ~ **lavage** lavado de la sangre; ~ **reaction** reacción generalizada *f*

systole, sístole *f*; **aborted** ~ sístole abortada; **anticipated** ~ sístole anticipada; extrasístole *f*; latido prematuro; sístole prematura; **arterial** ~ sístole arterial; **auricular** ~ sístole auricular; **ventricular** ~ sístole ventricular

systolic, sistólico *adj*; ~ **discharge** volumen sistólico *m*

---

[2] This is new vocabulary, not necessarily listed nor yet recognized by the Royal Academy of Spanish Grammar. It is understood that this vocabulary is primarily slang. Unless otherwise indicated, the gender of nouns is assumed to be obvious.

[3] For pronunciation purposes, the masculine definite and indefinite articles, *el* and *un*, not *la* or *una*, are used when the article immediately precedes the feminine singular noun which begins with stressed *a* or any other that begins with stressed *ha*.

[4] Current English street terminology for *seconals* includes: bullets, devils, M & M, red devils, and reds.

[5] In Spanish the word *herpes* is often used in the plural form.

[6] Part of the Drug Abuse Vocabulary.

[7] English words that have an initial *ps* now may be spelled either with or without the *p* in Spanish. In either case, the *p* is silent when the Spanish word is pronounced. This dictionary will show such words with a parenthesis around the *p*.

[8] Use the Spanish pronunciation of these letters.

T

tabacism/tabagism, tabacosis *f*; tabaquismo; **tabagism syndrome** asma[3] de los fumadores; síndrome respiratorio de los fumadores *m*

tabes, tabes *f*

table, mesa; **examining ~** mesa de exámenes; mesa de exploración; mesa de reconocimientos (médicos); **~ of stains** lista de colorantes; **operating ~** mesa de cirugía; mesa de operaciones; **tilt ~** mesa basculante; **to get up on the ~** subir a la mesa

tablespoonful, cucharada

tablet, comprimido; pastilla; tableta; trocisco

taboo, tabú *m*

taboparalysis, taboparálisis *f*

tachycardia, palpitación *f*; taquicardia *form*; **atrial ~** taquicardia auricular; **auricular ~** taquicardia auricular; **nodal ~** taquicardia nodal; **paroxysmal ~** taquicardia paroxística; (*See paroxysmal tachycardia.*); **sinus ~** taquicardia sinusal

tachycardiac, taquicardíaco *adj*

tactile, táctil *adj*; **~ sensibility** sensibilidad táctil *f*

tail, cola; apéndice *m*; rabo; **~ bone** cóccix *m*; cócciz *m*; colita; rabadilla

take, to, tomar; **~** (*drugs*) administrarse; ingerir (ie); injerir (ie); tomar; **~** (*vaccination/transplant*) prender (una vacuna/un transplante); **~ a deep breath** respirar profundo; **~ a hit** (*to take a puff from a joint*)[4] quemar[2]; tronarse[2]; tronársela[2]; **~ a swab** hacer un frotis; **~ advantage of** aprovecharse de; **~ care of** cuidar; **~**

charge of encargarse de; **~ hold** agarrar; **~ marijuana** amarihuanarse[2]; engrifarse[2]; enmarihuanarse[2]; **~ off** (*to undress*) quitarse; **~ out** (*to remove*) extraer; quitar; sacar; **~ place** tener lugar; **~ precautions** precaucionar(se); **~ to the hospital** encamar *CA, Mex*; **~ up** elegir(i) (una actividad); (*See take a hit, to.*)

taken internally, not to be, para uso externo

takeout food eaten at home, fiambrera

talc/talcum, talco; **~ powder** polvos de talco

talipes, talipes *m, form*; talismo; pie contrahecho *m*; pie talo; pie zambo *m*; pie zopo *m*

tall, alto *adj*; **~ person** palma *PR*; **~ woman with skinny legs** garza *PR*

Tampax, tampax *m*

tampon, ta(m)pón *m*

tamponade, tamponamiento; **cardiac ~** tamponamiento cardíaco

tan, bronceado *adj*; **to get a ~** broncearse

tandem kidney, riñón alargado *m*

tangle, to, enredar

tangled, enredado *adj*

tank, tanque *m*; **septic ~** tanque séptico

tantrum, berrinche *m, fam*; **temper ~** pataletas

tap, golpeteo; punción (quirúrgica) *f, Surg*; **spinal ~** punción lumbar; **~ water** agua[3] del grifo

tap, to, hacer una punción; puncionar *form*

tape, (*for bandages, etc.*) cinta; tela; **measuring ~** cinta métrica

taper, to, disminuir progresivamente (*un tratamiento*)

tapeworm, tenia *form;* (gusano) cestodo; solitaria

tar, alquitrán *m;* brea; ~ **acne** acné por alquitrán *f;* **coal** ~ brea de hulla; ~**like stools** disposiciones negras *f;* heces alquitranadas *f;* ~ **wart** verruga de brea

tarantula, tarántula

tarsal, tarsal *adj;* tarsiano *adj;* tarso

tarsus, (*pl, tarsi*) tarso *m, Anat*

tartar, sarro; **dental** ~ saburra; sarro; tártaro

tartaric acid, ácido tartárico; ácido tártrico

task, labor *m;* tarea

taste, gusto; sabor *m;* gustativo *adj;* **after**~ dejo; **bad** ~ **in one's mouth** mal sabor de boca; ~ **cells** células gustativas; ~ **sensitivity** sensibilidad gustativa *f*

taste, to, ~ (*to savor*) saborear; ~ **good (bad)** tener buen (mal) sabor; ~ (*to try*) ensayar; probar (ue); ~ **like** saber a

tastebud, botón gustativo *m;* papila gustativa *Anat*

tasteless, desabrido *adj;* insípido *adj;* sabrío *adj, PR*

tattoo(ing), tatuaje *m*

Tay-Sachs disease, enfermedad de Tay-Sachs *f;* idiocia amaurótica

TB, bacilo tuberculoso; tuberculosis *f*

td/ter die/three per day, tres veces al día

tea, té *m;* ~[4] mariguana[1]; **Texas** ~[4] cigarrillo de mariguana; **arnica flower** ~ (*used to treat internal blows, bronchitis, pneumonia, and as a muscular tonic*) té de arnica *ethn;* **black sage** ~ (*used to treat parasites, indigestion, and colic*) té de estafiate *ethn;* **borage** ~ (*used to treat coughs, to help urination and perspiration, and to help eliminate infection in childhood diseases such as chicken pox, measles, etc.*) té

de borraja; **camomile** ~ (*used to regulate menstruation and to treat children's diarrhea*) agua[3] de manzanilla *f, ethn;* té de manzanilla *ethn;* **cinnamon** ~ (*used for coughs and as a tonic for anemia, and to aid digestion and to prevent gas*) té de canela *ethn;* **corn tassel** ~ (*used to treat kidney problems, gallstones, and for swollen legs caused by advanced pregnancy or by gout*) té de barba de elote *ethn;* **croton** ~ té de pionillo *ethn;* **damiana** ~ (*used either as tea or a vaginal douche to treat a "cold womb." Also helps with diabetes, inflammation of the kidneys, and bladder problems*) té de damiana *ethn;* **desert milkweed** ~ (*used for kidney disorders*) té de hierba del indio *ethn;* **elderberry** ~ (*used to treat colic*) té de negrita *ethn;* **elderberry and lavender** ~ (*used to treat measles and fever*) té de flor de sauz y hojas de alhucema *ethn;* **fennel** ~ (*used to treat gas, infants' colic, vomiting*) té de hinojo *ethn;* **herb rose** ~ (*used to treat colic, "empacho" as well as a purge, and as an eyewash to treat conjunctivitis*) té de rosa de castilia *ethn;* **limberbush** ~ (*used to treat anemia*) té de sangre de drago *ethn;* **linden** ~ (*used to calm nerves, fitful coughs, and fevers caused by infections*) té de flores de tilo *ethn;* **mallow** ~ (*used to treat dysentery and children's stomach aches*) té de malva *ethn;* **medicinal** ~ té de maví *ethn, PR;* **medicinal** ~ (*used to treat colds*) té de careaquillo *ethn, PR;* **medicinal** ~ (*used to treat diabetes*) té de quinino de pobre *ethn, PR;* **medicinal** ~ (*used to treat indigestion and stomach disorders*) té de sacabuche *ethn, PR;* **medicinal** ~ (*used to help people with kidney stones*) té de baqueña *ethn, PR;* **medicinal** ~ tisana; "**Mormon**" ~

(*used to treat anemia*) té de cañutillo (del campo) *ethn*; **orange blossom** ~ (*used for heart and nerve conditions*) té de azahar *ethn*; **orange leaves** ~ (*used to treat colic*) té de naranja *ethn*; **parsley** ~ (*used to help cure kidney infections*) té de oshá; **rosemary** ~ (*used to regulate menstruation and stimulate digestion*) té de romero *ethn*; **rue** ~ (*used to alleviate high blood pressure, headaches, for menstrual problems, difficult deliveries, and abortions*) té de ruda; **sarsaparilla** ~ (*used to treat kidney problems*) té de cocolmeca; **spasm herb** ~ (*used to treat "pasmo"*) té de hierba del pasmo *ethn*; **spearmint** ~ (*used to treat colic*) té de yerbabuena *ethn*; **spider milkweed** ~ té de inmortal *ethn*; **strong** ~ té cargado; té fuerte; **swamp root** ~ (*used to treat stomach aches*) té de hierba del manzo *ethn*; **tansy mustard herb** ~ té de pamita *ethn*; **wild marjoram** ~ (*used to fight intestinal infections, dysentery, as well as to regulate menstruation*) té de orégano *ethn*; **wormseed** ~ (*used to treat parasites, and to help menstruation*) té borde *ethn*; té de epazote *ethn*; té de México *ethn*

teach, to, enseñar

teacupful, taza de té

team, equipo; ~ **effort** trabajo de equipo; ~ **of technicians** equipo de técnicos; **~work** trabajo en equipo; cooperación íntima *f*

tear, ~ (*from crying*) lágrima; **~drop** lágrima; ~ **duct** conducto lacrimal; ~ **gas** gas lacrimógeno *m*; ~ **gland** glándula lagrimal; **crocodile ~s** lágrimas de cocodrilo; **~stain** mancha de lágrima; **to burst into ~s** echarse a llorar; **to dissolve into ~s** deshacerse en lágrimas; **to hold back one's ~s**

tragarse las lágrimas; ~ (*split*) desgarramiento; desgarro; rasgón *m*; rotura; rajo *SpAm*

tear, to, ~ (*to shed tears*) derramar lágrimas; ~ (*to rip*) desgarrar; rasgar(se); romper; ~ **to pieces** (*paper*) rasgar; (*the flesh*) herir (ie); lacerar; ~ (*a muscle, ligament*) distender (ie)

tear-off, trepado *adj*; ~ **slip** cupón trepado *m*

teaspoonful, cucharadita; **level** ~ cucharadita llena al ras

technical, técnico *adj*

technician, técnico; especialista *m/f*; **laboratory** ~ ayudante de laboratorio *m/f*

technique, técnica; método; **flush** ~ técnica de enrojecimiento; **time diffusion** ~ técnica de tiempo de difusión

technology, tecnología

teenager, joven (*de 13 a 19 años m/f*; adolescente *m/f*

teeth, (*pl of tooth*) (*See* tooth.); dientes *m*; mazorca *sg, slang*; ~ **clattering** castañeteo de los dientes; **even** ~ dientes parejos; **fused** ~ dientes fusionados; **hag**[6] ~ dientes de bruja; **lacking** ~ chimuelo *adj, Chicano*; **mandibular** ~ dientes mandibulares; **maxillary** ~ dientes maxilares; **metal insert** ~ dientes con inserción metálica; **milk** ~ dientes de leche; **natal** ~ dientes natales; **primary** ~ dientes primarios; **rake** ~ dientes separados *m*; **row of widely spaced** ~ peineta *PR*; **stained** ~ dientes manchados *m*; **temporary** ~ dientes temporales; **white** ~ dientes blancos; **with one's** ~ a dentelladas; **to have bad** ~ tener mala dentadura

teethe, to, dentar (ie); echar dientes; endentecer

teething, dentición *f*; salida de los dientes

telepathy, telepatía
telephone, teléfono; ~ **call** llamada telefónica; **car** ~ teléfono móvil
telephone, to, llamar por teléfono; telefonear
telescope, telescopio
television, televisión *f*
tell, to, (*to say*) decir
telltale sign, indicio revelador
temper, disposición *f*; genio; humor *m*; **bad** ~ chicha *CA, Ec*; estrillo *Peru, Riopl*
temperament, temperamento
temperate, benigno *adj*; templado *adj*
temperature, calentura[10]; fiebre[10] *f*; temperatura; **basal body** ~ temperatura corporal basal; **body** ~ temperatura del cuerpo; ~ **chart** gráfico de la temperatura; **internal ~ of the human body** temperature interna del cuerpo humano; **room** ~ temperatura ambiente; temperatura de la habitación
temple, sien *f*; hueso temporal
temporomandibular, temporomandibular *adj*
temporomaxillary, temporomaxilar *adj*
temporooccipital, temporooccipital *adj*
temporary, temporal *adj*; temporero *adj*; transitorio *adj*; ~ **filling** empaque *m, Chicano*; empaste provisional *m*
temporate, moderado *adj*
tempt, to, tentar (ie)
tempting, tentador *adj*
tenacious, tenaz *adj*
tenancy, inquilinato
tenant, inquilino
tendency, tendencia; ~ **to(ward)** predisposición(a) *f, Med*
tender, sensible *adj*; ~ (*sore*) adolorido *adj*; dolorido *adj*; doloroso *adj*

tenderness, dolor a la presión *m*; dolorimiento; sensibilidad *f*; terneza
tendon, tendón *m*; **Achilles** ~ tendón de Aquiles; ~ **jerk** reflejo tendinoso; ~ **reflex** reflejo tendinoso
tenesmus, pujo; tenesmo *form*; **anal** ~ tenesmo anal; **rectal** ~ tenesmo rectal; **vesical** ~ tenesmo vesical
tennis elbow, codo de tenis *fam*; epicondilitis humeral *f, form*; epicondilalgia del húmero
tense, tenso *adj*
tense, to, poner tenso (*los músculos*); ~ **up** ponerse tenso
tension, tensión *f*; **blood** ~ tensión de la sangre; **arterial blood** ~ tensión de la sangre arterial; **capillary blood** ~ tensión de la sangre capilar; **venous blood** ~ tensión de la sangre venosa; ~ **headache** cefalea por tensión nerviosa; dolor de cabeza por tensión nerviosa *m*; **nervous** ~ tensión nerviosa
tent, tienda; **oxygen** ~ tienda de oxígeno; **steam** ~ tienda de vapor
tentative diagnosis, diagnóstico de presunción; diagnóstico de probabilidad
tepid, tibio *adj*
term, término; **at** ~ a término
terminal, terminal *adj*; ~**ly ill patient** paciente en fase terminal *m/f*
terminology, terminología
Terramycin, terramicina
tertiary, terciario *adj*; del tercer nivel *prep phr*; ~ **syphillis** sífilis terciaria *f*
test, prueba; ~ (*lab*) examen *m*; prueba; ~ (*of blood, urine, etc.*) análisis *m, inv*; **angiography** angiografía; radiografía de los vasos sanguíneos; **blood** ~ prueba

de sangre; **cardiac function** ~ prueba de función cardíaca; ~ **dose** dosis de prueba *f, inv*; **eye** ~ examen de la vista *m*; **glucose tolerance** ~ prueba de tolerancia a la glucosa; **hearing** ~ prueba de la audición; ~ **meal** comida de prueba; ~ **of learning capacity** prueba de la capacidad de aprendizaje; ~ **of time** prueba del tiempo; **patch** ~ prueba del parche; **pregnancy** ~ prueba de embarazo; **pulmonary function** ~ prueba de función pulmonar; ~ **results** resultados de pruebas; **serology** ~ prueba serológica; **sputum** ~ análisis de esputos; **stress** ~ prueba de esfuerzo; ~ **strip** tira reactiva; **TB** ~ prueba de la tuberculosis; **thematic apperception** ~/**TAT** test de apercepción temática *m*; **therapeutic** ~ prueba terapéutica; **treadmill** ~ prueba de la fuerza; ~ **tube** tubo de ensayo; **tuberculin** ~ tuberculina; **urinalysis** ~ análisis de la orina; prueba de la orina; urinálisis *m*

test, to, examinar; poner a prueba; probar (ue)

testicle, blanquillo *slang, Chicano*; bolas *f, pl, slang, common*; cojones *m, pl, vulg, slang*; compañones *m, pl, slang*; cuates *m, pl, slang*; güebos *m, pl, vulg*; huevos *m, pl, vulg*; lerenes *m, pl, vulg*; pelotas *f, pl, vulg*; testículo *form*; **undescended** ~ testículo no descendido

testicular, testicular *adj*

testing chamber, cámara de prueba

testing of vision, examen de la vista *m*

testosterone, testosterona

tetanus, mal de arco *m, slang*; pasmo *Med*; pasmo seco *fam*; pasmazón *m, Med, CA, Mex, PR*; tétano(s); trimo; **drug** ~ tétano

medicamentoso; ~ **infantum** tétano del recién nacido; moto *slang, Mex*; mozusuelo *Mex*; siete (7) días *m*

tetracycline, tetraciclina

tetralogy, tetralogía; ~ **of Fallot** tetralogía de Fallot

tetraplegia, cuadriplejía; tetraplejía

tetravalent, tetravalente *adj*

texture, textura

thalamus, tálamo; tálamo óptico

thalassemia/thalassanemia, talasanemia; talasemia; ~ **major** anemia de Cooley; anemia mediterránea; enfermedad de Cooley *f*; talasemia mayor; ~ **minima** talasemia menor

thalassotherapy, talasoterapia *form*; tratamiento por baños de mar

thalidomide, talidomida

thallium, talio

thanatognomonic, tanatognomónico *adj*; que indica la proximidad de la muerte

thank you, gracias

thaw, to, descongelar

theatre/theater staff, personal del quirófano *m, Surg*

theophylline, teofilina

theory, teoría; **atomic** ~ teoría atómica; **germ** ~ teoría germinal

therapeutic, terapéutico *adj*; ~ **test** prueba terapéutica

therapeutics, terapéutica; **alimentary** ~ terapéutica alimenticia

therapist, terapeuta *m/f, form*; psicoterapista[11] *m/f, fam*; terapista *m/f*

therapy, terapéutica *form*; terapia; tratamiento; **electroshock** ~ electroterapia por choque; **electroconvulsive** ~/**ECT** terapia electrochoque/TEC[12]; terapia electroconvulsiva/TEC[12]; **group** ~ terapia de grupo; **immunization** ~ terapia inmunizante; **massive drip intravenous** ~ terapia masiva por gota a gota intravenosa; **occupational** ~ terapia ocupacional; **physical** ~ terapéutica física; terapia física; **radiation** ~ radioterapia; **respiratory** ~ te-rapia respiratoria; **speech** ~ terapia del habla; **x-ray** ~ radioterapia

thermal, termal *adj*; térmico *adj*; ~ **burn** quemadura térmica; ~ **equilibrium** calor equilibrado *m*

thermalgesia, termalgesia; dolor producido por aplicación de calor *m*

therm(o)analgesia, term(o)analgesia

thermodynamics, termodinámica

thermometer, termómetro; **Celsius** ~ termómetro de Celsius; **centigrade** ~ termómetro centígrado; **clinical** ~ termómetro clínico; **oral** ~ termómetro bucal; termómetro oral; **rectal** ~ termómetro rectal; **surface** ~ termómetro de superficie

thermoresistant, termorresistente *adj*

thermostat, termostato; termorregulador *m*

thermotherapy, termoterapia

thiabendazole, tiabendazol *m*

thiamine, tiamina; ~ **chloride** cloruro de tiamina; ~ **hydrochloride** hidrocloruro de tiamina

thick, ~ (*consistency*) espeso *adj*; ~ (*dimension*) grueso *adj*; ~ **necked** pescozudo *adj*

thicken, to, espesar

thickness, ~ (*consistency*) espesura; viscosidad *f*; ~ (*dimension*) espesor *m*; grosor *m*

thigh, muslo; pierna *fam*; ~ **bone** fémur *m*; ~ **joint** articulación femorocoxal *f*

thighed, thick, de muslos voluminosos *prep phr*

thighed, thin, de muslos pequeños *prep phr*

thin, delgado *adj*; flaco *adj*; ~ (*hair*) ralo *adj*; **to become** ~ **(and weak)** enflaquecerse; **to become** ~ (*slim*) adelgazarse; **to get** ~ espicharse *Cu, Mex*; **to get** ~ (*to waste away*) chuparse *Med*

think, to, pensar (ie)

thinner, to get, adelgazar

thinner, blood, anticoagulante *m*

thinness, desmedro *Med*; ~ (*of the voice*) debilidad *f*; ~ (*of a person*) delgadez *f*; flaqueza *f*; magrez *f*; ~ (*of hair*) escasez *f*

third, tercer(o), -ra; ~ **molar** muela del juicio; ~ **nerve** nervio oculomotor; ~ **stage** tercer período de alumbramiento

thirst, sed *f*

thirsty, to be, tener sed *f*

thoracentesis (*pleural tap*), toracentesis *f*

thoracic, torácico *adj*; ~ **cage**/**cavity** caja torácica; ~ **duct** conducto torácico

thoracotomy, toracotomía

thorax, tórax *m*; pecho *fam*; **barrel-shaped** ~ tórax en tonel; **chickbreast** ~ tórax en quilla

thorn, espina; pincho

thorough, completo *adj*; minucioso *adj*; ~ **medical exam** examen médico minucioso *m*

thrashing, chinga *Mex*

thread, hilo; ~ (*filament*) filamento; ~**like** filamentoso *adj*; ~**like pulse** pulso filiforme; pulso ondulante

threatened abortion, aborto inminente; amenaza de aborto

three, tres *adj, inv*; ~ **times a day** tres veces al día; ~**-day fever** dengue *m*; fiebre rompehuesos *f*; ~**-day measles** rubeola; rubéola *form*; sarampión de tres días *m, fam*

threshold, umbral *m*; comienzo; ~ **of consciousness** umbral de conciencia; **to be on the** ~ **of life** estar en el umbral de la vida

throat, garganta; tragadero *fam*; gargüero *SpAm*; guari *Chi*
throaty, gutural *adj*
throb, ~ (*of heart*) latido; palpitación *f*; ~ (*of pulse*) pulsación *f*; ~ (*of pain*) punzada *f*
throb, to, vibrar; ~ (*with pain*) dar punzadas; ~ (*heart, pulse*) latir; pulsar
throbbing, pulsátil *adj*; ~ (*heart*) palpitante *adj*; ~ (*pain*) punzante *adj*; ~ **headache** cefalea pulsátil; dolor de cabeza pulsátil *m*
throes, *pl*, angustias; ansias; dolores *m*; ~ **of childbirth** dolores del parto; ~ **of death** ansias de la muerte
thrombocyte, trombocito
thrombogen, trombógeno
thrombogenic, trombógeno *adj*
thrombophlebitis, flebitis *f*; tromboflebitis *f*, *form*
thrombosis, trombosis *f*
thrombus, coágulo; cuajarón *m*; cuajo; trombo
throw, to, arrojar; ~ **away** botar; ~ **up** arrojar *fam*; basquear *fam*; deponer *Mex*, *fam*; devolver (ue) *fam*; dompear *Chicano*; gomitar *fam*; tener basca; tirar las tripas; vomitar
throw-back, salto atrás
thrush, afta; algodoncillo *fam*; candidiasis bucal *f*, *form*; muguet *m*; sapo *PR*, *SD*; ubrera *Med*
thrust, empujón *m*; hincada *Col*, *Cu*, *Perú*, *PR*, *Ven*
thrust, to, empujar
thumb, dedo gordo *fam*; dedo pulgar; pulgar *m*; ~-**sucking** succión del pulgar *f*; **tennis** ~ pulgar de tenista
thump, precordial, golpe torácico *m*
thyme, tomillo
thymus, timo; **accessory** ~ timo accesorio; **persist** ~ timo persistente
thyroid, tiroideo *adj*; tiroides *m/f*;

bocio *fam*; **aberrant** ~ tiroides aberrante; ~ **cartilage** cartílago tiroideo; ~ **gland** glándula tiroidea; glándula tiroides; ~ **storm** crisis tiroidea *f*, *inv*; ~ **therapy** terapia tiroidea
thyroidectomy, tiroidectomía
thyrotropin, tirotropina
TIA/transient ischemic attack, ataques isquémicos transitorios *m*
tibia, tibia; **saber** ~ tibia en sable; ~ **valga** tibia valga; ~ **vara** tibia vara
tic, tirón *m*; tic *m*; sacudida; ~ **degenerative** ~ tic degenerativo; ~ **douloureux** tic doloroso de la cara *m*; **laryngeal** ~ tic laríngeo; **psychomotor** ~ tic psicomotor
tick, (*insect*) garrapata; **American dog** ~ garrapata americana del perro; **cattle** ~ garrapata de los bovinos; ~ **fever** fiebre de las Montañas Rocosas *f*; **Pacific coast** ~ garrapata de las costas del Pacífico; **Rocky Mountain** ~ garrapata de las Montañas Rocosas
tickle, cosquillas; cosquilleo
tickle, to, hacer cosquillas
ticklish itch, picor *m*
tick-tack sounds, ritmo fetal
t.i.d./ter in die/three times a day, tres veces al día
tidal, ~ **air** aire respiratorio *m*; ~ **drainage** drenaje por irrigación *m*; ~ **volume** volumen corriente en reposo *m*; volumen respiratorio *m*
tie, to, amarrar; atar; ligar *Med*; ~ **one on** (*to get drunk*) ajumar(se) *PR*; guayar(se) *PR*; jender(se) *PR*; ~ **the tubes** amarrar los tubos; ligar trompas; ligar los tubos de Falopio; ligar los tubos uterinos; ~ **together** ligar
tight, apretado *adj*
tighten, to, apretar (ie)
tightness of the chest, opresión *f*, *Med*

tilted position, posición inclinada *f*
tilt-table, mesa basculante
time, tiempo; **(secondary) bleeding** ~ tiempo de hemorragia (secundaria); **circulation** ~ tiempo de circulación; **clot retraction** ~ tiempo de retracción del coágulo; **clotting** ~ tiempo de coagulación; **half-life** ~ tiempo de semidesintegración; **time lag** ~ tiempo de latencia; **partial thromboplastin** ~/**PTT** tiempo parcial de tromboplastina; **prothrombin** ~ tiempo de protrombina; **reaction** ~ tiempo de reacción; ~ **schedule** régimen horario *m*; **sedimentation** ~ tiempo de sedimentación; **thermal death** ~ tiempo de muerte térmica
timed release, difusión regulada *f*
tincture, tintura; **gentian** ~ **compound** tintura de genciana compuesta; ~ **of iodine** tintura de yodo
tinea, (*ringworm*) tinea; tiña; polilla; ~ **capitis** tiña de la cabeza; ~ **corporis** tiña del cuerpo; ~ **cruris** tinea de la pierna; tiña inguinal; ~ **pedis** tiña del pie
tingle, hormigueo; comezón *m*; picazón *m*
tingle, to, hormiguear
tingling, hormigueo; ~ **sensation** hormigueo
tinkle, retintín *m*
tinnitus, tinitus *m*; zumbido del oído
tip, punta; **finger** ~ punta del dedo; yema del dedo; ~ **of nose** punta de la nariz; ~ **of tongue** punta de la lengua
tire, to, cansar(se)
tired, cansado *adj*; **to be** ~ estar como un guanime *PR*; **to get** ~ cansarse
tiredness, cansancio; fatiga
tissue, tejido; ~ (*paper*) pañuelo de papel; **adipose** ~ tejido adiposo;

bony ~ tejido óseo; **connective** ~ tejido conectivo; tejido conjuntivo; ~ **culture** cultivo de tejido; ~ **diagnosis** diagnóstico histológico; **erectile** ~ tejido eréctil; **facial** ~ kleenex *m*; **nerve** ~ tejido nervioso; **scar** ~ tejido cicatrizal; **soft** ~ tejido blando; **toilet** ~ papel de baño *m*; ~ **plasminogen activator/TPA** activador del plasminógeno tisular *m*
titanium, titanio
titer/titre, dosificación *f*; título
titratable, titulable *adj*
titrate, titrato
titration, titulación *f*
t.i.w., tres veces a la semana
to and fro, ~ **movement** movimiento de vaivén; ~ **murmur** ruce pericárdico *m*
tobacco, tabaco; **chewing** ~ tabaco de mascar; hilao *slang, PR*; **wad of chewing** ~ mascaura *slang, PR*
tocologist, tocólogo; (*See obstretrician.*)
tocology, tocología; obstetricia
today, hoy
toddle, to, andar a tatas
toe, dedo (del pie); **big** ~ dedo grueso; **hammer** ~ dedo del pie en martillo; **pigeon** ~ dedo del pie de pichón
toeing in, desviación hacia dentro de los dedos del pie *f*
toeing out, desviación hacia fuera de los dedos del pie *f*
toenail, uña (de los dedos del pie)
toilet, baño; común *m*; excusado; inodoro; privado; retrete *m, Sp*; servicios; ~ **bowl** taza del excusado; taza del inodoro; ~ **paper** papel de excusado *m*; papel higiénico; papel sanitario
toke of marijuana or hashish[4], jalá[2] *PR*; jalaita[2] *PR*; pase[2] *m, PR*; toque[2] *m, Chicano*
tolerance, tolerancia; **acquired** ~ tolerancia adquirida
tolerate, to, aguantar; tolerar

tomogram, tomograma *m*
tomograph, tomógrafo
tomography, tomografía; **comput(eriz)ed ~/CT** tomografía computada/TC; **computerized axial ~/CAT** tomografía axial computarizada/ TAC; **positron emission ~/PET** tomografía por emisión de positrones/TEP[12]
tomorrow, mañana; **day after ~** pasado mañana
tone, tono; **~ gap** laguna auditiva; **heart ~s** tonos cardíacos; **muscle ~** tono muscular; **~ of voice** tono de la voz
tongs, pinzas; tenazas
tongue, lengua; **baked ~** lengua tostada; **black hairy ~** lengua negra peluda; **~ blade** depresor lingual *m*; **burning ~** lengua quemante; **coated ~** lengua cubierta; **~ depressor** bajalenguas *m*; depresor de la lengua *m*; paleta *fam*; pisalenguas, *inv*; abatelenguas *m, inv, Mex*; **furred ~** lengua saburral; **~ tied** premioso *adj*; tartajoso *adj*; que tiene frenillo *Med*
tonic, tónico
tonsil, amígdala; agalla *fam*; anginas *fam, Mex,Ven*; tonsil(s) *m, Chicano*; tonsila
tonsillectomy, tonsilotomía; amigdalectomía; amigdalotomía
tonsillitis, amigdalitis *f*; tonsilitis *f, Chicano*
tooth, diente *m*; dentadura *fam*; **acrylic resin ~** diente de resina acrílica; **anterior ~** diente anterior; **artificial (false) ~** diente postizo; **azzle ~** diente molar; **baby ~** diente de leche; diente mamón; **back ~** muela; **bicuspid ~** bicúspide *m*; premolar *m*; **buccal ~** diente bucal; **canine ~** (*eyetooth*)[7] diente canino; canino; colmillo *fam*; **cuspid** diente cuspídeo; **cuspless ~** diente acus-

pídeo; **~ decay** caries *f, inv*; dientes podridos; odontonecrosis *f*; **deciduous ~** diente de leche; diente caduco; diente temporal; **devitalized ~** diente desvitalizado; **eye ~** (*term refers especially to a canine tooth of the upper jaw*); **false ~** diente postizo; **front** (*incisor*) **~** incisivo; **impacted ~** diente impactado; **incisor** diente incisivo *form*; **large, misshapened ~** diente de ajo *fam*; **loose ~** diente flojo; **lower ~** diente inferior; **milk ~** (*See tooth, deciduous.*); **missing ~** diente ausente; **molar** molar *m*; **mottled ~** diente moteado; **neck of ~** cuello; **peg ~** diente en clavija; **permanent ~** diente permanente; **posterior ~** diente posterior; **premolar** (*See tooth, bicuspid.*); **pulpless ~** diente sin pulpa; **~ socket** alvéolo; **supernumerary ~** diente supernumerario; **temporary ~** diente temporal; **third molar** tercer molar *m*; **unerupted ~** diente retenido; **upper ~** diente superior; **vital ~** diente vital; **wisdom ~** muela cordal *f*; muela del juicio *f*; **to fill a ~** empastar
toothache, dolor de dientes *m*; dolor de muelas *m*; odontalgia
toothbrush, cepillo de dientes
toothed forceps, pinzas dentadas
toothless, desdentado *adj*; huaco *adj, SpAm*
toothpaste, dentífrico; crema dental; pasta de dientes; pasta dentífrica
toothpick, escarbadientes *m, inv*; mondadientes *m, inv*; palillo de dientes
top, **~** (*direction*) punta; vértice *m*; **~ of head** vértice de la cabeza; **~** (*lid*) tapa
topical, tópico *adj*
toric, tórico *adj*
torn, desgarrado *adj*

torsion, torsión *f;* ~ **fracture** fractura por torsión; ~ **spasm** espasmo por torsión

torso, torso

torticollis, (*stiff neck*) tortícolis *f, form*; **congenital** ~ tortícolis congénita; **intermittent** ~ tortícolis espasmódica

total, total *adj*; ~ **abstention** abstención total *f;* ~ **disorientation** desorientación total *f;* ~ **removal** ablación total *f;* ~ **retention** retención total *f*

touch, ~ (*sense*) tacto; **abdominal** ~ tacto abdominal; **double** ~ tacto vaginal y rectal simultáneos; **rectal** ~ tacto rectal; **vaginal** ~ tacto vaginal; ~ (*symptom, sign of*) amago *Med*; acceso; ~ (*light stroke*) toque *m*; ~ (*of pain*) punzada

touch, to, tocar; ~ (*taste*) probar (ue)

touch-and-go, arriesgado *adj*

touchy, sensitivo *adj*

tough, duro *adj*; fuerte *adj*; tenaz *adj*

Tourette's disease[8], enfermedad de Tourette *f*

tourniquet, liga; ligadura; torniquete *m*; **field** ~ torniquete de campo

towel, toalla; ~ **rack** toallero; **sanitary** ~ compresa; paño higiénico; **Turkish** ~ toalla de felpa

toxemia, toxemia; **eclamptic** ~ toxemia eclámptica; ~ **of pregnancy** intoxicación del embarazo *f*; toxemia del embarazo; toxemia gravídica

toxemic, toxémico *adj*

toxic, tóxico *adj*

toxicity, toxicidad *f;* ~ **rating** grado de toxicidad

toxicologist, toxicólogo

toxicology, toxicología

toxin, toxina; **bacterial** ~ toxina bacteriana; **staphylococcal** ~ toxina estafilocócica; **streptococcal** ~ toxina estreptocócica

toxoid, toxoide *m*; **diphtheria** ~ toxoide diftérico; **tetanus** ~ toxoide tetánico

toxoplasmosis, toxoplasmosis *f*

trace, indicio *Med*; ~ **element** oligoelemento

tracer, isótopo indicador; trazador *m*; **radioactive** ~ isótopo radioactivo

trachea, gaznate *m, fam*; tráquea

tracheitis, traqueítis *f*

tracheobronchial, traqueobronquial *adj*

tracheobronchitis, traqueobronquitis *f*

tracheoesophageal, traqueoesofágico *adj*

tracheolaryngeal, traqueolaríngeo *adj*

tracheopharyngeal, traqueofaríngeo *adj*

tracheoscopy, traqueoscopia

tracheostomy, traqueostomía

tracheotomy, traqueotomía; ~ **tube** tubo de traqueotomía

trachoma, tracoma *m*

tracing, trazado; registro; trazo

track, vestigio; vía; ~ **of bullet wound** trayecto del proyectil; ~ **marks**[4] (*See tracks.*)

tracks, (*marks and scars caused by use of hypodermic needles*)[4] marcas[2]; trakes[2] *Chicano*; traques[2] *Chicano*

tract, aparato *Anat*; fascículo; haz *m*; tracto; vías *f, pl*; **alimentary** ~ tracto alimenticio; tracto alimentario; **ascending** ~ haz ascendente; **biliary** ~ vías biliares; **corticospinal** ~ vía corticospinal; **descending** ~ fascículos descendentes; **digestive** ~ aparato digestivo; vías digestivas; **gastrointestinal** ~ tracto gastrointestinal; tubo digestivo; **genitourinary** ~ tracto genitourinario; **central ~ of auditory nerve** fascículo acústico central; **central ~ of thymus** haz central del timo; **central ~ of trigeminal nerve** vía central del trigémino; **respiratory ~** tracto respiratorio; vías respiratorias; **urinary ~** tracto urinario; vías urinarias

traction, tracción *f*

trade, to, cambiar

traffic, tráfico

traffic in drugs, to[4], dilear[2]; diliar[2]; traficar[2]

trafficker, (*of drugs, etc.*) traficante[2] *m/f*

tragus, (*pl, tragi*) trago *Anat*; pelo de la oreja

train, to, adiestrar; educar; entrenar(se)

trained reflex, reflejo condicionado

training, ~ (*education*) formación *f*; **vocational ~** formación profesional; **workers' ~** formación obrera; ~ (*in sports*) entrenamiento

trait, carácter hereditario *m*; característica; rasgo; toque *m*; **sickle cell ~** carácter de célula falciforme

trance, catalepsia *form*; trance *m*; **alcoholic ~** trance alcohólico; **hypnotic ~** trance hipnótico

tranquilize, to, tranquilizar

tranquilizer, ansiolítico; apaciguador *m*; calmante *m*; tranquilizante *m*

transection, transección *f*

transfer, transferencia; ~ **RNA** ARN de transferencia

transfer, to, transferir (ie); ~ (*a patient*) trasladar

transform, to, convertir (ie); transformar

transformation, transformación *f*

transfuse, to, hacer una transfusión; poner sangre *fam*

transfusion, transfusión *f*; **blood ~**

transfusión sanguínea; **direct ~** transfusión directa; **exchange ~** exanguinotransfusión *f*; desangrotransfusión *f*; **placental ~** transfusión placentaria; **to give a ~** hacer una transfusión; poner sangre *fam*

transient, transitorio *adj*

translate (into), to, traducir (al); ~ (*spoken language*) interpretar

translator, intérprete *m/f*; (*spoken*) / ~ (*written*) traductor, -ra *m/f*

translucent, traslúcido *adj*

transmission, transmisión *f*; ~ **by contact** transmisión mediante contacto; **droplet ~** transmisión por gotillas; **vector ~** transmisión mediante vector; ~ **vehicle** vehículo

transmit, to, tra(n)smitir

transmittable, tra(n)smisible *adj*; ~ **disease** enfermedad tra(n)smisible

transmitted through the blood, transmitido por vía sanguínea *adj*

transmitter (of), ~ vehículo (de) *Med*; ~ (*apparatus*) transmisor *m*; **ultrasouind ~** transmisor ultrasonido

transparent, transparente *adj*

transpiration, transpiración *f*; perspiración *f*; sudación *f*

transplant, trasplante *m*; **heart ~** trasplante de corazón

transplant, to, trasplantar

transplantation, transplantación *f*; tra(n)splante *m*

transport, to, transportar

transportation, transporte *m*

transsexual, transexual *m/f, adj*

transverse, transverso *adj*; ~ **muscle** músculo transverso

transvestite, transvestido; transvestista *m/f*

trapezius, trapecio

trauma, choque *m*; contusión *f*; golpe *m, fam*; susto *ethn*; trauma *m, form*; traumatismo; **birth ~** trauma del nacimiento; **psychic ~** trauma psíquico

traumatic, traumático *adj*; **~ experience** experiencia traumática

traumatism, traumatismo

traumatize, to, traumatizar

traumatologist, traumatólogo

traumatology, traumatología

tray, bandeja; charola *Mex*; **acrylic resin ~** bandeja de resina acrílica; **impression ~** bandeja para impresión *Dent*

tread, to, pisar; pisotear

treat, to, ~ (*a disease*) curar; tratar; **~** (*a patient*) atender (ie); **~ s.o. with a new drug** tratarle a uno con un nuevo fármaco

treatment, tratamiento; **x-ray ~** tratamiento con rayos x

tremble, to, temblar

tremor, temblor *m*; tremor *m*; tiritón *m, fam*

tremulous, tembloroso *adj*

trench fever, angina de Vicente; enfermedad de Vicente *f*; fiebre de las trincheras *f*; fiebre de los cinco días *f*

trend, tendencia

Trendelenburg's position[9], posición de Trendelenburg *f*

trepan, trépano

trial, ensayo; **~ diet** régimen de prueba *m*

triceps, tríceps *m*

trichinosis, triquinosis *f*

Trichomonas, tricomonas; **~ vaginalis** tricomonas vaginales

tricuspid, tricúspide *m, adj*; **~ valve** válvula tricúspide

trigeminal, trigémino *adj*; **~ neuralgia** neuralgia del trigémino

trigger, **~ area** zona reflexógena; **~ finger** dedo en gatillo; **~ point** punto doloroso; **~ zone** zona quimiorreceptora

trigger, to, provocar

triglicerides, triglicéridos

trimester, trimestre *m*

trip on drugs, gira[2], *PR*; tripeo[2], *Chicano*; viaje[2] *m*

trip, to, ~ (*fall*) dar un traspié; ~[4] tripear[2]; agarrar onda[2]; sonarse[2]

triplet, trillizo; tripleto

trismus, trismo

trivalent, trivalente *adj*

trochanter, trocánter *m*; **greater ~** trocánter mayor; **lesser ~** trocánter menor

troche, pastilla para chupar; trocisco

trots, the, (*diarrhea*) *slang* cagarreta *PR, vulg*; **to have ~** estar de carreritas *PR*; pintar a duco

troy ounce, unidad de peso igual a 480 gramos *f*

TRU/turbidity reducing unit, unidad reductora de enturbiamiento *f*

truncate, to, truncar; amputar

trunk, tronco; **~ of atrioventricular bundle** tronco del haz auriculoventricular

truss, braguero; faja (abdominal); **nasal ~** braguero nasal

trust, confianza

trust, to, confiar en; tener confianza en

try, to, probar (ue); **~ to** tratar de

tryptophan, triptófano

TSH/thyroid-stimulating hormone, hormona estimulante del tiroides

tsp/teaspoon, cucharadita

tub, bañera; tina de baño

tubal, tubario *adj*; tubárico *adj*; **~ abortion** aborto tubárico; **~ ligation** ligadura de trompas; ligadura de los tubos; ligazón de tubos *f*; **~ pregnancy** embarazo tubárico

tube, trompa *Anat*; tubo *Anat*; **air ~** tubo de aire; **capillary ~** tubo capilar; **digestive ~** tubo digestivo; aparato digestivo; **drainage ~** tubo de drenaje; **endotra-**

cheal ~ tubo endotraqueal; **esophageal** ~ tubo esofágico; **Eustachian** ~ trompa de Eustaquio; **Fallopian** ~ trompa de Falopio; tubo de Falopio; **intubation** ~ tubo de intubación; **stomach** ~ tubo gástrico; **test** ~ tubo de ensayo; **thoracostomy** ~ tubo de toracostomía; **thoracotomy** ~ tubo de toracotomía; **tracheotomy** ~ tubo de traqueotomía; **ventilating** ~ tubo de ventilación; ~ (*cannula*) cánula; ~ (*duct*) conducto *Anat*; **auditory** ~ conducto auditivo; tubo auditivo; ~ (*for feeding*) sonda; **feeding** ~ sonda para alimentación; **nasogastric** ~ sonda nasogástrica; ~-**fed** alimentado por sonda *adj*; ~ (*hose*) manguera; vaso *Med*

tubercular, afectado *adj*, *Chicano*; tuberculoso *m, adj*

tuberculin, tuberculina; ~ **reaction** tuberculinorreacción *f*

tuberculosis, tuberculosis *f*; afectado del pulmón *Chicano, Mex, fam*; hetiquencia *PR*; manchado del pulmón *Mex, fam*; paletero *Ec*; peste blanca *f*; tis *f, Chicano, fam*; tisis *f, fam*; tísico *fam*; **pulmonary** ~ tuberculosis pulmonar; **scrofula/scrophula** escrófula; **skin TB** tuberculosis de la piel; ~ **of bones and joints** tuberculosis de huesos y articulaciones; tuberculosis osteoarticular; ~ **of the intestines** tuberculosis intestinal; ~ **of the lungs** tuberculosis de los pulmones

tuberculous patient, tísico; tuberculoso

tuberosity, tuberosidad *f*

tubing, tubería

tubular, tubular *adj*

tubules, seminiferous, túbulos seminíferos

tumefaction, edema *m*; hinchazón *f*; tumefacción *f*

tumor, nacido; neoformación *f*; neoplasma *m*; postema *Med*; potro *SpAm, Med*; tlacote *m, Med*; tumor *m*; **benign** ~ tumor benigno; **connective tissue** ~ tumor de tejido conectivo; **fibroid** ~ tumor fibroideo; **granulosa cell** ~ tumor de células de la granulosa; **malignant** ~ tumor maligno; ~ **on the head** chiporra *Guat, Hond*; **sebaceous** ~ tumor sebáceo

tuning fork, diapasón *m*

tunnel, túnel *m*; **carpal** ~ túnel del carpo

turbid, turbio *adj*

turn, vuelta; **to take a** ~ **for the worse** dar un bajón

turn, to, darse vuelta; ~ (**over**) volverse (ue); ~ **around/over** darse (media) vuelta; voltearse; ~ **blue** ponerse azul; ~ **into** convertirse (ie) en; ~ **numb** ponerse dormido *adj*; ~ **off** apagar; ~ **on** (*lights, gas, TV, radio*) encender (ie); ~ **on** (*electric current*) conectar; ~ **on** (*water, etc.*) abrir; ~ **on one's side** ponerse de lado; ~ **out** resultar; ~ **out okay** salir bien; ~ **over** darse vuelta; virar; ~ **pale** palidecer; ponerse pálido *adj*; ~ **stiff** ponerse tieso

turpentine, esencia de trementina; trementina

tweezers, pinzas; pinza de cejas; tenacillas

twelfth nerve, nervio hipogloso

twice a day, dos veces al día

twilight, crepuscular *adj*; ~ **sleep** sueño crepuscular

twin, cuate *m/f, Mex*; gemelo; guares *m, pl*; jimagua *m/f, Cu*; mellizo; **fraternal** ~**s** gemelos fraternos; gemelos que no se parecen; **identical** ~**s** gemelos idénticos

twinge, dolor lancinante *m*; dolor punzante *m*; punzada

twist, to, ~ (*to bend*) bornear; ~ (*to turn*) torcer (ue)

twisted, torcido *adj*; zambo *adj*; chueco *adj*, *CA*, *Mex*, *Ven*

twitching, contracción espasmódica *f*; crispamiento; espasmo muscular; tics *m*, *pl*

two, dos; ~-**edged** de dos rebordes; ~-**stage operation** operación en dos tiempos; ~-**way catheter** catéter de dos ramas

tympanic, timpánico *adj*; ~ **artery** arteria timpánica; ~ **bone** hueso timpánico; ~ **cavity** caja del tímpano; ~ **membrane** membrana timpánica

tympanum, tímpano; caja del tímpano; caja del tambor

type, tipo; **athletic** ~ tipo atlético; **blood** ~ grupo sanguíneo *form*; tipo sanguíneo; tipo de sangre; **body** ~ tipo corporal; **unstable** ~ tipo inestable

type, to, escribir a máquina; ~ **blood** clasificar la sangre

typhoid fever, fiebre tifoidea *f*; (*See fever, typhoid.*)

typhus, tifus *m*; tifo *fam*; ~ **epidemic** fiebre de los campamentos *f*; tifus clásico *m*; tifus exantemático *m*; tabardillo; ~ **fever** fiebre abdominal *f*

typical, típico *adj*

typing, ~ (*classification*) tipificación *f*; ~ **of blood** tipificación de la sangre; ~ (*typewriting*) mecanografía

---

[1] I have followed the spelling given in the *Diccionario de la lengua española*, RAE, 21st edition, 1990. Spanish does recognize variations using *j* and *h*.

[2] This is new vocabulary, not necessarily listed nor yet recognized by the Royal Academy of Spanish Grammar. It is understood that this vocabulary is primarily slang. Unless otherwise indicated, the gender of nouns is assumed to be obvious.

[3] For pronunciation purposes, the masculine definite and indefinite articles, *el* and *un*, not *la* or *una*, are used when the article immediately precedes the feminine singular noun which begins with stressed *a* or any other that begins with stressed *ha*.

[4] Part of the Drug Abuse Vocabulary.

[5] When the word *tract* or *canal* is translated into Spanish, the word *conducto* is used when it refers to a closed tract or canal.

[6] Term is applied to upper centrals that are widely separated.

[7] Term refers especially to a canine tooth of the upper jaw.

[8] Neurological condition characterized by convulsions, lack of coordination, and verbal problems.

[9] Supine position on a table inclined at a 45° angle with the head below and the feet hanging over the extreme top of the table.

[10] The word *fiebre* is a more common choice of terms than *calentura*. *Calentura* is the word of choice when fever is sudden or especially high. *Calentura* is used especially by Mexican–Americans. For other Spanish speakers it often has sexual connotations. *Fiebre*, or *fever*, technically refers to an elevation of body temperature to a point higher than normal. In rural areas of Mexico, *fiebre* refers to a number of illnesses that cause a rise in body temperature: malaria, typhoid fever, typhus, pneumonia, rheumatic fever, postpartum fever, and brucellosis. *Fiebre* is generally used to refer to a specific disease, i.e., *fiebre reumática*—rheumatic fever. See David Werner, *Donde no hay doctor*, pp. 26–27, 4th ed. México: Editorial Pax–Mexico, 1980.

[11] English words that have an initial *ps* now may be spelled either with or without the *p* in Spanish. In either case, the *p* is silent when the Spanish word is pronounced. This dictionary will show words with a parenthesis around the *p*.

[12] Use the Spanish pronunciation of these letters.

U

ulcer, úlcera; ulceración *f*; pupa *Med*; chácara *CA, Chi, Col*; lacra *SpAm*; lamprea *Med*; ñácara *CA*; **concealed ~** úlcera oculta; **decubital ~** úlcera por decúbito; **duodenal ~** úlcera duodenal; **gastric ~** úlcera gástrica; **hard ~** úlcera dura; (*See chancre.*); **indolent ~** úlcera indolente; **inflamed ~** úlcera inflamada; **intractable ~** úlcera rebelde; **peptic ~** úlcera péptica; úlcera redonda; **perforating ~** úlcera perforante; **stress ~** úlcera de estrés

ulna, cúbito

ultramicroscope, ultramicroscopio

ultrasonoscopy, ultrasonoscopia

ultrasonography, ultrasonografía

ultrasound, ultrasonda; ultrasonido

ultrasonotherapy, ultrasonoterapia

ultraviolet, ultravioleta; **~ lamp** lámpara de rayos ultravioletas

umbilical, umbilical *adj*; **~ band** faja umbilical; **~ cord** cordón del ombligo *m*; cordón umbilical *m*; **to have an ~ hernia** estar desombligado

umbilicated, umbilicado *adj*; **~ vesicles**, vesículas umbilicadas

umbilicus, ombligo

unbotton, to, desabotonar; desabrochar

uncomfortable, incómodo *adj*; **to make ~** empachar *Med*

unconscious, inconsciente *adj*; insensible *adj, Med*; naqueado *adj, Chicano*

unconsciousness, falta de conocimiento; pérdida de conocimiento; inconsciencia; insensibilidad *f*

undernourished, desnutrido *adj, fam*; estrasijao *adj, fam, PR*

underpants, calzoncillos; **men's ~** pantaloncillos

undershirt, camiseta

underside, superficie inferior *f*

undersigned, abajo firmado *adj*

understand, to, comprender; entender (ie)

underwear, ropa interior

underweight, falta de peso; peso escaso; de peso insuficiente *prep phr*; **to be ~** no pesar bastante

underwriter, asegurador, -ra *m/f*

undress, to, desnudarse; desvestirse (i); encuerarse *Chicano*; veringuearse *Col*; quitar la venda de

uneasy, inquieto *adj*; intranquilo *adj*

unemployed, desempleado *adj*; parado *adj*; sin trabajo *prep phr*

unerupted tooth, diente retenido *m*

uneven, irregular *adj*

uneventful, sin complicaciones

unguent, pomada; ungüento

unhappy, infeliz *adj*

unhealthy, enfermizo *adj*; **~ (a wound)** pasmado *adj, SpAm*; **~ (a place)** insalubre *adj*; **~-looking (a person)** pasmado *adj, SpAm*

uniform, uniforme *m, adj*

uninterrupted suture, sutura continua

unit, unidad *f*; elemento; aparato; **medical ~** equipo médico; **~ of blood** unidad de sangre

universal, universal *adj*; **~ antidote** antídoto universal

unknown, desconocido *adj*

unload one's troubles, to, desahogarse *fam*

unpleasant, desagradable *adj*; chocante *adj, Mex*

unripe, inmaduro *adj*; ~ **cataract** catarata inmadura
unstable, deleznable *adj*
unsuccessful, infructuoso *adj*; sin éxito *prep phr*
untie, to, desatar
untreated, no tratado *adj*
unusual, atípico *adj*; raro *adj*
unwell, indispuesto *adj*
upper, superior *adj*; ~ **jaw** maxilar *m*; mandíbula superior; ~ **lid** párpado superior; ~ **tooth** diente superior *m*
upright position, posición erecta *f*
upset, agitado *adj*; alterado *adj*; desarreglo *Med*; disgustado *adj*; enojado *adj*; inquieto *adj*; molesto *m, adj*; perturbado *adj*; perturbación *f, Med*; trastorno; ~ (*emotional*) mortificado *adj*; **bowel** ~ desbaratamiento (de vientre) *Med*; ~ **stomach** desarreglos estomacales; estómago revuelto; estómago trastonado; jaleo *PR*; trastorno estomacal; **to be** ~ estar perturbado; sentirse (ie) molesto; renegar (ie) *Mex, Perú, Ríopl*; **to get** ~ perturbarse
upset, to, trastornar; entripar *Arg, Col, Ec*; indisponer *Med*; ~ (*stomach*) hacer daño (a) *Med*; trastornar; ~ (*spill*) derramas; ~ (*emotionally*) perturbar; ~ **oneself** acongojarse
urea, urea
uremia, intoxicación de orín *f*; uremia
ureter, uréter *m*
ureteritis, ureteritis *f*
ureterolithotomy, ureterolitotomía
ureteropyelitis, ureteropielitis *f*
ureterostomy, ureterostomía
urethra, canal urinario *m*; caño urinario; uretra
urethrocele, uretrocele *m*
urethroscope, uretroscopio
urethroscopy, uretroscopia
urethrotomy, uretrotomía

urge, ~ (*impulse*) impulso; ~ (*persistent desire*) vivo deseo
urgency, urgencia
urgent, urgente *adj*
URI/upper respiratory infection, infección de las vías respiratorias superiores *f*
uric, úrico *adj*; ~ **acid** ácido úrico
urinal, orinal *m*; bacineta; bacinica; bacinilla; urinario
urinalysis, (*pl, urinalyses*) análisis de la orina *m, inv*; análisis de los orines *m, inv*; examen de orina *m*; urinálisis *m, inv*
urinary, urinario *adj*; ~ **bladder** vejiga de la orina; vejiga urinaria; ~ **cylinder** cilindro urinario; ~ **output** excreción urinaria *f*; ~ **problem** mal de orín *m*; problema de las vías urinarias *m*; ~ **stream** chorro de orina; ~ **tract** vías urinarias
urinate, to, hacer agua[3] *Chicano*; hacer (la) chi(s) *Chicano, vulg*; hacer (la) pipi/pipí; mear; orinar; tirar (el) agua *slang*
urination, acto de orinar; micción *f*; urinación *f*; **burning sensation upon** ~ ardor al orinar *m*; quemazón al orinar; **precipitant** ~ micción imperiosa; **stuttering** ~ micción intermitente
urine, "aguas menores" *f*; chi *f, vulg*; orín *m*; orina; orines *m, pl*; ~ **acidifiers** acidificantes de la orina *f*; **blood in the** ~ sangre en la orina *f*; **collection of the** ~ **specimen** acumulación de la muestra *f*; toma de la muestra; recolección de la muestra *f*; ~ **color: straw-colored** de paja *prep phr*, ~ **color: yellow-colored** amarilla *adj*; ~ **constituents** componentes de orina *m*; **acetone** acetona; **albumin** albúmina; **ammonia** amoníaco; **bile** bilis *f*; **bilirubin** bilirrubina; **blood** sangre *f*; **calcium** calcio; **chlorides** cloruro; **creatine** crea-

tina; **creatinine** creatinina; **crystal(s)** cristal(es) *m*; **glucose** glucosa; **phosphate** fosfato; **solids** sólidos *m*; **total nitrogen** nitrógeno total; **total sulfur** azufre total *m*; **urea** urea; **urobilin** urobilina; urobilirrubina; **frequent urinating/urination** meadera *Chicano*; orinar muy de seguido; ~ **specimen** muestra de la orina

urobilinogen, urobilinógeno

urogenital, urogenital *adj*; ~ **apparatus** aparato urogenital

urologist, urólogo

urology, urología

urticaria, urticaria

urticarial, urticariforme *adj*; urticariano *adj*

use, uso

use, to, usar

used up, agotado *adj*; **to be ~** acabarse

useful, útil *adj*

useless, inútil *adj*; incachable *adj*, *SpAm*

user[4], adicto; adicto a drogas; drogadicto; tecato[2]; toxicómano[2]; yeso[2]; ~ **of marijuana/cocaine/morphine** maricocaimorfi[2]; ~ **of morphine** morfiniento[2], ~ **of pills**[4] pildoriento

usual, usual *adj*

uterine, uterino *adj*; ~ **anteflexion** antedesviación uterina *f*; anteflexión uterina *f*; ~ **anteversion** anteversión uterina *f*; ~ **cavity** cavidad uterina *f*; ~ **curettage** legado uterino; raspado uterino; vaciado uterino; ~ **deviations** desviaciones uterinas *f*; ~ **invagination** invaginación uterina *f*; ~ **neck** cuello uterino; ~ **retroflexion** retroflexión uterina *f*; ~ **retroversion** retroversión uterina *f*

uterosalpingography, uterosalpingografía

uterus, matriz *f*; útero; **polyp in the ~** fibroma en el útero *m*; pólipo en el útero; **prolapse of the ~** caída de la matriz; prolapso de la matriz; prolapso del útero

uvula, campanilla *fam*; galillo *fam*; úvula

uvular, uvular *adj*

uvulitis, uvulitis *f*

[2] This is new vocabulary, not necessarily listed nor yet recognized by the Royal Academy of Spanish Grammar. It is understood that this vocabulary is primarily slang. Unless otherwise indicated, the gender of nouns is assumed to be obvious.
[3] For pronunciation purposes, the masculine definite and indefinite articles, *el* and *un*, not *la* or *una*, are used when the article immediately precedes the feminine singular noun which begins with stressed *a* or any other that begins with stressed *ha*.
[4] Part of the Drug Abuse Vocabulary.

V

VA/Veterans Administration, Administración de Veteranos *f*
VA/visual acuity, agudeza visual
vacancy, vacío; hueco
vacant, vacante *adj*
vaccinal, vacunal *adj*; vaccìneo *adj*; ~ **prophylaxis** vacunal profilaxis *f*; vacunoprofilaxis *f*
vaccinate, to, vacunar
vaccination, inoculación *f*; chot *m*, *Chicano*; vacuna; vacunación *f*; **booster** ~ refuerzo; **DPT** ~ triple *f*
vaccine/immunization, inmunización *f*; vacuna; **anthrax** ~ vacuna anticarbuncosa; **bacterial** ~ vacuna bacteriana; **cholera** ~ vacuna anticolérica; **inactivated measles virus** ~ vacuna de virus sarampionoso inactivado; **live attenuated measles virus** ~ vacuna de virus sarampionoso vivo atenuada; **mumps** ~ vacuna contra parotiditis; vacuna contra las paperas; **polyvalent** ~ polivacuna; **rabies** ~ vacuna contra la rabia; **Sabin's oral polio** ~ gotas para polio; vacuna de Sabin por vía bucal; vacuna oral contra polio; **smallpox** ~ vacuna contra la viruela
vaccinotherapy, vacunoterapia
vacillate, to, ~ (*to fluctuate*) fluctuar; ~ (*to hesitate*) titubear; vacilar
vacillation, fluctuación *f*; vacilación *f*
vacuole, vacuola; **air** ~ alveolo pulmonar; vacuola de aire; **food** ~ vacuola alimenticia
vacuum, vacío; ~ **chamber** aspirador *m*; ventosa; **high** ~ alto vacío; **in a** ~ en vacío; ~ **pump** bomba neumática
vagal, vagal *adj*

vagina, agujero *vulg*, *Chicano*; panocho *slang*; papaya *Cu*, *PR*, *Ven*, *vulg*; raja *vulg*; tajo *vulg*; tostón *m*, *vulg*, *PR*; vagina *form*; ~ **prolapse** prolapso de la vagina; vaginopexia
vaginal, vaginal *adj*; (**non-bloody**) ~ **discharge** desecho vaginal; secreción vaginal *f*; ~ **spermicide** espermaticida vaginal *m*; ~ **suppositories** óvulos *m*, *pl*
vaginalitis, vaginalitis *f*
vaginitis, vaginitis *f*, *inv*
vaginismus, vaginismo
vaginodynia, vaginodinia; dolor en la vagina *m*
vaginoperineotomy, vaginoperineotomía
vagotomy, vagotomía; **complete** ~ vagotomía completa; **medical** ~ vagotomía médica; **surgical** ~ vagotomía quirúrgica
vagrant, vagabundo *adj*
vague, vago *adj*
vagueness, vaguedad *f*
vagus, nervio neumogástrico; vago *form*
valgus, valgo *adj*
validity, grado de validez
valley fever, (*coccidioidomycosis*) coccidioidomicosis pulmonar primaria *f*; fiebre del valle *f*
valuable, valioso *adj*
value, valor *m*; precio; **globular** ~ valor globular; **hematocrit** ~ valor hematócrito
valva, valva; **aortae** ~ válvula sigmoidea aórtica; valva aórtica
valve, válvula; **anal** ~s válvulas anales; **left atrioventricular** ~ válvula auriculoventricular izquierda; **right atrioventricular** ~ válvula auriculoventricular derecha; **bicuspid** ~ válvula

bicúspide; **cardiac** ~s válvulas cardíacas; **coronary** ~ válvula coronaria; ~ **of coronary sinus** válvula del seno coronario; ~ **of the inferior vena cava** válvula de la vena cava inferior; **mitral** ~ válvula mitral; **tricuspid** ~ válvula tricúspide; **pulmonary** ~ válvula pulmonar; **pyloric** ~ válvula pilórica

valvotomy, valvotomía

valvula, (*pl,* *valvulae*) válvula; válvula pequeña

valvular, valvular *adj*

valvulitis, valvulitis *f*

V and T/volume and tension, (*refers to the pulse*) volumen y tensión

vanish, to, desaparecer; ~ (*to fade away*) esfumarse; desvanecerse

vanishing lung, distrofia pulmonar

vapor, vapor *m*; ~ **bath** baño de vapores; ~ **pressure** presión del vapor *f*; **water** ~ vapor de agua

vaporize, to, vaporizar

vaporizer, vaporizador *m*

vapotherapy, vapoterapia

variability, variabilidad *f*

variable, variable *f, adj*

variance, variación *f*; **to be at** ~ **with** estar en desacuerdo con

variant, ~ (*changeable*) variable *f, adj*; ~ (*differing*) variante *f, adj*

variation, variación *f*; ~ **width** amplitud de la variación *f*

varicella, varicela; viruela loca

varicocele, varicocele *m*

varicose, varicoso *adj*; ~ **veins** várices *f, pl*; varices *f, pl*; variz *m*; venas varicosas; **stockings for** ~ **veins** medias para várices

varicosity, varicosidad *f*

varicotomy, resección de una vena varicosa *f*; varicotomía

varied, variado *adj*

variety, variedad *f*

variolous, (*pockmarked*) picado de ciruelas *adj*; varioloso *adj, form*

varix, (*pl,* *varices*)[5] várice *f*; **esophageal varices** várices esofágicas

varnish, barniz *m*

varus, dirigido hacia dentro *adj*; varo *adj*; varus *adj*; **tibia** ~ pie contrahecho *m*; tibia dirigida hacia dentro

vary, to, variar

vas deferens, (*pl,* *vasa deferentia*) conducto deferente

vascular, vascular *adj*; ~ **markings** trama vascular *m*; ~ **ring** anillo vascular; ~ **spiders** circulación colateral *f*; ~ **tissue** tejido vascular

vasculature, (árbol) sistema vascular *m*; vascularización *f*; vasculatura

vasectomy, vasectomía

vaseline, vaselina

vasoconstriction, vasoconstricción *f*

vasoconstrictor, vasoconstrictor *m, adj*

vasodepression, vasodepresión *f*

vasodepressor, vasodepresor *m, adj*

vasodilation, vasodilatación *f*

vasodilator, vasodilatador *m, adj*

vasography, radiografía de vasos sanguíneos; vasografía

vasomotion, vasomotilidad *f*; vasomoción *f*; vasomovimiento

vasomotor, vasomotor *m, adj*

vasoreflex, vasorreflejo

vasostimulant, vasoestimulante *m, adj*

VC/vital capacity, capacidad vital *f*

VD/venereal disease, enfermedad venérea *f*; (*See venereal disease.*)

VDA/visual discriminatory acuity agudeza visual discriminatoria

V.D.H./valvular disease of the heart, cardiopatía valvular

VDRL/Venereal Disease Research Laboratory Laboratorio de Investigación de Enfermedades Venéreas

vegetable, legumbre *f*; vegetal *m*; verdura; ~ **jelly** pectina

vegetarian, vegetariano *m, adj*

vegetative, vegetativo *adj*

vehicle, excipiente *m, Med*; vehículo

veil, velo; ~ **humeral** velo humeral

veil, to, velar

vein, vena; vaso venoso; **accompanying** ~ vena satélite; **afferent** ~ vena aferente; ~ **anesthesia** anestesia venosa; **anterior (posterior) auricular** ~ vena auricular anterior (posterior) del pabellón de la oreja; **azygos** ~ vena ácigos; **brachial** ~ vena humeral; **cardiac** ~s venas del corazón; **(great) (small) cardiac** ~ vena coronaria (mayor) (menor); **(anterior) (inferior) (internal) cerebral** ~ vena cerebral (anterior) (inferior) (profunda); **(superior) cerebral** ~s venas cerebrales ascendentes internas y externas; **deep** ~ vena profunda; **deep lingual** ~s venas profundas de la lengua; **deep** ~s **of penis** venas profundas del pene; **enlargement of the** ~s agrandamiento de las venas; **(anterior) (common) (posterior) facial** ~ vena facial (anterior) (común) (posterior); *(deep)* **facial** ~ vena facial profunda ; **(deep) femoral** ~ vena femoral (profunda); **fibular** ~s venas peroneas; **(common) (dorsal) (palmar) digital** ~s **of the foot** venas digitales (comunes) (dorsales) (palmares) del pie; **frontal** ~s venas anteriores del cráneo; **left gastric** ~ vena coronaria estomáquica; **right gastric** ~ vena pilórica; **short gastric** ~s venas gástricas cortas; **(internal) (external) iliac** ~ vena ilíaca (interna) (externa); **jugular** ~ vena yugular; **(anterior) (posterior) labial** ~s venas (ante-

riores) (posteriores) de los labios mayores y menores; **(inferior) (superior) labial** ~s venas del labio inferior (superior); **ascending lumbar** ~ vena lumbar ascendente; **external mammary** ~s venas costoaxilares; **internal mammary** ~s venas mamarias internas; **maxillary** ~s venas maxilares internas; **median** ~ **of elbow** vena mediana basílica; **median** ~ **of forearm** vena mediana del antebrazo; **perforating** ~s venas perforantes; **descending pharyngeal** ~ vena faríngea descendente; **portal** ~ vena portal; **posterior** ~ **of left ventricle** vena posterior del ventrículo izquierdo; **(right/left) (inferior/superior) pulmonary** ~ vena pulmonar (inferior derecha/izquierda) (superior derecha/izquierda); **(inferior) (middle) (superior) rectal** ~s venas hemorroidales (inferiores) (medias) (superiores); **renal** ~s venas renales; **(accessory) (great) (small) saphenous** ~ vena safena (accesoria) (interna) (externa); **striated** ~s venas estriadas; **subclavian** ~ vena subclavia; **(deep) (middle) (superficial) temporal** ~ vena temporal (profunda) (media) (superficial); **(internal) (lateral) thoracic** ~ vena mamaria (interna) (externa); **transverse facial** ~ vena transversal de la cara; **transverse of neck** ~s venas escapulares posteriores y cervicales transversas; **ulnar** ~s venas cubitales; **umbilical** ~s venas umbilical; **uterine** ~s venas uterinas; ~ **stripping** extracción de várices *f*

vellus hair, vello

velum, velo del paladar *Anat*

vena, (*pl, venae*) vena; **(inferior)**

(superior) ~ cava vena cava (inferior) (superior)

vending machine, distribuidor automático *m*

venereal, venéreo *adj*; **~ disease** enfermedad venérea *f*; secreta *slang*; **AIDS** SIDA *m*; (*See AIDS.*); **canker sore** postemilla; úlcera gangrenosa; **chancre** chancro; grano; **hard ~** chancro duro; chancro sifilítico; **noninfecting ~** chancro blando; chancro simple; **chlamydia** clamidia; **cold sore** fuego en la boca; fuego en los labios; herpes[4] labial *m*; **conduloma** condiloma *m*; **genital wart** verruga genital; verruga venérea; **gonorrhea** blenorragia; chorro *euph, Chicano*; gonorrea *form*; gota *slang*; mal de orín *m, slang*; purgaciones *f, pl, slang*; **herpes** herpe(s)[4] *m/f*, [*Ú.m.c.m.*]; **herpes genitalis** herpes[4] genital; **herpes menstrualis** herpes[4] menstrual; **herpes zoster** herpes[4] zoster; **lymphogranuloma venereum** bubones *m*; linfogranuloma venéreo *m*; **moniliasis** algodoncillo; boquera; candidiasis *f*; moniliasis *f*; muguet *m*; **nongonococcal urethritis** uretritis no gonococal *f*; **nonspecific urethritis** uretritis inespecífica *f*; uretritis no específica *f*; **sexually transmitted diseases/STD** enfermedades pasadas sexualmente *f*; **syphilis** infección de la sangre *f, euph*; sangre mala *f, slang*; sífilis *f, form*; **trichomonas** tricomonas; **~ lesion** chancro; grano; úlcera venérea; **vesicular eruption** erupción vesicular *f*

venereologist, especialista en enfermedades venéreas *m/f*; venereólogo

venereology, venereología

venepuncture, (*See venipuncture.*)

venesection, venesección *f*; (*See phlebotomy.*)

venipuncture, punción quirúrgica de una vena *f*; venepuntura; venipuntura

venisection, (*See venesection and phlebotomy.*)

venogram, venograma *m*; radiografía de las venas; ~ (*phlebography*) flebografía; flebograma *m*; ~ (*phlebogram*) flebograma *m*

venom, ponzoña; veneno

venomous, venenoso *adj*

venous, venoso *adj*; **~ cutdown** disección de una vena *f*

vent, ~ (*hole, passsage*) abertura; agujero; ~ (*air hole*) respiradero; agujero de ventilación; ~ (*tube*) tubo de ventilación; conducto de ventilación; ~ (*grille in a wall, etc.*) rejilla de ventilación

vent one's feelings, to, desahogarse

ventilate, to, ventilar; ~ (*blood*) oxigenar

ventilation, ventilación *f*; **downward ~** ventilación descendente; **~ duct** conducto de ventilación; **exhausting ~** ventilación por escape; **natural ~** ventilación natural; **pulmonary ~** ventilación pulmonar; **~ shaft** pozo de ventilación; **upward ~** ventilación ascendente; ~ (*of blood*) oxigenación *f*

ventilator, ventilador *m*

ventricle, ventrículo; **~ of the brain** ventrículo del cerebro; **(first) (lateral) (second) (third) ~ of cerebrum** ventrículo (primero) (lateral) (segundo) (tercero) del cerebro; **~ of the cord** ventrículo de la médula espinal; **~ of the heart** ventrículo del corazón

ventricular, ventricular *adj*; **~ escape** extrasístole ventricular *f*

ventriculogram, radiografía de los ventrículos cerebrales; ventriculograma *f, form*

ventriculography, radiografía de los ventrículos del cerebro, inyectando aire después de extraer líquido cefalorraquídeo de ellos; radiografía de los ventrículos del corazón, inyectando previamente en ellos un medio de contraste; ventriculografía *form*

ventriculostomy, ventriculostomía

venture, to, arriesgar

verbal, verbal *adj*; ~ **communication** comunicación verbal *f*

verge, ~ (*border*; *edge*) borde *m*; **on the ~ of** al borde de *prep*; **on the ~ of tears** a punto de echarse a llorar; **to be on the ~ of something** estar en un hilo *PR*

verge on, to, rayar en

vermicide, vermicida *m*

vermifuge, antihelmíntico *m, adj*; que expulsa los gusanos intestinales; vermifugo *m, adj*

vermin, solitary, verme solitario *m*

vernix caseosa, vernix caseosa *f*

verrucous, verrugoso *adj*

verruga, verruga; (*See wart.*)

version, versión *f*; ~ (*of fetus*) versión *f*

vertebra, (*pl, vertebrae*) vértebra; huesos *fam*; **cervical ~** vértebra cervical; **coccygeal ~s** vértebras coccígeas; **dorsal ~s** vértebras dorsales; **lumbar ~s** vértebras lumbares; **sacral ~s** vértebras sacras

vertebral, vertebral *adj*; ~ **column** columna vertebral; ~ **discs** discos vertebrales

vertex, vértice *m*

vertigo, vértigo; **aural ~** vértigo auricular; **height ~** vértigo de la altura

vesicant, vesicante *m, adj*

vesicle, ampolla; vesícula

vessel, vaso; **blood ~s** vasos sanguíneos

vestibule, vestíbulo; ~ **of aorta** vestíbulo de la aorta; **buccal ~** vestíbulo bucal; **labial ~** vestíbulo labial; ~ **of larynx** vestíbulo de la laringe; ~ **of pharynx** vestíbulo de la faringe; ~ **of vagina** vestíbulo de la vagina

vestige, rastro; vestigio

veteran, veterano *m, adj*

veterinarian, veterinario

veterinary, veterinario *adj*; ~ **medicine** veterinaria; ~ **surgeon** veterinario

VF/visual field, campo visual

viable, viable *adj*

vial, ampolla pequeña; botella; frasco; vial *m*

vibrate, to, vibrar; ~ (*to swing to and fro*) oscilar

vibrating, vibrante *adj*; vibratorio *adj*; ~ **movement** movimiento vibratorio; **voice ~ with emotion** voz vibrante de emoción *f*

vibration, vibración *f*

vibrator, vibrador *m*

vibromassage, vibromasaje *m*

vice, vicio

vicinity, vecindad *f*

vicious, ~ (*characterized by vice*) vicioso *adj*; ~ (*person*) perverso *adj*; ~ (*crime*) atroz *adj*; ~ (*blow*) cruel *adj*

victim, víctima *f*; ~ (*of an accident, etc.*) siniestrado

view, vista

viewpoint, punto de vista

vigil, vigilia; **to keep ~** velar

vigilance, insomnio *Med*

vigorous, enérgico *adj*; vigoroso *adj*; ~ **man** un hombre vigoroso; ~ **massage** un masaje enérgico

villus, (*pl, villi*) vello; vellosidad *f*; **chorionic ~** vellosidad coriónica *f*; **pericardial ~** vellosidad pericárdica; **villi of small intestine** vellosidades del intestino delgado

vinegar, vinagre *m*

vinyl, vinilo; ~ **acetate** acetato de vinilo; ~ **chloride** cloruro de vinilo

violate, to, (*a woman*) violar

violation, (*of a woman*) violación *f*

violence, violencia
violent, violento *adj*
violet, violeta *adj*
violinist's cramp, calambre de los violinistas *m*; (*See cramps.*)
viper, víbora
viral, viral *adj*; **~ infection** infección viral *f*; monga *PR*; (*See infection.*)
virgin, virgen *f*
virginal, virginal *adj*
virginity, virginidad *f*
viril, varonil *adj*; viril *adj*; **~ member** miembro viril *Anat*
virility, virilidad *f*
virology, virología
virucide, virucida *m, adj*
virulence, virulencia
virulent, virulento *adj*
virus, virus *m*; **Colorado tick fever ~** virus de la fiebre de garrapata del Colorado; **Epstein-Barr ~/EBV** virus de Epstein-Barr/VEB[6]; **hepatitis ~** virus de la hepatitis; **human immunodeficiency ~/HIV** virus de inmunodeficiencia humana/VIH[6]; **masked ~** virus enmascarado; **tick-borne ~** virus transmitido por garrapatas
viscera, vísceras *f, pl*
visceral, visceral *adj*
viscometer, viscómetro
viscosity, viscosidad *f*
viscus, (*pl, viscera*) víscera
visibility, visibilidad *f*
visible, visible *adj*
visibly, visiblemente *adv*
vision, visión *f*; vista; **(a)chromatic ~** visión (a)cromática; **binocular ~** visión binocular *f*; **blurred ~** visión borrada; visión borrosa; vista borrosa; visión emborronada; vista empañada; vista nublada; **central ~** visión central; **day ~** visión diurna; **double ~** visión doble; vista doble; **foggy ~** vista empañada;

monocular ~ visión con un solo ojo; visión monocular; **night ~** visión nocturna; vista nocturna; **ocular ~** visión ocular; **peripheral ~** visión periférica; **tunnel ~** visión en túnel; **twilight ~** visión crepuscular; **~s** visiones *f, pl*; **within the range of ~** al alcance de la vista; **to have good ~** tener la buena vista; **to have normal ~** tener la vista normal
visit, visita
visit, to, visitar
visiting, de visita; visitante *adj*; **~ hours** horas de visita; **~ nurse** enfermera ambulante; enfermera visitadora; enfermera visitante
visitor, visita; visitante *m/f*
visual, visual *adj*; **~ aids** medios visuales; **~ field** campo visual; **~ purple** pigmento purpúrico visual; púrpura visual
visualization, imagen mental *f*
visualize, to, imaginar
vital, vital *adj*; **~ capacity** capacidad vital *f*; **~ dye** colorante vital *m*; **~ functions** funciones vitales *f*; **~ organs** órganos vitales; **~ parameters** parámetros vitales; **~ signs** signos vitales; **~ statistics** estadísticas demográficas; estadísticas vitales; **~ statistics (of a woman)** mensuraciones
vitamin, vitamina; **~ B$_1$** tiamina; **~ B$_2$** riboflavina; **~ B$_6$** piridoxina; **~ C** ácido ascórbico; **calcium** calcio; **~ deficiency** avitaminosis *f, inv*; deficiencia de vitaminas; **enriched with ~s** vitaminado *adj*; vitamínico *adj*; **fat-soluble ~** vitamina liposoluble; **iron** hierro; sulfato ferroso; **niacin** ácido nicotínico; niacina; **water-soluble ~** vitamina hidrosoluble
vitaminology, vitaminología
vitiligo, ciricua *fam*; jiricua *slang*; vitíligo

vitreous, vítreo *adj*; ~ **body** cuerpo vítreo; ~ **chamber** cámara vítrea; cápsula vítrea; ~ **humor** humor vítreo *m*

vitropression, vitropresión *f*

vivacious, vivaz *adj*

vivaciousness, vivacidad *f*

vivid, vivo *adj*; ~ (*color*) intenso *adj*; ~ (*description*) gráfico *adj*; ~ (*impression*) fuerte *adj*

viviparous, vivíparo *adj*

vivisection, vivisección *f*

vizor, visera

vocabulary, vocabulario

vocal, vocal *adj*; ~ **cord** cuerda vocal

vocation, vocación *f*

vodka, vodca *m*; vodka *f*

vogue, moda; boga; **to be in** ~ estar de moda; estar en boga

voice, voz *f*; ~ **box** galillo *PR*; **whispered** ~ voz cuchicheada; **to hear ~s** oír voces; **to lose one's** ~ perder (ie) la voz; **to strain one's** ~ forzar (ue) la voz

voiceless, afónico *adj*

voicelessness, mudez *f*; mutismo

void, ~ (*empty*) vacío *m*, *adj*; desocupado *adj*; ~ (*position*) vacante *adj*

void, to, orinar; vaciar la vejiga

voiding, micción *f*; ~ **cystogram** cistograma excretorio *m*

volatile, volátil *adj*

volt, voltio

voltage, voltaje *m*; tensión *f*; **high** ~ alta tensión

volubility, volubilidad *f*; locuacidad *f*

volume, volumen *m*; **atomic** ~ volumen atómico; **blood** ~ volumen sanguíneo; ~ **control** botón del volumen *m*; **expiratory reserve** ~ volumen de reserva espiratoria; **inspiratory reserve** ~ volumen de reserva inspiratoria; ~ **receptor** receptor de volumen *m*; **tidal** ~ volumen de ventilación pulmonar; **to turn down the** ~ bajar el volumen

voluntary, voluntario *adj*

volunteer, voluntario

voluptuous, voluptuoso *m*, *adj*

volvulus, vólvulo

vomit/vomitus, vómito; arrojadera *vulg*; arrojos *fam*; basca(s) *fam*; vasca(s) *fam*; **bilious** ~ vómito bilioso; **black** ~ fiebre amarilla *f*; vómito negro; **bloody** ~ vómito de sangre; **coffee-ground** ~ vómito en poso de café

vomit, to, vomitar; arrojar *fam*; basquear *fam*; deponer *Mex*, *fam*; devolver (ue) *fam*; dompear *Chicano*; gomitar *fam*; parir *PR*; revulsar *Mex*; tener basca *fam*; tirar las tripas; trasbocar *Arg*, *Chi*, *Col*; ~ **violently** echar las tripas

vomiting, vómito; ~ **blood** vómitos de sangre; **dry** ~ vómitos secos; **hysterical** ~ vómito histérico; **morning** ~ vómitos matutinos; **nervous** ~ vómito nervioso; ~ **of pregnancy** vómitos del embarazo

vomitive, emético *m*, *adj*; vomitivo *m*, *adj*

voodoo, vudú *m*

voracious, voraz *adj*; ávido *adj*; insaciable *adj*

voucher, vale *m*; ~ (*piece of evidence*) prueba

voyeurism, voyurismo

VP/venous pressure, presión venosa *f*

VRI/viral respiratory infection, infección respiratoria viral *f*

VSD/ventricular septal defect, comunicación interventricular /CIV *f*

VT/tidal volume, volumen de ventilación pulmonar *m*

vulnerable, vulnerable *adj*

vulnerability, destructibilidad *f*

vulva, vulva
vulvitis, vulvitis *f*

vulvovaginitis, vulvovaginitis *f*
V.W./vessel wall, pared vascular *f*

---

[4] In Spanish the word *herpes* is often used in the plural form.
[5] English almost always uses the plural form. (En inglés casi siempre se usa la forma plural.)
[6] Use the Spanish pronunciation of these letters.

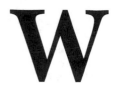

wad, borra; guata

waddle, anadeo; marcha de ánade

waddle, to, anadear

wailing, llanto; gemidos; ~ (*of a newborn infant*) vagidos *m, pl*

waist, cintura; talle *m, Anat*; **from the ~ down** de la cintura para abajo; **from the ~ up** de la cintura para arriba

wait, espera; ~ (*pause*) pausa

wait (for), to, esperar

waiting, espera; ~ **list** lista de espera; ~ **room** cuarto de estar; sala de espera; sala de estar

waiver, ~ (*of a right*) renuncia voluntaria; ~ (*of a claim*) desistimiento

wake, to, ~ (*a corpse*) velar; ~ **up** (*from sleep*) despertar (ie); ~ **oneself up** despertarse (ie)

wakefulness, desvelo; insomnio

walk, to, andar; caminar; ~ **back** volver (ue) andando; ~ **in one's sleep** andar dormido; ~ **with bowed head** samurar *Ven*

walker, andador *m*; andadera *f*; **baby ~** pollera

walking cane, bastón de paseo *m*

wall, pared *f*; ~ **of the blood vessels** pared de los vasos sanguíneos; ~**s of the digestive system** paredes del sistema digestivo

Walther's canal, conducto de Walther (*conducto de la glándula salival sublingual*)

wamble, to, tener náuseas

wandering, errante *adj*; migratorio *adj*; ~ **pain** dolor errático *m*

want, to, (*to love*) querer (ie)

wants, deseos

ward, crujía *form*; cuarto múltiple; pabellón *m*; sala *form*; ~ **clerk** secretaria de sala; **to walk the ~s** hacer práctica de clínica

warm, templado *adj*; tibio *adj*; **to be ~** (*person*) tener calor; **to feel ~** sentir (ie) calor

warm up, to, calentar (ie); encender (ie); ~ (*before exercising*) hacer calentamiento

warmer, calentador *m*; más caliente *adv*

warmth, calor *m*

warn, to, advertir (ie); avisar (de)

warning, aviso; ~ **light** lámpara indicadora; ~ **sign** signo de advertencia; señal de peligro *f*; señal premonitoria *f*; ~ **symptom** síntoma de advertencia *m*; síntoma premonitorio *m*; **without ~** sin avisar

warrant, to, hacer certificación

wart, mezquino *Mex*; verruga *form*; pisporra *CA*; **genital ~** verruga genital; **plantar ~** verruga plantar *form*; ojo de pescado *fam*

wash, to, lavar; higienizarse *Arg*; ~ **oneself** lavarse

washable, lavable *adj*

washbasin/washbowl, basija; jofaina; lavabo; lavacara *Col, Ec*; lavador *m, Arg, Para*; palangana *Mex*; ponchera *CA, Col, Mex, Ven*; tacho *Ríopl*; taza, *Chi*

washcloth, paño de lavarse; toallita

wasp, avispa; ~ **nest** avispero; ~ **sting** picadura de avispa

Wassermann's reaction, reacción de Wassermann (*prueba de la sífilis*) *f*

waste, desecho; ~ **basket** papelera; ~**s** *pl* desechos; desperdicios; residuos; **hazardous ~** desechos peligrosos; **industrial ~ products** residuos industriales; **metabolic ~** desechos metabólicos; **radioactive ~**

desechos radiactivos; **toxic** ~ desechos tóxicos

waste, to, desechar; malgastar; ~ **away** consumirse; chuparse *Med*; deshacerse *Med*; desmejorarse *Med*

watch, reloj *m*; **wrist~** reloj de pulsera; reloj de muñeca

watch, to, ~ (*to care for*) cuidar; ~ (**closely**) vigilar (de cerca)

water, agua³; **bag of** ~ bolsa de aguas; **distilled** ~ agua destilada; **fresh** ~ agua dulce; **hard** ~ agua con alto contenido de minerales; **mineral** ~ agua mineral; ~ **on the brain** (*hydrocephalus*) agua en el cerebro; ~ **on the knee** derrame sinovial *m*; ~ **pill** diurético; **purified** ~ agua purificada; **running** ~ agua corriente; **salt** ~ agua salada; **soft** ~ agua con poco contenido de minerales; **tap** ~ agua de la llave; agua del grifo; **~-borne** transmitido por el agua *adj phr*

water, to (*eyes*) lagrimear

wateriness, acuosidad *f*

waterpick, limpiador de agua a presión *m*

watery, acuoso *adj*; aguoso *adj*; blandito *adj*; ~ **eyes** ojos blandos *fam*; ojos llorosos

watt, vatio

wave, ola; onda; **brain** ~ onda cerebral; **~length** longitud de onda *f*

wax, (*cerumen*) cera; cerumen *m*

waxy, de cera

way, manera; ~ **of life/living** modo de vivir

WBC/white blood count, NGB⁶; numeración de glóbulos blancos *f*

weak, débil *adj*; inválido *adj*; endeble *adj*, *Med*; enteco *adj*; enclenco *adj*, *Col*, *PR*; engerido *adj*, *Col*, *Ven*; ñango *adj*, *Mex*; pachaco *adj*, *CA*; revejido *adj*, *Col*; timbebe *adj*, *Chi*; tere *adj*, *Col*; telenque *adj*, *Chi*; ~ **blood**

fam slang anemia *form*; sangre débil *f*, *fam*; sangre pobre *f*, *fam*

weaken, to, debilitar; depauperar *Med*; desmejorar *Med*; postrar *Med*

weakened, debilitado *adj*

weakening, debilitación *f*; decaimiento; depauperación *f*, *Med*; debilitante *adj*

weakness, debilidad *f*; desmedro *Med*; **muscular** ~ debilidad muscular *f*; **organic** ~ decaimiento orgánico; **resultant** ~ reliquias *f*, *pl*, *Med*

weal, (*large welt*) cardenal *m*; remalazo; verdugo; verdugón *m*

wean, to, destetar; quitarle el pecho al bebé; quitar la teta a; despechar *Chi*, *Hond*, *PR*

weaning, destete *m*; despecho *Chi*, *Hond*, *PR*

wear, to, llevar; ~ **off** pasar

weariness, cansancio; fastidio; fatiga

wedge, cuña

weed, hierba; hierbajo; ~⁷ *slang* mariguana¹; matojo²; **to blow** ~⁷ (*to smoke marijuana*) motear²; motiar²; tronar²

week, semana; **~end** fin de semana *m*; **~ly** cada ocho días; cada semana; semanalmente

weep, to, ~ (*to cry*) llorar; ~ (*a wound*) rezumar; supurar; ~ (*to mourn*) lamentarse

weeping, ~ (*crying*) lloroso *adj*; ~ (*oozing*) rezumante *adj*; supurante *adj*

weepy, tere *adj*, *Col*

weigh, to, pesar

weight, peso; ~ **at birth** peso al nacer; peso al nacimiento; **excess** ~ sobrepeso; **human body** ~ peso del cuerpo humano; ~ **loss** enflaquecimiento; magrez *f*; pérdida de peso; **~s and measures** pesos y medidas; **to gain** ~ aumentar de peso; **to lose** ~ bajar de peso; perder (ie) peso

welfare, asistencia pública; asistencia social; bienestar público *m*; salud *f, fig*

well, bien *adj/adv*; ~ **on** bien avanzado; **to get** ~ aliviarse; curarse

well-being, bienestar *m*; salud *f, fig*

well-timed, oportuno *adj*

welt, verdugo; patacón *m, Chi*; verdón *m, Arg*

wen, lobanillo; lupia; chibola *CA*; chibolo *Col, Ec, Hond, Perú*

wet, húmedo *adj*; mojado *adj*; ~ **cough** tos productiva *f*; ~ **nurse** nodriza

wet, to, humedecer; mojar; **to get** ~ mojarse

what, qué; ~ **amount?** ¿qué proporción?

wheal, cardenal *m*; grano; habón *m*; pápula; roncha; verdugón *m*

wheelchair, silla de ruedas; sillón de ruedas *m*

wheeze, resuello ruidoso; respiración sibilante *f*; resoplido

wheeze, to, chiflar; respirar asmáticamente; respirar con dificultad; resollar; silbar

whey, suero de leche

whimper, sollozo

whimper, to, sollozar

whiplash, contusión de la columna vertebral *f*; golpe en la nuca *m*; latigazo; lesión de latigazo *f*

whiskers, patillas

whiskey, whisk(e)y *m*

whisper, cuchicheo

whisper, to, cuchichear

whistle, silbido

whistle, to, chiflar; silbar

whistling rale, estertor sibilante *m*

white, blanco *n, adj*; ~ (*of an egg*) clara; ~ **blood corpuscles** glóbulos blancos; leucocitos *form*; ~ **cell count** recuento de leucocitos; ~ **hemogram** fórmula leucocitaria; ~ **lie** mentira piadosa; ~ **of the eye** blanco del ojo; ~ **spots** hilachas blancas

whitehead, grano

WHO/World Health Organization, OMS[6]/Organización de la Salud *f*

whole, conjunto; totalidad *f*; completo *adj*; entero *adj*; ~ (*unbroken*) sano *adj*; ~ **blood** sangre completa *f*; ~ **milk** leche entera *f*; ~ **wheat** trigo entero

wholesome, sano *adj*

whooping cough, (*pertussis*) tos ferina[4]; coqueluche *f*; tos ahogona *f*; tosferina[4]

wide, amplio *adj*

widen, to, ensanchar; hacer más ancho

widespread, difuso *adj*

widow, viuda; **recently widowed** recién viuda

widower, viudo

widowhood, viudez *f*

wife, esposa; mujer *f*

wig, peluca

will, ~ (*testament*) testamento; **to make one's** ~ hacer testamento; ~ (*volition*) voluntad *f*; **to have a strong** ~ tener mucha voluntad; **of (one's) own free** ~ por (su) propia voluntad; ~ **power** fuerza de voluntad; ~ **to live** la voluntad de vivir

wince, to, reaccionar

wind, viento; ~ (*flatus in youngsters*) flato; ~ (*flatus, gas in adults*) gases *m, pl*; ~ (*to leave without breath*) dejar sin aliento; ~ (*to roll*) enrollar; ~ (*a watch, clock, etc.*) dar cuerda a; ~ **down** (*a window*) bajar; ~ **up** (*to conclude*) concluir; terminar; **to have** ~ tener gases

windburn, resequedad de la piel causada por el viento *f*

window, ventana

windpipe, gaznate *m*; tráquea

wine, vino

winged, alado *adj*

winking, guiño

wipe, limpión *m*

wipe, to, ~ (*dry*) enjugar; ~ **one's**

brow enjugarse la frente; ~ **one's eyes** enjugarse las lágrimas; ~ **s.o.'s eyes** enjugar las lágrimas a alguien; ~ **one's nose** (*to blow nose*) sonarse las narices; ~ (*to clean*) limpiar; ~ **o.s.** (**after a B.M.**) asearse; limpiarse

wire, alambre *m*

wire, to, atar con alambre; **to be wired**[7] (*See inject oneself with drugs, to.*)

wisdom tooth, diente de juicio *m*; cordal *m*; muela de juicio

witch, brujo

witchcraft, hechicería

witch hazel, agua[3] de hamamelis

withdraw, to, retirarse; ~ (*sexually*) salirse

withdrawal, retirada; supresión *f*; (*sexual*) ~ coitus interruptus *form*

withering, marchito *adj*

withhold one's consent, to, negarse (ie) a dar su consentimiento

within, por dentro *prep*

withstand, to, aguantar; padecer

witness, testigo

witness, to, presenciar

wobble, bamboleo

wobble, to, balancearse; vacilar

woman, mujer *f*; ~ **in labor** parturienta; ~ **who has just given birth** parturienta; **women's (bath)room** baño para mujeres

womb, matriz *f*; útero; ~ (*pelvic cavity*) vientre *m*; **fallen** ~ descenso del utero *Med*

wood, madera; ~ **alcohol** alcohol de madera *m*; alcohol metílico *m*

woolsorter's disease, ántrax *m*

work, empleo; trabajo

work, to, trabajar; mostrarse (ue) activo (un medicamento); obrar[5]; ~ **out** hacer ejercicio

worker, trabajador, -ra *m/f*

workup, diagnóstico diferencial; marcha diagnóstica

world, mundo

worm, gusano; lombriz *f*; **bladder** ~ cisticerco; **pork** ~ gusano del cerdo; triquina

worn out, gastado *adj*; ~ (*exhausted*) rendido de fatiga *adj*

worried, preocupado *adj*; intranquilo adj; **to get** ~ intranquilizarse

worrisome, preocupante *adj*

worry, pena; preocupación *f*; subsidio *Col, Ec*; **worries** agonizos *m, pl, Mex*

worry, to, preocuparse; afligarse; apenarse *Chicano*; intranquilizar

worse, peor *adj, adv*

worsen, to, empeorar

worsening, empeoramiento

wound, herida; lastimadura; llaga; coco; chira *CA*; cholla *CA*; estacada *SpAm*; tajarrazo *CA, Mex*; tarrajazo *Guat*; yaya *m, CA, Col*; **abrasion** abrasión *f*; **bullet** ~ herida de bala; plomazo *CA, Mex*; **chafe** rozadura; **cut** cortadura; **incised** ~ herida incisa; **incision** cisura; incisión *f*; **knife** ~ cuchillada; filorazo *Chicano*; puntazo *SpAm*; **laceration** laceración *f*; **open** ~ lora *Col, Ec, PR, Ven*; **open skin** ~ grano; **puncture** ~ herida penetrante; herida por punción; herida punzante; **ragged** ~ herida anfractuosa; **scrape** raspadura; **slight** ~ yaya *m, Chi, Col, Cu Perú*; **stab** ~ puñalada; puntazo *SpAm*; **tear** (*torn* ~) desgarro

wound, to/to hurt, herir (ie); lastimarse; estacar *Ven*; puyar *SpAm*; victimar *SpAm*

W.R./Wassermann Reaction, R.W.[6]/ reacción de Wassermann *f*

wrap up, to, abrigar(se); envolver(se) (ue)

wrapping in a cold (wet) sheet, empacamiento en sábana fría (mojada)

wrench, torcedura
wrench, to, torcer (ue)
wring (one's hands), to, tallarse
wrinkle, arruga
wrinkle, to, arrugar(se)
wrist, muñeca
write, to, escribir

writer's spasm, calambre de los escribientes *m*
writhe in pain, to, retorcerse (ue) de dolor
writing, escritura
wryneck, tortícolis *f*

---

[1] I have followed the spelling given in the *Diccionario de la lengua española*, RAE, 21st edition, 1990. Spanish does recognize variations using *j* and *h*.

[2] This is new vocabulary, not necessarily listed nor yet recognized by the Royal Academy of Spanish Grammar. It is understood that this vocabulary is primarily slang. Unless otherwise indicated, the gender of nouns is assumed to be obvious.

[3] For pronunciation purposes, the masculine definite and indefinite articles, *el* and *un*, not *la* or *una*, are used when the article immediately precedes the feminine singular noun which begins with stressed *a* or any other that begins with stressed *ha*.

[4] This term, also spelled *tosferina*, commonly refers to any persistent cough that children have.

[5] This verb also means *to have a bowel movement*.

[6] Use the Spanish pronunciations of these letters.

[7] Part of the Drug Abuse Vocabulary.

X chromosome, cromosoma X *m*

xanthoma, manchas de color amarillo; nódulos de color amarillo; xantoma *m, form*

xanthosis, decoloración amarillenta de la piel *f*; xantosis *f, form*

xerosis, resequedad de los ojos *f*; xerosis *f, inv, form*

xerox copy, xerografía *fam*

X-linked, ligado al cromosoma X *adj*

x-ray, ~ (*film*) radiografía; retrato del x-ray *Chicano*; ~ (*Roentgen ray–one picture*) rayo equis/ rayo x; **chest** ~ radiografía del pecho; radiografía del tórax; rayo equis del pecho; ~ **examination** examen con rayos x *m*; examen radiológico *m*; ~ **therapy** radioterapia

x-ray, to, ~ (*on a fluorescent screen*) examinar con rayos x; tratar con rayos x; ~ (*to take an x-ray photo of*) radiografiar; tomar una radiografía (de)

Y chromosome, cromosoma Y *m*
yage[4], ayahuasca
yam, ñame *m*; camote *m*, *SpAm*
yank, tirón *m*
yank, to, dar un tirón a; ~ **a tooth** sacar un diente de un tirón
yard, (*measurement*) yarda
yawn, bostezo
yawn, to, bostezar
yaws, frambesia; pian *m*
year, año; **all the ~ round** durante todo el año; **XX times a ~** XX veces al año; **~ly** anual *adj*; anualmente *adv*; cada año *adv*
yeast, clase de hongos *f*; fermento; levadura; **brewer's ~** levadura de cerveza; ~ **fungus** saca-romiceto *form*; ~ **infection** infección por candida *f*; infección vaginal causada por una clase de hongos *f*
yell, aullido; grito
yell, to, aullar; gritar; ~ **for help** pedir (i) auxilio a gritos; ~ **with pain** gritar de dolor
yellow, amarillo *adj*; ~ **body** cuerpo lúteo; ~ **fever** fiebre amari-lla *f*; ~ **fibers** fibras elásticas; ~ **skin** (*jaundice*) piel amarilla *f*, (*See jaundice.*); **~ish** amarillento *adj*
yelp, to, ladrar; gañir
Yemen ulcer, úlcera del Yemen; forúnculo oriental
yes, sí
yesterday, ayer
yield, to, (*to give in*) ceder; ~ (*to give back*) devolver (ue); ~ (*to give, produce*) producir; ~ (*to admit defeat*) rendir(se)
yodel, to, cantar a la tirolesa
yoga, yoga *m*
yogurt, yogur *m*
yolk, vitelo; **egg ~** yema del huevo; ~ **sac** membrana vitelina; saco vitelino
you, ~ *form, sg* usted (*abbr Vd./Ud.*); ~ *form, pl* ustedes (*abbr Vds./Uds.*)
young person, joven *m/f*
youth, juventud *f*; mocedad *f*; **~ful** juvenil *adj*; ~ **hostel** albergue para jóvenes *m*

---

[4] The current English street terminology for *yage* includes: ayahuasca, caapi, drug, jungle drug.

Z

zero, cero
zinc, cinc *m*; zinc *m*; ~ **oxide** óxido de cinc; radióxido de zinc
zip code, zona postal; código postal
zip, to, cerrarse (ie) con cremallera
zipper, cierre *m*; ziper *m*, *Chicano*; cremallera; ~ (*pants*) bragueta

zodiac, zodíaco
zone, zona; **ciliary ~** zona ciliar
zonked, to be ~ (*See blasted, to be.*); **to get ~** ajumar(se)[2]; guayear(se)[2]
zoology, zoología
zoster, zona; zoster *m*, *f*
zygote, zigoto; cigoto

---

[2] This is new vocabulary, not necessarily listed nor yet recognized by the Royal Academy of Spanish Grammar. It is understood that this vocabulary is primarily slang. Unless otherwise indicated, the gender of nouns is assumed to be obvious.

ARTERY	ARTERIA
inferior alveolar artery	arteria dentaria inferior
descending thoracic aorta artery	arteria aorta torácica descendente
ascending aorta artery	arteria aorta ascendente
arcuate artery of the foot	arteria dorsal del metatarso
arcuate arteries of the kidney	arterias arciformes del riñón
deep auricular artery	arteria auricular profunda
axillary artery	arteria axilar
basilar artery	arteria basilar
brachial artery	arteria humeral
bronchial arteries	arterias bronquiales
buccal artery	arteria bucal
capsular artery	arteria capsular
caroticotympanic artery	ramos caroticotimpánicos
(common) (external) (internal) carotid artery	arteria carótida (primitiva) (externa) (interna)
caudal artery	arteria sacra media
central artery of retina	arteria central de la retina
cerebellar artery	arteria cerebelosa
cerebral artery	arteria cerebral
ascending cervical artery	arteria cervical ascendente
anterior choroidal artery	arteria coroidea anterior
long posterior ciliary arteries	arterias ciliares largas posteriores
posterior circumflex artery	arteria circunfleja posterior
dorsal artery of the clitoris	arteria dorsal del clítoris
posterior conjunctival arteries	arterias conjuntivales posteriores
coronary artery	arteria coronaria
descending posterior coronary artery	arteria interventricular posterior
left coronary artery of stomach	arteria coronaria estomáquica
right coronary artery of stomach	arteria pilórica derecha
left coronary artery of heart	arteria coronaria izquierda
right coronary artery of heart	arteria coronaria derecha
cremasteric artery	arteria funicular
deferential artery	arteria deferente
dental artery	arteria dental
diaphragmatic artery	arteria diafragmática inferior
duodenal artery	arteria pancreaticoduodenal inferior
external epigastric artery	arteria circunfleja ilíaca
inferior esophageal arteries	ramos cardioesofágicos
transverse facial artery	arteria facial transversa; arteria transversal de la cara
fallopian artery	arteria uterina
femoral artery	arteria femoral
fibular artery	arteria peronea
short gastric arteries	vasos cortos del estómago
gastroduodenal artery	arteria gastroduodenal

inferior gluteal artery	arteria isquiática
superior gluteal artery	arteria glútea
common iliac artery	arteria ilíaca primitiva
internal iliac artery	arteria ilíaca interna
inguinal arteries	ramas de las arterias pudendas externas
highest/superior intercostal artery	arteria intercostal superior
anterior interventricular artery	arteria interventricular anterior
jejunal arteries	arterias yeyunales
inferior labial artery	arteria coronaria inferior
lingual artery	arteria lingual
lowest/fifth lumbar artery	quinta arteria lumbar
(external) (internal) mammary artery	arteria mamaria (externa) (interna)
superficial medial artery of foot	ramos superficiales de la arteria plantar interna
anterior meningeal artery	arteria meníngea anterior
dorsal metacarpal arteries	arterias interóseas dorsales
obturator artery	arteria obturatriz
occipital artery	arteria occipital
ophthalmic artery	arteria oftálmica
perforating arteries	arterias perforantes
peroneal artery	arteria peronea
popliteal artery	arteria poplítea
pubic artery	arteria suprapúbica
external pudendal arteries	arterias pudendas externas superior e inferior
pulmonary artery	arteria pulmonar
quadriceps artery of femur	arteria del cuadríceps
radial artery	arteria radial
ulnar recurrent artery	arteria recurrente cubital
renal artery	arteria renal
lateral sacral arteries	arterias sacras laterales
dorsal scapular artery	arteria cervical transversa profunda
sigmoid arteries	arterias sigmoideas
anterior spinal artery	arteria espinal anterior
splenic artery	arteria esplénica
subclavian artery	arteria subclavia
sublingual artery	arteria sublingual
lateral tarsal artery	arteria dorsal del tarso
deep posterior temporal artery	arteria temporal profunda posterior
testicular artery	arteria espermática
lateral thoracic artery	arteria torácica inferior; arteria mamaria externa
tibial artery	arteria tibial
tympanic artery	arteria timpánica
ulnar artery	arteria cubital
umbilical artery	arteria umbilical

urethral artery	arteria uretral
uterine artery	arteria uterina
vaginal artery	arteria vaginal
vertebral artery	arteria vertebral

LIGAMENT — LIGAMENTO

acromioclavicular ligament	ligamento acromioclavicular
acromiocoracoid ligament	ligamento acromiocoracoideo
adipose ligament of the knee	ligamento adiposo de la rodilla
alar ligaments	ligamentos alares de la odontoides
alveolodental ligament	ligamento alveolodental
annular ligament of base of stapes	ligamento anular de la base del estribo
annual ligament of radius	ligamento anular del radio
anococcygeal ligament	ligamento anococcígeo
apical odontoid ligament	ligamento occipitoodontoideo medio; ligamento suspensorio de la apófisis odontoides
apendiculo-ovarian ligament	ligamento apendiculoovárico
arcuate ligament, lateral	arco del cuadrado lumbar
arcuate ligament, median	arco del psoas
arcuate ligament, pubic	ligamento arqueado de la sínfisis púbica
brachiocubital ligament	ligamento lateral interno de la articulación del codo
brachioradial ligament	ligamento lateral externo de la articulación del codo
broad ligament of uterus	ligamento ancho
calcaneocuboid ligament, plantar	ligamento calcaneocuboideo inferior
calcaneofibular ligament	ligamento peroneocalcáneo
calcaneonavicular ligament, plantar	ligamento calcaneoescafoideo inferior
capsular ligament	cápsula articular
carpometacarpal ligament, dorsal	ligamento dorsal de las articulaciones carpometacarpianas
carpometacarpal ligaments, interosseous	ligamento interóseo carpometacarpiano
carpometacarpal ligaments, volar	ligamentos palmares de la articulación carpometacarpiana
caudal ligament	ligamento caudal
cheek ligaments of axis	ligamentos alares de la odontoides
coracoclavicular ligament	ligamento coracoclavicular
coracohumeral ligament	ligamento coracohumeral
coronary ligament of knee	ligamento coronario de la rodilla
coronary ligament of liver	ligamento coronario del hígado

costocentral ligament	ligamento costocentral
costoclavicular ligament	ligamento costoclavicular
costocoracoid ligament	ligamento costocoracoideo
costopericardiac ligament	ligamento costopericárdico
costotransverse ligaments	ligamentos costotransversos
costovertebral ligament	ligamento costovertebral
cricoarytenoid ligament, posterior	ligamento cricoaritenoideo posterior
cricosantorinian ligament	ligamento yugal
cruciate ligament of atlas	ligamento cruciforme
cruciate ligaments of knee	ligamentos cruzados de la rodilla
cruciate ligament of leg	ligamento anular anterior del tarso
crural ligament	arco crural
cuneonavicular ligaments	ligamentos tranversos del metatarso
cuneonavicular ligaments, plantar	ligamentos escafoidocuneales
deltoid ligament	ligamento deltoideo
denticulate ligament	ligamento dentado
diaphragmatic ligament	ligamento diafragmático
fallopian ligament	ligamento de Falopio
gastrocolic ligament	epiplón gastrocólico; epiplón mayor
gastrohepatic ligament	epiplón menor; ligamento gastrohepático
gastrolienal ligament	epiplón gastrosplénico
gastropancreatic ligament	ligamento gastropancreático
gastrophrenic ligament	ligamento frenogástrico; ligamento gastrofrénico
glenohumeral ligaments	ligamentos glenohumerales
hamatometacarpal ligament	ligamento hamatometacarpiano
ligament of head of femur	ligamento redondo de la cabeza del fémur
hyaloideocapsular ligament	ligamento hialoideocapsular
iliofemoral ligament	ligamento iliofemoral
iliolumbar ligament	ligamento iliolumbar
iliopectineal ligament	ligamento iliopectíneo; cinta iliopectínea
iliopubic ligament	ligamento iliopúbico
inguinal ligament	arco crural
interarticular ligament	ligamento interarticular
intercarpal ligaments, dorsal	ligamentos dorsales de las articulaciones carpianas
intercarpal ligaments, interosseous	ligamentos interóseos carpianos
intercarpal ligaments, palmar	ligamentos palmares de las articulaciones carpianas
interclavicular ligament	ligamento interclavicular
intercostal ligaments	ligamentos intercostales
intercuneiform ligaments, dorsal	ligamentos intercuneales dorsales
intercuneiform ligaments, plantar	ligamentos plantares de las articulaciones cuneales

intermetatarsal ligaments, transverse dorsal	ligamentos dorsales de las articulaciones intermetatarsianas
interosseous ligaments of tarsus	ligamentos interóseos del tarso
interosseous metatarsal ligaments	ligamentos interóseos de las articulaciones intermetatarsianas
interspinal ligaments	ligamentos interespinosos
intertransverse ligaments	ligamentos intertransversos
interureteral ligament	ligamento interureteral
intra-articular ligament of costovertebral joints	ligamento interóseo de las articulaciones costovertebrales; ligamento intraarticular de la articulación costovertebral
ischiofemoral ligament	ligamento isquiofemoral
ischioprostatic ligament	aponeurosis perineal profunda
lateral ligament of knee	ligamento lateral externo de la articulación de la rodilla
lateral ligaments of liver	ligamentos triangulares del hígado
lateral ligament of wrist	ligamento lateral externo de la articulación de la muñeca
Lauth's ligament	ligamento transverso del atlas
longitudinal ligament, anterior	ligamento vertebral común anterior
longitudinal ligament, posterior	ligamento vertebral común posterior
Luschka's ligament	ligamento esternopericardíaco superior
Mackenrodt's ligament	ligamentos uterorrectosacros
medial ligament of elbow joint	ligamento lateral interno de la articulación del codo
medial ligament of knee joint	ligamento lateral interno de la articulación de la rodilla
medial ligament of wrist	ligamento lateral interno de la articulación de la muñeca
metacarpal ligaments	ligamentos transversos del metacarpo
metacarpophalangeal ligaments, palmar	ligamentos palmares de las articulaciones metacarpofalángicas
nephrocolic ligament	ligamento nefrocólico
oblique ligaments of carpometacarpal joint of thumb	ligamentos oblicuos de la articulación carpometacarpiana del pulgar
oblique posterior ligament of knee	ligamento poplíteo oblicuo de la articulación de la rodilla
odontoid ligaments	ligamentos odontoideos; ligamentos alares de la apófisis odontoides
orbicular ligament of the radius	ligamento anular del radio
pancreaticosplenic ligament	epiplón pancreaticosplénico
patellar ligament	ligamento rotuliano
perineal ligament, transverse	ligamento transverso de la pelvis
phrenocolic ligament	ligamento frenocólico

pisohamate ligament	ligamento inferior de la articulación pisipiramidal
plantar ligaments	ligamentos plantares
plantar ligament, long	ligamento calcaneocuboideo inferior
popliteal ligament, arcuate	ligamento poplíteo arqueado
pterygomandibular ligament	aponeurosis buccinatofaríngea; ligamento pterigomaxilar
pubic ligament, inferior	ligamento inferior de la sínfisis púbica; ligamento arqueado; ligamento subpúbico
pubic ligament, superior	ligamento superior de la sínfisis del pubis
pubofemoral ligament	ligamento pubiofemoral
pulmonary ligament	ligamento triangular del pulmón
radial ligament	ligamento radial
radiate ligament	ligamento anterior de la articulación costovertebral
radiocarpal ligaments	ligamentos radiocarpianos
radiocarpal ligament, dorsal	ligamento posterior de la articulación de la muñeca
radiocarpal ligament, palmar	ligamento anterior de la articulación de la muñeca
rhomboid ligament	ligamento romboidal
round ligament	ligamento redondo
sacrococcygeal ligament, deep dorsal	fascículo profundo del ligamento sacrococcígeo posterior
sacrococcygeal ligament, superficial dorsal	fascículo superficial del ligamento sacrococcígeo posterior
sacrococcygeal ligaments, lateral	ligamentos sacrococcígeos laterales
sacrococcygeal ligament, dorsal (or posterior)	ligamento sacrococcígeo posterior
sacrococcygeal ligament, ventral (or anterior)	ligamentos sacrococcígeos anteriores
sacroiliac ligaments, anterior	ligamentos sacroiliacos anteriores
sacroiliac ligaments, dorsal	ligamentos sacroiliacos posteriores
sacroiliac ligaments, interosseous	ligamentos sacroiliacos interóseos
sacrosciatic ligaments	ligamentos sacrociáticos
sacrospinous ligament	ligamento sacrociático menor
sacrotuberous ligament	ligamento sacrociático mayor
scaphocuneiform ligaments, dorsal	ligamentos escafoidocuneales dorsales
sphenomandibular ligament	ligamento esfenomaxilar
spinoglenoid ligament	ligamento espinoglenoideo
splenophrenic ligament	ligamento frenosplénico
spring ligament	ligamento calcaneoescafoideo inferior

stapedial ligament	ligamento anular de la base del estribo
stellate ligament	ligamento estrellado; ligamento radiado de las articulaciones costovertebrales
subflavous ligament	ligamentos amarillos
subpubic ligament	ligamento subpúbico
suprascapular ligament	ligamento coracoideo
supraspinous ligament	ligamento supraespinoso
suspensory ligament of axilla	ligamento suspensorio de la axila
suspensory ligament of lens	ligamento suspensorio del cristalino
talocalcaneal ligament, interosseous	ligamento interóseo de la articulación astragalocalcánea
talocalcaneal ligament, posterior	ligamento calcaneoastragalino posterior
talofibular ligament, anterior	ligamento peroneoastragalino anterior
talofibular ligament, posterior	ligamento peroneoastragalino posterior
talonavicular ligament	ligamento astragaloescafoideo
talotibial ligament, anterior	haz anterior de la capa superficial del ligamento deltoideo
talotibial ligament, posterior	haz posterior de la capa superficial del ligamento deltoideo
temporomandibular ligament	ligamento lateral externo de la articulación temporomaxilar
tensor ligament	ligamento anterior del martillo
tibiofibular ligaments	ligamentos anterior y posterior de la articulación peroneotibial inferior
tibiofibular ligament, interosseous	ligamento interóseo de la articulación peroneotibial inferior
tibionavicular ligament	ligamento tibioescafoideo
transverse humeral ligament	ligamento humeral transverso de Gordon Brodie
transverse ligament of acetabulum	ligamento transverso del acetábulo
transverse ligament of knee	ligamento yugal de la rodilla
transverse metacarpal ligament	ligamento transverso del metacarpo
transverse metatarsal ligament	ligamento transverso del metatarso
transverse ligament of pelvis	ligcamento transverso de la pelvis
transverse perineal ligament	ligamento transverso del perineo
trapezoid ligament	ligamento trapezoideo
triangular ligament	ligamento triangular; diafragma urogenital
triangular ligaments of the liver	ligamentos triangulares del hígado
umbilical ligament, lateral	cordón fibroso de la arteria umbilical
umbilical ligament, median	uraco

utero-ovarian ligament	ligamento uteroovárico; ligamento del ovario
uteropelvic ligaments	ligamentos uteropélvicos
uterorectosacral ligaments	ligamentos uterorrectosacros
uterosacral ligament	ligamento uterosacro
ventricular ligament	ligamento tiroaritenoideo superior
vertebropleural ligament	ligamento vertebropleural
vesicopubic ligament	ligamento pubiovesical
vesico-umbilical ligament	uraco
vesico-uterine ligament	ligamento vesicouterino
vestibular ligament	ligamento tiroaritenoideo superior
vocal ligament	ligamento tiroaritenoideo inferior
xiphoid ligaments	ligamentos costoxifoideos

MUSCLE	MÚSCULO
abductor muscle	músculo abductor
articular muscle of the elbow	fascículos tensores de la sinovial del codo
articular muscle of the knee	músculo tensor de la sinovial de la rodilla
arytenoid muscle	músculo aritenoideo
auricular muscle	músculo auricular
biceps muscle of the arm	músculo bíceps braquial
biceps muscle of the thigh	músculo bíceps crural
brachial muscle	músculo braquial anterior
buccopharyngeal muscle	músculo bucofaringeo
chin muscle	músculo del mentón o de la barba
ciliary muscle	músculo ciliar
coccygeal muscle	músculo isquiococcígeo
constrictor muscle of the pharynx	músculo constrictor de la faringe
cremaster muscle	músculo cremáster
deltoid muscle	músculo deltoides
depressor muscle of the angle of the mouth	músculo triangular de los labios
diaphragmatic muscle	diafragma
dilator muscle	músculo dilator
erector muscle of the penis	músculo isquiocavernoso
erector muscle of the spine	músculos espinales o de la masa común
extensor muscle	músculo extensor
muscles of the eye	músculos del ojo
femoral muscle	músculo crural
fibular muscle	músculo peroneo lateral
fixator muscle of base of stapes	músculo del estribo
flexor muscle	músculo flexor
glossopharyngeal muscle	músculo faringogloso

gluteal muscle	músculo glúteo
intermediate great muscle	músculo crural
iliac muscle	músculo ilíaco
intercostal muscles	músculos intercostales
dorsal interosseous muscles	músculos interóseos dorsales
interspinal muscles	músculos interespinosos
intertransverse muscles	músculos intertransversos
joint muscle	músculo articular
levator muscle	músculo elevador
long muscle of the head	músculo recto anterior mayor de la cabeza
long muscle of the neck	músculo largo del cuello
longitudinal muscle of the tongue	músculo lingual
external oblique muscle of the abdomen	músculo oblicuo mayor del abdomen
superior oblique muscle of the eyeball	músculo oblicuo mayor del ojo
obturator muscle	músculo obturador
occipital muscle	músculo occipital
opposing muscle	músculo oponente
orbital muscle	músculo orbitario
palmar muscle	músculo palmar
anterior papillary muscle of the left ventricle	músculo papilar anterior del ventrículo izquierdo
septal papillary muscles of the right ventricle	músculos papilares internos del ventrículo derecho
pectoral muscle	músculo pectoral
popliteal muscle	músculo poplíteo
quadrate muscle	músculo cuadrado
rectococcygeal muscle	músculo rectococcígeo
rectouterine muscle	músculo rectouterino
rotator muscles	músculos rotatorios
long rotator muscles	músculos rotadores largos
sphincter muscle	músculo esfínter
spinal muscle	músculo espinoso
splenius muscle	músculo esplenio
subclavius muscle	músculo subclavio
subscapular muscle	músculo subescapular
tarsal muscle	músculo palpebral
temporal muscle	músculo temporal
tibial muscle	músculo tibial
transverse muscle	músculo transverso
trapezius muscle	músculo trapecio
triceps muscle	músculo tríceps
vocal muscle	músculo vocal; fascículo propio de la cuerda vocal

VEIN	VENA
accompanying vein	vena satélite
afferent vein	vena aferente
anterior auricular vein	vena auricular anterior del pabellón de la oreja
posterior auricular vein	vena auricular posterior del pabellón de la oreja
azygos vein	vena ácigos
brachial vein	vena humeral
cardiac veins	venas del corazón
great cardiac vein	vena coronaria magna; vena coronaria mayor
small cardiac vein	vena coronaria menor; vena coronaria derecha
(anterior) (inferior) (internal) cerebral vein	vena cerebral (anterior) (inferior) (profunda)
superior cerebral veins	venas cerebrales ascendentes internas y externas
deep vein	vena profunda
deep veins of penis	venas profundas del pene
(common) (dorsal) (palmar) digital veins of the foot	venas digitales (comunes) (dorsales) (palmares) del pie
enlargement of the veins	venas agrandadas *fam*
anterior common facial vein	vena facial anterior común
posterior facial vein	tronco temporomaxilar
deep femoral vein	vena femoral profunda
fibular veins	venas peroneas
frontal veins	venas anteriores del cráneo
left gastric vein	vena coronaria estomáquica
(internal) (external) (common) iliac vein	vena ilíaca (interna) (externa) (primitiva)
jugular *n*; jugular vein	vena yugular
anterior labial veins	venas anteriores de los labios mayores y menores
(inferior) (superior) labial veins	venas del labio (inferior) (superior)
posterior labial veins	venas posteriores de los labios mayores y menores
deep lingual veins	venas profundas de la lengua
ascending lumbar vein	vena lumbar ascendente
external mammary veins	venas costoaxilares
internal mammary/internal thoracic vein	vena mamaria interna
maxillary veins	venas maxilares internas
median vein of the elbow	vena mediana basílica
median vein of the forearm	vena mediana del antebrazo
perforating veins	venas perforantes
descending pharyngeal vein	vena faríngea descendente
(right/left) (inferior/superior) pulmonary vein	vena pulmonar(derecha/izquierda) (inferior/superior)

(inferior) (middle) (superior) rectal veins   venas hemorroidales (inferiores) (medias) (superiores)

renal veins   venas renales

right gastric vein   vena pilórica

short gastric veins   venas gástricas cortas

(accessory) (great) (small) saphenous vein   vena safena (accesoria) (interna) (externa)

striate veins   venas estriadas

subclavian vein   vena subclavia

(deep) (middle) (superficial) temporal vein   vena temporal (profunda) (media) (superficial)

internal thoracic veins   venas mamarias internas

lateral thoracic vein   vena mamaria externa

transverse facial vein   vena transversa de la cara

transverse veins of neck   venas escapulares posteriores y cervicales transversas

ulnar veins   venas cubitales

umbilical vein   vena umbilical

uterine veins   venas uterinas

varicose veins   venas varicosas

(inferior) (superior) vena cava   vena cava (inferior) (superior)

posterior vein of left ventricle   vena posterior del ventrículo izquierdo

Skeleton/Esqueleto
Anterior View/Vista Anterior

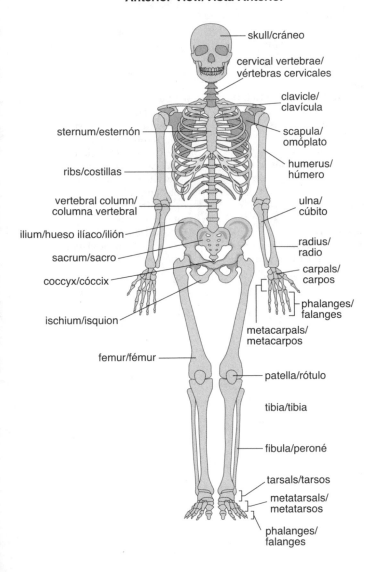

skull/cráneo

cervical vertebrae/
vértebras cervicales

clavicle/
clavícula

sternum/esternón

scapula/
omóplato

ribs/costillas

humerus/
húmero

vertebral column/
columna vertebral

ulna/
cúbito

ilium/hueso ilíaco/ilión

radius/
radio

sacrum/sacro

carpals/
carpos

coccyx/cóccix

phalanges/
falanges

ischium/isquion

metacarpals/
metacarpos

femur/fémur

patella/rótulo

tibia/tibia

fibula/peroné

tarsals/tarsos

metatarsals/
metatarsos

phalanges/
falanges

Skeleton/Esqueleto
Posterior View/Vista Posterior

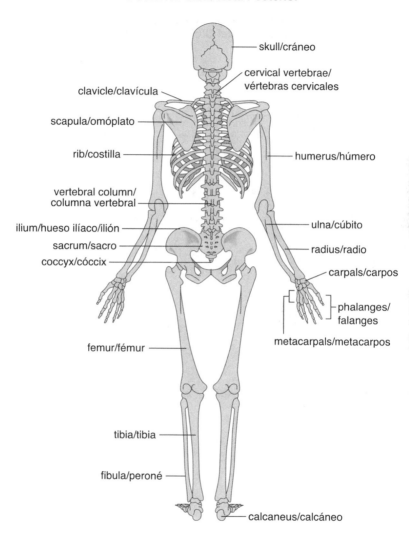

skull/cráneo

cervical vertebrae/
vértebras cervicales

clavicle/clavícula

scapula/omóplato

rib/costilla

humerus/húmero

vertebral column/
columna vertebral

ilium/hueso ilíaco/ilión

sacrum/sacro

coccyx/cóccix

ulna/cúbito

radius/radio

carpals/carpos

phalanges/
falanges

metacarpals/metacarpos

femur/fémur

tibia/tibia

fibula/peroné

calcaneus/calcáneo

Structures of the Eye
Estructuras del Ojo

Lateral View of the Eyeball Interior
Vista Lateral del Globo del Ojo Interior

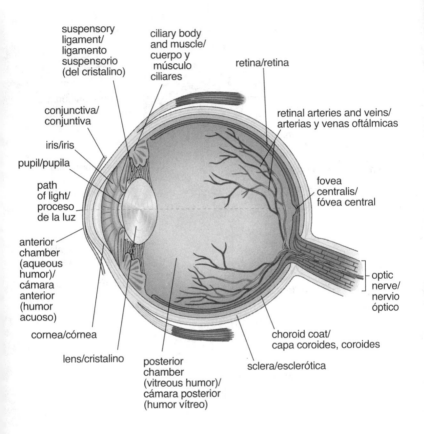

suspensory ligament/ ligamento suspensorio (del cristalino)

ciliary body and muscle/ cuerpo y músculo ciliares

retina/retina

conjunctiva/ conjuntiva

iris/iris

pupil/pupila

path of light/ proceso de la luz

anterior chamber (aqueous humor)/ cámara anterior (humor acuoso)

cornea/córnea

lens/cristalino

posterior chamber (vitreous humor)/ cámara posterior (humor vítreo)

retinal arteries and veins/ arterias y venas oftálmicas

fovea centralis/ fóvea central

optic nerve/ nervio óptico

choroid coat/ capa coroides, coroides

sclera/esclerótica

Structures of the Ear
Estructuras del Oído

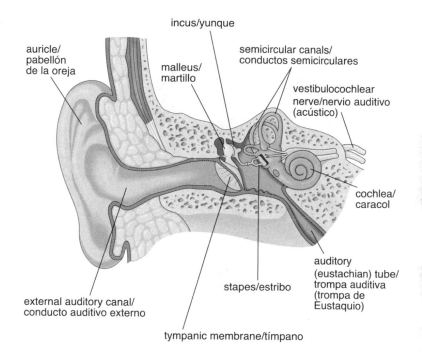

incus/yunque

auricle/
pabellón
de la oreja

malleus/
martillo

semicircular canals/
conductos semicirculares

vestibulocochlear
nerve/nervio auditivo
(acústico)

cochlea/
caracol

auditory
(eustachian) tube/
trompa auditiva
(trompa de
Eustaquio)

stapes/estribo

external auditory canal/
conducto auditivo externo

tympanic membrane/tímpano

Structures of the Mouth
Estructuras de la Boca

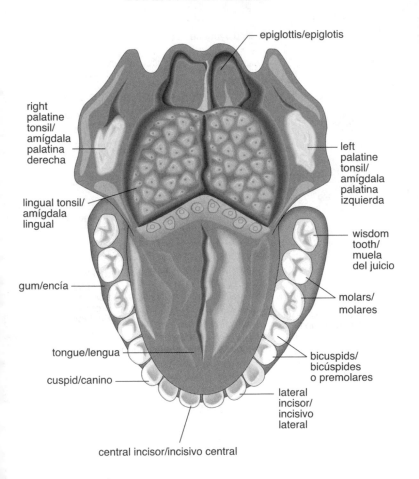

epiglottis/epiglotis

right palatine tonsil/ amígdala palatina derecha

left palatine tonsil/ amígdala palatina izquierda

lingual tonsil/ amígdala lingual

wisdom tooth/ muela del juicio

gum/encía

molars/ molares

tongue/lengua

bicuspids/ bicúspides o premolares

cuspid/canino

lateral incisor/ incisivo lateral

central incisor/incisivo central

Digestive System
Aparato o Sistema Digestivo

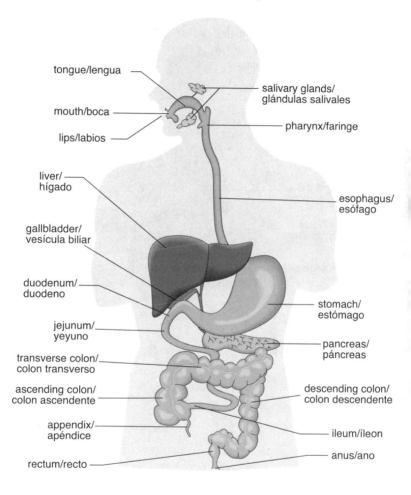

tongue/lengua

salivary glands/
glándulas salivales

mouth/boca

pharynx/faringe

lips/labios

liver/
hígado

esophagus/
esófago

gallbladder/
vesícula biliar

duodenum/
duodeno

stomach/
estómago

jejunum/
yeyuno

pancreas/
páncreas

transverse colon/
colon transverso

ascending colon/
colon ascendente

descending colon/
colon descendente

appendix/
apéndice

ileum/íleon

rectum/recto

anus/ano

Respiratory System
Aparato o Sistema Respiratorio

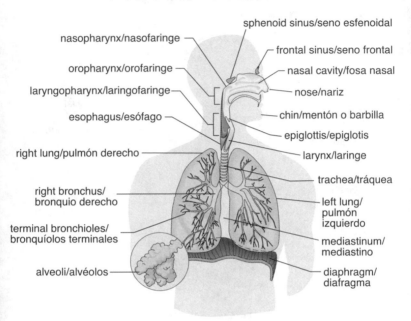

sphenoid sinus/seno esfenoidal

nasopharynx/nasofaringe

oropharynx/orofaringe

laryngopharynx/laringofaringe

esophagus/esófago

right lung/pulmón derecho

right bronchus/
bronquio derecho

terminal bronchioles/
bronquíolos terminales

alveoli/alvéolos

frontal sinus/seno frontal

nasal cavity/fosa nasal

nose/nariz

chin/mentón o barbilla

epiglottis/epiglotis

larynx/laringe

trachea/tráquea

left lung/
pulmón
izquierdo

mediastinum/
mediastino

diaphragm/
diafragma

General or Systemic Circulation
Circulación General o Sistemática

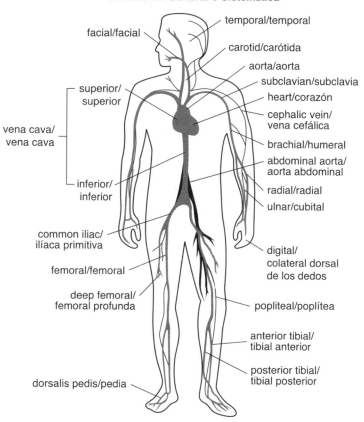

facial/facial

temporal/temporal

carotid/carótida

aorta/aorta

subclavian/subclavia

superior/
superior

heart/corazón

cephalic vein/
vena cefálica

vena cava/
vena cava

brachial/humeral

abdominal aorta/
aorta abdominal

inferior/
inferior

radial/radial

ulnar/cubital

common iliac/
ilíaca primitiva

digital/
colateral dorsal
de los dedos

femoral/femoral

deep femoral/
femoral profunda

popliteal/poplítea

anterior tibial/
tibial anterior

posterior tibial/
tibial posterior

dorsalis pedis/pedia

Urinary System
Sistema Urinario o Aparato Urinario

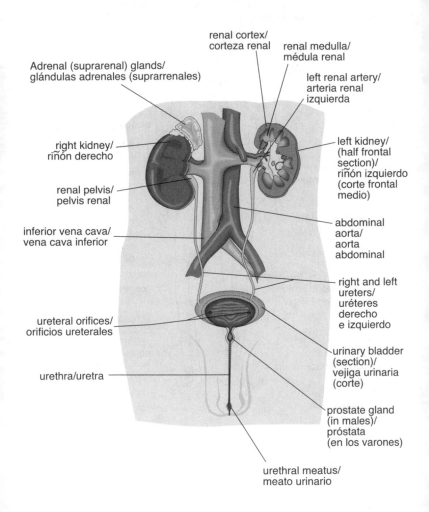

renal cortex/
corteza renal

renal medulla/
médula renal

Adrenal (suprarenal) glands/
glándulas adrenales (suprarrenales)

left renal artery/
arteria renal
izquierda

right kidney/
riñón derecho

left kidney/
(half frontal
section)/
riñón izquierdo
(corte frontal
medio)

renal pelvis/
pelvis renal

inferior vena cava/
vena cava inferior

abdominal
aorta/
aorta
abdominal

right and left
ureters/
uréteres
derecho
e izquierdo

ureteral orifices/
orificios ureterales

urinary bladder
(section)/
vejiga urinaria
(corte)

urethra/uretra

prostate gland
(in males)/
próstata
(en los varones)

urethral meatus/
meato urinario

ARTERIA	ARTERY
arteria aorta ascendente	ascending aorta artery
arteria aorta torácica descendente	descending thoracic aorta artery
arterias arciformes del riñon	arcuate arteries of the kidney
arteria auricular profunda	deep auricular artery
arteria axilar	axillary artery
arteria basilar	basilar artery
arterias bronquiales	bronchial arteries
arteria bucal	buccal artery
arteria capsular	capsular artery
arteria carótida (primitiva) (externa) (interna)	(common) (external) (internal) carotid artery
arteria central de la retina	central artery of retina
arteria cerebelosa	cerebellar artery
arteria cerebral	cerebral artery
arteria cervical ascendente	ascending cervical artery
arteria cervical transversa profunda	dorsal scapular artery
arterias ciliares largas posteriores	long posterior ciliary arteries
arteria circunfleja ilíaca	external epigastric artery
arteria circunfleja posterior	posterior circumflex artery
arterias conjuntivales posteriores	posterior conjunctival arteries
arteria coroidea anterior	anterior choroidal artery
arteria coronaria	coronary artery
arteria coronaria derecha	right coronary artery of heart
arteria coronaria estomáquica	left coronary artery of stomach
arteria coronaria inferior	inferior labial artery
arteria coronaria izquierda	left coronary artery of heart
arteria cubital	ulnar artery
arteria deferente	deferential artery
arteria del cuadríceps	quadriceps artery of femur
arteria dental	dental artery
arteria dentaria inferior	inferior alveolar artery
arteria diafragmática inferior	diaphragmatic artery
arteria dorsal del clítoris	dorsal artery of the clitoris
arteria dorsal del metatarso	arcuate artery of the foot
arteria dorsal del tarso	lateral tarsal artery
arteria espermática	testicular artery
arteria espinal anterior	anterior spinal artery
arteria esplénica	splenic artery
arteria facial transversa	transverse facial artery
arteria femoral	femoral artery
arteria funicular	cremasteric artery
arteria gastroduodenal	gastroduodenal artery
arteria glútea	superior gluteal artery
arteria humeral	brachial artery
arteria ilíaca interna	internal iliac artery
arteria ilíaca primitiva	common iliac artery
arteria intercostal superior	highest/superior intercostal artery
arterias interóseas dorsales	dorsal metacarpal arteries

arteria interventricular anterior	anterior interventricular artery
arteria interventricular posterior	descending posterior coronary artery
arteria isquiática	inferior gluteal artery
arteria lingual	lingual artery
quinta arteria lumbar	lowest/fifth lumbar artery
arteria mamaria (externa) (interna)	(external) (internal) mammary artery
arteria meníngea anterior	anterior meningeal artery
arteria obturatriz	obturator artery
arteria occipital	occipital artery
arteria oftálmica	ophthalmic artery
arteria pancreaticoduodenal inferior	duodenal artery
arterias perforantes	perforating arteries
arteria peronea	fibular artery; peroneal artery
arteria pilórica derecha	right coronary artery of stomach
arteria poplítea	popliteal artery
arteria pulmonar	pulmonary artery
arterias pudendas externas superior e inferior	external pudendal arteries
arteria radial	radial artery
arteria recurrente cubital	ulnar recurrent artery
arteria renal	renal artery
arterias sacras laterales	lateral sacral arteries
arteria sacra media	caudal artery
arterias sigmoideas	sigmoid arteries
arteria subclavia	subclavian artery
arteria sublingual	sublingual artery
arteria suprapúbica	pubic artery
arteria temporal profunda posterior	deep posterior temporal artery
arteria tibial	tibial artery
arteria timpánica	tympanic artery
arteria torácica inferior	lateral thoracic artery
arteria transversal de la cara	transverse facial artery
arteria umbilical	umbilical artery
arteria uretral	urethral artery
arteria uterina	uterine artery; fallopian artery
arteria vaginal	vaginal artery
arteria vertebral	vertebral artery
arterias yeyunales	jejunal arteries
ramos cardioesofágicos	inferior esophageal arteries
ramos caroticotimpánicos	caroticotympanic artery
ramos de las arterias pudendas externas	inguinal arteries
ramos superficiales de la arteria plantar interna	superficial medial artery of foot
vasos cortos del estómago	short gastric arteries

LIGAMENTO	LIGAMENT
aponeurosis buccinatofaríngea	pterygomandibular ligament
aponeurosis perineal profunda	ischioprostatic ligament
arco crural	crural ligament; inguinal ligament
arco del cuadrado lumbar	lateral arcuate ligament
arco del psoas	median arcuate ligament
cápsula articular	capsular ligament
cinta iliopectínea	iliopectineal ligament
cordón fibroso de la arteria umbilical	lateral umbilical ligament
diafragma urogenital	triangular ligament
epiplón gastrocólico	gastrocolic ligament
epiplón gastrosplénico	gastrolienal ligament
epiplón mayor	gastrocolic ligament
epiplón menor	gastrohepatic ligament
epiplón pancreaticosplénico	pancreaticosplenic ligament
fascículo profundo del ligamento sacrococcígeo posterior	deep dorsal sacrococcygeal ligament,
fascículo superficial del ligamento sacrococcígeo posterior	superficial dorsal sacrococcygeal ligament
haz anterior de la capa superficial del ligamento deltoideo	anterior talotibial ligament
haz posterior de la capa superficial del ligamento deltoideo	posterior talotibial ligament
ligamento acromioclavicular	acromioclavicular ligament
ligamento acromiocoracoideo	acromiocoracoid ligament
ligamento adiposo de la rodilla	adipose ligament of the knee
ligamento alveolodental	alveolodental ligament
ligamento ancho	broad ligament of uterus
ligamento anococcígeo	anococcygeal ligament
ligamento anterior de la articulación costovertebral	radiate ligament
ligamento anterior de la articulación de la muñeca	palmar radiocarpal ligament
ligamento anterior del martillo	tensor ligament
ligamento anular anterior del tarso	cruciate ligament of leg
ligamento anular de la base del estribo	annular ligament of base of stapes; stapedial ligament
ligamento anular del radio	annular ligament of radius; orbicular ligament of the radius
ligamento apendiculoovárico	apendiculo-ovarian ligament
ligamento arqueado	inferior pubic ligament
ligamento arqueado de la sínfisis púbica	pubic arcuate ligament
ligamento astragaloescafoideo	talonavicular ligament
ligamento calcaneoastragalino posterior	posterior talocalcaneal ligament
ligamento calcaneocuboideo inferior	plantar calcaneocuboid ligament; long plantar ligament

ligamento calcaneoescafoideo inferior	plantar calcaneonavicular ligament; spring ligament
ligamento caudal	caudal ligament
ligamento coracoclavicular	coracoclavicular ligament
ligamento coracohumeral	coracohumeral ligament
ligamento coracoideo	suprascapular ligament
ligamento coronario de la rodilla	coronary ligament of knee
ligamento coronario del hígado	coronary ligament of liver
ligamento costocentral	costocentral ligament
ligamento costoclavicular	costoclavicular ligament
ligamento costocoracoideo	costocoracoid ligament
ligamento costopericárdico	costopericardiac ligament
ligamento costovertebral	costovertebral ligament
ligamento cricoaritenoideo posterior	posterior cricoarytenoid ligament
ligamento cruciforme	cruciate ligament of atlas
ligamento de Falopio	fallopian ligament
ligamento del ovario	utero-ovarian ligament
ligamento deltoideo	deltoid ligament
ligamento dentado	denticulate ligament
ligamento diafragmático	diaphragmatic ligament
ligamento dorsal de las articulaciones carpometacarpianas	dorsal carpometacarpal ligament
ligamento esfenomaxilar	sphenomandibular ligament
ligamento espinoglenoideo	spinoglenoid ligament
ligamento esternopericardíaco superior	Luschka's ligament
ligamento estrellado	stellate ligament
ligamento frenocólico	phrenocolic ligament
ligamento frenogástrico	gastrophrenic ligament
ligamento frenosplénico	splenophrenic ligament
ligamento gastrofrénico	gastrophrenic ligament
ligamento gastrohepático	gastrohepatic ligament
ligamento gastropancreático	gastropancreatic ligament
ligamento hamatometacarpiano	hamatometacarpal ligament
ligamento hialoideocapsular	hyaloideocapsular ligament
ligamento humeral transverso de Gordon Brodie	transverse humeral ligament
ligamento iliofemoral	iliofemoral ligament
ligamento iliolumbar	iliolumbar ligament
ligamento iliopectíneo	iliopectineal ligament
ligamento iliopúbico	iliopubic ligament
ligamento inferior de la articulación pisipiramidal	pisohamate ligament
ligamento inferior de la sínfisis púbica	inferior pubic ligament
ligamento interarticular	interarticular ligament
ligamento interclavicular	interclavicular ligament

ligamento interóseo carpometacarpiano	interosseous carpometacarpal ligament
ligamento interóseo de la articulación astragalocalcánea	interosseous talocalcaneal ligament
ligamento interóseo de la articulación peroneotibial inferior	interosseous tibiofibular ligament
ligamento interóseo de las articulaciones costovertebrales	intra-articular ligament of costovertebral joints
ligamento interureteral	interureteral ligament
ligamento intraarticular de la articulación costovertebral	intra-articular ligament of costovertebral joints
ligamento isquiofemoral	ischiofemoral ligament
ligamento lateral externo de la articulación del codo	brachioradial ligament
ligamento lateral externo de la articulación de la rodilla	lateral ligament of knee
ligamento lateral externo de la articulación de la muñeca	lateral ligament of wrist
ligamento lateral externo de la articulación temporomaxilar	temporomandibular ligament
ligamento lateral interno de la articulación del codo	brachiocubital ligament; medial ligament of elbow joint
ligamento lateral interno de la articulación de la muñeca	medial ligament of wrist
ligamento lateral interno de la articulación de la rodilla	medial ligament of knee joint
ligamento nefrocólico	nephrocolic ligament
ligamento occipitoodontoideo medio	apical odontoid ligament
ligamento peroneoastragalino anterior	anterior talofibular ligament
ligamento peroneoastragalino posterior	posterior talofibular ligament
ligamento peroneocalcáneo	calcaneofibular ligament
ligamento poplíteo arqueado	arcuate popliteal ligament
ligamento poplíteo oblicuo de la articulación de la rodilla	oblique posterior ligament of knee
ligamento posterior de la articulación de la muñeca	dorsal radiocarpal ligament
ligamento pterigomaxilar	pterygomandibular ligament
ligamento pubiofemoral	pubofemoral ligament
ligamento pubiovesical	vesicopubic ligament
ligamento radiado de las articulaciones costovertebrales	stellate ligament
ligamento radial	radial ligament
ligamento redondo	round ligament
ligamento redondo de la cabeza del fémur	ligament of head of femur
ligamento romboidal	rhomboid ligament
ligamento rotuliano	patellar ligament

ligamento sacrociático mayor	sacrotuberous ligament
ligamento sacrociático menor	sacrospinous ligament
ligamento sacrococcígeo posterior	dorsal (or posterior) sacrococcygeal ligament
ligamento subpúbico	inferior pubic ligament; subpubic ligament
ligamento superior de la sínfisis del pubis	superior pubic ligament
ligamento supraespinoso	supraspinous ligament
ligamento suspensorio de la apófisis odontoides	apical odontoid ligament
ligamento suspensorio de la axila	suspensory ligament of axilla
ligamento suspensorio del cristalino	suspensory ligament of lens
ligamento tibioescafoideo	tibionavicular ligament
ligamento tiroaritenoideo inferior	vocal ligament
ligamento tiroaritenoideo superior	ventricular ligament; vestibular ligament
ligamento transverso de la pelvis	transverse perineal ligament; transverse ligament of pelvis
ligamento transverso del acetábulo	transverse ligament of acetabulum
ligamento transverso del atlas	Lauth's ligament
ligamento transverso del metacarpo	transverse metacarpal ligament
ligamento transverso del metatarso	transverse metatarsal ligament
ligamento transverso del perineo	transverse perineal ligament
ligamento trapezoideo	trapezoid ligament
ligamento triangular	triangular ligament
ligamento triangular del pulmón	pulmonary ligament
ligamento uteroovárico	utero-ovarian ligament
ligamento uterosacro	uterosacral ligament
ligamento vertebral común anterior	anterior longitudinal ligament
ligamento vertebral común posterior	posterior longitudinal ligament
ligamento vertebropleural	vertebrópleural ligament
ligamento vesicouterino	vesico-uterine ligament
ligamento yugal	cricosantorinian ligament
ligamento yugal de la rodilla	transverse ligament of knee
ligamentos alares de la odontoides	alar ligaments; cheek ligaments of axis
ligamentos alares de la apófisis odontoides	odontoid ligaments
ligamentos amarillos	subflavous ligament
ligamentos anterior y posterior de la articulación peroneotibial inferior	tibiofibular ligaments
ligamentos costotransversos	costotransverse ligaments
ligamentos costoxifoideos	xiphoid ligaments
ligamentos cruzados de la rodilla	cruciate ligaments of knee

ligamentos dorsales de las articulaciones carpianas	dorsal intercarpal ligaments
ligamentos dorsales de las articulaciones intermetatarsianas	transverse dorsal intermetatarsal ligaments
ligamentos escafoidocuneales	plantar cuneonavicular ligaments
ligamentos escafoidocuneales dorsales	dorsal scaphocuneiform ligaments
ligamentos glenohumerales	glenohumeral ligaments
ligamentos intercostales	intercostal ligaments
ligamentos intercuneales dorsales	dorsal intercuneiform ligaments
ligamentos interespinosos	interspinal ligaments
ligamentos interóseos carpianos	interosseous intercarpal ligaments
ligamentos interóseos de las articulaciones intermetatarsianas	interosseous metatarsal ligaments
ligamentos interóseos del tarso	interosseous ligaments of tarsus
ligamentos intertransversos	intertransverse ligaments
ligamentos oblicuos de la articulación carpometacarpiana del pulgar	oblique ligaments of carpometacarpal joint of thumb
ligamentos odontoideos	odontoid ligaments
ligamentos palmares de la articulación carpometacarpiana	volar carpometacarpal ligaments
ligamentos palmares de las articulaciones carpianas	palmar intercarpal ligaments
ligamentos palmares de las articulaciones metacarpofalángicas	palmar metacarpophalangeal ligaments
ligamentos plantares	plantar ligaments
ligamentos plantares de las articulaciones cuneales	plantar intercuneiform ligaments
ligamentos radiocarpianos	radiocarpal ligaments
ligamentos sacrociáticos	sacrosciatic ligaments
ligamentos sacrococcígeos anteriores	ventral (or anterior) sacrococcygeal ligaments
ligamentos sacrococcígeos laterales	lateral sacrococcygeal ligaments
ligamentos sacroiliacos anteriores	anterior sacroiliac ligaments
ligamentos sacroiliacos interóseos	interosseous sacroiliac ligaments
ligamentos sacroiliacos posteriores	dorsal sacroiliac ligaments
ligamentos transversos del metacarpo	metacarpal ligaments
ligamentos transversos del metatarso	cuneonavicular ligaments
ligamentos triangulares del hígado	lateral ligaments of liver; triangular ligaments of the liver
ligamentos uteropélvicos	uteropelvic ligaments
ligamentos uterorrectosacros	Mackenrodt's ligament; uterorectosacral ligaments
uraco	median umbilical ligament; vesico-umbilical ligament

MÚSCULO	MUSCLE
diafragma *m*	diaphragmatic muscle
fascículos tensores de la sinovial del codo	articular muscle of the elbow
músculo abductor	abductor muscle
músculo aritenoideo	arytenoid muscle
músculo articular	joint muscle
músculo auricular	auricular muscle
músculo bíceps braquial	biceps muscle of the arm
músculo biceps crural	biceps muscle of the thigh
músculo braquial anterior	brachial muscle
músculo bucofaríngeo	buccopharyngeal muscle
músculo ciliar	ciliary muscle
músculo constrictor de la faringe	constrictor muscle of the pharynx
músculo cremáster	cremaster muscle
músculo crural	femoral muscle; intermediate great muscle
músculo cuadrado	quadrate muscle
músculo largo del cuello	long muscle of the neck
músculo del estribo	fixator muscle of base of stapes
músculo del mentón o de la barba	chin muscle
músculo del ojo	muscles of the eye
músculo deltoides	deltoid muscle
músculo dilator	dilator muscle
músculo elevador del párpado superior	levator muscle of the upper eyelid
músculo esfínter	sphincter muscle
músculo espinoso	spinal muscle
músculos espinales o de la masa común	erector muscle of the spine
músculo esplenio	splenius muscle
músculo extensor	extensor muscle
músculo faringogloso	glossopharyngeal muscle
músculo flexor	flexor muscle
músculo glúteo	gluteal muscle
músculo ilíaco	iliac muscle
músculos intercostales	intercostal muscles
músculos interespinosos	interspinal muscles
músculos interóseos dorsales	dorsal interosseous muscles
músculos intertransversos	intertransverse muscles
músculo isquiocavernoso	erector muscle of the penis
músculo isquiococcígeo	coccygeal muscle
músculo lingual	longitudinal muscle of the tongue
músculo oblicuo mayor del abdomen	external oblique muscle of the abdomen
músculo oblicuo mayor del ojo	superior oblique muscle of the eyeball
músculo obturador	obturator muscle
músculo occipital	occipital muscle

músculo oponente	opposing muscle
músculo orbitario	orbital muscle
músculo palmar	palmar muscle
músculo palpebral	tarsal muscle
músculo papilar anterior del ventrículo izquierdo	anterior papillary muscle of the left ventricle
músculos papilares internos del ventrículo derecho	septal papillary muscles of the right ventricle
músculo pectoral	pectoral muscle
músculo peroneo lateral	fibular muscle
músculo poplíteo	popliteal muscle
músculo recto anterior mayor de la cabeza	long muscle of the head
músculo rectococcígeo	rectococcygeal muscle
músculo rectouterino	rectouterine muscle
músculos rotadores largos	long rotator muscles
músculos rotatorios	rotator muscles
músculo subclavio	subclavius muscle
músculo subescapular	subscapular muscle
músculo temporal	temporal muscle
músculo tensor de la sinovial de la rodilla	articular muscle of the knee
músculo tibial	tibial muscle
músculo transverso	transverse muscle
músculo trapecio	trapezius muscle
músculo triangular de los labios	depressor muscle of the angle of the mouth
músculo tríceps	triceps muscle
músculo vocal o fascículo propio de la cuerda vocal	vocal muscle

VENA	**VEIN**
tronco temporomaxilar	posterior facial vein
vena ácigos	azygos vein
vena aferente	afferent vein
venas agrandadas *fam*	enlargement of the veins
venas anteriores de los labios mayores y menores	anterior labial veins
venas anteriores del cráneo	frontal veins
vena auricular anterior del pabellón de la oreja	anterior auricular vein
vena auricular posterior del pabellón de la oreja	posterior auricular vein
vena cava (inferior) (superior)	(inferior) (superior) vena cava
vena cerebral (anterior) (inferior) (profunda)	(anterior) (inferior) (internal) cerebral vein
venas cerebrales ascendentes internas y externas	superior cerebral veins
vena coronaria derecha	small cardiac vein

vena coronaria estomáquica	left gastric vein
vena coronaria magna	great cardiac vein
vena coronaria mayor	great cardiac vein; left coronary vein
vena coronaria menor	small cardiac vein
venas costoaxilares	external mammary veins
venas cubitales	ulnar veins
venas del corazón	cardiac veins
venas del labio (inferior) (superior)	(inferior) (superior) labial veins
venas digitales (comunes) (dorsales) (palmares) del pie	(common) (dorsal) (palmar) digital veins of the foot
venas escapulares posteriores y cervicales transversas	transverse veins of neck
venas estriadas	striate veins
vena facial anterior común	anterior common facial vein
vena faríngea descendente	descending pharyngeal vein
vena femoral profunda	deep femoral vein
venas gástricas cortas	short gastric veins
venas hemorroidales (inferiores) (medias) (superiores)	(inferior) (middle) (superior) rectal veins
vena humeral	brachial vein
vena ilíaca (interna) (externa) (primitiva)	(internal) (external) (common) iliac vein
vena lumbar ascendente	ascending lumbar vein
vena mamaria interna	internal mammary/internal thoracic vein
vena mamaria externa	lateral thoracic vein
venas maxilares internas	maxillary veins
vena mediana basílica	median vein of the elbow
vena mediana del antebrazo	median vein of the forearm
venas perforantes	perforating veins
venas peroneas	fibular veins
vena pilórica	right gastric vein
venas posteriores de los labios mayores y menores	posterior labial veins
vena posterior del ventrículo izquierdo	posterior vein of left ventricle
vena profunda	deep vein
venas profundas de la lengua	deep lingual veins
venas profundas del pene	deep veins of penis
vena pulmonar (derecha/izquierda) (inferior/superior)	(right/left) (inferior/superior) pulmonary vein
venas renales	renal veins
vena safena (accesoria) (interna) (externa)	(accessory) (great) (small) saphenous vein
vena satélite	accompanying vein
vena subclavia	subclavian vein

vena temporal (profunda) (media) (superficial)   (deep) (middle) (superficial) temporal vein

vena transversal de la cara   transverse facial vein

vena umbilical   umbilical vein

venas uterinas   uterine veins

venas varicosas   varicose veins

vena yugular   jugular *n*; jugular vein

A

a[1], *slang*, amphetamines
a corto plazo, short-term
a cuenta, on account
a la derecha, on/to the right
a la izquierda, on/to the left
a lo largo, long-term
a menudo, often
a prueba de ácidos, acid-proof
a veces, occasionally
abandonar, to abandon
abertura, opening (*hueco*)
abdomen, *m*, abdomen; ~ **agudo** acute abdomen; appendicitis *slang*
abdominal, *adj*, abdominal
abierto, *adj*, open
abnegación, *f*, self-denial
abnegado, *adj*, self-sacrificing
abofetear, to slap (*golpear*)
abombar(se), to begin to spoil; to stink; ~(**se**) *PR*, to smell bad
abortar, to abort
aborto, abortion; ~ **espontáneo** spontaneous abortion; ~ **inducido** induced abortion; ~ **inminente** threatened abortion; ~ **provocado** induced abortion; ~ **terapéutico** therapeutic abortion; ~ **tubárico** tubal abortion
abreviar, to shorten (*reducir*)
abreviatura, abbreviation
abrigo, overcoat
abrir, to open
abrumador, *adj*, overpowering
abrumar, to overpower; to overwhelm (con trabajo, etc.)
absceso, abscess; ~ **en la mama** milk abscess
absorbencia, absorbency
absorbente, *adj*, absorbent; ~ **higiénico**, *m*, sanitary napkin
absorber, to absorb
abstención, *f*, abstention

abstenerse, to abstain; ~ **de las relaciones sexuales** to abstain from sexual relations
abstraerse, to absorb
abundante, *adj*, abundant
abuja[1], spike (*aguja hipodérmica*)
abusar de, to abuse; to over-indulge in
abuso, abuse; ~ **del alcohol** alcohol abuse; ~ **habitual del opio** opium habit; ~ **infantil** child abuse
acabar, to experience orgasm
acceso, access; *Med*, onset; seizure; fit; attack (*de locura, tos, etc.*); ~ **para silla de ruedas** wheelchair access
accidente, *m*, accident; ~ **cerebral** (cerebrovascular) stroke; ~ **de aviación** airplane accident; ~ **de carretera** highway accident; ~ **de circulación** traffic accident; ~ **de coche** car accident; ~ **de trabajo** industrial accident
acción, *f*, action
aceite, *m*, oil; acid[2]; LSD *slang;* ~ **de algodón** cottonseed oil; ~ **de almendras amargas** bitter almond oil; ~ **de cártamo** safflower oil; ~ **de castor** castor oil; ~ **de comer** cooking oil; ~ **de gaulteria** oil of wintergreen; ~ **de hígado de bacalao** cod liver oil; ~ **de linaza** linseed oil; ~ **de maíz** corn oil; ~ **de oliva** olive oil; ~ **de ricino** castor oil; ~ **de mineral blanco** mineral oil; ~ **para niños** baby oil
aceituna, olive
aceleración, *f*, acceleration
aceptar, to accept
acera, sidewalk
acercar(se) a, to approach
acero inoxidable, stainless steel

acetaminofén, *m*, acetaminophen
achacoso, *adj*, ailing; sickly (*persona*)
achaque, *m*, affliction (*de la vejez*); sickliness
aciclovir, *m*, acyclovir
acidez, *f*, acidity
ácido, acid; ~ **acético (puro)** acetic acid; ~ **acetilsalicílico** acetylsalicylic acid; ~ **arsénico** arsenic acid; ~ **ascórbico** ascorbic acid; ~ **bórico** boric acid; ~ **carbólico** carbolic acid; ~ **cianhídrico** cyanhydric acid; ~ **desoxirribonucleico/ADN** deoxyribonucleic acid/DNA; ~ **fólico** folic acid; ~ **fosfórico** phosphoric acid; ~ **gástrico** gastric acid; ~ **graso** fatty acid; ~ **inosínico** inosinic acid; ~ **láctico** lactic acid; ~ **oleico** oleic acid; ~ **oxálico** oxalic acid; ~ **paramino salicílico** p-aminosalicylic acid/PAS; ~ **prúsico** cyanhydric acid; ~ **ribonucleico/ARN** ribonucleic acid/RNA; ~ **salicílico** salicylic acid; ~ **sulfúrico** sulfuric acid; ~ *sg*, acid[2]; LSD *slang;* amphetamines
acné, *f*, acne; ~ **rosácea** *f*, acne rosacea
acoger, to shelter (*pobre, etc.*)
acondicionador de aire, *m*, air conditioner
aconsejar, to advise
acordar (ue), to agree
acortar, to shorten (*reducir*)
acrílico, *adj*, acrylic
actitud, *f*, attitude; outlook
activar, to activate
actividad, *f*, activity; ~ **fuerte** strenuous activity; ~ **óptica** optical activity; ~ **sexual** sexual activity
activo, *adj*, active
acto, act; action; ~ **carnal** sexual intercourse; ~ **impulsivo** acting-out; ~ **reflejo** reflex action
actual, *adj*, actual; current; present
acuclillarse, to squat
acumulación, *f*, accumulation

acupuntura, acupuncture
adaptable, *adj*, adjustable
adaptarse, to adjust
adecuado, *adj*, adequate
adelantado, *adj*, advanced
adelanto, advancement
adelfa, oleander
adenoidectomía, adenoidectomy
adenoide, *f*, adenoid
adenoideo, *adj*, adenoid
adenoma, *m*, adenoma
adherencia, adhesion; synechia
adherir (ie), to attach
adhesivo, *adj*, adhesive
adicción, *f*, (drug) addiction
adicional, *adj*, added
adictivo, *m, adj*, addictive
adicto, *m, adj*, (drug) addict; addicted; ~ **a cocaína** snow bird[2], *slang;* ~ **a droga(s)** (drug) addict; ~ **a heroína** sleep walker[2]; ~ **a las drogas narcóticas** (drug) addict
adiposo, *adj*, adipose; fatty *Anat*
administrativo, *adj*, administrative
admisión, *f*, admitting; admission (*al hospital*)
adolescencia, adolescence
adolescente, *m/f*, adolescent
adopción, *f*, adoption
adoptar, to adopt
adoptivo, *adj*, adoptive
adormido, *adj*, asleep
adquirir (ie), to obtain
adrenalina, adrenalin(e)
adulto, adult
adverso, *adj*, adverse
adyacente, *adj*, adjoining
aeróbicos, *m, pl*, aerobics
aerofagia, aerophagia
aerosol, *m*, aerosol
afasia, aphasia
afección, *f*, affection *Med*; complaint; disease
afectar, to affect; to shake (*empeorar*)
afecto, affection
afectuoso, *adj*, affectionate
afeitar(se), to shave
afilado, *adj*, sharp

aflicción, *f*, affliction *Med*, illness; sore; ~ (*pesar*) sorrow

afligido, *adj*, sorry (*triste*)

afligir, to afflict

afonía, aphonia; hoarseness

afuera, *adv*, outside

agarrotamiento, stiffness (*de los músculos*)

agarrotar(se), to stiffen (*músculos*)

agente, *m*, agent

agitado, *adj*, agitated

agitar, to agitate; to shake (*líquido*); ~**se** to become agitated; **agítese bien antes de usar** shake well before using

agobiante, *adj*, oppressive (*carga mental*)

agobiar (de), to overburden

agonía, agony

agonizar, to agonize

agotamiento, strain (*extenuada*)

agotar, to overexert; to overfatigue; ~ **los nervios** to strain

agravar, to aggravate

agraviar, to injure

agravio, outrage (*a los sentimientos propios*)

agregar, to add

agresión, *f*, aggression

agresivo, *adj*, aggressive

agridulce, *adj*, sweet-and-sour

agriera, *SpAm*, heartburn

agrietado, *adj*, chapped

agrietar, to split (*la piel, los labios*); ~(**se**) to crack (*la piel, los labios*); ~**se** to chap

agrio, *adj*, bitter (*amargo*); sour

agruras del estómago, *fam*, heartburn

agua[3], *f*, water; ~**s** bag of waters; ~ **con alto contenido de minerales** hard water; ~ **con azúcar** glucose water; ~ **con mostaza** mustard water; ~ **con poco contenido de minerales** soft water; ~ **con sal** saline solution; ~ **corriente** running water; ~ **de hamamelis** witch hazel; ~ **de la llave** tap water; ~ **de lluvia** rain

water; ~ **de manzanilla** camomile tea; ~ **del amnios** amniotic fluid; ~ **del grifo** tap water; ~ **destilada** distilled water; ~ **dulce** fresh water; ~ **en el cerebro** water on the brain (*hidrocefalia*); ~ **en los sesos** hydrocephalus; ~ **ferruginosa** iron water; ~ **jabonosa** soapy water; ~**s mayores** *pl*, *euph*, bowel movement; ~ **mayores** *fam*, feces; ~**s menores** *pl*, *euph*, urine; ~ **mineral** mineral water; ~ **oxigenada** hydrogen peroxide; peroxide; sodium peroxide; ~ **potable** drinking water; ~ **purificada** purified water; ~ **salada** salt water; ~ **salina** saline solution; ~ **yodurada** iodine water

aguantar, to bear (*tolerar*); to endure; to last; to tolerate; to withstand; ~ **la respiración** to hold one's breath

aguar, to dilute

aguardiente de caña, *m*, rum

agudeza, acuity; ~ **visual** visual acuity/VA ; ~ **visual discriminatoria** visual discriminatory acuity/VDA

agudizarse, to become more acute

agudo, *adj*, acute; keen; high-pitched; severe; sharp (*afilado*)

aguijar, *PR*, to goad

aguijón, *m*, stinger (*de abeja, avispa, etc.*)

aguja, needle; ~[1] nail[2] (*aguja para una inyección de droga*); spike[2] (*aguja hipodérmica*); ~ **aspiradora** aspirating needle; ~ **de aneurisma** aneurysm needle; ~ **de insulina** diabetic needle; ~ **hipodérmica** hypodermic needle; ~ **hueca** hollow needle

agujero, hole; vent (*hoyo, pasaje*); *vulg*, *Chicano*, anus; vagina; ~ **de trépano** drill hole; ~ **de ventilación** vent (*respiradero*)

agujetas en las piernas, *f*, *pl*, stiff-

ness of legs (*después de hacer ejercicio*)
aguoso, *adj*, watery
aguzar el oído, to strain one's ears
ahijado, godchild
ahogamiento, drowning
ahogar(se), to suffocate; to choke (*debido a la falta de aire*); to drown
ahogo, choking; suffocation; **~s** shortness of breath
ahoguijo, congestion of the chest; shortness of breath
ahoguío, congestion of the chest; *fam*, shortness of breath; *fam*, *Mex*, asthma
ahora, *adv*, now; **~ mismo** *adv*, right away; right now
ahorcadura, hanging
ahorcamiento, hanging
ahorcar, to hang (*el cuello*)
ahorita, *fam*, right now
ahorrar, to save (*electricidad, dinero, etc.*)
aire, *m*, air; flatus; *slang*, gas (*pedo*); **~ acondicionado** air conditioning; **~ ambiente** room air; **~ en el ojo**, *fam*, conjunctivitis; pinkeye; **~ fresco** fresh air; **~ puro** fresh air; **~ respiratorio** tidal air; **~ viciado** foul air
airear, to air (*ventilar*)
aislamiento, isolation; **~ por cuarentena** isolation
aislar, to isolate; **~ en cultivos bacterianos** to grow out a culture
ají, *m*, chili pepper
ajo, garlic
ajumao, *adj*, intoxicated
ajumar(se), to get drunk; to get zonked *slang*; *PR*, to tie one on (*emborracharse*)
ajustable, *adj*, adjustable
ajustador, *m*, *Cu*, brassiere
ajustar, to correct; to fit (*gafas, zapatos*)
ajuste, *m*, adjustment
al, at the; to the; **~ aire libre** outdoors; **~ alcance de la mano** within reach; at one's elbow; **~ alcance**

de la vista within the range of vision; **~ anochecer** at dusk; **~ atardecer** at dusk; **~ azar** at random; **~ contado** cash over the counter; **~ lado de** next to; **~ mes** monthly; per month; **~ ras** level
alado, *adj*, winged
alambre, *m*, wire; **~ de acero inoxidable** stainless steel wire; **~ de contacto** electrical lead wire; **~ de púas** barbed wire
alambrito, coil (*anticonceptivo*); loop (*anticonceptivo*)
alargar, to lengthen
alarido, howl (*de dolor*)
alarma, alarm; **~ generalizada** generalized fear
alarmante, *adj*, alarming
alarmarse, to become alarmed (*asustado*)
alarmista, *m/f*, alarmist
alazor, *m*, safflower
albaricoque, *m*, apricot
albayalde, *m*, (*syn. para hormiguilla brava*) insect
albergue para jóvenes, *m*, youth hostel
albino, *m*, *adj*, albino
albornoz, *m*, bathrobe
alboroto, excitement (*desorden*)
albumen, *m*, albumen
albúmina, albumen; albumin
álcali, *m*, alkali
alcalino, *adj*, alkaline
alcalizar, to alkalize
alcance, *m*, reach; scope (*extensión*)
alcanfor, *m*, camphor
alcanzamiento, overreaching
alcanzar, to reach; **~ su pleno desarrollo** to reach full growth
alcohol, *m*, alcohol; **~, abuso del** alcohol abuse; **~, consumo del** alcohol consumption; **~ de madera** wood alcohol; **~ desnaturalizado** denatured alcohol; **~ etílico** ethyl alcohol; **~ metílico** methyl alcohol; **~ para fricciones** rubbing alcohol
alcohólico, *m*, *adj*, alcoholic

Alcohólicos Anónimos, AA; Alcoholics Anonymous
alcoholismo, alcoholism
alcohómetro, alcoholometer; breathalyser; breathalyzer
ALD[1], LSD
aldilla, inguinal region; *fam*, groin
aleación, *f*, alloy
alegrarse (de), to be glad
alegre, *adj*, cheerful; jolly (*jovial*)
alergeno/alergénico, allergen
alergia, allergy; hay fever
alérgico, *adj*, allergic
alergista, *m/f*, allergist
alergólogo, allergist
alerta, *adj*, [Ú.t.c.s.m.] alert; *adv*, on the alert
alertar, to alert
aleta, flange *Dent*; ~ **bucal** buccal flange *Dent*; ~ **de dentadura** denture flange *Dent*; ~ **labial** labial flange *Dent*
aletargado, *adj*, lethargic
aletargamiento, lethargy
aleteo, flutter
alfalfa[1], marijuana
alferecía, *fam*, convulsion resulting from fever
alfiler, *m*, pin; ~ **de seguridad** safety pin
alfombra, carpet; rug; *PR*, *Chicano*, rash; ~ **de baño** bath mat
alfombría, *Chicano*, German measles; rubella; rash
alga[3], alga
algodón, *m*, cotton; ~ **absorbente** absorbent cotton; ~ **estéril** sterile cotton; ~ **hidrófilo** absorbent cotton
algodoncillo, moniliasis; *fam*, thrush
alguna vez, *adv*, ever
alianza, wedding ring
aliento, breath; ~ **feo** halitosis
alifafe, *m*, *slang*, chronic complaint
aligeramiento, lightening (*nacimiento*)
alimentación, *f*, feeding; nourishment; ~ **al seno** breast feeding;

~ **artificial** artificial feeding; ~ **equilibrada** balanced diet; ~ **por sonda** feeding by tube; ~ **por vía intravenosa** intravenous feeding; ~ **suplementaria** supplementary feeding
alimentado por sonda, *adj*, tube-fed
alimentar, to feed; to nourish
alimenticio, *adj*, alimentary; nutritional
alimento, aliment; food; nourishment
alineamiento, alignment
alinear, to line up; ~(se) to align
aliñado, *adj*, constipated
aliñamiento, constipation
alivianado[1], *adj*, high on (*drogas narcóticas*)
aliviane[1], cocaine
aliviar, to allay; to alleviate; to cure; to ease; to make better; to relieve; to subdue (*dolor*); ~(se) to dull (*reducir el dolor*); ~se to get well; to loosen up (*toser*); to recover (*de una enfermedad*); ~se *Chicano*, *Mex*, *fam*, to deliver; ~se *Mex*, *fam*, to give birth
alivio, relief
alma[3], *f*, soul
almacenaje, *m*, storage
almacenar, to store
almeja, mussel
almíbar, *m*, syrup (*culinario*)
almidón, *m*, starch
almidonado, *adj*, starchy; stiff (*con almidón*)
almohada, cushion
almohadilla, cushion; pad; pillow; ~ **caliente eléctrica** electric heating pad; ~ **eléctrica** heating pad; ~ **higiénica** sanitary napkin; ~ **neumática en forma de anillo** pillow (*una cámara de goma*)
almohadita, nursing pad
almorranas, *fam*, hemorrhoids; *f*, *pl*, piles
almorzar (ue), to eat lunch; to have lunch
almuerzo, lunch

áloe, *m*, aloe
alojamiento, quarters
alojarse (en), to take up quarters
alquitrán, *m*, tar
alrededor de la cintura, around the middle/waist
alta[3] **de un enfermo**, discharge from the hospital
altavoz, *m*, loud-speaker
alteración, *f*, alteration
alterado, upset
alterar, to disturb (*de paz*; *planes*)
alternancia, alternation
alternar, to alternate
alternativa, alternative
alterno, *adj*, alternate
alto, *adj*, tall; high; ~ **riesgo** high risk; **alta presión** *f*, hypertension (*alta presión arterial*); **alta tensión** *f*, high voltage; ~ **vacío** high vacuum
altura, height; ~ **cuspídea** cusp height; ~ **en posición de pie** standing height; ~ **en posición sentada** sitting height; ~ **promedio** average height
alucinación, *f*, hallucination; ~ **auditiva** auditory hallucination; ~ **del muñón** stump hallucination; ~ **depresiva** depressive hallucination; ~ **gustativa** gustatory hallucination; ~ **olfativa** olfactory hallucination; ~ **refleja** reflex hallucination; ~ **táctil** tactile hallucination; ~ **visual** visual hallucination
alucinante, *m*, *adj*, hallucinogen; ~**s**[1] LSD
alucinar, to hallucinate
alucinatorio, *adj*, hallucinatory
alucine, *m*, cocaine
alucinógeno, drug hallucinogenic; hallucinogen
alumbrado, *adj*, *slang*, *Chicano*, drunk; ~ **de neón** *adj*, neon lighting
alumbramiento, afterbirth; birth; childbirth; confinement; ~ **con**

fórceps forceps assisted delivery; ~ **múltiple** multiple birth
alumbrao, *adj*, *PR*, knowledgeable
alumbrar, to give birth
alveolar, *adj*, alveolar
alveolo/alvéolo, alveolus (*pl*, *alveoli*); socket (*de un diente*); tooth socket; ~ **pulmonar** air sack; air vacuole
alzar, to elevate (*los ojos*, *la voz*)
ama[3], lady of the house; housekeeper; ~ **de casa** housewife; HW; ~ **de cría** baby nurse; wet nurse; ~ **de leche** foster mother; wet nurse
amable, *adj*, kind; sympathetic (*generoso*)
amago, touch *Med*
amalgama, amalgam
amamantamiento, nursing
amamantar, *form*, to breast feed; to nurse; to suckle
amapola, poppy; ~[1] (*término usado en las cárceles y prisiones*) marijuana
amargo, *m*, bitters; ~ **de Angostura** Angostura bitters; *adj*, bitter
amarihuanar[1], to administer marijuana to s.o.; ~**se**[1] to take marijuana
amarillas[1], nebbis[2]
amarillento, *adj*, yellowish
amarillo, *adj*, yellow
amarrar, to bind (*atar*); to tie; ~ **los tubos** to tie the tubes
amarre de las trompas, *m*, *fam*, tubal ligation
amasadura, kneading
amasamiento, kneading
amasar, to caress; to knead; to mix (cemento, harina, etc.)
ambiental, *adj*, environmental
ambiente, *m*, environment; ~ **y herencia** environment and heredity/E & H
ambliopia/ambliopía, amblyopia; lazy eye
ambulancia, ambulance
ambulatorio, clinic (*lugar para*

ayuda médica gratis); *adj*, ambulatory

ameba, amoeba

amenaza de aborto, threatened abortion

amenorrea (*falta de menstruación*), amenorrhea

amiba, amoeba; ~[1] PCP

amígdala, tonsil

amigdalectomía, tonsillectomy

amigdalitis, *f*, glandular fever; tonsillitis; ~ **supurativa** quinsy (*dolor de garganta*)

amigdalotomía, tonsillectomy

amigo, friend

amiláceo, starchy

aminoácido, amino acid

aminoglucósido, aminoglycoside

amnesia, amnesia; loss of memory; memory loss

amnésico, *m*, *adj*, amnesic

amniocentesis, *f*, amniocentesis

amnios, amnion

amniótico, *adj*, amniotic

amodorrado, *adj*, drowsy (*dormido*)

amogollao, *adj*, *PR*, sticky (*pegadizo*)

amogollar(se), *PR*, to become complicated

amoníaco/amoniaco, ammonia

amontonarse, to crush into

amor, *m*, love; ~ **propio** self-esteem; ~[1] heroin

amoratado, *adj*, black and blue; bruised (*en una área*); *fam*, cyanotic

amordazar, to gag (*para evitar que hable*)

amortiguado, *adj*, buffered

amortiguador, *m*, buffer

amortiguamiento, buffering

amortiguar(se), to dull (*sonidos*)

amoxacilina, amoxacillin

ampicilina, ampicillin

ampliación, *f*, enlargement

ampliar, to enlarge (*hacer más grande*)

amplificación, *f*, amplification

amplificado, *adj*, amplified

amplificador, *m*, magnifier

amplificar, to amplify; to magnify

amplio, *adj*, wide; ~ **espectro** broad-spectrum; (*Vea antibiótico.*)

amplitud, *f*, range; ~ **de la variación** variation width

ampolla, bleb; blister (*en la piel*); cartridge; vesicle; vial; ~**s** *pl*, *fam*, herpes; ~ **en los labios** fever blister

ampollar(se), to blister

ampolleta, ampoule/ampule; bulb (*de un termómetro*)

ámpula, ampoule/ampule

amputación, *f*, amputation; ~ **a colgajos** flap amputation; ~ **a doble colgajo** double flap amputation; ~ **sin colgajo** flapless amputation

amputar, to amputate; to cut off; to truncate

anabolismo, constructive metabolism

anadear, to waddle

anadeo, waddle

anafilaxia, anaphylaxis

analfabetismo, illiteracy

analfabeto, *adj*, illiterate

analgesia, analgesia; ~ **caudal continua** continuous caudal analgesia; ~ **de superficie** surface analgesia; ~ **por infiltración** infiltration analgesia

analgésico, *m*, *adj*, analgesic; pain killer

análisis, *m*, *sg/pl*, analysis; test (*de sangre, orina, etc.*); ~ **cromosómico** karyotyping; ~ **cualitativo** qualitative analysis; ~ **cuantitativo** quantitative analysis; ~ **de (la) sangre** blood analysis; blood chemistry; blood test; hematology; ~ **de esputos** sputum test; ~ **de la orina** urinalysis test; urinalysis; ~ **de laboratorio** laboratory test; ~ **de los orines** urinalysis; ~ **oclusal** occlusal analysis

analizador del oxígeno de la sangre, *m*, blood oxygen analyzer analizar, to analyze

anaranjado, *adj*, orange (*color*)

anatomía, anatomy

anatómico, *adj*, anatomic; anatomical

anca, buttock

anciana, old woman

anciano, elderly (*hombre*); old man; *adj*, aged; ~ de más edad/mayor elder

andadera, *f*, walker

andador, *m*, walker

andar, to walk; ~ (+ *adj*)[1], to be high[2]; ~ a tientas to grope; ~ andando to be up and about after an illness; ~ bombo *slang*, to be/get drunk; ~ botando[1] to be blasted[2]; to be high[2]; to get high[2]; ~ carga[1] to be carrying narcotic drugs; ~ cargado[1] to be carrying narcotic drugs; ~ con los hombros caídos y la cabeza inclinada to slouch (*mala postura*); ~ con paso vacilante to be shaky on one's legs; ~ con rodeos to avoid the issue; ~ crudo[1] to have a hangover; ~ derecho[1] to be clean[2] (*de drogas*); ~ desgarbado to slouch (*mala postura*); ~ dormido to walk in one's sleep; ~ eléctrico *slang*, to be/get drunk; ~ elevado a-mil[1] to be blasted[2]; to be high[2]; ~ en la línea *slang*, to be/get drunk; ~ enfermo[1] to be in need; ~ hasta las manitas[1] to be blasted[2]; to be high[2]; ~ hasta las manos[1] to be blasted[2]; to be high[2]; ~ hypo[1] to be blasted[2]; to be/get high[2]; ~ limpio[1] to be clean[2] (*de drogas*); ~ loco[1] to be blasted[2]; to be/get high[2]; *slang*, to be/get drunk; ~ locote[1] to be blasted[2]; to be/get high[2]; ~ pasado[1] to be blasted[2]; to be/get high[2]; ~ prendido[1] to be blasted[2]; to be/get high[2]; ~ servido[1] to be blasted[2]; to be/get high[2]; ~ subido a-mil[1] to be blasted[2]; to be high[2]; ~ volado *fam*, to be distracted; to go berserk; ~ volando to berserk

andén, *m*, *Ven*, *Col*, *CA*, sidewalk

anemia, anemia; weak blood *slang*; ~ (aguda) febril (acute) febrile anemia; ~ (atrófica) aplástica (atrophic) aplastic anemia; ~ de células falciformes sickle cell anemia; ~ de Cooley thalassemia major; ~ drepanocítica sickle cell anemia; ~ ferropénica/ferropriva *form*, iron deficiency anemia; ~ hemolítica (aguda) (acute) hemolytic anemia; ~ mediterránea thalassemia major; ~ perniciosa pernicious anemia; iron deficiency anemia; ~ por deficiencia de hierro iron deficiency anemia

anémico, *adj*, anemic

anestesia, anesthesia; ~ caudal caudal anesthesia; ~ de bloque block anesthesia; ~ en silla de montar saddleblock anesthesia; ~ epidural epidural anesthesia; ~ equilibrada balanced anesthesia; ~ espinal spinal anesthesia; ~ general general anesthesia; ~ local local anesthesia; ~ por compresión compression anesthesia; ~ por inhalación inhalation anesthesia; ~ raquídea spinal anesthesia; ~ regional regional anesthesia; ~ total general anesthesia; ~ venosa vein anesthesia

anestesiar, to anesthetize

anestesiología, anesthesiology

anestesiólogo, anesthesiologist

anestético, *m*, *adj*, anesthetic

aneurisma, *m/f*, [*Ú.m.c.m.*], aneurysm; ~ abdominal abdominal aneurysm; ~ aórtico aortic aneurysm; ~ arteriovenoso arteriovenous aneurysm; ~ cardíaco cardiac aneurysm; ~ cirsoideo cirsoid aneurysm; ~

disecante dissecting aneurysm; ~ **embólico** embolic aneurysm; ~ **espurio** false aneurysm; ~ **falso** false aneurysm; ~ **fusiforme** fusiform aneurysm; ~ **micótico** mycotic aneurysm; ~ **ramificado** branching aneurysm; ~ **saculado** sacculated aneurysm; ~ **silencioso** silent aneurysm; ~ **ventricular** ventricular aneurysm; ~ **verdadero** true aneurysm

aneurismograma, *m*, aneurysmogram

anfetamina, amphetamine; **~s** bennies/benz/benzies[2]

anfiteatro, dissecting room

angina, angina; ~ **abdominal** angina abdominis; ~ **aguda** acute angina; ~ **de pecho** angina pectoris; cardiac neuralgia; ~ **de Vicente** trench fever; trench mouth; Vincent's angina; ~ **estreptocócica** strep throat; angina streptococcus; ~ **falsa** mock angina; ~ **folicular** follicular angina; ~ **herpética** canker sore; ~ **inestable** unstable angina; ~ **péctoris** angina pectoris; quinsy (*garganta dolorida*); **~s** *Mex, Ven, fam*, tonsils

angiocardiografía, angiocardiography

angiocardiopatía, angiocardiopathy

angiografía, angiogram; angiography; angiography test

angiograma, *m*, angiogram

angioma, *m*, angioma; ~ **elevado**; raspberry mark; strawberry mark

angioplastia, angioplasty; ~ **transluminal percutánea (coronaria)** percutaneous transluminal (coronary) angioplasty

ángulo, angle; bend; ~ **coronal** coronary angle; ~ **costal** costal angle; ~ **cuspídeo** cusp angle; ~ **de abertura** angle of aperture; ~ **de convergencia** angle of convergence; ~ **de desviación** angle of deviation; ~ **de elevación** elevation angle; ~ **de incidencia** angle of incidence; ~ **de la mandíbula** angle of the jaw; ~ **de polarización** angle of polarization; ~ **de porte** carrying angle; ~ **de reflexión** angle of reflection; ~ **del ojo** corner of the eye; ~ **mandibular** angle of the jaw; ~ **óptico** optic angle; ~ **visual** visual angle

angustia, agony; anguish (*mental*); distress (*congoja*); heartache; *fam*, anxiety; **~s** throes *pl*

angustiar, to distress (*congoja*); **~se** to agonize

angustioso, *adj*, distressing (*doloroso*)

anhelo, longing

anhídrido carbónico, carbon dioxide

aniarse, *PR*, to go to bed

anillo, ring; ring (*DIU, anticonceptivo*); ~ **de compromiso** *Mex*, engagement ring; ~ **de oclusión** *Dent*, occlusion ring; ~ **de prometida** engagement ring; ~ **para vaciado** *Dent*, casting ring; ~/**sortija de boda** wedding ring; ~/**sortija de casamiento** wedding ring; ~/**sortija de matrimonio** wedding ring; ~ **vascular** vascular ring

animal, *m, adj*, animal

animar, to become animated; to encourage; **~(se)** to liven up

ánimo, spirit

ano, anus

anoche, *adv*, last night

anomalía, anomaly; ~ **congénita** congenital anomaly; developmental anomaly

anonadar, to be crushed by (*abrumador*)

anorexia, anorexia; ~ **mental** anorexia nervosa; ~ **nerviosa** anorexia nervosa

anormal, *adj*, abnormal

anquilosado, *adj*, stiff (*Med: articulación*)

anquilosamiento, stiffness (*de una articulación*)
anquilosar(se), to stiffen (*una articulación*)
ansia, anxiety (*ansiedad*); ~s throes, *fam*, anxiety; ~ de la muerte throes of death; ~ matutinas morning sickness; tener ~s to feel sick
ansiedad, *f*, anxiety
ansiolítico, tranquilizer
ansioso, *adj*, anxious
antagonista, *f*, *adj*, antagonist
antaño, *adv*, long ago
anteayer, day before yesterday
antebrazo, forearm
antecedente tromboplástico del plasma, *m*, plasma thromboplastic antecedent/PTA
antedatar, to backdate
anteojos, *m*, *pl*, eyeglasses; glasses; spectacles; ~ oscuros sunglasses
antepié, *m*, *fam*, ball of the foot
anterobius, *m*, piperazine
antiácido, *m*, *adj*, antacid
antibiótico, *m*, *adj*, antibiotic; ~ de alcance amplio broad-spectrum antibiotic; ~ de alcance reducido limited-spectrum antibiotic; ~ de espectro amplio broad-spectrum antibiotic; ~ de espectro reducido limited-spectrum antibiotic
anticoagulante, *m*, *adj*, anticoagulant; blood thinner
anticolinérgico, *m*, *adj*, anticholinergic
anticoncepción, *f*, contraception
anticoncepcionismo, birth control
anticonceptivo, *m*, *adj*, contraceptive
anticongelante, *m*, antifreeze
anticonvulsivo, *m*, *adj*, anticonvulsant
anticuado, *adj*, obsolete; outdated
anticuerpo, antibody; ~ (in)completo (in)complete antibody; ~ anafiláctico anaphylactic antibody; ~ bloqueador blocking antibody; ~ inhibidor inhibiting antibody; ~ neutralizante neutralizing antibody; ~ sensibilizante sensitizing antibody
antidepresivo, *m*, *adj*, antidepressant
antídoto, antidote; ~ fisiológico physiological antidote; ~ mecánico mechanical antidote; ~ químico chemical antidote; ~ universal universal antidote
antiemético, *m*, *adj*, antiemetic
antiespasmódico, *m*, *adj*, antispasmodic
antiespástico, *m*, *adj*, antispasmodic
antifármaco, antidote
antiflogístico, *m*, *adj*, antiphlogistic
antigénico, *adj*, antigenic
antígeno, antigen
antihelmíntico, *m*, *adj*, vermifuge
antihemorrágico, *adj*, antihemorrhagic
antihipertensivo, *m*, *adj*, antihypertensive
antihistamínico, *m*, antihistamine; *adj*, *PR*, antihistaminic
antiinflamatorio, *m*, *adj*, anti-inflammatory; ~ no esteroide nonsteroidal anti-inflammatory drug
antipalúdico, *adj*, antimalarial
antipatía, dislike
antipático, *adj*, disagreeable
antipirético, *m*, *adj*, *Med*, antipyretic; fever reducing agent
antipirina, antipyrine
antiséptico, *m*, *adj*, *Med*, antiseptic
antitetántico, *adj*, *Med*, antitetanic; anti-tetanus
antitóxico, *adj*, antitoxic; *m*, antitoxin
antitoxina, antitoxin
antojo, craving
ántrax, *m*, anthrax; carbuncle; woolsorter's disease
antro mastoideo, mastoid antrum
anual, *adj*, annual; *adv*, yearly
anucleado, *adj*, non-nucleated
anudar, to knot; to cancel
anular, to repeal (*rescindir*)
anuria, anuria; renal blockade

añadir, to add

añiao, *adj*, hole(d) up in one's house; *adj*, *PR*, spoiled (*mimado*)

año, year

añoranza, homesickness

añublo, mildew (*en una planta*)

aojadura, evil eye

aojar, to cast the evil eye on

aorta, aorta

aórtico, *adj*, aortic

apacible, *adj*, even (*plácido*); gentle

apaciguador, *m*, tranquilizer

apagar, to dull (*sonidos*); to turn off; to quench (*la sed*); ~se to go out (*cerillas, la luz, etc.*)

aparatito, coil (*anticonceptivo*); *Chicano*, IUD

aparato, apparatus; appliance; device; equipment; machine; *Anat*, system; tract; *Chicano*, buttock; ~ afilador knife sharpener; ~ auditivo hearing aid; ~ cardiocinético pacemaker; ~ cardiovascular cardiovascular system; ~ circulatorio circulatory (*hematológico*) system; ~ de compresión consecutiva sequential compression device; ~ digestivo digestive system; digestive tract; digestive tube; ~ endocrino endocrine system; ~ gastrointestinal gastrointestinal system; ~ genitourinario genitourinary system; ~ hematológico circulatory system; ~ intrauterino intrauterine device/IUD; ~ nervioso autónomo autonomic nervous system; ~ nervioso central central nervous system; ~ ortodóntico braces *Dent*; ~ ortopédico calliper; orthopedic brace; ~ para la sordera hearing aid; ~ para medir la glucosa glucose monitor; ~ para medir la presión *fam*, blood pressure cuff; ~ para prolongar la vida life support device; ~ para sordos hearing aid; ~

prótesis prosthetic apparatus; ~ respiratorio respiratory system; ~s ortopédicos braces

aparente, *adj*, ostensible

aparición, *f*, apparition

apariencia, appearance (*externa*)

apartado postal, post office box

apartar, to isolate; ~ la mirada to look away; ~se de to stand clear of

apatía, apathy; listlessness

apático, *adj*, apathetic; listless (*desinteresado*)

apellido, family name; last name; surname

apenado, *adj*, sorry (*triste*)

apenarse, *Chicano*, to worry

apendejao, *adj*, *vulg*, *PR*, cautious

apéndice, *m*, appendix; tail

apendicitis, *f*, appendicitis

apendis, *m*, *fam*, appendicitis; appendix

apendix, *f*, appendix

apertura, opening (*término general*)

apestillar(se), to cuddle

apestoso, *adj*, foul-smelling

apetito, appetite

aplastante, *adj*, crushing (*dolor*)

aplastar, to crush (*despachurrar*); to smash

aplatanao, *adj*, *PR*, indecisive

aplicación, *f*, application; ~ de hielo empaquetado ice pack; ~ de un injerto grafting; ~ de ventosas cupping; aplicaciones calientes, *pl*, hot compresses

aplicador, *m*, applicator

aplicar(se), to apply (*a uno mismo*); ~ una ligadura to ligate

apnea, apnea; ~ del sueño sleep apnea

apodo, nickname

apófisis, *f*, *Anat*, process; ~ del hueso temporal mastoid process; ~ mastoides mastoid process

apoplejía, apoplexy (*ataque*); (cerebrovascular) stroke

apósito, dressing (*tirita*); gauze pad; ~ **absorbente adhesivo** adhesive absorbent bandage; ~ **enyesado** plaster cast; ~ **femenino** sanitary napkin; ~ **ligado con vendas** bandage (*vendaje*)

apostema, (*var. de postema*) abscess

apostemado, *adj*, abscessed

apostemar, to form abscess; ~**se** to abscess (*llenarse*)

apostillarse, *Med*, to scab over

apoyar, to support (*para evitar caerse*); ~**se contra** to lean against; ~**se en** to lean upon/against

apoyo, support; ~ **de la cabeza** headrest; ~ **moral** moral support; ~ **para la cabeza** headrest

apreciar, to appreciate

aprender, to learn

aprendizaje, *m*, learning

aprensión, *f*, qualm (*duda*)

apresurarse, to hurry

apretado, *adj*, tight

apretar (ie), to bind (*ropa, etc.*); to press (*empujar*); to squeeze; to tighten; ~ **los dientes** to bite down *Dent;* to clinch one's teeth; to grit one's teeth (*con determinación*); ~ **los labios** to screw up/to seal one's lips; ~ **los puños** to clench one's fists

apretón, *m*, press (*de la mano*)

apropiado, *adj*, appropriate

aprovecharse de, to take advantage of

aproximadamente, *adv*, approximately

aptitud, *f*, fitness

apto, *adj*, able-bodied

apuntar, to record (*anotar*)

apuñalar, to stab (*con un puñal*)

aquillado, *adj*, keel-shaped

araña capulina, black widow spider

arañado, *adj*, skinned (*rasguñado*)

arañar, to scratch (*herir*)

arañazo, nail-scratch; scratch (*en la piel*)

árbol *m*, tree; ~ **genealógico** family tree; ~ **vascular** vasculature

arca, *Mex*, armpit

arcada, retching

archivar, to file (*clasificar*)

archivo, file (*carpeta*)

arcilla, clay

arco, arc; arch; ~ **crural profundo** deep femoral arc; ~ **del pie** arch of the foot; ~ **dental** cope *Dent;* ~ **facial** face-bow *Dent*

arder, to burn (*picar*); *Mex, CA, Ríopl*, to smart

ardiente, *adj*, burning; hot blooded

ardor, *m*, burning sensation; ~ **al orinar** burning on urination; burning sensation when urinating; ~ **del estómago** heartburn; ~ **epigástrico** heartburn; *Mex, CA, Ríopl*, smarting (*sensación*); ~[1] heroin

área[3], area

arena, sand

arenilla, gravel *Med*

arete, *m*, earring (*que no cuelga*)

argolla, parts of *SpAm*, ring

armadura, frame (*de una cama, etc.*)

armazón, *f*, frame (*de un edificio, máquina, etc.*); framework; skeleton; ~ **de calentamiento** warming crib; ~ **para cuadripléjicos** quadriplegic standing frame

ARN de transferencia, transfer RNA

ARN mensajero, messenger RNA

arpon[1], *m*, heroin

arponazo[1], cocaine; heroin

arquear, to retch

arrancar, to start out; ~**se los ojos de lágrimas** to film with tears

arrebatao[1], *adj*, stoned on marijuana

arrebato, fit

arreglado, *adj*, orderly

arreglar, to arrange; to fix; ~[1] to fix up[2] (*calentar y mezclar heroína*)

arreglo, arrangement

arremangarse, to roll up one's sleeve

arrematao, *adj*, crazy

arrepentido, *adj*, sorry (*lamentación*)

arrepentir(se) (ie), to repent

arriesgado, *adj*, touch-and-go
arriesgar, to hazard (*poner en peligro*); to venture
arriñonado, *adj*, kidney-shaped
arritmia, arrhythmia; irregular heartbeat; ~ **cardíaca** cardiac arrhythmia
arrodillarse, to kneel
arrojadera, *vulg*, vomit
arrojar, to hurl; to spit; to throw; *fam*, to barf *vulg* (*vomitar*); to throw up; to vomit
arrojos, *fam*, vomit
arrollador, *adj*, devastating
arroz, *m*, rice
arruga, fold; line; wrinkle
arrugar(se), to wrinkle
arruinado, *adj*, broken (*salud*)
arrullar, to lull to sleep (*cantándole a un niño a adormecer*)
arseniato de bario, barium arsenate
arsénico, arsenic
arteria, artery; ~ **aorta ascendente** ascending aorta artery; ~ **aorta torácica descendente** descending thoracic aorta artery; ~ **carotida (primitiva)** (common) carotid artery; ~ **coronaria** coronary artery
arterial, *adj*, arterial
arteriosclerosis, *f*, arteriosclerosis
arteriosclerótico, *adj*, arteriosclerotic
arteriovenoso, *adj*, arteriovenous
articulación, *f*, articulation; joint; ~ **coxofemoral** hip joint; ~ **de la cadera** hip joint; ~ **de la rodilla** knee joint; ~ **de movimiento anormal** flail joint; ~ **de rótula** ball and socket joint; ~ **envarada** stiff joint (*anquilosada*); ~ **esférica** ball and socket joint; ~ **femorocoxal** thigh joint; ~ **inmóvil** immovable joint; ~ **irritable** irritable joint; ~ **suelta/flácida** flail joint; ~ **trabada** stiff joint (*anquilosada*); ~ **trocoide** rotatory joint

articular, *adj*, articular
artificial, *adj*, artificial
artritis, *f*, arthritis; ~ **reumatoide** rheumatoid arthritis; ~ **reumatoidea** rheumatoid arthritis
artrograma, *m*, arthrogram
artroscopia, arthroscopy
artrosia, arthrosis
asa, loop (*anticonceptivo*); handle; loop
asado, *adj*, broiled; roast
asaltar, to assault
asalto, assault; ~ **con lesión** assault and battery
asar, to roast
asbesto, asbestos
ascáride, *f*, *form*, ascaris; roundworm
ascaris, *f*, ascaris; roundworm
ascendente, *adj*, ascending
ascender, to ascend
ascensor, *m*, elevator
asco, disgust; nausea
asearse, to wipe oneself (*después de evacuar*)
asegurador, -ra, *m/f* underwriter
aseguranza, *Chicano*, life insurance
asegurar, to assure; to insure; ~**se** to make sure; ~**se de** to make certain of
asentir (ie), to nod
aseo, cleanliness; ~ **bucal** oral hygiene; ~ **personal** personal hygiene
aséptico, *adj*, germ free; sterile
asesor genético, genetic counselor
asexual, *adj*, asexual
asfixia, asphyxia; suffocation
asfixiar(se), to asphyxiate; to choke (*debido a la falta de aire*)
así, *adv*, like this; ~ **como** the same as
asidero, handgrip
asiento, seat; ~**s** *slang*, diarrhea
asignado, *adj*, assigned
asilo, asylum; shelter (*para los pobres, los vagabundos, los ancianos*); ~ **de ancianos** nursing

home; ~ **de dementes** hospital for the insane; ~ **de locos** hospital for the insane

asimilación, *f*, constructive metabolism (*anabolismo*)

asintomático, *adj*, asymptomatic; symptomless

asistencia, assistance; help; ~ **a los enfermos** nursing (*para los enfermos*); ~ **médica** medical aid; medical attention; ~ **pública** welfare; ~ **social** welfare

Asistencia Médica, Medicaid

asistenta, attendant

asistente, *m/f*, aide; assistant; attendant; *m/f*, *adj*, assisting; attending; ~ **de enfermera** nurse's aide; ~ **de enfermeras** orderly; ~ **en cirugía** surgical assistant; ~ **médico** orderly

asistir, to doctor (*proveer cuidados médicos*); to attend; to treat; ~ **al parto** to deliver (*alguien a un bebé*)

asma, *m*, asthma; ~ **bronquial** bronchial asthma; ~ **de los fumadores** tabagism syndrome

asmático, *m*, *adj*, asthmatic

asociación, *f*, association; ~ **de práctica individual** I.P.A.

asociado, *adj*, associated

asoleada, *SpAm*, sunstroke

asomarse a, to lean out of; to look out of

asorocharse, *Bol, Chi, Ec, Perú*, to get mountain sickness

aspecto, appearance; aspect; looks; (*No me gusta el aspecto de la herida. I don't like the looks of the wound.*)

aspereza, harshness

áspero, *adj*, rough (*piel, superficie*); scratchy (*tono*)

aspiración, *f*, aspiration; suction; ~ **con aguja** needle aspiration

aspirador, *m*, aspirator; vacuum chamber

aspirar, to aspirate; to inhale (*inhalar*); ~ **cocaína** to blow snow[2]; ~ **cola**[1] to inhale glue; to sniff glue; ~ **narcóticos**[1] to scoop[2] *slang*; ~ **narcóticos por la nariz** to snort[2] (*sorber restos de narcóticos en polvo por la nariz*)

aspirina, aspirin; ~ **para niños** children's aspirin

asqueo, morning nausea

asqueroso, *adj*, filthy; foul; vile

astenia, asthenia

astenopía, *form*, eyestrain

astigmatismo, astigmatism

astilla, chip; sliver; splinter (*de madera, etc.*); ~ **ósea** bone splinter; ~ (**de metal**) bur/burr *Dent*

astillar(se), to chip; to crack (*un hueso*)

astrágalo, ankle bone; astragal

astringente, *m*, *adj*, astringent

asumir, to assume

asunto, matter (*negocio*)

asustado, *adj*, frightened

asustar, to frighten; to scare; ~**se** to become frightened; to get scared

atacado de mal de altura, *adj*, air sick

atacado de vértigo, *adj*, feeling of dizziness

atacar, to rape

atadura, restraint (*física*)

ataque, *m*, attack; fit; onset *Med*; seizure; spell (*de una enfermedad*); *fam*, convulsion; heart attack; ~ **al corazón** heart attack; myocardial infarction; ~ **asmático** asthmatic attack; ~ **cardíaco** heart attack; ~ **cerebral** (cerebrovascular) stroke; ~ **de epilepsia** epileptic attack; ~ **de nervios** a fit of nerves; *fam*, hysteria; hysterics; ~ **del corazón** heart attack; ~ **epiléptico** epileptic attack; ~ **fulminante** (cerebrovascular) stroke; ~ **histérico** hysterics; ~ **vesicular** gallbladder attack; ~**s isquémicos transitorios** transient ischemic attack/TIA

atar, to bind (*liar*); to fasten; to tie; ~ **con alambre** to wire; ~ **con correa** to strap (*liar*)

atarantado, *adj*, dizzy

atarantarse, to become dizzy

atascar, to clog (*obstruir*)

atemorizado, *adj*, afraid

atención, *f*, care; notice; ~ **del primer nivel** primary care; ~ **médica** health care/healthcare; ~ **médica subsecuente** follow-up care; ~ **prenatal** prenatal care; ~ **primaria** primary care

atender (ie) (a), to doctor (*proveer cuidados médicos*); to follow (*encargarse de un paciente*); to look after; to take care of; to treat (*a un enfermo*); ~ **el suicidio** to attempt suicide; ~ **un parto** to deliver (*alguien a un bebé*)

atento, *adj*, attentive

atenuado, *adj*, attenuated

aterido, *adj*, numb; stiff with cold

aterrorizador, *adj*, frightening

atestado, *adj*, overcrowded (*de gente*)

atestamiento, overcrowding

atezado, *adj*, swarthy

atiesar, to stiffen (*poner tieso*)

atípico, *adj*, atypical; unusual

atleta, *m/f*, athlete

atómico, *fam*, chronic alcoholic

atomización, *f*, nebulization

atomizador, *m*, nebulizer

atomizar, to nebulize

atontado, *adj*, bewildered

atorarse, to choke

atóxico, *adj*, nontoxic

atragantarse, to choke on (*comida, etc.*)

atrasado, *adj*, backward; in arrears; late (*entrega*); overdue (*avión, etc.*) retarded; ~ **mentalmente** *adj*, mentally retarded

atrasar, to delay; ~**se** to be slow (*un reloj*); *Arg, Col, Ur*, to suffer a setback (*de salud*)

atraso, delay; slowness (*un reloj*); ~ **mental** backwardness; ~**s** in arrears

atravesar (ie), to pass over

atribuir, to attribute

atrioventricular, *adj*, atrioventricular/A.V.

atrocidad, *f*, outrage (*ultraje*)

atrofia, atrophy; ~ **muscular peronea** peroneal muscular atrophy; ~ **óptica** optic atrophy

atrofiarse, to atrophy

atropellar, to knock down or over

atropina, atropine

aturdido, *adj*, in a daze; dazed; dizzy

aturdimiento, daze

aturdir, to daze (*atolondrar*)

audición, *f*, hearing

audífono, hearing aid

audiograma, *m*, audiogram

audiología, audiology

audiólogo, audiologist

audiometría, audiometry

audiómetro, audiometer

audioscopio, earscope

auditivo, *adj*, auditory

aullar, to yell

aullido, yell

aumentar, to augment; to build up (*resistencia propia*); to gain; to increase; to magnify; ~ **de peso** to fill out (*engordar*); to gain weight

aumento, gain; increase; magnification; rise (*proporción, presión, etc.*); ~ **de la excreción urinaria de potasio** kaluresis

aurícola, (*var. de aurícula*) external ear

aurícula, auricle (*del corazón o de la oreja*)

auricular, *adj*, atrial

auriculoventricular/A.V., *adj*, atrioventricular/A.V.

auscultar, to sound (*con un estetoscopio*)

ausencia, absence

ausente, *adj*, missing (*perdido*)

auténtico, *adj*, positive (*definido*)

autismo, autism

autista, *m/f*, autistic

autístico, *adj*, autistic

auto exploración de las mamas, *f*, breast self-examination

autoclave, *m*, autoclave

autocontrol, *m*, self-control

autocrítica, insight; self-criticism

autodefensa, self-defense
autodidacta, *adj*, *inv*, self-taught
autodisciplina, self-discipline
autoexamen (mensual) de los senos, *m*, (monthly) breast self-examination
autoinmune, *adj*, autoimmune
autoinmunidad, *f*, autoimmunity
autopsia, autopsy; postmortem; ~ **médico-legal** obduction; ~ **parcial** limited autopsy
autorecetarse, to prescribe for oneself
autoritario, *adj*, overbearing (*dominante*)
autorización, *f*, authorization
autorizado, *adj*, official; authorized; legal
autorizar, to authorize
autorregulación, *f*, feedback; self-regulation
autosuficiente, *adj*, self-sufficient
auxiliar, *m/f*, aide; ~ **de enfermeras** nurses' aide; ~ **en enfermeras** nurses' aide
auxilio, aid; help
avance, *m*, advance
avándaro[1], LSD
avanzado, *adj*, advanced
avariosis, *f*, *SpAm*, syphilis
avena, oatmeal
aventado, *adj*, bloated
aventurar, to hazard (*creer*)
avergonzar, to shame (*causar vergüenza*); ~**se** to be embarrassed
averiguar, to find out
aversión, *f*, aversion; dislike
ávido, *adj*, voracious
avión, *m*, plane
avisar, to inform (*decir*); to warn
aviso, advice; warning sign; warning

avispa, wasp
avispón, *m*, hornet
axila, armpit
ayahuasca, yage
ayer, *adv*, yesterday
ayuda, aid; assistance; *Med*, enema; help; ~ **médica** medical care
ayudante, *m/f*, aide; assistant; ~ **de enfermeras** nurses' aide; ~ **médico** orderly
ayudar, to aid; to help; to relieve; ~ **al parto** to deliver (*alguien a un niño*)
ayunar, to fast
ayunas, en, *adv*, fasting; without breakfast
ayuno, fast (*abstinencia*); fasting
azafrán, *m*, saffron
azogue, *m*, quicksilver
azotaina, spanking
azotar, to pound (*el mar*); to spank; to smack (*a los niños*)
azote, *m*, lash (*golpe con un látigo*); slap (*en las posaderas*)
azúcar, *m/f*, sugar; ~[1] *m*, acid[2] (LSD); (green) barrels/(the) beast[2]; cocaine; heroin; LSD; ~[1] *m*, *Arizona*, *Texas*, boy[2] (*heroína*); H[2] (*heroína*); ~ **de almidón** starch sugar; ~ **de caña** cane sugar; ~ **de remolacha** beet sugar; ~ **de uva** grape sugar; dextrose; ~ **en el orín** diabetes; ~ **en terrones** lump sugar; ~ **morena** brown sugar; ~ **negro** brown sugar; ~ **refinada** refined sugar; ~ **sanguínea** blood sugar
azucarado, *adj*, sugary
azufre, *m*, sulfur; ~[1] heroin; ~ **total** total sulfur
azul, *adj*, blue (color)

---

[1] Este vocabulario es nuevo y todavía no se encuentra en el *Diccionario de la lengua española*, publicado por la Real Academia Española. Forma parte del argot o la lengua de la calle. Se supone que el género es obvio a menos que sea indicado.
[2] Forma parte del vocabulario inglés actual de los drogadictos.
[3] Se emplean el artículo definido e indefinido masculinos en español delante de esta palabra con la *a* inicial acentuada aunque se usan adjetivos calificativos femeninos para modificarla.

B

baba, dribble; drool (*de niños*); slobber (*de adultos*)

babear, to drool

babeo, drooling

babero, bib

baby, *m*, Chicano, baby (*infante*)

bacalaito, fried or fritter codfish

bacalao, *PR*, skinny person

bacha[1], roach[2] (*colilla de un cigarrillo de mariguana*); marijuana

bachica, (*esp. mariguana*)[1] cigarette butt

bachilla[1], roach[2] (*colilla de un cigarrillo de mariguana*)

bacilo, bacillus (*pl, bacilli*); rod (*bacteria*); ~ **de Calmette-Guérin/BCG** Bacillus Calmette-Guérin/BCG; ~ **gaseoso** gas bacillus; ~ **tuberculoso** TB

bacín, *m*, bedpan

bacineta, urinal

bacinete, *m*, basin; pelvis *Anat*

bacinica, urinal

bacinilla, bedpan; urinal

bacitracina, bacitracin

bacteremia, bacteremia (*presencia de bacterias patógenas en la sangre*); septicemia

bacteria, bacterium; ~s bacteria; ~ **(superior) (inferior)** (higher) (lower) bacterium; ~ **acidorresistente** acid-fast bacterium; ~ **infecciosa** infectious bacterium; ~ **parásita** parasitic bacterium; ~ **patógena** pathogenic bacterium; ~ **tóxica** toxic bacterium; ~ **virulenta** virulent bacterium

bacteriano, *adj*, bacterial

bactérico, *adj*, bacterial

bacteriología, bacteriology; ~ **higiénica** hygienic bacteriology; ~ **patológica** pathological bacteriology; ~ **sanitaria** sanitary bacteriology; ~ **sistemática** systematic bacteriology

bacteriólogo, bacteriologist

bacterioscopia, bacterioscopy (*estudio microscópico de las bacterias*)

báculo, cane

bailarina[1], marijuana

baile, *m*, dance; ~ **de San Guido** chorea; ~ **de San Vito** chorea; ~ **de zambito** *fam*, epileptic attack

baja, drop (*de temperatura*); fall (*de temperatura, presión, etc.*); ~ **de batalla** battle casualty; ~ **por enfermedad** sick leave

bajada, drop (*caída*); descent (*descendimiento*)

bajado, *adj*, drooping (*ojos*)

bajalenguas, *m*, *inv*, tongue depressor

bajar, to droop (*los párpados*); to drop (*los ojos, la voz, etc.*); to ease off/up; to go down (*temperatura*); to lower; ~ **de peso** to lose weight; ~ **el nivel del colesterol** to lower the cholesterol count; ~ **el volumen** to turn down the volume; ~ **la cabeza** to bend one's head down; ~ **la escalera** to go down the stairs; ~ **la mirada** to look down (*bajar los ojos*); ~ **la regla** to flow (*menstrual*); ~ **los ojos** to look down (*bajar la mirada*); ~**(se)** to come down; to fall (*la temperatura, una fiebre, la voz*); ~**(se)** *vulg*, to go soft (*erección*); to lose an erection

bajo, *adj*, low; short (*persona*); small (*estatura*)

bajón[1], *m*, letdown[2]

bala, bullet

balance, *m*, balance (*de una cuenta*); equilibrium; ~ **acidobásico** acid-base balance; ~ **de enzi-**

mas enzyme balance; ~ **líquido** fluid balance

balanceado, *adj*, balanced

balancearse, to wobble

bálano, glans (*del pene*)

balanza, balance (*para pesar*); scale (*instrumento para pesar*)

balazo, bullet wound; shot (*que causa una herida*)

balbucear, to babble; to falter; to lisp; to stammer

balbucencia, stuttering

balbuceo, babble (*de un nene*); lisp (*de un niño*); stammer

baldado, *adj*, maimed

balde, *m*, bucket

balísticas, ballistics; ~ **de las heridas** wound ballistics

balístico, *adj*, ballistic

balón, *m*, balloon (*de un catéter, etc.*); ~ **de oxígeno** oxygen cylinder

balone, *m*, *Chicano*, penis

bálsamo, balm; balsam; salve

bamboleo, wobble

bambú, *m*, bamboo

banco, bank; ~ **de arterias, huesos, ojos, piel** arteries, bone, eye, skin bank; ~ **de sangre** blood bank

banda, band; ~ **de absorción** absorption band; ~ **de metal** metal strap

bandeja, basin; tray; ~ **de resina acrílica** *Dent*, acrylic resin tray; ~ **para impresión** *Dent*, impression tray; ~ **para los cubitos de hielo** ice cube tray

bandillera[1], heroin

bandita, *PR*, Bandaid

banqueta, *Mex*, sidewalk

bañadera, *Cu*, bathtub

bañado, *adj*, bathed; ~ **en sangre** drenched in blood; ~ **en sudor** dripping with perspiration

bañar, to bathe; ~**se** to bathe oneself; to take a bath

bañera, bathtub; tub

baño, bath; lavatory; restroom; toilet; ~ **ácido** acid bath; ~ **aromáti-**co herb bath; ~ **caliente** hot bath; ~ **de aceite** oil bath; ~ **de agua** water bath; ~ **de aire** air bath; ~ **de aire caliente** warm air bath; ~ **de alcohol** alcohol bath; ~ **de almidón** starch bath; ~ **de asiento** sitz bath; ~ **de azufre** sulfur bath; ~ **de brea** tar bath; ~ **de esponja** sponge bath; ~ **de harina de avena** oatmeal bath; ~ **de leche** milk bath; ~ **de mostaza** mustard bath; ~ **de permanganato de potasio** potassium permanganate bath; ~ **de pies** foot bath; ~ **de regadera** *Chicano*, shower bath; ~ **de salvado** bran bath; ~ **de sodio** sodium bath; ~ **de sudor** sweat bath; ~ **de toalla** *Chicano*, sponge bath; ~ **de torbellino** whirlpool bath; ~ **de vapor** steam bath; ~ **de vapor(es)** vapor bath; ~ **emoliente** emollient bath; ~ **fresco** cool bath; ~ **frío** cold bath; ~ **medicamentoso** medicated bath; ~ **medicinal** medicated bath; ~ **medio (de las caderas y las piernas)** half bath; ~ **ocular** eye bath; ~ **para mujeres** women's (bath)room; ~ **químico** chemical bath; ~ **salino** saline bath; ~ **sulfuroso** sulfur bath; ~ **tibio** tepid bath

baqueña, *PR*, herb

baranda, bedrail

barandal, *m*, bedrail; siderail

barba, beard; chin; ~**s** thick, bushy beard

barbilla, chin; mentum

barbital, *m*, barbital; ~ **sódico** sodium barbital; ~ **soluble** soluble barbital

barbiturato, barbiturate

barbitúrico, *m*, *adj*, barbiturate; ~ candy[2] (*barbiturato*)

barbudo, *adj*, bearded

bario, barium

barniz, *m*, varnish

barra, bar; stick (*de chicle, chocolate,*

etc.); ~ **en arco** arch bar *Dent*; **~s paralelas** *pl*, parallel bars

barreño, basin (*para lavarse*)

barrera, barrier; ~ **hematocefálica** blood-brain barrier/BBB; ~ **placentaria** placental barrier; ~ **sanguíneo-cerebral** blood-brain barrier/BBB

barriga, belly; stomach; *fam*, abdomen

barrigón, *adj*, *fam*, big-bellied

barril, *m*, barrel (*de una jeringa*)

barrillo, pimple

barrio, neighborhood

barro, mud; pimple; blackhead (*granillo*); **~s** *fam*, acne

basal, *adj*, basal

basarse, to be based

basca, nausea; retching; **~s** qualm *Med*; **~(s)** *fam*, vomit/ vomitus

báscula, scale (*instrumento para pesar*)

base, *f*, base *Chem*, *Pharm*, *etc.*; ~ **de dentadura** denture base; ~ **de estudio** baseplate *Dent*; ~ **del cráneo** base of the cranium; ~ **metálica** metal base

básico, *adj*, basic

basija, washbowl; washbasin

basófilos, basophiles

basquear, *fam*, to throw up; to vomit

bastante, *adj*, enough; *adv*, plenty (*suficiente*); quite; sufficient

bastón, *m*, cane; stick (*para apoyarse*); ~ **de paseo** walking cane

bastoncillo, rod (*del ojo*); **~s** rod epithelium; **~s de la retina** rod cells

bastoncito, rod (*del ojo*)

basura, garbage; litter (*en la calle*); rubbish

bata, gown; nightgown; robe; white coat (*de médicos, etc.*); ~ **de baño** bathrobe

bate, *m*, cribsheet

batería, battery

baumanómetro, blood pressure cuff

bazo, spleen

bazofia, *fam*, swill; leftovers (*de comida*)

bebé, *m*, baby (*infante*)

bebedor, -ra, *m/f*, *adj*; drinker (hard) drinking

beber, to drink; ~ **mucho** to drink plenty of

bebida, drink; ~ **alcohólica** booze *vulg*; **~s alcohólicas** alcohol

beca, grant; scholarship

bellacar(se), *slang*, to excite sexually

belladona, belladonna

bencedrina, benzedrine

benceno, benzene

beneficio, benefit

beneficioso, *adj*, beneficial

benigno, *adj*, benign; temperate; mild (*enfermedad*)

benjuí, *m*, benzoin

benzedrinas, bennies/benz/benzies[2] (*anfetaminas*)

benzodiazapina, benzodiazepine

benzoína, benzoin

béquico, cough suppressant

beriberi, *m*, beriberi

bermejizo, *adj*, reddish (*pelo*)

berrear, to howl (*como llora y grita un niño*); ~ **hasta dormirse** to scream oneself to sleep

berrido, howl (*de un niño llorono*)

berrinche, *m*, *fam*, tantrum

besito, *PR*, candy (*hecho de coco rallado*)

beta, beta; ~ **bloqueador/betabloqueador** *m*, beta blocker; **bloqueante adrenérgico** ~ beta blocker; ~ **hemolítico** *adj*, beta-hemolytic

bi, *m/f*, bisexual

bianual, *adj*, biennial

biberón, *m*, baby bottle; nursing bottle

bicarbonato, bicarbonate; ~ **(sódico)** baking soda; ~ **de soda** bicarbonate of soda; ~ **de sosa** baking soda; ~ **sanguíneo** blood bicarbonate

biceps, *m*, *Chicano*, biceps

bicúspide, *m, adj*, bicuspid
bicho, bug (*insecto*); *vulg, PR*, penis
bidé, *m*, bidet
bien, *m*, benefit; *adj, adv*, well; ~ **afeitado** *adj*, close-shaven; ~ **avanzado** well on
bienestar, *m*, well-being; ~ **materno** maternal welfare; ~ **público** welfare
bifocales, *m, pl*, bifocals
bifurcación, *f*, bifurcation
bifurcado, *adj*, bifurcate; forked
bigote, *m*, moustache
bilateral, *adj*, bilateral
bilharzia, schistosoma (*parásito*)
biliar, *adj*, bile; biliary
biliario, *adj*, biliary
bilingüe, *adj*, bilingual
bilioso, *adj*, bilious
bilirrubina, bilirubin
bilis, *f*, bile; cholecystitis; gall; gallbladder disease; ~[4] *ethn*, irritability
bimba, punch (*puñetazo*); *Mex*, drunkenness
bimbazo, blow (*golpe*)
biodegradable, *adj*, biodegradable
bioestadística, biostatistics; vital statistics
biofísica, biophysics
biología, biology; ~ **molecular** molecular biology
biológico, *adj*, biological
biólogo, biologist
biometría hemática, blood count
biopsia, biopsy; ~ **aspirativa** suction biopsy; ~ **con aguja** needle biopsy; ~ **de sacabocado** punch biopsy; ~ **por aspiración** aspiration biopsy; ~ **por succión** suction biopsy
bioquímica, biochemistry
bioquímico, *adj*, biochemical
biorretroalimentación, *f*, biofeedback
bióxido de carbono, carbon dioxide
bípara, *f, adj*, bipara
biper, *m, Chicano*, beeper

bíper, *m, Chicano*, pager
bipolar, *adj*, bipolar
bisabuelo/bizabuelo, great-grandfather
bisexual, *adj*, bisexual
bisnieto/biznieto, great-grandson
bisojo, *adj*, cross-eyed; squint-eyed
bisturí, *m*, scalpel
bisulfato de quinina, quinine bisulfate
bisulfito de calcio, calcium bisulfite
bizcar, to look cross-eyed; to squint
bizco, *adj*, cross-eyed; squint-eyed; *CA*, strabismus
bizcorneado, *SD*, (*Vea bizco*.)
bizcornear, *Cu, PR*, to look cross-eyed; to squint
bizcorneto, *Col, Mex*, (*Vea bizco*.)
bizquear, to squint
bizquera, cross-eyes; *Col, PR*, squint
blanca[1], heroin; ~ **nieves**[1] *f* cocaine; ~**s**[1] bennies/benz/benzies[2] (*anfetamina*)
blanco, *adj*, fair (*tez*); white (*color, piel, raza*); ~ **del ojo** white of the eye; ~[1] heroin; ~ **de España**[1] LSD
blandito, *adj*, watery
blando, *adj*, soft; ~ **de carnes** flabby
blanducho, flabbiness
blanqueador, *m*, bleach; ~ **de ropa** sodium hypochlorite (*blanqueo, lejía*)
blanquear(se), to bleach
blanqueo, bleach
blanquillo, *slang, Chicano*, testicle
blastodermo, blastoderm
blefaritis, *f*, blepharitis (*inflamación de los párpados*)
blenorragia, gonorrhea
blindaje contra la radiación, *m*, radiation shield
blondo, *adj*, blond; fair; *Arg, Mex*, curly; *Guat*, lank; *SpAm*, soft; smooth
bloqueador, *m*, blocker; obturator; ~ **adrenérgico** adrenergic

blocker; **~(es) beta** beta blocker(s); **~ de los canales de calcio** calcium channel blocker; **~ neuronal** neuronic blocker; *adj*, blocking

bloquear, to block *Pharm*

bloqueo, block *Pharm*; blocking; obstruction; **~ cardíaco** cardiac/heart block; heart blockage; heart stoppage; **~ de la trompa** ear blockage; **~ de rama** bundle branch block/BBB; **~ de un pasaje** obturation; **~ del corazón** heart blockage; **~ del nervio** nerve block; **~ nervioso** nerve block; **~ neuromuscular residual** residual neuromuscular block

blusa, shirt (*femenina*)

boba, *PR*, insect (*tipo de insecto*)

bobas, *fam*, chicken pox

bobito, eye gnat; *Chicano*, gnat

boca, oral cavity; mouth; pit (*del estómago*); **~ abajo** face down; on one's stomach; **~ arriba** face up; on one's back; **~ de trinchera** trench mouth; **~ del estómago** epigastrium; gullet; pit of stomach; *fam*, esophagus

bocadillo, snack

bocado, bite (*mordisco*); gulp (*de comida*); morsel; mouthful; snack; **~ de Adán** Adam's apple

bocal, *m*, mouthpiece

bocanada, mouthful (*de vino, etc.*); puff (*de humo, aire, etc.*)

bochorno, flash; hot flashes

bochornoso, *adj*, muggy (*el tiempo*)

bocio, goiter; *fam*, thyroid; **~ aberrante** aberrant goiter; **~ cístico** cystic goiter; **~ fibroso** fibrous goiter; **~ nodular** nodular goiter; **~ quístico** cystic goiter; **~ simple** simple goiter; **~ sofocante** suffocative goiter; **~ retrosternal** substernal goiter; **~ tóxico** toxic goiter

bofe, *m*, *Chicano*, *SpAm*, lung

bofetada, slap (*guantada*)

boga, vogue

bola, ball (*esfera*); bump; lump; *pl, Chicano*, knot *Med*, (*nudo*); mumps; *pl, slang, common*, testicles; *vulg*, balls *vulg* (*testículos*)

bolígrafo, ball point pen

bolita, bump; induration; lump; *slang*, clitoris; **~ de algodón** cotton ball

bolo, *adj*, *CA*, drunk

bolones, *m, pl, vulg*, balls (*testículos*)

bolsa, bag; purse; sac; bursa; **~ (debajo de los ojos)** bag under the eye; **~ amniótica** amniotic sac; **~ de aguas** *fam*, amniotic sac; **~ de agua caliente** hot water bag; **~ de caucho para hielo** ice bag/pack; **~ de hielo** ice bag; **~ de lágrimas** tear sac (*del ojo*); **~ de las aguas** bag of waters; **~ de los testículos** scrotum; **~ de papel** paper bag; **~ membrosa** bag of waters; **~ para enemas** enema bag; **~ para la compra** shopping bag; **~s de pus** *fam*, cyst

bolsita[1], bindle[2] (*cantidad de mariguana u otra droga narcótica*)

bomba, pump; **~ aspirante** suction pump; **~ de inyección** injection pump; **~ de ordeñar** breast pump; **~ estomacal** stomach pump; **~ gástrica** stomach pump; **~ neumática** vacuum pump; **~**[1] LSD; *slang*, rubber *slang* (*condón*)

bombiao[1], *adj*, extremely high on[2] (*drogas narcóticas*); stoned on marijuana

bombido[1], amphetamines

bombilla, bulb *Elect*

bombillo, *CA*, *Col*, bulb *Elect*

bombita[1], amphetamines

bombo, *Ur*, buttock

bombón, *m*, candy (*dulces*)

boqueada, gasp (*antes de morir*)

boquear, to gasp; to be at one's last gasp

boquera, oral lesion; moniliasis

boquilla, cigarette holder; mouthpiece; *fam*, cheilosis (*llaga en la comisura de la boca*)

boquineta, *m*, *Chicano*, cleft palate; harelip

bórax, *m*, borax

borde, *m*, border; edge; margin; lip (*de una herida*); ~ **ciliar** ciliary margin; ~ **de dentadura** denture border; ~ **de las uñas** nail fold; ~ **gingival** gingival margin; ~ **pupilar** pupillary margin

bornear, to twist (*doblar*)

borujo, lump

borujón, *m*, large lump

borra, wad; ~ **blanca**[1] heroin

borrachera, binge; drunken fit; drunkenness

borracho, *m*, *adj*, drunk; intoxicated

borradura, effacement

borrar, to efface; ~**se (la vista)** to blur (*la visión*)

borroso, *adj*, blurred; blurry; dim

bostezar, to yawn

bostezo, yawn

bota, boot

botánica, botany; herb shop; spiritist store; ~ **médica** medical botany

botánico, herbalist

botar, to throw away; ~ **aire** *Carib*, *SpAm*, *fam*, to breathe out

bote, *m*, can; *slang*, *Chicano*, baby bottle

botella, bottle; baby bottle; vial

botellero, *fam*, chronic alcoholic

botica, drugstore; pharmacy

boticario, druggist; pharmacist

botiquín *m*, ambulance box; kit; medicine chest; ~ **de emergencia** emergency kit; ~ **de primeros auxilios** first aid kit; ~ **de urgencia** first aid kit

botón, *m*, button; ~ **gustativo** tastebud/taste bud

botulismo, botulism

bóveda ósea del paladar, hard palate

bradicardia, bradycardia

braga, diaper; ~**s** *pl*, panty/panties

braguero, brace (*ortopédico*); truss; ~ **nasal** nasal truss

bragueta, fly *slang* (*cremallera*); zipper (*de pantalones*)

Braille, *m*, Braille

brasiere, *m*, brassiere

brazalete, *m*, arm band; ~ **para identificación** identification bracelet

brazo, arm; ~ **de barra de gancho** bar clasp arm; ~ **de pájaro** bird-arm; ~ **de retención** retention arm *Dent*; ~ **portaelectrodo** electrode supporting arm

brea, tar; ~ **de hulla** coal tar

brebaje, *m*, draught; potion *Pharm*

brecha, gap (*boquete*); gash; head wound

bretear, *PR*, to do something illicit

breve, *adj*, brief; short (*corto*)

brida amniótica, amniotic band

brillante, *m*, *adj*, diamond; bright; brilliant

brillo, brightness; light; sheen (*del cabello, una superficie, etc.*); sparkle (*de los ojos*)

brincacharcos, *m*, *pl*, high water pants

brincar, to jump

broca, dental drill

broco, *adj*, *PR*, amputated

bromo, bromine

bromocriptina, bromocriptine

bromuro, bromide; ~ **de cadmio** cadmium bromide; ~ **de demecario** demecarium bromide; ~ **de etilo** ethyl bromide

bronceado, suntan; *adj*, suntanned; tan

broncearse, to get a tan

bronco, *adj*, rough (*voz*)

bronco(e)spasmo, bronchospasm

broncología, bronchology

bronconeumonía, bronchopneumonia/broncho-pneumonia

broncoscopia/broncoscopía, bronchoscopy

broncoscopio, bronchoscope

broncospirometría, bronchospirometry

bronquial, *adj*, bronchial

bronquio, bronchus (*pl, bronchi*)

bronquiodilatador, *m*, bronchodilator

bronquíolo, bronchiole; ~ **alveolar** alveolar bronchiole; ~ **respiratorio** respiratory bronchiole; ~ **terminal** terminal bronchiole

bronquitis, *f*, bronchitis; ~ **aguda** acute bronchitis; ~ **crónica** chronic bronchitis; ~ **crupal** croupous bronchitis; ~ **exudativa** exudative bronchitis; ~ **productiva** productive bronchitis; ~ **secundaria** secondary bronchitis

brotar, to break out; to issue forth (*sangre, líquido*)

brote, *m*, outbreak (*de una epidemia*)

brucelosis, *f*, Malta fever

brujo, witch

brumoso, *adj*, foggy

bruscamente, *adv*, cold turkey

brusco, *adj*, sharp (*cambio de temperatura*); short; sudden (*repentina*)

búa, bubo (*pl, buboes*)

buba, pimple

bubón, (*pl, bubones*), *m*, bubo (*pl, buboes*); pustule; ~ **tropical** lymphogranuloma venereum; ~**es** lymphogranuloma venereum /LGV

bubonocele, *m*, inguinal hernia

bucal, *adj*, buccal; oral *Dent*

buche, *m*, *slang*, goiter; *vulg*, *Chicano*, buttock; *Mex*, mumps

bucolingual, *adj*, buccolingual *Dent*

bueno, *adj*, sound (*salud, consejo, carácter, etc.*); **buen carácter** *m*, sound character; **buena salud** *f*, fitness; sound health; **buenos días** *m*, *pl*, good morning

bufanda, scarf

bufar de cólera, to howl with anger

bujía, candle

bulbo, bulb; ~ **auditivo** auditory bulb; ~ **dental** tooth bulb; ~ **gustativo** gustatory bulb; taste bud; ~ **olfatorio** olfactory bulb; ~ **raquídeo** brainstem; medulla oblongata

bulimia, bulimia

bulímico, *adj*, bulimic

bulla, blister

bulto, bump (*chichón*); growth (*tumor*); knob (*nudo*); lump (*protuberancia*); swelling (*hinchazón*)

burbuja, blister (*en una superficie*); bubble

burlarse de, to make fun of

bursitis, *f*, bursitis; ~ **aquiliana** Achilles bursitis; ~ **prerrotuliana** housemaid knee

burundanga, hodgepodge

burro[1], dope pusher; peddler[2] (*vendedor de drogas narcóticas*)

buscar, to look for; ~ **a tientas** to grope for

buscatoques[1], *sg*, *m/f*, addict in search of a fix

búster, *m*, *Chicano*, booster shot

busto, *slang*, breast; bust

Butazolidina, Butazolidin

butón, *m*, *slang*, pimple

bypass, *m*, *Chicano*, by-pass (*coronario*)

---

[1] Este vocabulario es nuevo y todavía no se encuentra en el *Diccionario de la lengua española*, publicado por la Real Academia Española. Forma parte del argot o la lengua de la calle. Se supone que el género es obvio a menos que sea indicado.

[2] Forma parte del vocabulario inglés actual de los drogadictos.

[4] Esta *enfermedad* no tiene nada que ver con la verdadera *bilis*. Se dice que las personas que son muy corajudas sufren de *bilis*. Muchas mujeres de la edad de menopausia muchas veces sufren de bilis a causa de la menopausia.

C

ca-ca[1], heroin

caballete de la nariz, *m*, bridge of the nose

caballo[1], boy[2] (*heroína*); H[2] (*heroína*); heroin; runner[2] (*portador de drogas*)

caballón[1], *adj*, high[2] (*en drogas narcóticas*)

cabecear, to nod (*por estar dormido*)

cabecera, head (*de la cama, mesa*); headboard

cabecita de vena, *Chicano*, angiomate (*puntos rojos en la piel*)

cabello, *fam*, hair; **~s** hair (*de la cabeza*)

cabestrillo, arm sling; halter; sling

cabete, *m*, shoelace

cabeza, head; *fam*, brain; *slang*, glans (*pene*); **~ en declive** head down

cabezal, *m*, compress

cabo, strand; stump (*del lápiz, vela, etc.*)

cabra, goat

cabrear, *fam*, to be very active

cabro, *Chi*, child; kid

caca, *fam*, *juv*, bowel movement; excrement; *fam*, number two *euph*; *slang*, feces; **~ aguada** *slang*, mushy stool

cacahuete, *m*, peanut; **~**[1] *m*, *slang*, barbiturate

cácara, *Chicano*, acne

cacaraña, *Mex*, *Guat*, pock

cacha, cheek (*of buttock*); **~s** *PR*, buns *slang;* buttocks (*nalga*)

cachete, *m*, *fam*, cheek

cachipa, fibrous covering of coconut

cachucha[1], cap[2] (*cápsula*); drug supply; heroin capsule

cada, each; *adj*, every; **~ cuatro horas** *q.q.h./quater quarta horas*/every 4 hours; **~ día** *q.d./quaque die*/every day; **~ dos días** every other day; **~ dos días/en días alternos** on alternate days; **~ hora** *q.h./quaque hora*/every hour; **~ dos horas** *q.2h./quaque secunda hora*/every two hours; **~ tres horas** *q.3h./quaque tertia hora*/every 3 hours; **~ mañana** *o.m./omni mane*/every morning; **~ noche** *o.n./omni nocte*/every night; **~ ocho días** once a week; weekly; **~ semana** each week; weekly

cadáver, *m*, cadaver; corpse; dead body; deceased

cadavérico, *adj*, deathlike

cadena, chain; **~ de seguridad** safety catch (*de joyas*)

cadera, hip; **~ dislocada de nacimiento** congenital hip

cadmio, cadmium

caducado, *adj*, outdated (*medicamento*)

caducidad, *f*, obsolescence

caduquez, *f*, senility

caer, to fall; to fall down; **~(se)** to fall; **~se** to collapse; to droop (*párpados*); to drop; to fall down; **~ de cansancio** to drop from exhaustion; **~ enfermo** to be taken ill; **~ mal** to disagree with one (*mal efecto*); **~ muerto** *adj*, to drop dead; **~ bien** to agree with one; **~ con algo** to come down with (+ *una enfermedad*); to catch (+ *una enfermedad*); **~ de rodillas** to drop on one's knees; **~ en el error** to lapse (*equivocarse*); **~ en un sueño profundo** to fall into a deep sleep; **~ enfermo de** to go down with (*una enfermedad*); **~ mala** to have the (monthly) curse

café, *m*, coffee; **~ caliente** hot coffee; **~ molido** coffee grounds; **~**

ralo *PR,* bad coffee; ~ **soso** *PR,* unsweetened coffee; ~ **término** *PR,* unsweetened coffee with some milk; ~[1] LSD; marijuana

cafeína, caffeine

cafetería, cafeteria

caftán, *m,* caftan

cagada, *vulg,* bowel movement; feces; ~[1] *vulg,* heroin

cagadera, *vulg, Chicano,* diarrhea

caída, dip; droop (*de párpados*); dropping; (*de temperatura, etc.*); fall; ~ **de la matriz** prolapse; prolapse of the uterus; ~ **de la mollera**[4] fallen fontanel

caído, *adj,* drooping (*orejas, espaldas, etc.*)

caja, box; cage; cashier's office/window; dish; ~ **costal** rib cage; ~ **de los costillas** rib cage; ~ **de la escalera** stairwell; ~ **del cráneo** braincase; skull; ~ **del tímpano** barrel of the ear; tympanic cavity; ~ **encefálica** braincase; skull; ~ **torácica** thoracic cage/cavity

cajero, cashier

cajetilla, pack of cigarettes

cajetuda, *Chicano,* headache

cajita de píldoras, pillbox

cajón, *m,* drawer

cal, *f,* lime *Chem;* ~ **clorurada** chlorinated lime; ~ **sodada** soda lime; ~ **sulfurada** sulfurated lime; ~ **viva** quicklime

cala, suppository

calabaza, squash

calambre, cramp; menstrual cramp; muscular cramp; ~**s abdominales** abdominal cramps; ~ **de los cortadores de caña** cane-cutter's cramp; ~ **de los escribientes** writers' cramp; writers' spasm; ~ **de los escritores** graphospasm (*calambre de los escribientes*); ~ **de los violinistas** violinists' cramp; ~ **intermitente** intermittent cramp; ~ **por calor** heat cramp; ~ **profesional** occupational cramp; ~ **térmico** heat cramp

calamina, calamine

calar, to drench (*empapar*); to soak through

calavera, *Chicano,* skull

calcañal/calcañar/calcaño, *m,* heel

calceta, stocking (*hasta la rodilla*); ~ **compresiva** surgical stocking; ~ **elástica** elastic stocking

calcetín, *m,* sock (*media*); stocking (*calceta que llega a la mitad de la pantorrilla*)

calcificación, *f,* calcification

calcificar(se), to calcify

calcio, calcium; calcium vitamin

calcular, to calculate

cálculo, calculation; estimate; calculus; stone; ~ **biliar** gallstone; ~ **dental** dental calculus; ~ **en el riñón** kidney stone; ~ **en la vejiga** gallstone; ~ **renal** kidney stone; ~ **urinario** kidney stone

caldo, bouillon; broth; ~ **de carne** meat infusion; ~ **de cultivo** culture medium

calentador, *m,* warmer

calentar (ie), to heat (up); to scald (*leche*); to warm up

calentura[5], fever; temperature

calibrador, *m,* calibrator; gauge; ~ **de sondas** catheter gauge

calibrar, to calibrate

calidad, *f,* quality (*carácter, genio*); ~ **de la vida** quality of life

caliente, *adj,* hot (*temperatura; sexualmente*)

calificación, *f,* qualification (*experiencia*)

calificado, *adj,* qualified (*preparado*)

calilla, suppository

calistenia, calisthenics

calisténica, calisthenics

callado, *adj,* closemouthed; quiet (*carácter de una persona*)

callarse, to be quiet

calle, *f,* street

callista, *m/f,* chiropodist

callo, callus; corn (*en el pie*); ~ **envolvente** ensheathing callus

callosidad, *f*, callus; keratoma
calloso, *adj*, calloused; rough (*manos*)
calma, calm
calmante, *m*, *adj*, depressant; ~[1] calmative; downer[2] (*barbiturato*); tranquilizer; pain killer; sedative; ~ **para la tos** cough suppressant
calmar, to allay; to alleviate; to calm; to quell; ~**se** to calm down; to quiet down; to relax; to subside
calmoso, calm
calofrío, *Chicano*, hot flashes (*de la menopausia*)
calo(s)fríos, *slang*, chills
calor, *m*, heat; ~**es** *fam*, *pl*, hot flashes; ~ **apoplético** heat apoplexy; ~ **atómico** atomic heat; ~ **corporal** body heat; ~ **de conducción** conductive heat; ~ **de convección** convective heat; ~ **en la vejiga**[6] "heat in" bladder; ~ **equilibrado** thermal equilibrium; *cult*, body heat; ~ **radiante** radiant heat; ~ **seco** dry heat
caloría, calorie
calórico, *m*, *adj*, caloric
calostro, colostrum
calote, *m*, cast
caluresis, *f*, kaluresis
calva, bald patch
calvicie, *f*, baldness
calvo, *adj*, bald; hairless
calzado, footwear; ~ **ortopédico** orthopedic shoes
calzoncillos, panty/panties; shorts (*ropa interior de hombres*); underpants
cama, bed; ~ **de agua** waterbed; ~ **de partos** labor bed; ~ **neumática** air bed; ~ **quirúrgica** surgical bed
cámara, chamber; feces; innertube; *fam*, bowel movement; *slang*, diarrhea; ~ **anterior del cerebro** anterior chamber of cerebrum; ~ **de aire** air chamber; ~**s del corazón** chambers of the heart; ~ **de oxígeno** oxygen tent; ~ **de prueba** testing chamber; ~ **hiperbárica** hyperbaric chamber; ~**s oculares** chambers of the eye; ~ **posterior del cerebro** posterior chamber of cerebrum; ~ **pulpar** pulp chamber *Dent*; ~ **vacía** air chamber *Dent*
camarones, *m*, *pl*, shrimp
cambiador, *m*, *adj*, exchanger; ~ **de calor** heat exchanger
cambiar, to change; to shift; to trade; ~ **el pañal** to diaper; ~ **de** to change; ~ **de color** to change color; ~ **de costumbres** to change one's habits; ~ **de idea** to change one's mind; ~**(se) de ropa** to change one's clothes; to get changed
cambio, change (*modificación*); shift (*de sitios*); ~ **de apetito** appetite change; change in appetite; ~ **de personalidad** personality change; ~ **de peso** change in weight; ~ **de vida** change of life; menopause; ~ **en el libido** change in libido
camilla, litter (*para enfermos*); stretcher; ~ **calentadora de niño** warming crib; ~ **de niño** crib
camillero, litter bearer; orderly; stretcher bearer
caminar, to walk; ~ **arrastrando los pies** to walk with a shuffle
camisa, jacket; shirt (*de hombre*); ~ **de fuerza** strait jacket; ~ **de noche** nightgown
camiseta, undershirt
camisón, *m*, nightgown (*hospital*)
camonear, to hoof it (*ir andando; bailar*)
campanilla, *fam*, uvula
campaña contra el ruido, noise abatement
campechana verde[1], marijuana
campo, area; country (*rural, no ciudad*); field; range; ~ **auditivo**

auditory field; ~ **de fijación** field of fixation; ~ **de la conciencia** field of consciousness; ~ **del microscopio** field of a microscope; ~ **eléctrico** electric field; ~ **eléctrico visual** electrical field of vision; ~ **magnético** magnetic field; ~ **visual** field of vision; range of vision; VF (*campo visual*); visual field; ~ **visual excedido** overshot field of vision

cana(s), gray/grey hair

canabis[1], marijuana

canal[7], *m*, canal; channel; duct *Anat*; groove; ~ **auditivo** auditory canal; ~ **basilar** basilar groove; ~ **costal** subcostal groove; ~ **de la oreja** *fam*, external ear canal; ~ **de la raíz** root canal; ~ **del parto** birth canal; ~ **del subclavio** subclavian groove; ~ **lagrimal** lacrimal canal; tear duct; ~ **neural** neural canal; ~ **radicular** root canal; ~ **urinario** urethra

canas (verdes), *f, pl*, (premature) gray hair

canastilla de niño, layette

cancelar, to cancel

cáncer[8], *m*, cancer; malignant disease; ~ **cerebral** brain cancer; ~ **cutáneo** skin cancer; ~ **de la mama** *form* breast cancer; ~ **de la piel** skin cancer; ~ **de la próstata** prostate cancer; ~ **de la sangre** leukemia; ~ **del cerebro** brain cancer; ~ **del ovario** ovarian cancer; ~ **del pecho** breast cancer; ~ **del pulmón** lung cancer; ~ **del seno** breast cancer; ~ **ovárico** ovarian cancer

canceroso, cancer patient; *adj*, cancerous

candela, candle; sexually active girl

candidato, candidate

candidiasis, *f*, candidiasis; moniliasis; ~ **bucal** *form*, thrush

caneca, hip flask

caneco, *adj, Arg, Bol*, drunk

canelo, *vulg, PR*, semen

canería, cannery

cangrena, gangrene

canicas, marbles

canijo, *adj*, infirm

canilla, longbone; shin

canino, eyetooth; canine tooth (*colmillo*)

canoso, *adj*, gray/grey haired

cansado, *adj*, tired; strained (*ojos, corazón*)

cansancio, fatigue (*fatiga*); tiredness; weariness; ~ **excesivo** overstrain

cansar, to fatigue (*fatigar*); to strain one's eyes; to strain (*corazón*); ~**(se)** to tire; ~**se** to get tired

cantar a la tirolesa, to yodel

cantazo, *fam*, blow (*al cuerpo de una persona, coche*); ~ [1]a fix of heroin; hit of cocaine or heroin

cantidad, *f*, quantity; ~ **suficiente** q.s./*quantum satis*/sufficient quantity

cánula, cannula; probe; ~ **nasal** nasal cannula

caña, haft (*de un hueso*)

cáñamo[1], marijuana

cañinga de mono[1], *PR*, extremely high on[2] (*drogas narcóticas*)

caño urinario, urethra

cañones, *m*, stubble (*de una barba*)

capa, film (*capa fina*); layer; stratum; ~[1] heroin capsule; ~ **de conos y bastones** layer of rods and cones; ~ **de fibras nerviosas** nerve fiber layer; ~ **germinal** germ layer; ~ **social** social stratum

capacidad, *f*, capacity; qualification (*competencia*); ~ **carga** load-carrying capacity; ~ **invasora** invasiveness; ~ **pulmonar total** total lung capacity; ~ **vital** VC/vital capacity

capaz, (*pl, capaces*) *adj*, capable

capear, to fight the disease; ~[1] to put heroin in capsules

caperucita en carnada, *slang*, rubber (*condón*)

capiar[1], to put heroin in capsules
capilar, *m*, capillary
capilaria, capillary
capón, *adj*, Chicano, infertile
cápsula, cap; capsule; pill; ~ **para ablandar evacuaciones** stool softener; ~ **vítrea** vitreous chamber
cápsulas[1], LSD; ~ **de drogas** goofballs[2] (*sedantes, especialmente barbitúricos*)
capuchón cervical, *m*, cervical cap
cara, face; ~ **de pájaro** bird-face; ~ **desfigurada por la enfermedad** face ravaged by disease; ~ **inexpresiva** expressionless face
caracol, *m*, *fam*, cochlea
carácter, *m*, character; makeup (*temperamento*); manner; ~ **de célula falciforme** sickle cell trait; ~ **dominante** dominant character; ~ **hereditario** trait; ~ **ligado al sexo** sex-linked character; ~ **recesivo** recessive character; ~ **sexual primario** primary sex character
característica, characteristic; hallmark; trait; ~ **distintiva** distinguishing feature; ~**s físicas** features
característico, *adj*, characteristic
caracterizar, to characterize; ~**se** to be characterized
carátula, *slang*, Chicano, face
carbohidrato, carbohydrate
carbón, *m*, charcoal; ~ **activado** activated charcoal
carbonato, carbonate; ~ **de calcio** calcium carbonate; ~ **de magnesio** magnesium carbonate; ~ **de sodio** sodium carbonate
carbono, carbon
carbunclo, boil; carbuncle
carbunco, boil; carbuncle
carcajada, howl of laughter; loud laugh
carcinoide, *m*, *adj*, carcinoid
carcinoma, *m*, carcinoma; ~ **agudo** acute carcinoma; ~ **basocelular** basal cell carcinoma; ~ **de células escamosas** squamous cell

carcinoma; ~ **de células pequeñas** small cell carcinoma; ~ **espinocelular** squamous cell carcinoma
cardenal, *m*, bruise (*en el cuerpo*); weal (*verdugón*); wheal; *fam*, ecchymosis
cardíaco/cardiaco *adj*, cardiac
cardialgia, heartburn
cardiogénico, *adj*, cardiogenic
cardiógeno, *adj*, cardiogenic
cardiograma, *m*, cardiogram; ~ **esofágico** esophageal cardiogram
cardioinhibidor, cardio-inhibitory
cardiología, cardiology
cardiólogo, cardiologist
cardiomiopatía, cardiomyopathy; ~ **dilatada** dilated cardiomyopathy; ~ **hipertrófica** hipertrophic cardiomyopathy; ~ **restrictiva** restrictive cardiomyopathy
cardiopatía, heart disease; ~ **reumática** rheumatic heart disease; ~ **valvular** V.D.H. (*enfermedad de la válvula del corazón*)
cardiorrespiratorio, *adj*, heart-lung
cardioscopio, cardioscope
cardiovascular, *adj*, cardiovascular
carencia, deficiency; deprivation; lack
carga[1], big C^2 (*cocaína*); boy[2] (*heroína*); candy[2] (*cocaína*); cocaine; H^2 (*heroína*); heroin; load of narcotics
cargar, to carry; ~[1] to be carrying narcotic; ~ **la calentura** Chicano, to increase/continuar (*fiebre*)
caricortao, *adj*, PR, scar-faced
caries, *f*, *inv*, *form*, caries; cavity *Dent*; decay *Dent*; tooth decay
cariño, affection
cariñoso, *adj*, affectionate
caritativo, *adj*, charitable
carnal, *m/f*, blood relative; *adj*, carnal
carne, *f*, flesh; meat; ~ **asada** roast beef; ~ **cruda** raw meat; ~ **de animal sacrificado según la ley**

judía kosher meat; ~ **de gallina** goose pimples; goose flesh; ~ **de puerco** pork; ~ **de res** beef; ~ **y hueso** flesh and blood

carnosidad, *f, fam*, pterygium

caro, *adj*, expensive

caroteno, carotene

carótido, *adj*, carotid

carpeta, file (*archivo*)

carraspear, to clear one's throat; to be hoarse

carraspera, *fam*, hoarseness

carrasposo, *adj*, chronically hoarse

carrete, *m*, coil *Elect*

carretilla, handcart

carrillo, cheek

carrujo[1], marijuana

carta, chart; letter; ~ **de examen visual** eye chart; ~ **de personería** power of attorney; ~ **de Snellen** Snellen chart

cártamo, safflower

cartel, *m*, poster

cartelón, *m*, chart; ~ **de Snellen** Snellen chart

cartera, purse

cartero, mailman

cartílago, cartilage; ~ **tiroideo** thyroid cartilage

cartucho[1], marijuana

casa, home; house; ~ **de correos** post office; ~ **de maternidad** maternity hospital

casado, *adj*, married

casamiento, marriage

casarse (con), to get married; ~**(se) por detrás de la iglesia** to live with someone in common-law marriage

cascar, to crack (*la voz*)

cáscara, peel (*peladura de las naranjas, patatas, etc.*); rind; ~ **de huevo** eggshell; ~ **de nuez** nutshell; ~[1] heroin

cascarrabias, *m/f, inv*, grouch (*persona que fácilmente riñe, se enoja o demuestra enfado*)

casco, scalp

cascorvo, *adj*, bow-legged

caseína, casein

caseinato de calcio, calcium caseinate

caso, case; ~ **de fuerza mayor** Act of God; ~ **desesperado** hopeless case; ~ **límite** borderline case; limiting case; ~ **precedente** leading case; ~ **urgente** emergency

caspa, dandruff

casquivano, *adj*, light-headed (*atolondrado*)

castañetear, to chatter

castañeteo de los dientes, teeth chattering

castración, *f*, castration; ~ **masculina** emasculation

castrado, *adj*, emasculated

castrar, to castrate; to sterilize

casual, *adj*, chance

catabolismo, destructive metabolism

catalepsia, *form*, trance

catalizador, *m*, catalyst

cataplasma, cataplasm; plaster *Med*; poultice (*pasta medicinal*); ~ **de mostaza** mustard plaster

catarata, cataract; ~ **adherente** adherent cataract; ~ **congénita** congenital cataract; ~ **diabética** diabetic cataract; ~ **hipermadura** overripe cataract; milky cataract; ~ **incipiente** incipient cataract; ~ **inmadura** immature cataract; unripe cataract; ~ **lechosa** milky cataract; ~ **madura** ripe cataract; ~ **por fulguración** electric cataract; ~ **por radiación** irradiation cataract; ~ **primaria** primary cataract

catarro, catarrh; *fam*, cold (*enfermedad*); ~ **constipado** *Chicano*, hay fever

catársis, *f*, catharsis

catártico, *adj*, purgative

catatonía/catatonia, catatonia

catatónico, *adj*, catatonic

catéter, *m*, catheter; ~ **central** central line; ~ **de dos ramas** two-way catheter; ~ **de Hickman** Hickman catheter; ~ **de Tenckhoff** Tenckhoff catheter; ~ **permanente** dwelling catheter

cateterismo, catheterization; ~ **cardíaco** cardiac catheterization

cateterizar, to catheterize

catgut, *m*, catgut; ~ **fino** fine catgut

catrueca, *fam*, head

caucasiano, *adj*, caucasian

caucho, rubber

causa, cause; ~ **de muerte** cause of death; ~ **inmediata** leading cause; ~**s naturales** natural causes

causar, to bring on; to cause; ~ **dolor** to hurt (*producir dolor*); ~ **moretones** to bruise

cauteloso, *adj*, precautious

cauterización, *f*, cauterization

cauterizar, to cauterize; to sear *Med*

cavernoso, *adj*, hollow (*voz*)

cavidad, *f*, cavity; chamber; ~ **dental** cavity *Dent*; ~ **abdominal** abdominal cavity; ~ **bucal** mouth cavity; ~ **del diente** nerve cavity; ~ **dental** caries; ~ **medular** medullary canal; ~ **nasal** nasal cavity; ~ **pulpar** nerve cavity; ~ **uterina** uterine cavity; ~**es cardíacas** cardiac chambers

cayado de la aorta, arc of the aorta

cc/centímetro cúbico, cc/cubic centimeter

cebada, barley; ~ **perlada** pearl barley

cebolla, onion

cecear, to lisp

ceceo, lisp (*defecto de habla*)

ceder, to ease off (*el dolor*); to give way; to yield (*no poder resistir*)

cefalalgia, *form*, headache

cefalea, *form*, headache; ~ **por acúmulos** cluster headache; ~ **por tensión nerviosa** tension headache; ~ **pulsátil** throbbing headache

cefálico, *adj*, cephalic

cegato, *adj, fam*, shortsighted

ceguedad, *f*, blindness

ceguera, blindness; ~ **del río** river blindness (*oncocerciasis*); ~ **diurna** day blindness/dayblindness; ~ **funcional** functional blindness; ~ **nocturna** *fam*, night blindness (*nictalopia*); ~ **para los colores** *fam*, color blindness; ~ **por eclipse** eclipse blindness; ~ **de objetos** objectblindness

ceja, brow (*del ojo*); eyebrow

celíaca, celiac disease

celiaquía, celiac disease

celoso, *adj*, jealous

célula, cell; ~ **B** B cell; ~ **cancerosa** cancerous cell; ~ **ciliada** ciliated cell; ~ **de revestimiento** encasing cell; ~ **falciforme** sickle cell; ~ **fotoeléctrica** electric eye; ~ **grasa** fat cell; ~**s gustativas** taste cells; ~ **huésped** host cell; ~ **insular** islet cell; ~**s mastoideas** mastoid cells; ~ **medular** marrow cell; ~ **nerviosa** nerve cell; ~ **nucleada** nucleated cell; ~**s parietales** parietal cells; ~ **plasmática** plasma cell; ~ **sanguínea** blood cell; ~ **T** T cell; ~ **viviente** living cell

celular, *adj*, cellular

celulitis, *f*, cellulite; ~ **pélvica** pelvic cellulitis

cemento, cement; cementum; ~ **dentario** tooth cement

cena, dinner; supper

cenar, to eat dinner/supper; to have dinner

cenicero, ashtray

cenizas, *f, pl*, dust (*restos mortales*)

centeno, rye

centígrado, Centigrade

centímetro, centimeter; ~ **cúbico** cubic centimeter

central, *adj*, central

centro, center; core; head (*de un absceso*); ~ **de aprendizaje** learning center; ~ **de salud** health care center; health center (*generalmente subvencionado por el gobierno*); ~ **de salud** health department; ~ **del lenguaje** motor speech area; ~ **médico polivalente** multicare health facility; ~ **nervioso** nerve center; ~ **para víctimas de quemaduras** burn center

ceñido, *adj*, narrow-waisted

ceñir (i), to girdle; **~se el cinturón de seguridad** to buckle up

ceño, frown

cepa, strain (*Med: grupos de microorganismos dotados de propiedades específicas*)

cepillado, brushing

cepillar, to brush; **~se el pelo** to brush one's hair; **~se los dientes** to brush one's teeth

cepillo, brush; comb; ~ **de dientes** toothbrush

cera, wax; ~ **de los oídos** earwax (*cerumen*); ~ **del oído** cerumen; ~ **para vaciado** casting wax

cercano, *adj*, close; near

cerdo, pork

cerebelo, cerebellum (*pl*, *cerebella*)

cerebral, *adj*, cerebral

cerebro, brain; cerebrum; occiput; ~ **medio** midbrain

cerebrovascular, *adj*, cerebrovascular

cerilla, earwax; match

cero, zero

cerrado, *adj*, closed

cerrar (ie), to close; ~ **el puño** to make a fist

certificado, certificate; ~ **de aptitud** certificate of fitness; ~ **de defunción** certificate of death; death certificate; ~ **de nacimiento** birth certificate; ~ **para no trabajar** work excuse

certificar, to certify

cerumen, *m*, earwax; wax (*del oído*)

cerveza, beer

cervical, *adj*, cervical

cervix, *f*, cervix

cerviz, *f*, cervix; back of the neck

cesárea, *f*, Caesarean

cesáreo, *adj*, Caesarean

cesariano, *adj*, Caesarean

cesio, cesium

cesta, basket

cetoacidosis, *f*, ketoacidosis

cetógeno, *adj*, ketogenic

cetólisis, *f*, ketolysis

cetona, ketone

cetónico, *adj*, ketotic

cetonuria, ketonuria

cetosis, *f*, ketosis

cetosuria, ketosuria

chácara, *CA*, *Col*, *Chi*, sore; ulcer

chale, *m*, *vulg*, *Chicano*, penis

chalito, *vulg*, *Chicano*, penis

chamaca, *Mex*, girl

chamaco, *Mex*, boy; child; kid

chamarra, *Mex*, jacket

chamarrero, *Ven*, quack doctor

chambón, *m*, tennis shoe

chamorro, *fam*, *Chicano*, calf (*pl*, *calves*) (*parte de la pierna*)

champiñón, *m*, mushroom

champú, *m*, shampoo

chancleta, *PR*, *SpAm*, baby girl, newborn

chancro, chancre; venereal lesion; ~ **blando** soft chancre; noninfecting chancre; ~ **duro** hard chancre; ~ **sifilítico** hard chancre; ~ **simple** noninfecting chancre

chancroide, *f*, chancroid

changa, thigh

chanza, *Chicano*, mumps

chapa, *PR*, bottle cap

chaparro, *adj*, *Mex*, *CA*, short (*persona*); *adj*, *Mex*, *CA*, *Ec*, *Perú*, *Bol*, squat

chapurreado, *adj*, broken (*lenguaje*)

chaqueta, jacket; jacket of a woman's suit

chara[1], marijuana

charlatán, *fam*, quack

charlatanería, quackery

charlatanismo, quackery

charola, *Mex*, tray

charuto[1], *esp. Arg*, jive stick[2] (*cigarrillo de mariguana*); joint[2] (*cigarrillo de mariguana*); nail[2]; reefer[2]

chasquido, click
chata, bedpan
chato, *slang*, crab louse
chaucha, *adj, Chi, Ec*, premature (*nacimiento*)
chavalongo, *Arg, Chi*, fever; sunstroke; drowsiness
chavar(se), to harass; to irritate (*molestar*)
chaveta, *fam*, head
chechén, *m*, poison ivy
cheque, *m*, check
chequeo, *Chicano*, check-up; examination; ~ **general médico** *Chicano*, check-up
chester[1], marijuana
cheuto, *adj, Chi*, harelip
chévere, *interj, adj, PR*, excellent
chi, *f, vulg*, urine
chibola, *CA*, bump; swelling; wen
chibolo, *Col, Ec, Hond, Perú*, bump; swelling; wen
chicha, *Ríopl*, blood; *CA, Ec*, bad temper; **estar de ~** *CA, Ec*, to be in a bad mood
chíchara[1], marijuana
chícharo, pea
chicharra, *PR*, buzzer
chichas, *CR*, breast
chiche, *f*, breast; *m, Mex, Guat*, breast (*de una nodriza*); *f, Mex*, nursemaid
chichi, *f, Mex*, breast; *f, Arg, slang*, nipple (*del seno de una mujer*); *f, fam, Guat, Mex*, wet nurse
chichigua, *vulg, SpAm*, wet nurse
chicho, handle around waistline (*love handle*)
chichón, *m*, boil; bump (*causado por trauma, esp. a la cabeza o la frente*); lump on the head; lump (*contusión*); swelling (*contusión*); *fam*, hematoma
chicle, *m*, gum (*goma de masticar*)
chiclona[1], marijuana
chico, *Cu, Pan*, child; kid
chicote, *m, slang*, penis
chiflado, *adj*, crazy
chiflar, to wheeze; to whistle

chile, *m*, hot pepper
chillar, to scream
chillido, scream
chimar, *CA*, to scratch; *Mex, Nic*, to annoy; to bother
chimbomba, balloon[2] (*drugs*)
chimpa, *Chicano*, hair
chimuelo, *adj, Chicano*, lacking teeth
chinaloa[1], *slang*, opium
chinche, *f*, bedbug
chincual, *m, Mex, Chicano*, diaper rash
chinga, *Ven*, drunkenness; *Mex*, thrashing; *vulg, common*, sexual intercourse
chingar, *vulg*, to have sexual intercourse; *Mex, PR*, to screw *slang*
chino, *Mex*, fine-toothed comb; *Chicano*, curl of hair; *adj, CA, Cu*, angry; furious; **estar ~** to be angry; *m, Arg, CA, Cu*, anger; **tener un ~** to be angry
chipe, *m/f, CA, Col, Mex*, baby
chipear[1], to chip[2] (*usar drogas narcóticas de vez en cuando*); to jolly pop[2] (*usar drogas narcóticas de vez en cuando*); to joy pop[2] (*usar drogas narcóticas de vez en cuando*)
chipiar[1], to chip[2] (*usar drogas narcóticas de vez en cuando*); to jolly pop[2] (*usar drogas narcóticas de vez en cuando*); to joy pop[2] (*usar drogas narcóticas de vez en cuando*); to use occasionally (*normalmente heroína*)
chiporra, *Guat, Hond*, tumor on the head
chiquero, *Ríopl*, sty
chira, *CA*, wound; sore; *Col*, rag; ~[1] marijuana
chiringa, kite
chirlo, cut (*en la cara*); slash
chiste, *m*, joke
chiva[1], boy[2] (*heroína*); H[2] (*heroína*); heroin; horse[2]; junk[2]; Mexican brown[2]; scag[2]; smack[2]; stuff[2] (*refiere a otras drogas también, como el opio*)

chivo, *PR*, small imperfection

Chlamydia, Chlamydia

chocante, *adj*, noteworthy; odd; *adj*, *Arg*, offensive; *adj*, *Mex*, unpleasant; *adj*, *SpAm*, annoying

chochera, dotage

chochez, *f*, dotage; *vulg*, senility

chochos[1], LSD

choco, *adj*, *Chi*, *Ec*, curly; curly-haired; *adj*, *Bol*, *Col*, *Ec*, *Ríopl*, swarthy; chocolate-colored

chola, *fam*, head

cholenco, *adj*, *Chicano*, sickly

cholla, *CA*, wound; sore

chompeta, *fam*, head

chopetear, *slang*, to have sexual relations

choque, *m*, impact; knock; shock; trauma; ~ **alérgico** *fam*, anaphylactic shock; ~ **anafiláctico** anaphylactic shock; ~ **asmático** *m*, asthmatic seizure; ~ **eléctrico** *m*, electroshock; ~ **emocional** emotional shock; ~ **nervioso** nervous breakdown; nervous shock; ~ **pericárdico** pericardial knock

choquezuela, kneecap (*rótula*)

chorcha, *CA*, goiter

chorizo, sausage

chorreando sudor, *adj*, sweltering (*persona*)

chorrear, to stream (*sangre*)

chorrillo, *slang*, diarrhea

chorro, gush (*de un líquido*); jet (*de sangre, agua, gas, un caudal muy pequeño, etc.*); stream (*común: de agua, sangre.*); *euph*, *Chicano*, gonorrhea; *fam*, gonorrhea; *slang*, diarrhea; ~ **de orina** urinary stream

chot, *m*, *Chicano*, injection; shot; vaccination

chuchín, *adj*, *PR*, excellent

chucho, *SpAm*, *Med*, chill; *SpAm*, *Med*, fever; *Arg*, *Chi*, malarial fever

chueca, *Anat*, rounded bone; round head of a bone

chueco, *adj*, crooked; **andar** ~[1] to deal in illegal transactions; *adj*, *SpAm*, knock-kneed; *adj*, *Arg*, *Perú*, pigeon-toed; *adj*, *Col*, lame; *adj*, *Mex*, one-armed; one-legged

chula, *adj*, *PR*, cute; excellent

chuleta de puerco, pork chop

chulón, *adj*, *CA*, naked

chuma, *adj*, *Ec*, *Ríopl*, drunkenness

chumarse, *Ec*, *Ríopl*, to get drunk

chupa, *SpAm*, drunkenness

chupado, *adj*, gaunt; emaciated

chupar, to suck; ~**se** *Med*, to waste away; to get thin

chupe[1], marijuana

chupeta, nipple (*para niños*); pacifier

chupete, *m*, nipple (*para niños*); pacifier

chupo, *SpAm*, *Med*, boil

chupón, *m*, hickey; nipple (*de un biberón*); pacifier; *m*, *Col*, boil

churrias, *f*, *pl*, *Col*, *Guat*, *RD*, diarrhea

churriento, *adj*, *SpAm*, *Med*, loose

churrusco, *adj*, *Col*, *Pan*, curly; kinky (*pelo*)

churus[1], marijuana

chutazo[1], cocaine; heroin

CIA/comunicación interauricular, *f*, ASD/atrial septal defect

cianhídrico, *adj*, hydrocyanic

cianosis, *f*, cyanosis

cianótico, *adj*, cyanotic

cianuro, cyanide; ~ **de potasio** potassium cyanide

ciática, sciatica

ciático, *adj*, sciatic

cicatriz, (*pl, cicatrices*), *f*, scar; ~ **filtrante** filtering scar; ~**es radiadas** radiating scars

cicatrizado, *adj*, scarred

cicatrizarse, to close (*una herida*); to scar

ciclamato, cyclamate; ~ **cálcico** calcium cyclamate; ~ **sódico** cyclamate, sodium

cíclico, *adj*, cyclic; cyclical

ciclo, cycle; ~ **biológico** life history; ~ **cardíaco** cardiac cycle; ~ **ciego** dead-end cycle; ~ **menstrual** menstrual cycle; ~ **ovulatorio** ovulatory cycle; ~ **reproductivo** reproductive cycle; ~ **reproductor** reproductive cycle; ~ **vital** life cycle

cicuta, poison hemlock

ciego, cecum (*pl*, *ceca*); *adj*, blind

cielo de la boca, palate; roof of the mouth

ciempiés, *m, inv*, centipede

ciencia, science; ~ **médica** medical science

científico, scientist; *adj*, scientific

cientopiés, *m, inv*, centipede

cierre, *m*, zipper; ~ **defectuoso de la válvula** mitral valve prolapse/mitral MVP; ~ **renal** renal shut-down

cierto, *adj*, certain

cifosis, *f*, kyphosis

cigarrera, cigar case

cigarrillo, cigarette; ~ **de marihuana**[1] Texas tea[2]

cigarro, cigarette; ~ **de mariguana**[1] jive stick[2]; joint[2]; ~ **puro** cigar

cilindro, cast (*molde de un órgano hueco, como el tubo renal*); ~ **adiposo** fatty cast; ~ **hemático** blood cast; ~ **purulento** pus cast; ~ **urinario** urinary cast

cilosis, *f*, kyllosis

cimbomba[1], *slang*, balloon[2] (*de heroína*)

cinc, *m*, zinc

cincha, band

cinemática, kinematics

cinesia, car sickness (*cinetosis*); kinetosis

cinestesia, kinesthesia

cinetosis, *f*, car sickness (*cinesia*); kinetosis

cinta, band; ribbon; tape (*para tiritas, etc.*); ~ **adhesiva** adhesive strip; adhesive tape; ~ **métrica** measuring tape

cintura, binder; girdle; waist; ~ **escapular** shoulder girdle; ~

pélvica pelvic girdle; ~ **torácica** thoracic girdle

cinturón, belt; ~ **de seguridad** seat/safety belt

cipote, *m, El Sal*, child; kid

circuito, circuit; ~ **abierto** open circuit; ~ **corto** short circuit; ~ **reflejo** reflex circuit

circulación, *f*, circulation; blood flow; ~ **colateral** vascular spiders; ~ **cruzada** cross circulation; ~ **extracorpórea** cardiac bypass; ~ **fetal** fetal circulation; ~ **hepática** liver circulation; ~ **mayor** systemic circulation; ~ **pulmonar** pulmonary circulation; ~ **sanguínea** blood circulation; blood flow; ~ **sistémica** systemic circulation

circular, *adj*, circular; ~ **del cordón** circular of the umbilical cord

circular, to circulate; to flow (*la sangre en el cuerpo*)

circulatorio, *adj*, circulatory

círculo, circle

circuncidar, to circumcise

circuncisión, *f*, circumcision

circundante, *adj*, encircling

circundar, to surround

circunvolución, *f*, convolution

ciricua, *fam*, vitiligo

cirrosis, *f*, cirrhosis; ~ **del hígado** cirrhosis of the liver; ~ **hepática** cirrhosis of the liver; ~ **pulmonar** cirrhosis of the lung

ciruela, plum; ~ **pasa** prune

cirugía, surgery (*trabajo del cirujano*); ~ **artroscópica** arthroscopic surgery; ~ **cardíaca** cardiac surgery; ~ **clínica** clinical surgery; ~ **conservadora** conservative surgery; ~ **cosmética** cosmetic surgery; ~ **de corazón abierto** open-heart surgery; ~ **electiva** elective surgery; ~ **estética** cosmetic surgery; plastic surgery; ~ **general** general surgery; ~ **mayor**

major surgery; ~ **menor** minor surgery; ~ **ortopédica** orthopedic surgery; ~ **plástica** plastic surgery; ~ **plástica del oído** otoplasty surgery; ~ **radical** radical surgery; ~ **reconstructiva** reconstructive surgery; ~ **reparadora** reconstructive surgery; ~ **torácica** chest surgery

cirujano, surgeon; ~ **asistente** house surgeon; ~ **auxiliar** assisting surgeon; ~ **ortopédico** orthopedic surgeon

cisticerco, bladder worm; cysticercus

cístico, *adj*, cystic (*relativo a una vejiga*); **conducto** ~ cystic duct

cistitis, *f*, cystitis; ~ **crónica** chronic cystitis

cistocele, *m*, cystocele

cistografía, cystography

cistograma, *m*, cystogram; ~ **excretorio** voiding cystogram

cistoscopia/cistoscopía, cystoscopy

cistoscópico, *adj*, cystoscopic

cistoscopio, cystoscope

cisura, fissure; wound incision; ~ **del ano** anal fissure

cita, appointment; date (*entre chico y chica*); meeting; quotation

citoblasto, cytoblast

citología, citology; cytology

citólogo, cytologist

citoplasma, *m*, cytoplasm

citosis, *f*, cytosis

citrato, citrate

ciudad, *f*, city

clamidia, Chlamydia

clamp, *m*, clamp

clara, white (*de un huevo*); bald patch (*en el cráneo*); ~ **de huevo** egg white

claro, *adj*, bright; clear; fair (*la tez*)

clase, *f*, category; class; ~ **de** kind; ~ **de hongos** yeast; ~ **social** social class

clasificación, *f*, categorization; classification

clasificar, to categorize; ~ **la sangre** to blood type

claustrofobia, claustrophobia

clavar, to fix (*ojos*); to stash[2] (*esconder un suministro de drogas*); to stick (*un puñal, puñetazo, etc.*); ~**se**[1] to fix[2] (*inyectarse drogas*); to hit up[2]; to inject oneself with drugs; ~**se**[1] *fam*, to bang[2] (*drogas*)

clave, *f*, key (*código*)

clavícula, collar bone; clavicle

clavija, peg; ~ **de contacto** electrical plug

clavo, nail (*larga pieza metálica*); pin *Ortho*

cleptomanía, kleptomania

cleptómano, kleptomaniac

climatérico, menopause

clínica, clinic (*lugar de consulta privada*); private hospital; surgery (*lugar de consulta privada*); ~ **de consulta externa** outpatient clinic; ~ **de reposo** nursing home; ~ **dental** dental office; ~ **privada** private clinic

clínico, clinician; general practitioner/GP; ~ **principal** leading practitioner; *adj*, clinical

clip, *m*, clip

clítoris, *m*, clitoris

cloasma, mask of pregnancy; chloasma (*descoloración de la piel, máscara del embarazo*)

cloración, *f*, chlorination

clorado, *adj*, chlorinated

cloranfenicol, *m*, chloramphenicol

clorhidrato, hydrochloride; ~ **de hidralacina** hydralazine hydrochloride; ~ **de quinina y urea** quinine and urea hydrochloride; ~ **de Demerol** Demerol hydrochloride

clorhídrico, *adj*, hydrochloric

cloro, bleach; chlorine

clorofila, chlorophyll

cloroformo, chloroform

cloromicetín/cloromycetín, *m*, chloromycetin

cloroquina, chloroquine
clorpropamide, chlorpropamide
cloruro, chloride; ~ **de bario** barium chloride; ~ **de etilo** ethyl chloride; ~ **de metilo** methyl chloride; ~ **de tiamina** thiamine chloride; ~ **de vinilo** vinyl chloride; ~ **mercúrico** bichloride of mercury
coagulante, *m, adj*, coagulant
coagular(se), to clot (*la sangre en las arterias*); to set (*la sangre en una herida*)
coágulo, clot (*de sangre*); thrombus; ~ **de sangre** blood clot; ~ **sanguíneo** blood clot
coaltar, *m*, coal tar
cobalto, cobalt
cobayo, guinea pig
cobertizo, lean-to
cobija, *CA, Mex, Ven, Col*, blanket
cobrar, to charge; ~ **un precio excesivo (a)** to overcharge
cobre, *m*, copper
cobro, charge; payment; ~ **detallado** itemized charge
coca[1], big C[2] (*cocaína*); candy[2] (*cocaína*); cocaine
cocacola[1], cocaine
cocada[1], cocaine
cocaína, big C[2]; candy[2]; cocaine
cocazo[1], cocaine
coccidioidomicosis pulmonar primaria, *f*, valley fever; coccidioidomycosis
coccígeo, *adj*, caudal
cóccix, *m*, tail bone
cócciz, *m*, tail bone; *Chicano, fam*, coccyx
cocer, to boil (*comida*); to cook; ~ **en el horno** to bake
cochornis[1], marijuana
cocido, *adj*, cooked
cociente, *m*, quotient; ~ **calórico** caloric quotient; ~ **de crecimiento** growth quotient; ~ **de inteligencia** intelligence quotient/IQ; ~ **de realización** achievement quotient; ~ **espinal** spinal quotient; ~ **intelectual** intelligence quotient; ~ **proteínico** protein quotient; ~ **raquídeo** rachidian quotient; ~ **respiratorio** respiratory quotient; ~ **sanguíneo** blood quotient
cocinar, to cook
cóclea, *form*, cochlea
coco, coconut; coconut palm; grub; larva; worm (*de frutas*); wound; *fam*, brain; *fam*, head; *fam*, hurt; *fam*, injury; ~[1] cocaine
cócono[1], person high on drugs
cocopelao, *adj, PR*, bald
cocotazo, blow (*en la cabeza*)
codazo, jab (*con el codo*)
codeína, codeine
código, code; ~ **de ética** code of ethics; ~ **genético** genetic code
codo, elbow; ~ **de golf** golfer's elbow; ~ **de lanzador** baseball pitcher's elbow; ~ **de los mineros** miners' elbow; ~ **de tenis** *fam*, tennis elbow
coeficiente, *m*, coefficient
coercitivo, restraining device
coffee[1], marijuana
coger, to take hold of; to lift (*tomar*); *vulg, Arg, PR, Mex*, to have sexual relations; ~**lo suave** *PR*, to take it easy; ~ **hora para** to make an appointment with; ~ **pela** *fam*, to be badly beaten; ~ **una borrachera** to be/get drunk
cogioca, *PR*, graft
cogote, *m*, scruff (*del cuello*); *fam*, Adam's apple; nape (*del cuello*)
cohabitación, *f*, cohabitation
cohesión, *f*, cohesion
cohete[1], *m*, boy[2] (*heroína*); H[2] (*heroína*); heroin; LSD
cohibido, *adj*, inhibited; self-conscious
coil, *m, Chicano*, coil (*anticonceptivo*)
coito, coitus; sexual relations; ~ **interrumpido** coitus interruptus; ~ **interruptus** *form*, withdrawal (*sexual*)

cojear, to limp to (*andar inclinando el cuerpo más a un lado que a otro*)
cojera, lameness; limp
cojín, *m*, pad; ~ **eléctrico** electric heating pad
cojincillo, pad
cojo, *adj*, crippled; crippled in the foot; lame
cojones, *m*, *pl*, *vulg*, *slang*, testicle; balls *slang*
coka[1], cocaine
cola, line (*de gente*); queue; tail; *slang*, glue[2]
colado, casting; *adj*, strained
colágena, collagen
colágeno *adj*, collagen
colangiografía, cholangiogram; cholangiography; ~ **transhepática** percutaneous cholangiography
colangiograma, *m*, cholangiogram
colapsado, *adj*, broken down
colapsarse, to collapse (*un pulmón*)
colapso, breakdown; collapse; nervous breakdown; ~ **de pulmón** collapsed lung; ~ **físico** physical collapse; ~ **nervioso** nervous breakdown; ~ **renal** renal shut-down
colar (ue), to strain (*vegetales, macarrones, etc.*)
colcha, quilt
colchón, *m*, mattress; ~ **de aire** air mattress; ~ **de viento** air mattress
coleccionar, to save
colecistectomía, cholecystectomy
colecistograma, *m*, cholecystogram
colecistopatía, gallbladder disease
colectomía, colectomy
colelitiasis, *f*, gallstone
cólera, anger; fury; *Med*, cholera
colesterina, cholesterol
colesterol, *m*, cholesterol; fat in the veins; ~ **elevado** high cholesterol
colgajo, flap; ~ **cutáneo** skin flap
colgar (ue), to hang; to sag (*la carne*); ~ (*las piernas*) to dangle (*dejarlas colgadas*)

cólico, bellyache; *fam*, abdominal cramp; ~ **menstrual** menstrual cramp; *m*, *adj*, colic
colilla, roach[2] (*resto de un cigarrillo de marijuana*); stump (*de un cigarrillo*)
colirio, eye drops; eye salve; ~ **graso** eye ointment; ~ **seco** eye powder
colita, tail bone; *fam*, coccyx
colitis, *f*, colitis; ~ **mucosa** mucous colitis; ~ **ulcerosa** ulcerative colitis; diverticulitis
collar, *m*, necklace; ~ **cervical** cervical collar
collarín, *m*, cervical collar
colmar de honores, to overwhelm with honors
colmillo, eyetooth; fang; *fam*, cuspid; *fam*, canine tooth
colocar, to place (*poner*)
coloide, *m*, colloid
colombiana[1], Acapulco gold[2] (*mariguana*); marijuana
colon, *m*, colon; ~ **ascendente** ascending colon; ~ **descendente** descending colon; ~ **inestable** irritable colon; ~ **irritable** irritable colon; ~ **espástico** spastic colon
colonia, colony
colonoscopia/colonoscopía, colonoscopy
colonoscopio, colonoscope
color, *m*, color
coloración, *f*, stain (*colorante*); ~ **acidorresistente** acid-fast stain; ~ **anormal** discoloration; ~ **de azul de metileno** methylene blue stain; ~ **de Giemsa** Giemsa's stain; ~ **de Gram** Gram's stain; ~ **de Papanicolaou** Pap stain; ~ **de Wright** Wright's stain
colorada, *slang*, *Chicano*, blood; ~[1], seconal; seconal capsule; *slang*, barbiturate; ~**s**[1] devils[2] (*seconal; barbituratos*)
colorado, *adj*, hued; red
colorante, *m*, dye; stain(ing) (*para el estudio con el microscopio*); ~ **de**

Ziehl-Neelsen   Ziehl-Neelsen stain; ~ **selectivo** selective stain; ~ **vital** vital dye; **~s y métodos de coloración** stains and staining methods

colorar, to dye

colorete, *m*, rouge

colorines[1], LSD

colostomía, colostomy

colposcopia/colposcopía, colposcopy

columna, column;   *fam*, backbone; ~ **adiposa** fat column; ~ **vertebral** backbone; vertebral column; spinal column; spine; vertebral column

coma, *m*, coma; ~ **alcohólico** alcoholic coma; ~ **diabético** diabetic coma

comadrona/comadrón, midwife (*empírica, sin formación profesional*)

comatoso, *adj*, comatose

combatir, to combat

combinación, *f*, combination; slip (*ropa interior*); ~ **de PCP y LSD** Product IV[2]

comedón, *m*, blackhead

comenzar (ie), to begin; to start

comer, to eat; ~ **demasiado** to eat too much; **~se las palabras** *fam*, to slur (*palabras*); **~se las uñas** to bite one's nails

comestible, *adj*, eatable; edible

comezón, *m*, tingle; *f*, itch (*sensación*); ~ **intensa** pruritus (*picazón aguda*)

comida, food; meal; *Mex*, lunch; ~ **balanceada** balanced meal; ~ **de prueba** test meal; ~ **para niños** baby food; **~s llevadas al domicilio** Meals on Wheels

comido de la luna, *fam*, harelip

comienzo, beginning; onset; threshold

comisura, commisure; suture; ~ **de los labios** corner of the mouth

comité, *m*, committee

como, *adv*, like; as; ~ **pepa jobo** *PR*, having long, dirty hair

comodidad, *f*, comfort; **~es** *f*, *pl*, restroom

cómodo, *adj*, comfortable; easy (*vida*); *Mex*, bedpan

compadecerse (de), to sympathize (with)

compañía, company; ~ **de seguro(s)** insurance company; ~ **aseguradora** insurance company

compañones, *m*, *pl*, *slang*, testicle

compás, *m*, calliper

compasión, *f*, compassion

compasivo, *adj*, sympathetic (*mostrando pena*)

compatible, *adj*, compatible

compensación, *f*, compensation; ~ **excesiva** overcompensation; ~ **rota** broken compensation

compensar, to compensate; to make up (*una pérdida*)

competencia, competence; qualification (*capacidad*); scope (*habilidad*)

competente, *adj*, competent; qualified (*apto*)

competir (i), to compete

complejidad, *f*, complexity

complejo, complex; ~ **de Edipo** Oedipal complex; ~ **de inferioridad** inferiority complex; ~ **relacionado con el SIDA** AIDS related complex/ARC; ~ **sintomático** syndrome

complemento, complement

completamente desarrollado, *adj*, full-blown

completo, *adj*, complete; full; thorough; whole

complicación, *f*, complication

complicado, *adj*, complicated; compound (*fractura*)

complicar, to complicate; to embarrass (*dificultar*)

componente, *m*, component; **~s de orina** urine constituents; ~ **de sangre** blood component; ~ **sanguíneo** blood component; ~

tromb. plástico del plasma plasma thromboplastic component
componer, to compose; to constitute; to fix; ~ **una fractura** to set a fracture; ~**(se)** to mend; ~**se**[1] to fix[2] (*inyectar drogas*); to hit up[2]; to inject oneself with drugs; ~**se**[1] *fam*, to bang[2] (*drogas*)
comportamiento, behavior; manner
comportarse, to behave
comprender, to understand; ~ **mal** to misunderstand
comprensión auditiva, *f*, listening comprehension
comprensivo, *adj*, sympathetic; understanding
compresa, compress; dressing (*tirita*); pack *Med*; sanitary towel; ~ **de gasa** gauze swab; ~ **fría** cold compress; cold pack
compresión, *f*, compression; ~ **del cerebro** compression of the brain; ~**es torácicas** chest compressions
comprimido, lozenge; pill (*sólido*); tablet
comprimir, to compress
compuesto, compound; ~ **(in)saturado** (un)saturated compound; ~ **graso** fatty compound
compulsión, *f*, compulsion
compulsivo, *adj*, compulsive
computador digital, *m*, digital computer
computadora, computer
común, *m*, toilet; *Mex*, buttock
comunicación, *f*, communication; ~ **interauricular/CIA** atrial septal defect/ASD; ~ **interventricular/CIV** ventricular septal defect/VSD; ~ **verbal** verbal communication
comunicar, to communicate
comunicativo, *adj*, communicative
comunidad, *f*, community
comunitario, *adj*, community
con, with; ~ **agujetas** *adj*, stiff *Med*, (*después de hacer ejercicio*); ~ **articulaciones dobles** *adj*, double

jointed; ~ **cuidado** carefully; ~ **el pecho aplanado** flat bosomed; ~ **el tiempo** eventually; ~ **exactitud** accurately; ~ **facilidad** easily; ~ **fluidez** fluently (*en escritura*); ~ **frecuencia** frequently; often; ~ **granos** spotty *Med* (*tumorcillos*); ~ **la cabeza descubierta** *adj/adv*, bareheaded; ~ **(las) piernas arqueadas** bandy-legged; bow-legged; ~ **los nervios destrozados** overwrought (*extenuado*); ~ **manchas** mottled (*piel*); spotty *Med* (*de infección*); ~ **náuseas** queasy; ~ **permiso** excuse me (*permisión*); ~ **regularidad** *adv*, regularly; ~ **retraso** late (*después de decidir una hora*); ~ **seguridad** safely; ~ **soltura** fluently (*hablando*); ~ **voz ronca** *adv*, huskily (*voz*)
concebir (i), to conceive
concentrado, concentrate
concentración, *f*, concentration; ~ **de iones de hidrógeno** hydrogen ion concentration
concentrar(se), to concentrate
concepción, *f*, conception
concernir (ie), to concern; to involve
conciencia, awareness; conscience
concluir, to conclude
conclusión, *f*, conclusion
concurso, assistance
concusión, *f*, concussion; ~ **de la médula espinal** concussion of the spine; ~ **del cerebro** concussion of the brain
condado, county
condición, (*pl, condiciones*), *f*, condition; shape; ~**es de vida** living conditions
condicionamiento, conditioning; ~ **del aire** air conditioning
cóndilo, condyle; ~ **occipital** occipital condyle
condiloma, *m*, conduloma
condimento, condiment; seasoning
condón, *m*, condom; prophylactic; rubber (*cubierta anticonceptiva*)

condriosoma, *m*, mitochondria
condrosarcoma, *m*, chondrosarcoma
conducción,   *f*,   conduction;   ~
nerviosa nerve conduction; ~
retardada delayed conduction
conducir, to drive
conducta, behavior; ~ **automática**
automatic behavior; ~ **(in)vari-
able** (in)variable behavior
conducto, canal; channel; duct
Anat; tube; ~ **a seguir** management; ~ **alimentario** alimentary
canal; ~ **alveolar** alveolar duct; ~
arterioso arterial duct; ~ **auditivo** auditory duct; auditory tube;
~ **auditivo externo** external
acoustic meatus; external ear
canal; ~ **auriculoventricular** auriculoventricular channel; ~**(s)
biliar(es)** bile duct(s); ~ **biliar
interlobulillar** interlobular biliary canal; ~ **coclear** cochlear
canal; cochlear duct; ~ **colédoco** common bile duct; ~ **de la
pulpa** pulp canal; ~ **de ventilación** airway; vent (*tubo*); ventilation duct; ~ **de Walther**
(*conducto de la glándula salival
sublingual*) Walther's canal; ~
deferente vas deferens (*pl, vasa
deferentia*); ~ **dental** alveolar
canal; ~ **eyaculador** ejaculatory
duct; ~ **galactóforo** milk duct; ~
hepático hepatic duct; ~ **inguinal** abdominal canal; ~
lacrimal eye-tear duct; tear
duct; ~ **linfático derecho** right
lymphatic duct; ~ **mamario** milk
duct; ~ **meato auditivo external**
acoustic duct; ~ **nasal** nasal
canal; ~ **ovárico** ovarian duct; ~**s
prostáticos** prostatic ducts; ~
radicular root canal; ~**s salivales**
salivary ducts; ~ **semicircular**
semicircular canal; ~ **semicircular óseo** bony canal of the ear; ~
torácico alimentary duct; left
lymphatic duct; thoracic duct; ~
venoso venosum ligamentum

conectar, to connect
conejo, rabbit; *slang, Chicano*, biceps
conexión, *f*, connection
conexionar, to connect
confesar (ie), to confess
confianza, confidence; faith; trust;
~ **en sí mismo** self-confidence
confiar (en), to rely (on/upon); ~
en to trust
confidencial, *adj*, private; privileged
confinamiento, confinement
confinar en una institución, to
confine in an institution
conflicto, conflict
confortable, *adj*, comfortable
confrontación, *f*, confrontation
confrontar, to confront
confundido, *adj*, baffled
confundir, to confuse; to perplex;
~**se** to become confused
confusión, *f*, confusion; ~ **mental**
obfuscation
confuso, *adj*, baffled; confused
congelación, *f*, frostbite
congelado en seco, *adj*, freeze-
dried
congelar, to freeze
congénito, *adj*, congenital; inborn
congestión, *f*, *fam*, congestion; ~
mamaria *fam*, caked breast; ~
nasal nasal congestion; sinus
congestion; ~ **pasiva** passive
congestion
congestionado,   *adj*,   stuffy
(*taponado*)
congoja, anguish; distress (*angustia*); grief (*tristeza*); heartache
cónico, *adj*, conical
coniforme, *adj*, cone-shaped
conjuntiva, conjunctiva
conjuntivitis,   *f*,   conjunctivitis;
pinkeye; ~ **aguda contagiosa**
acute contagious conjunctivitis;
~ **catarral aguda** conjunctivitis;
pinkeye
conjunto, set (*de cosas diversas*);
whole
conmoción nerviosa, *f*, shock

cono, cone; ~ **arterioso** arterial cone; ~ **luminoso** cone of light; **~s y bastones** rods and cones
conocer, to know (*gente, lugares*); to meet; to have sexual relations
conocido, *adj*, familiar
conocimiento, awareness; consciousness; knowledge
consciente, *adj*, conscious
consecuencia, consequence; **~s** after-effects
conseguir (i), to get; to obtain
consejero, counselor; ~ **médico** medical adviser
consejo, advice; ~ **médico** doctor's advice; medical advice; **~s acerca de la salud** health counseling
consentimiento, consent
consentir (ie), to consent; ~ **en** to consent to
conservación de la energía, *f*, conservation of energy
conservar, to conserve
conservativo, *adj*, conservative
consistencia de las heces, stool character
consola central, central console
consolar (ue), to comfort; to console
consolidación, *f*, knitting (*de una fractura*)
constante, *f*, *adj*, constant; lasting (*temor, etc.*); steady (*continuo*)
constipación, *f*, *fam*, constipation; ~ **nasal** stopped-up nose
constipado, congestion; head cold; "stopped-up" head; *adj*, congested (*taponado*)
constitución, *f*, makeup (*estructura*); system
constituir, to constitute
constituyente, *m/f*, *adj*, constituent
constricción, *f*, constriction; stricture
constrictor, *m*, *adj*, constrictor
consulta, advice; consultation; ~ **particular** private practice
consultar, to consult; ~ **algo con la almohada** to sleep on something
consultor, *m*, *adj*, consultant

consultorio, doctor's office; medical office; ~ **del dentista** dentist's office; ~ **dental** dental office; ~ **externo** outpatient clinic
consumir, to consume; to exhaust; **~(se)** to burn out
consumo, consumption; ~ **del alcohol** alcohol consumption
consunción, *f*, consumption; phthisis
consuntivo, *adj*, consumptive
contacto, contact; **~s de balance** balancing contacts *Dent*; ~ **directo** direct contact; ~ **inicial** initial contact; ~ **inmediato** immediate contact; ~ **sexual** sexual intercourse; sexual contact
contagiar, to communicate a disease; to give (*infectar*); to infect
contagio, contagion; contamination (*de una enfermedad*)
contagioso, *adj*, communicable; contagious
contaminación, *f*, contamination (*de una enfermedad*); pollution; ~ **del agua** water pollution; ~ **del aire** air pollution
contaminante, *m*, polluting agent
contaminar, to contaminate (*enfermedad, ambiente*); **~se** to become contaminated
contar (ue), to count
contener, to contain; to hold back (*emociones, etc.*); ~ **la respiración** to hold one's breath
contenido, *m*, *adj*, content; ~ **gástrico** gastric content
contento, *adj*, content; happy
contexto, context
contigüidad, *f*, contiguity
contiguo, *adj*, adjoining
continuado, *adj*, continuous
continuamente, *adv*, continuously
continuar, to continue
continuo, *adj*, continual; continuous
contorneado, *adj*, contoured
contorno, contour; ~ **gingival** gingival contour *Dent*

contracción, *f*, contraction; ~ **auricular prematura** premature atrial contraction/PAC; ~ **de hambre** hunger pain; ~**es de la matriz** contractions *Obst*; ~ **espasmódica** jerking movement; twitching; ~**es expulsivas** bearing down; expulsive pression; ~ **isométrica** isometric contraction; ~ **isotónica** isotonic contraction; ~ **muscular** muscular contraction; spasm; ~ **súbita** jerk (*movimiento repentino; sacudida*); ~**es uterinas** contractions *Obst*; ~ **ventricular automática** automatic ventricular contraction; ~ **ventricular prematura** premature ventricular contraction/PVC
contracepción, *f*, contraception
contraceptivo, *m*, *adj*, contraceptive
contradictorio, *adj*, conflicting
contraer(se), to contract; ~ **una enfermedad** to catch a disease
contrahecho, *adj*, deformed
contraído, *adj*, contracted
contraindicación, *f*, contraindication; ~ **de tratamiento** inadvisability of treatment
contraveneno, antidote; antitoxin
contribución, *f*, contribution
contribuir, to contribute
control, *m*, control; ~ **de la calidad** quality control; ~ **de la natalidad** birth control; ~ **del ritmo cardíaco** cardiac monitoring
controlable, *adj*, controllable
controlar, to control
contusión, *f*, *form*, bruise; contusion; trauma; ~ **de la columna vertebral** whiplash
contusionado, *adj*, bruised
convalecencia, aftercare; convalescence
convalecer(se), to convalesce; to get better (after); to recover (from)
convaleciente, *m/f*, *adj*, convalescent

conveniente, *adj*, convenient
convergencia, convergence
convertir (ie), to convert; to transform; ~**se** to evolve; to turn into
convexo, *adj*, convex
convolución, *f*, convolution
convoluto, *adj*, convolute
convulsión, *f*, convulsion; epileptic attack; fit; seizure
conyugal, *adj*, conjugal; marital
coñac, *m*, cognac
cooperación íntima, *f*, teamwork
cooperar, to cooperate
cooperativo, *adj*, cooperative
coordinación, *f*, coordination
coordinar, to coordinate
copa, cup; glass; drink; ~ **graduada** measuring glass; ~ **ocular** eye cup
coprocultivo, coproculture; stool culture
coqueluche, *f*, whooping cough; pertussis
coquetas, *Mex*, mumps
coquito, *PR*, coconut drink
coraje, *m*, *fam*, emotional shock; anger
corajudo, *adj*, *fam*, angry
coramina, Coramine
corazón, *m*, heart; ~ **arterial** left heart; ~ **atlético** athletic heart; ~ **fibroide** fibroid heart; ~ **grande** enlarged heart; ~ **graso** fatty heart; ~ **irritable** irritable heart
corchete, *m*, hook (*en un vestido*)
corcova, humpback (*joroba*); hunch (*giba*)
corcovado, *m/f*, hunchback; humpback (*persona*); *adj*, hunchbacked; humpbacked
cordal, *m*, wisdom tooth
cordero, lamb
cordón, *m*, cord; ~ **del ombligo** umbilical cord; ~ **dental** dental floss; ~ **espermático** spermatic cord; ~ **nervioso** nerve cord; ~ **umbilical** umbilical cord
cordura, sanity (*estado de cuerdo*)
corea, chorea; ~ **de Huntington**

Huntington's chorea; ~ **epidémica** dancing disease

corino, *PR*, clubfoot

coriza, rhinitis

córnea, cornea; ~ **opaca** sclera

coroides, *f, inv*, choroid;chorioid

corona, cap *Dent;* corona; crown; ~ **acrílica** acrylic jacket crown; ~ **anatómica** anatomical crown; ~ **de porcelana** porcelain jacket crown; ~ **en cáscara** jacket crown; ~ **en cáscara de porcelana** porcelain jacket crown *Dent*

coronamiento, crowning *Obst*

coronar, to crown

coronario, *adj*, coronary

corporal, *adj*, corporal

corpulento, *adj*, large; obese

corpúsculo, corpuscle; ~ **blanco** white blood corpuscle; ~ **de la sangre** blood corpuscle; ~ **esferoidal** ball; ~ **rojo** red blood corpuscle

corral, *m*, pen (*para animales de granja*)

correa, strap (*tira de cuero*)

corrección, *f*, adjustment; ~ **oclusal** occlusal correction

correctivo, *adj*, corrective

correcto, *adj*, correct

corredera, *Chicano*, diarrhea

corredizo, *adj*, sliding (*parte*)

corregir (i), to correct; to emend

correlación, *f*, correlation

correo, mail

correr, to flow (*lágrimas; sangre de una herida*); to run; to slide (*un objeto*); to stream (*líquido*); ~ **riesgo** to hazard (*poner en peligro*); ~**se** *vulg*, to climax (*sexualmente*); to come (*tener orgasmo*); ~**se** *vulg, PR*, to ejaculate

corriente, *f*, current stream (*de agua, sangre*); ~ **alterna** alternating current; ~ **alternativa** alternating current; ~ **centrífuga** centrifugal current; ~ **continua** constant current; ~ **de alta frecuencia** high-frequency current; ~ **directa** direct current; ~ **eléctrica** electric current; ~ **electrostática** electrostatic current; ~ **estática** static current; ~ **galvánica** battery current; ~ **invertida** reversed current; ~ **sanguínea** bloodstream; ~ **sinusoidal** sine wave current; *adj*, current; average

corroer, to corrode; to erode

corrosión, corrosion; rust

corrosivo, *adj*, corrosive

corsé, *m*, corset; *m, fam*, brace; *m/f*, jacket; ~ **enyesado** plaster-of-Paris jacket

cortada, incision; laceration; *SpAm*, cut

cortadura, cut (*herida pequeña*); cutting; wound

cortante, *adj*, cutting (*afilada*); sharp

cortaplumas, *m, inv*, penknife

cortapuros, *m, inv*, cigar cutter

cortar, to amputate; to bite (*frío, viento*); to cut; ~ **el tendón de la corva** to hamstring (*desjarretar*); ~ **la fiebre** to bring down the fever; ~**se** to cut oneself; ~ **el pelo** to cut one's hair; to get a haircut; ~ **el vicio**[1] to clear up; to kick the habit; ~ **las uñas** to cut one's nails

cortauñas, *m, inv*, nail clippers

corte, *m*, cut (*incisión*); section; ~ **de las partes** episiotomy; ~ **de parafina** paraffin section; ~ **de pelo** haircut; ~**s en serie** serial section; ~ **frontal** frontal section; ~ **microscópico** microscopic section; ~ **por congelación** frozen section; ~ **sagital** sagittal section; ~ **transversal** cross-section

cortedad de la vista, myopia; nearsightedness

corteza, bark; cortex; ~ **cerebral** cerebral cortex; mantle

corticosteroide, *m*, corticosteroid

cortisona, cortisone

corto, *adj*, little (*distancia*); short (*de poca duración; distancia*); ~ **circuito** by-pass; shunt; ~ **de oído** hard of hearing; ~ **de respiración** dyspneic; shortness of breath; ~ **de vista** nearsighted

corva, back of knee; bend of the knee; ham *Anat*

corvo, bow-legged

cosa[1], marijuana

coser, to suture; to sew

cosmético, *m*, *adj*, cosmetic; **~s** makeup

cosmetología, cosmetology

cósmico, *adj*, cosmic

cosquillas, *f*, *pl*, tickle

cosquilleo, tickling (sensation)

costado, flank; side

costal de huesos, *m*, *fam*, bag of bones

costar (ue), to cost

costarricense, *m/f*, *adj*, Costa Rican

costear, to meet (*deuda*)

costilla, rib; ~ **cervical** cervical rib; ~ **falsa** false rib; ~ **flotante** floating rib; ~ **verdadera** true rib; **~s asadas** pork ribs

costo, charge; ~ **de vida** cost of living

costoso, *adj*, expensive

costra, crust; scab; scale *Med* (*de piel*); ~ **láctea** cradle cap; milk crust

costroso, *adj*, scabby

costumbre, *f*, custom; habit; menstruation; ~ **dañina** harmful habit

costura, sewing

cotidiano, *adj*, daily

cotita, *PR*, shirt (*de un bebé*)

cotorear[1], to be on the nod[2] (*bajo la influencia de heroína*)

cotorra[1], cocaine

coxis, *m*, coccyx

coyuntura, articulation; *esp. CA*, *Mex*, joint

crack[1], *m*, crack[2] (*cocaína*)

craneal, *adj*, cranial

craneano, *adj*, cranial

cráneo, cranium; head; skull

craqueo, *adj*, *Chicano*, crazy

craquear(se), *Chicano*, to crack up

craso, *adj*, gross (*manifiesto*)

creatina, creatine

creatinina, creatinine

crecer, to grow (*aumentar de talla*)

creciente, *m*, *adj*, crescent

crecimiento, growth; ~ **nuevo** new growth

credibilidad, *f*, credibility

creencia, belief

creer, to believe

crema, cream; lotion; ointment; ~ **de cacahuete** peanut butter; ~ **dental** toothpaste; ~ **hidratante** moisturizing cream; ~ **para el sol** suntan lotion; ~ **para las manos** hand lotion; ~ **vaginal** vaginal cream (*anticontraceptiva*)

cremación, *f*, cremation

cremáster, *m*, cremaster

cremastérico, *adj*, cremasteric

crematorio, crematory

cremoso, *adj*, creamy

crepuscular, *adj*, twilight

crepúsculo, dusk; twilight

cresa, maggot (*larva*)

cresta, crest; **~s endocárdicas** endocardial ridges

creta pulvorizada en agua, ground chalk in water

cretinismo, cretinism

criada, maid

criar, to raise (*niños*); ~ **a los pechos** to nurse; ~ **con pecho** *Chicano*, to breastfeed

criatura, baby (*bebé*); infant

criceto, hamster

criocirugía, cryosurgery

criógeno, *m*, *adj*, cryogen

crioterapia, cryotherapy

cripta, crypt

cris[1], marijuana

crisis, *f*, *inv*, crisis (*pl*, *crises*); seizure; ~ **asmática** asthmatic seizure; ~ **de ausencia** absence seizure; ~ **de histeria** hysterics; ~ **de identidad** identity crisis; ~ **de la edad madura** midlife crisis; ~ **del haut mal** grand mal seizure; ~ **del pequeño mal** petit mal seizure; ~ **epiléptica** epileptic seizure; ~ **nerviosa** anxiety attack; nervous breakdown; ~ **tiroidea** thyroid storm

crisol, *m*, melting-pot

crispamiento, twitching

cristal, *m*, crystal; glass (*de una ventana*); ~**(es)** crystal(s) (*componente de orina*); ~**es hemáticos** blood crystals; ~ **opalino** frosted glass; ~**es**[1] heroin; LSD

cristalino, crystalline; lens (*parte anatómica del ojo*); ~ **artificial** artificial lens; ~ **opaco** opaque lens

criterio, criterion (*pl, criteria*)

crítico, *adj*, critical

cromo, chromium

cromosoma, *m*, chromosome

cromosoma Y, *m*, Y chromosome

crónicamente, *adv*, chronically

crónico, *adj*, chronic; lingering (*enfermedad*); long-standing

crótalo, rattlesnake

CRS/complejo relacionado al SIDA, ARC/AIDS related complex

crucial, *adj*, crucial

cruda[1], *fam*, hangover

crudo, *adj*, raw (*comida*); *Mex, adj*, hungover

cruento, *adj*, bloody

crujía, *form*, ward

crujir, to crack (*los nudillos*); to groan (*puerta, muelles, etc.*)

crup, *m*, croup

crusiar, *Chicano*, to seek a sexual partner

Cruz Roja, *f*, Red Cross

cruzado, *adj*, crossed

cruzar, to cross; ~ **la sangre** *fam*, to cross match; ~ **las manos** to fold one's hands; ~ **los brazos** to fold one's arms

cuadernillo de apuntes, scratch pad

cuadrángulo, quadrangle

cuadrante, *m*, quadrant

cuadríceps, *m, adj*, quadriceps

cuadricúspide, *adj*, quadricuspid

cuadrigémino, quadrigemina (*sg, quadrigeminum*); *adj*, quadrigeminal

cuadril, *m, Mex, Chicano*, hip

cuadrillizo, quadruplet

cuadrípara, *f, adj*, quadripara; quadriparous

cuadriplejía, quadriplegia; tetraplegia

cuadripléjico, *m, adj*, quadriplegic

cuadripolar, *adj*, quadripolar

cuadrisección, *f*, quadrisect

cuadro, picture; chart; table (*gráfico*); staff; ~ **de abreviaturas** table of abbreviation; ~ **florido** full-blown picture; ~ **médico** medical staff

cuádruple, *m/f*, quadruplet

cuadrúpleto, *adj*, quadruplet

cuajar, to clot

cuajarón, *m*, blood clot; clot; thrombus; ~ **de sangre** blood clot

cuajo, blood clot; thrombus

cualidad, *f*, quality (*característica*)

cualitativo, *adj*, qualitative

cuantificar, to quantify

cuantímetro, quantimeter

cuantitativo, *adj*, quantitative

cuáquero, Quaker

cuarentena[9], forty days following parturition; confinement; quarantine

Cuaresma, *f*, Lent

cuarteado, *adj*, chapped

cuarto, quart; quarter (*cuarta parte*); room; ~ **de baño** bathroom; restroom; ~ **de estar** waiting room; ~ **de los niños** nursery; ~ **doble** double room; ~ **múltiple** ward; ~ **privado** private room

cuarzo, quartz

cuasiorcor, *m*, kwashiorkor

cuate, *m/f, Mex*, twin; ~**s** *m, pl, slang*, testicle

cuatrillizo, quadruplet

cuatro veces al día, *q.i.d./quater in die/*4 times a day

cubano, *m, adj*, Cuban

cubeta, basin; jar
cubículo, cubicle
cubito de hielo, ice cube
cúbito, ulna
cubo, bucket; pail; ~ **de la basura** garbage can
cubre-bocas/cubrebocas, *m, inv,* surgical mask
cubrir, to cover; ~ **con** to film with (*una película, capa*); **~se de ampollas** to blister; **~se de** to film with (*algo*) (*una tela, nube, etc.*)
cucaracha, cockroach; roach[2] (*colilla de un cigarrillo de mariguana*)
cucarachear[1], *Chicano,* to hang around low-class places
cuchara, spoon
cucharada, spoonful; tablespoonful; ~ **de postre (10 cc)** dessert-spoonful
cucharadita, teaspoonful; tsp/teaspoon; ~ **colmada** heaping teaspoon; ~ **llena al ras** level teaspoonful; ~ **rasa** level teaspoon
cucharazo[1], cocaine
cuchichear, to whisper; *fam,* to mutter
cuchicheo, whisper
cuchilla, blade (*cuchillo*); pocket knife; ~ **cortante** curette; ~ **de afeitar** razor blade; razor
cuchillada, gash; knife wound
cuchillo, knife; ~ **eléctrico** endotherm knife
cuco, evil spirit
cucuy[1], *m,* angel dust[2] (*PCP*); dust[2] (*cocaína, PCP*)
cuello, collar; neck (*parte delantera de*); neck (*de un diente; la matriz*); neck of tooth; throat; ~ **de la matriz** *fam,* cervix; ~ **del útero** cervix; ~ **tieso** stiff neck; ~ **uterino** cervix
cuenca, socket (*de un ojo*); *Chicano,* collar bone/clavicle; ~ **de los ojos** eye socket
cuenta, account; bead; bill (*factura*); count; ~ **corriente** current account; ~ **directa de plaquetas** direct platelet count; ~ **en común** joint account; ~ **leucocitaria diferencial** differential blood count; ~ **sanguínea diferencial** differential blood count
cuentagotas, *m, inv,* medicine dropper; dropper; eye dropper/eyedropper
cuento, story (*historia*); ~ **de viejas** old wives' tale
cuerda, cord; string; ~ **vocal** vocal cord
cuerdo, *adj,* sound in mind; sane (*sano de juicio*)
cuerín, *m, Chicano,* scab
cuerito, *Chicano,* scab
cuerno, horn
cuero, hide; leather; *fam,* skin; ~ **cabelludo** scalp
cuerpo, body; *fam,* corpse; **~s acetónicos** acetone bodies; **~s de cáncer** cancer bodies; ~ **ciliar** ciliary body; ~ **esponjoso** spongy body; ~ **extraño** foreign body; ~ **lúteo** corpus luteum; yellow body; ~ **vitreo** vitreous body; vitreous humor
cuestión, *f,* matter (*asunto*); question (*tema*); ~ **secundaria** side issue
cuestionario, questionnaire
cuete, *adj,* drunken
cuidado, care; **~s auxiliares** nursing care; ~ **básico** primary care; ~ **cardíaco** cardiac care; ~ **en el hospital** hospital care; ~ **en los asilos** nursing home care; ~ **en un hospicio para ancianos** nursing home care; ~ **general** primary care; ~ **intensivo** intensive care; ~ **intenso** intensive care; ~ **posthospitalarios** follow-up care; ~ **postnatal** postnatal care; ~ **prenatal** prenatal care
cuidador, -ra, *m/f,* caregiver
cuidadosamente, carefully
cuidadoso, *adj,* careful; gentle

cuidar, to mind; to take care of; to watch (*asistir*); to nurse (*una herida*); ~ (a) to care for; ~se to take care of oneself; ~se la vista to save one's eyes

culco, hairlip

culebra, snake

culebrilla, *fam*, ringworm/tinea

culo, *fam*, *Arg*, buttock; *vulg*, anus; ass

culpa, blame (*responsabilidad*); guilt

culpabilidad, *f*, guilt; guiltiness

cultivar, to culture

cultivo, cultivation; culture; smear; ~ **bacteriano** bacterial culture; **caldo de** ~ culture medium; ~ **de materia fecal** stool culture; ~ **de tejido** tissue culture

culto, cult

cultura, culture

Cumadina, Coumadin

cumpleaños, *m*, *inv*, birthday

cumplir con, to meet (*obligaciones*)

cuna, cradle; crib

cunilinción, *f*, cunnilingus

cunilinguo, cunnilingus

cuña, bedpan; wedge

cuñada, sister-in-law (*pl*, *sisters-in-law*)

cuñado, brother-in-law (*pl*, *brothers-in-law*)

cuota, quota

cupón trepado, *m*, tear-off slip

cuquear[1], to fix up[2] (*calentar y mezclar heroína*)

cura, bandage (*vendaje*); cure; dressing (*tirita*); *m*, priest; ~ **abierta** air dressing; ~ **antiséptica** antiseptic dressing; ~ **de urgencia** first aid; ~ **protectora** protective dressing; ~ **seca** dry dressing; ~[1] fix[2] (*una inyección intravenosa de drogas*); heroin

curable, *adj*, curable

curación, *f*, cure; dressing (*tirita*); healing; ~ **casera** home cure; ~ **del nervio** *fam*, root canal work

curador, -ra, *m/f*, healer

curanderismo, faith healing; folk healing; folk medicine

curandero, faith-healer; healer

curao[1,] *adj*, high on[2] (*drogas narcóticas*); stoned on marijuana

curar, to cure; to heal; to treat (*una enfermedad*); ~ **espontáneamente una enfermedad** to grow out of (*de una enfermedad*); ~[1] to provide an addict with a fix; ~se to be cured; to get well; to recover (*de una enfermedad*); ~se **de . . . con la edad** to outgrow (*una enfermedad, etc.*); ~se[1] to fix[2] (*inyectarse drogas*); to inject oneself with drugs; to hit up[2]; ~se[1] *fam*, to bang[2] (*drogas*)

curare, *m*, curari

cureta, *form*, curette

curetaje, *m*, curettage

curioso, *adj*, quizzical

curita[1], anything that prolongs a high

Curita, (*trademark*) Bandaid (*una marca*)

cursera, *slang*, diarrhea

cursio, *fam*, dysentery

curso, progress (*de una enfermedad*)

curtido, leathery (*piel*)

curva, bend; curve; ~ **bucal** buccal curve; ~ **de compensación** compensating curve; ~ **de crecimiento** growth curve; ~ **de la temperatura** temperature curve; ~ **de oclusión** curve of occlusion; ~ **del pulso** pulse curve; ~ **dental** dental curve; ~ **térmica** temperature curve

curvatura, curvature; curve; ~ **anormal con prominencia dorsal de la columna vertebral** kyphosis; ~ **espinal** spinal curvature; ~ **mayor del estómago** greater curvature of stomach; ~ **menor del estómago** lesser curvature of stomach

cúspide, *f*, cusp; top *Dent* (*dirección*); ~ **canina** canine cusp

cuspídeo, *adj*, cuspid
cutáneo, *adj*, cutaneous
cutícula, cuticle; ~ **de la vaina radicular** cuticle of root sheath; ~ **del esmalte** enamel cuticle; ~ **dental** dental cuticle; ~ **desgarrada** hangnail

cutirreacción, *f*, scratch test; skin reaction
cutis, *m*, *inv*, complexion; skin of the face

---

[1] Este vocabulario es nuevo y todavía no se encuentra en el *Diccionario de la lengua española*, publicado por la Real Academia Española. Forma parte del argot o la lengua de la calle. Se supone que el género es obvio a menos que sea indicado.

[2] Forma parte del vocabulario inglés actual de los drogadictos.

[4] La mollera de los recién nacidos no se cierra normalmente durante el primer año y medio de vida, hasta que los huesos de la cabeza están formados completamente. Por eso, muchas madres temen *la caída de mollera* y saben que si se le cae la mollera durante este período, el niño está en peligro. En realidad hay muchas madres que piensan que están cayéndosele los sesos a su niño a causa de ella. A veces acuden a un curandero, a veces usan un remedio casero para "levantar la mollera." En los dos casos frecuentemente su tratamiento consiste en chupar la mollera, levantar el paladar con el dedo, y agarrarle al niño por los pies, dándole palmadas—todo para "levantarla" en vano. Sin embargo, *la caída de mollera* en los recién nacidos es seña de deshidratación, que quiere decir que el niño pierde más líquido de lo que toma— muchas veces debido a una diarrea, o diarrea con vómitos. El mejor tratamiento es darle mucho líquido al niño.

[5] En inglés la palabra *fever (fiebre)* refiere a una temperatura del cuerpo más alta que lo normal. En español, especialmente para los de origen mexicano, *la fiebre* es el nombre que se usa para las diferentes enfermedades que producen *calenturas* o fiebres. Entre estas enfermedades figuran: brucelosis, fiebre del parto, fiebre reumática, hepatitis, maleria o paludismo, pulmonía, tifo o tifoidea. Los mexicanos y los chicanos suelen usar la palabra *calentura* cuando los anglosajones usan *fiebre*. Para otros que hablan español, muchas veces *calentura* tiene sentido sexual.

[6] Muchas curaciones caseras existen, especialmente en el mundo hispanoamericano, para enfermedades. Hay gente que todavía cree que una enfermedad es causada por una falta de balance en el tracto gastrointestinal. Este concepto tiene origen con Hipócrates, pero se hace bien popular en Latinoamérica desde el siglo XVI. Según este concepto, para mantenerse en buena salud, hay que tomar un balance de comidas "calientes" y comidas "frías." Originalmente las comidas y medicinas se juzgaban por el efecto que tenían en el cuerpo. No tenía nada que ver físicamente con la temperatura de la comida. Por ejemplo, a causa de la erupción (roja –> calor) que puede causar, la penicilina se considera una medicina caliente. De la misma manera, el calcio que puede producir contracciones musculares, se considera frío. Poco a poco esta teoría se modifica para adoptarse con las ideas científicas modernas. El alcohol que se usa para frotar se considera "frío" y esto va mejor con la medicina moderna de usar baños frescos para reducir fiebres o calenturas altas.

Hoy en día la mayoría de las personas no saben nada de las enfermedades calientes y frías ni de las medicinas calientes y frías. Los que siguen la teoría generalmente suelen pensar en la temperatura de la comida y no en las calidades de calor y frío.

Hay muchos artículos escritos acerca de esta teoría. Se puede referir a los artículos de A. Harwood, "Hot–Cold Theory of Disease," *JAMA*, Vol. 216, No. 7, 1153–1158, o a N. Galli, "The Influence of Cultural Heritage on the Health Status of Puerto Ricans," *Journal of School Health*, Vol. 45, 10–16 o a R. L. Currier, "The Hot–Cold Syndrome and Symbolic Balance in Mexican and Spanish–American Folk Medicine," *Ethnology*, Vol. 5, 251–263.

[7] En español *canal* es un conducto abierto; cuando está cerrado es más propio hablar de *conducto*.

[8] En regiones rurales de habla español, y especialmente en México y Puerto Rico, los campesinos suelen nombrar cualquier enfermedad de la piel, y especialmente heridas infectadas y gangrena, *cáncer*.

[9] Se trata del período de cuarenta días inmediatamente después de dar a luz. Aunque todavía se observa por Latinoamérica, en los Estados Unidos del final del siglo XX solamente las nuevas madres bajo la supervisión bien estricta de su madre o suegra siguen todas las costumbres de *la dieta*. Para muchas mujeres de habla española, especialmente las mejicanas, este período, *la dieta cuarentena*, les provee con la oportunidad de guardar cama por largo rato, mucha libertad de las responsabilidades de la casa, y abstinencia del sexo. Durante este período se observa que muchas evitan "comida fría" para no obstruir la sangre que sale de la matriz. (Vea la nota acerca de la teoría de comida fría y caliente.)

D

D y L/dilatación y legrado, D & C/dilation and curettage

D y R/dilatación y raspado, D & C/dilation and curettage

dacriagogo, *m*, *adj*, dacryagogue

dacriocistitis, *f*, dacryocystitis

dacriocisto, dacryocist; dacryocystis

dactilograma, *m*, fingerprints; dactylogram

dactiloscopia, dactyloscopy

dado con el revés de la mano, *adj*, backhand (*deportes*)

dador, -ra, *m/f*, donor

dagazo, *Mex*, *PR*, stab wound

DAL, *f*, LSD

daltónico, *adj*, color blind

daltonismo, *form*, color blindness; daltonism; red-green blindness

dama, lady; ~ **blanca**[1] heroin

danza, dance; ~ **de San Guido** St. Guy's dance; ~ **de San Juan** St. John's dance; ~ **de San Vito** St. Vitus' dance;(*See chorea.*)

dañar, to abuse; to damage; to harm; ~ **por esfuerzo excesivo** to strain *Med*, (*exigir demasiado*); ~**se** to harm oneself

dañinear, *Chi*, (*Vea dañar.*)

dañino, *adj*, harmful; injurious

daño, damage; harm; **hacer** ~ *Med*, to upset (*estómago*); ~ **sufrido por causa de la helada** frostbite

dañoso, *adj*, bad (*nocivo*); harmful; injurious

dar, to donate (*sangre*); to give; ~ **a luz** to bear (*hijo*); to deliver; to give birth; ~ **al galillo** *slang*, to choke; ~ **alaridos** to howl (*con dolor*); ~ **alaridos de dolor** to howl with pain; ~ **ánimos** to encourage; ~ **cabezadas** to nod (*a causa de cansancio*); ~ **chiche** to breastfeed; ~ **de alta** to discharge from the hospital; to dismiss from the hospital; ~ **de comer** to feed; ~ **de mamar** to breastfeed; to nurse; ~ **de pecho** to breastfeed; ~ **del cuerpo** *Carib*, *fam*, to have a bowel movement; ~ **dentelladas a algo** to bite something; ~ **el pecho** to breastfeed; ~ **el pecho al niño** to nurse; ~ **golpes** to pound (*golpear*); ~ **información errónea** to misinform; ~ **la espalda a** to stand with one's back to; ~ **la luna** to have the curse (*mensualmente*); ~ **lugar a** to allow; to give it a chance; ~ **masajes (a)** to massage; ~ **metástasis** to metastasize; ~ **náusea(s)** to make nauseated; to gag; ~ **patadas en el suelo** to stamp one's foot; ~ **permiso** to give permission; ~ **picor** to itch (*escocer*); ~ **puntadas** to give stitches; ~ **puntos** to give stitches; ~ **punzadas** to throb (*con dolor*); ~ **rienda suelta (a)** to overindulge (*una pasión, etc.*); ~**le a uno una enfermedad** to catch a disease; ~ **seguridades** to reassure; ~ **subsidios a** to subsidize (*gente*); ~ **un bajón** to take turn for the worse; ~ **un codazo** to elbow; ~ **un codazo (a)** to nudge; to jab (*con el codo*); ~ **un empujón a** to jolt (*empujar*); ~ **un puñetazo (a)** to punch; to jab (*con el puño*); ~ **un sedante, calmante, sedativo o soporífero** to sedate; ~ **un tirón a** to jerk (*empujar*); ~ **un traspié** to trip (*caer*); ~ **una bofetada a uno** to slap someone on the face; ~ **una dosis ex-**

cesiva (a) to overdose; ~ **una navajazo** to stab (*con una navaja*); ~ **una oportunidad** to give it a chance; ~ **una sacudida a** to jerk (*sacudir*); ~ **una zurra a** to spank; ~ **unos toques (a)** to paint *Med*; ~ **unos toques de** to dab; **~se cuenta (de)** to realize; **~se la mano** to shake hands; **~(se) leche** *vulg*, to come (*culminación sexual*); to reach sexual climax; **~se leche** *vulg, PR*, to ejaculate; **~(se) patas** to put on airs; **~se prisa** to hasten; **~(se) un juanetazo** to take shot of straight liquor; **~se un piquete**[1] to inject oneself with drugs; **~(se) un tropezón** to stub one's foot; **~se una dosis excesiva** to take an overdose; **~se vuelta** to turn; to turn over; **~se (media) vuelta** to turn around

datos, *m, pl*, data (*sg, datum*)

de, of; from; ~ **acción prolongada** *adj*, long-acting; ~ **breve vida** short-lived; ~ **caucho** *adj*, rubber; ~ **cera** waxy; ~ **color amarillo** yellow-hued; ~ **crianza** *adj*, nursing; ~ **difusión prolongada** *adj*, sustained-release *Pharm*; ~ **difusión sostenida** *adj*, sustained-release *Pharm*; ~ **dos filos** double-edged; ~ **dos rebordes** two-edged; ~ **esta manera** in this manner; ~ **fibra óptica** fiberoptic; ~ **genio vivo** quick-tempered; ~ **goma** *adj*, rubber; ~ **guardia** on call; ~ **la bilis** *adj*, biliary; ~ **la buena**[1] marijuana; ~ **la cintura para abajo** from the waist down; ~ **la cintura para arriba** from the waist up; ~ **labios finos** thin-lipped; ~ **liberación prolongada** *adj*, sustained-release *Pharm*; ~ **mal genio** *adj*, bad-tempered (*constante*); ~ **mal humor** in a bad mood; *adj*, bad-tempered (*de vez en cuando*); ~ **mater-**

nidad *adj*, maternity; ~ **media jornada** *adj*, part-time; ~ **mediana edad** middle-aged; ~ **mediana estatura** middle-sized (*persona*); ~ **mejillas hundidas** hollow cheeked; ~ **miras estrechas** narrow-minded; ~ **modo definitivo** *adv*, permanently; ~ **mucho movimiento** busy (*lugar*); ~ **muslos pequeños** thin-thighed; ~ **muslos voluminosos** thick-thighed; ~ **nacimiento** natal; ~ **nariz aguileña** hawk nose; hook(ed) nose; ~ **niño** *adj*, babyish (*infantil*); ~ **noche** at night; ~ **ojos hundidos** hollow-eyed; ~ **ojos rasgados** almond-eyed; ~ **paja** *adj*, straw-colored; ~ **paso ligero** light-footed; ~ **pecho hundido** hollow-chested; ~ **pie** *adj*, standing; ~ **prisa** in a hurry; ~ **repente** suddenly; ~ **secreción interna** ductless *Anat*; ~ **servicio** on duty; ~ **tamaño descomunal** oversize (*muy grande*); ~ **tamaño mediano** middle-sized (*cosa*); ~ **tamaño natural** full-size(d); ~ **tono agudo** high-pitched; ~ **tono alto** high-pitched; ~ **turno** on duty; ~ **vacaciones** on holiday; ~ **valor incalculable** invaluable; ~ **veras** *adv*, really; ~ **visita** visiting

deambulación, *f*, saunter

deber, *m*, duty; obligation; ~ **médico** medical duty

deber, to ought to; to owe

débil, *adj*, faint; feeble; frail; infirm (*decaído físicamente*); weak

debilidad, *f*, debility; thinness (*de la voz*); weakness; infirmity (*decaimiento*); ~ **mental** feeble-mindedness; mental retardation; ~ **muscular** muscular weakness; ~ **senil** dotage

debilitación, *f*, weakening

debilitado, *adj*, debilitated; limp; weakened

debilitante[1], *m*, depressant; *adj*, debilitating; weakening

debilitar, to debilitate; to enfeeble; to exhaust; to fade; to weaken

débito cardíaco, cardiac output

decaer, to decay

decaído, *adj*, dejected; listless (*sin energía*)

decaimiento, abatement; decay; languor (*de interés*); weakening; *fam*, fatigue (*fatiga*); ~ **orgánico** organic weakness

decantar, to decant

decapitación, *f*, decapitation

decapitar, to decapitate

decente, *adj*, comfortable

decepción, *f*, disappointment

decibel, *m*, decibel

deciduo, *adj*, deciduous

decigramo, decigram

decilitro, deciliter

decimetro, decimeter

decir, to say; to tell; ~ **con voz trémula** to quaver (*voz*); ~ **entre dientes** to mumble; to mutter; ~ **tonterías** *fam*, to drivel; to talk nonsense

decisión moral, *f*, moral decision

declaración, *f*, flare up (*de una epidemia*); ~ **de voluntad de vida** living will declaration

declarar, to record; to register (*un nacimiento o una muerte*); ~**se** to break out; to flare up (*epidemia*); to start (*una enfermedad*); ~ **en quiebra** to go bankrupt

decocción, *f*, decoction

decolación, *f*, decapitation

decoloración amarillenta de la piel, *f*, xanthosis

decrépito, *adj*, enfeebled

decrepitud, *f*, decrepitude

decubación, *f*, decubation

dedo, finger; ~ **anular** ring finger; ~ **de beisbolista** baseball finger; ~ **de hule** finger cot; rubber finger; ~ **del corazón** middle finger; ~ **del medio** middle finger; ~ **del pie** toe; ~ **del pie de pichón** pigeon toe; ~ **del pie en martillo** hammer toe; ~ **en**

gatillo trigger finger; ~ **en martillo** mallet finger; ~ **en maza** clubbed finger; ~ **gordo** big toe; *fam*, thumb; ~ **gordo en martillo** hammertoe; ~ **grueso** big toe; ~ **índice** forefinger; ~ **medio** middle finger; ~ **muerto** dead finger; ~ **palmado** webbed finger; ~ **pulgar** thumb

deducir, to subtract

defecación, *f*, *form*, B.M./bowel movement; defecation; stool; ~ **colérica** rice water stool; ~ **fragmentaria** fragmentary defecation

defecar, to defecate; *form*, to have a bowel movement

defectivo, *adj*, lacking

defecto, defect; deficiency; ~ **congénito** congenital defect; ~ **congénito del corazón** congenital heart defect; ~ **de dicción** speech defect; ~**s de la audición** hearing defects; ~**s de la visión** visual defects; ~**s de la vista** visual defects; ~ **de nacimiento** birth defect; congenital malformation; ~ **del habla** speech defect; speech impediment; ~ **del lenguaje** speech defect; ~**s del oído** hearing defects; ~**s hereditarios** hereditary defects

defectuoso, *adj*, defective; imperfect

defensa, defense; ~**s naturales** natural defenses

defibrilador, *m*, defibrillator

deficiencia, deficiency; lack; ~ **de vitaminas** vitamin deficiency; ~ **mental** feeble-mindedness

deficiente, *adj*, defective; deficient

déficit, (*pl*, *déficits*), *m*, deficit; ~ **de oxígeno** oxygen deficit

definición poco exacta, *f*, loose definition

definido, *adj*, established

definitivo, *adj*, definite

deflexión, *f*, deflection

deflujo, defluxion
deformación, *f*, deformation (*del cuerpo*); deformity; disfigurement; malformation; ~ **congénita** congenital malformation; ~ **profesional** occupational idiosyncrasy
deformante, *adj*, deforming
deformar, to deface; to deform (*cuerpo*); to mangle (*una palabra*); to strain (*Med: exigir demasiado*)
deforme, *adj*, deformed (*miembro*)
deformidad, *f*, congenital malformation; deformation (*de un cuerpo*); deformity
defunción, *f*, death; decease
degeneración, *f*, degeneracy; degeneration; ~ **nerviosa** nerve degeneration
degenerado, degeneracy; ~ **inferior/superior** inferior/superior degeneracy
degenerar, to decay; to degenerate
degenerativo, *adj*, degenerative
deglución, *f*, swallowing
deglutir, to swallow
degolladero, *Anat*, throat; neck; throttle
dejar, to leave; to allow; to let; ~ **de** to stop; ~ **de** (+ *infinitive*) to give up (*parar*); ~ **de tomar** to discontinue (*un medicamento*); to miss (*una dosis de algo*); ~ **embarazada** to knock up *euph*; ~ **imposibilitado** to disable (*incapacitado físicamente*); ~ **mal sabor de boca** to leave nasty taste in the mouth; ~ **mentalmente incapacitado** *adj*, to disable
del, of the/from the; ~ **ambiente** *adj*, *PR*, gay; ~ **habla** speech; ~ **personal** staff; ~ **tercer nivel** tertiary
delantal, *m*, apron; ~ **de plomo** lead apron
deleción, *f*, deletion
deletéreo, *adj*, deleterious
deletrear, to spell (*letra por letra*); *Chi*, to look at in great detail

deleznable, *adj*, fragile; brittle; unstable
delgadez, *f*, thinness (*de una persona*)
delgado, *adj*, lank (*flaco*); lean (*persona*); slender; skinny; thin
delicado, *adj*, dainty; delicate; fragile (*salud*); *m*, *Anat*, *fam*, small intestine
delincuencia, delinquency
deliquio, faint; syncope; (*Vea desvanecimiento*.)
delirante, *adj*, delirious; raving
delirar, to be delirious
delirio, delirium (*pl, deliria*); delusion; ~ **agudo** acute delirium; ~ **alcohólico crónico** chronic alcoholic delirium; ~ **de grandeza** delusion of grandeur; ~ **de negación** delusion of negation; ~ **de persecución** delusion of persecution; ~ **depresivo** depressive delusion; ~ **no sistematizado** unsystematized delusion; ~ **sistematizado** systematized delusion; ~ **traumático** traumatic delirium
deltoides, *m*, deltoid
delusión, *f*, delusion
delusorio, *adj*, delusional
demacración, *f*, emaciation
demacrado, *adj*, emaciated; sickly
demarcación, *f*, demarcation
demasculinizado, *adj*, emasculated
demasiado, *adj*, too much; *adv*, too; too much; ~ **cauteloso** *adj*, overcautious; ~ **deseoso (de)** overanxious; ~ **grande** oversize (*muy grande*)
demencia, dementia; insanity; ~ **crónica** chronic dementia; ~ **epiléptica** epileptic dementia; ~ **precoz** dementia precox
demenciado, *adj*, demented
dementado, *adj*, demented
demente, *adj*, demented; insane; mad (*loco*)
demerol, *m*, demerol
demografía, demography; ~ **diná-**

mica dynamic demography; ~ **estática** static demography
demoniaco, *adj*, demoniac
demora, delay
demorar, to delay
demostrar (ue), to demonstrate (*mostrar*); to show
dengue, *m*, breakbone fever; dandy fever; dengue; dengue fever; three-day fever
densidad, *f*, density
dentado, *adj*, jagged
dentadura, teeth; a set of teeth; *fam*, tooth; ~ **artificial** artificial dentition; ~ **completa** complete denture; ~ **de inserción inmediata** immediate denture; ~ **parcial** partial denture plate; ~ **parcial de extensión distal** distal extension partial denture; ~ **parcial fija** fixed partial denture; ~ **parcial removible** removable partial denture; ~ **postiza** denture; denture plates; ~ **postiza completa** full denture; ~ **postiza parcial** partial denture; **tener mala** ~ to have bad teeth
dental, *adj*, dental
dentar (ie), to cut teeth; to jag; to teethe
dentellada, bite *Dent*; tooth mark; ~ **abierta** open bite *Dent*; ~ **cerrada** closed bite *Dent*
dentellado, *adj*, notched
dentición, *f*, dentition; teething; ~ **artificial** artificial dentition; ~ **caduca** deciduous dentition; ~ **permanente** permanent dentition; ~ **primaria** primary dentition; ~ **secundaria** secondary dentition
dentífrico, toothpaste; *m*, *adj*, dentifrice
dentina, dentin; dentine
dentinoma, *m*, dentinoma
dentista, *m/f*, dental practitioner; dental surgeon; dentist; odontologist; ~ **especialista de niños**

pedodontist; ~ **pediátrico** pedodontist/pediatric dentist
dentistería, dentistry
dentro, *adv*, inside
dentro de, *prep*, in; inside; within; ~ **de un vaso de vidrio** in vitro; ~ **del útero** in utero
departamento, department; ~ **de archivo clínico** medical records (department); ~ **de enfermedades mentales** mental health department; ~ **de salubridad** health department; ~ **de salud** health department; ~ **de salud pública** public health department
depauperación, *f*, *Med*, exhaustion; weakening
depauperar, *Med*, to exhaust; to weaken
depellejarse, to peel off (*la piel humana*); to be peeling
dependencia, dependence; dependency; ~ **farmacológica**[1] drug addiction
dependiente, *m/f*, clerk; dependent
depilación, *f*, depilation
depilado, *adj*, hairless
depilatorio, *m*, *adj*, depilatory
depleción, *f*, depletion
deponer, to defecate; to testify; to lay down; *CA*, *Mex*, to throw up; to vomit; *Mex*, *fam*, to barf *vulg* (*vomitar*); ~ **el estómago** to have nausea
deposición, *f*, feces; stool; ~**es** *SpAm*, *slang*, bowel movement; ~ **colérica** rice water stool; ~ **de agua de arroz** rice water stool; ~ **mucosa** mucous stool
depositar(se), to deposit
depósito, buildup; deposit (*sedimento*); pound (*para coches y animales*); ~ **de cadáveres** morgue; mortuary; ~ **de colesterol** cholesterol deposit; ~ **de sangre** bloodstock

depravación, *f,* depravation; ~ **mental** moral insanity

depravado, *adj,* depraved

depresión, *f,* depression; dip; ~ **nerviosa** nervous breakdown; ~ **nerviosa al pasar los efectos de un barbitúrico** hangover; ~ **reactiva** reactive depression; ~ **sistólica** systolic depression; ~ **ventricular** ventricular depression

depresivo, *adj,* depressive

depresor, *m,* blade (*lengua*); depressant; depressor(*en general*) *Med, Anat;* tongue depressor; ~ **de la lengua** tongue depressor; ~ **lingual** tongue depressor; tongue blade; *adj,* depressing

deprimente[1], *m, adj,* depressant; *adj,* depressing

deprimido, *adj,* depressed

deprimir, to depress/to press down; ~**se** to get depressed

depuración, *f,* clearance; purification; ~ **ureica** blood-urea clearance

deque[1], *m,* cap[2] (*cápsula*)

derecho, *m, adj,* right; straight; *adj,* erect; ~**s del/de la paciente** patient's rights

derivación, *f,* by-pass/bypass; derivation; lead; shunt; ~ **del flujo coronario** heart bypass; ~**es esofágicas** esophageal leads; ~**es precordiales** precordial leads; ~**es unipolares de los miembros** unipolar limb leads

derivativo, *m, adj,* derivative

dermabrasión, *f,* dermabrasion

dermatitis, *f,* dermatitis; ~ **alérgica** allergic dermatitis; ~ **amoniacal** diaper/napkin area dermatitis; ~ **calórica** calorica dermatitis; ~ **de contacto** contact dermatitis; ~ **industrial** industrial dermatitis; ~ **medicamentosa** medicinal rash; ~ **por contacto** contact dermatitis; ~ **por orugas** cater-pillar dermatitis; ~ **por pañal** diaper rash

dermatología, dermatology

dermatólogo dermatologist

dérmico, *adj,* skin; **enfermedad** ~ *f,* skin disease

derotomía, decapitation

derramar, to leak

derrame, *m,* discharge; bloody discharge; efflux; effusion; issue (*de sangre u otro líquido*); excess fluid (*que está presente en el cuerpo*); overflow; ~ **biliar** jaundice; ~ **cerebral** brain stroke; (cerebrovascular) stroke; ~ **de bilis** gallbladder attack; ~ **del cerebro** cerebral vascular accident; ~ **hemorrágico** hemorrhagic effusion; ~ **pericárdico** pericardial effusion; ~ **pleural** pleural effusion; ~ **sinovial** water on the knee

derrengado, *adj,* crippled; lame

derrengarse, to strain one's back

derretir (i), to melt (*cambiar a un líquido*)

DES/dietilestilbestrol, *m,* DES/diethylstilbestrol

desabotonar, to unbutton

desabrido, *adj,* tasteless

desabrochar, to unbutton

desaceleración, *f,* deceleration

desafinador, *m, slang,* rubber (*condón*)

desagüe, *m,* discharge (*líquido*); drainage

desahogarse, to vent one's feelings; *fam,* to unload one's troubles; *vulg,* to climax (*sexualmente*), to come (*tener orgasmo*); *PR, vulg,* to ejaculate

desahogo, outlet *Psych*

desahuciado, *adj,* past recovery

desahuciar (a un enfermo), to give up on (*un paciente*)

desajuste, *m,* maladjustment

desaldillado, *Mex, fam,* hernia

desalentado, *adj,* despondent; downhearted

desalentar (ie), to discourage; to dishearten; ~se to get/become discouraged

desaliento, breathlessness; despondency; dismay

desaliñado, *adj*, scruffy (*apariencia sucia*)

desangramiento, bleeding to excess; hemorrhage; **morir (ue) de ~** to bleed to death

desangrar, to bleed excessively (*una persona*); ~se to exsanguinate; to bleed to death; to lose a lot of blood

desangrotransfusión, *f*, exchange transfusion

desanimado, *adj*, despondent

desanimar, to discourage; to dishearten; ~se to become demoralized; to get/become discouraged

desánimo, despondency

desaojar, to cure from the evil eye

desaparecer, to go away; to vanish

desaparecido, *adj*, missing

desarreglo, derangement (*desorden*); ~ **nervioso** nervous breakdown; *Med*, upset; ~**s estomacales** stomach upset

desarrollarse, to develop; to grow

desarrollo, development; ~ **anómalo** maldevelopment; ~ **del embrión** embryonic development; ~ **del habla** speech development; ~ **del lenguaje** speech development; ~ **detenido** arrested development; ~ **embrionario** embryonic development; ~ **tardío** delayed development

desarticulación, *f*, dislocation

desasimilación, *f*, destructive metabolism (*catabolismo*); dissimilation

desastre, *m*, casualty; disaster

desatar, to untie

desatender (ie), to neglect

desayunar(se), to have breakfast; to eat breakfast

desayuno, breakfast

desazonarse, *Med*, to be out of sorts

desbaratamiento (de vientre), *Med*, bowel upset

desbridar, to debride

desburbujeador, *m*, debubbler

descalcificación, *f*, decalcification

descalcificado, *adj*, decalcified

descalcificar, to decalcify

descalzo, *adj/adv*, barefoot; *adj*, naked (*pies*); in one's stocking feet

descamar, to flake (*piel*)

descansar, to relax; to rest

descanso, recess; relaxation; rest

descarga, discharge (*líquido*); shock *Elect*; ~ **nerviosa** neural discharge

descargarse, to loosen up (*el vientre*)

descargo, release (*de una obligación, deber, etc.*)

descartar, to cast off; to dismiss; to rule out

descendente, *adj*, descending

descender (ie) (de), to issue (from); to drop (*una fiebre , etc.*); to go down

descendiente, *m/f*, *adj*, descendant

descendimiento, *Med*, dropping; prolapse *Med* (*de un órgano*)

descenso, *Med*, rupture; ~ **del útero** prolapse; fallen womb

descerebración, *f*, decerebration

descloruración, *f*, dechloridation

descoagulante, *adj*, decoagulant

descompensación, *f*, decompensation

descomponer, to break down

descomposición, *f*, rotting; decomposition (*acción de pudrirse*)

descompostura, displacement

descompresión, *f*, decompression

desconcertar (ie), to shake (*perturbar*); *Anat*, to sprain; to dislocate; ~se *Anat*, to be dislocated; to get out of joint

desconchabar, *SpAm*, to dislocate

desconcharse, to peel off (*una pared*)

desconfianza, mistrust (*falta de confianza*)

desconfiar de, to mistrust

descongelar, to thaw

descongestión, *f*, depletion *Med*

descongestionante, *m, adj*, decongestant

descongestionar, to deplete *Med*; to relieve congestion in

descongestivo, *m, adj*, decongestant; *adj*, decongestive

desconocido, *m, adj*, unknown

descontaminación, *f*, decontamination

descontinuar, to discontinue

descorazonado, *adj*, despondent

descorazonamiento, despondency

descorazonar, to discourage; to dishearten; ~se to get/become discouraged

descoyuntado, *adj*, dislocated/out of joint

descoyuntar, to dislocate

descremar, to skim

descrépito, *adj*, decrepit

describir, to describe

descubierto, *adj*, naked (*cabeza*); uncovered

descubrimiento, discovery; finding

descubrir, to detect; to find out; to find

descuidado, *adj*, careless (*negligente*); negligent

descuidar, to neglect

descuido, carelessness; neglect; oversight (*negligencia*)

desdentado, *adj*, toothless

desdoblamiento de la personalidad, split personality

desecación, *f*, dehydration

desecante, *m, adj*, desiccant; *adj*, drying

desecar, to desiccate

desechable, *adj*, disposable

desechar, to waste

desecho, debris; discharge (*líqui-do*); lochia; menstrual discharge; waste; ~ **vaginal** vaginal discharge (*sin sangre*); ~s wastes *pl*; ~ **peligrosos** hazardous wastes

desembarcarse, estar para, *fam*, to be about to give birth

desempeñar, to perform

desempleado, *adj*, unemployed

desencadenar, to release

desencajamiento, dislocation (*de la mandíbula*)

desencajar, *Anat*, to dislocate; ~se la **mandíbula** to dislocate one's jaw

desenconar, to reduce (*inflamación*)

desengaño, disappointment

desengrasado, *adj*, defatted

desenlace fatal, *m*, fatal outcome

desenredar, to extricate

desensibilización, *f*, desensitization

desensibilizar, to desensitize

desenterramiento, disinterment

desentumecer, to loosen up (*músculos*); ~se las piernas to stretch one's legs (*después de agarrotamiento o embotamiento*)

desenvolvimiento, development (*de una idea , etc.*)

deseo, desire; ~s wants

desequilibrio, imbalance; *Med*, psychological disorder; unbalanced mental condition

desesperación, *f*, anxiety

desesperado, *adj*, desperate; hopeless

desesperarse, to become desperate

desfallecer, to weaken (*perder las fuerzas*); to fail (*la voz*); to faint (*desmayarse*)

desfallecimiento, fainting spell; faintness

desfibrilación, *f*, defibrillation

desfibrilador, *m*, defibrillator

desfibrilar, to defibrillate

desfibrinación, *f*, defibrination

desfiguración, *f*, deformation (*de gente*)

desfigurado, *adj*, disfigured

desfigurar, to deface; to deform (*persona*)

desfloración, *f*, defloration

desganglionar, to deganglionate

desgarrado, *adj*, torn; lacerated

desgarradura, laceration

desgarramiento, tear (*de un músculo, ligamento, etc.*)

desgarrar, to lacerate; to tear; *Chicano*, *SpAm*, to cough up phlegm; ~**se un músculo**, to pull a muscle

desgarro, tear (*muscular*); tear wound; ~ **leve** pulled muscle; *SpAm*, sputum; phlegm

desgasificar, to degas

desgastarse, *Med*, to get weak

desgaste oclusal, *m*, occlusal wear

desgerminar, to degerm

desgonzarse, *fam*, to be anxious

desgracia, misery (*mala suerte*)

deshacer, (*la vista*) to damage; to harm; ~**se en lágrimas** to dissolve into tears; ~**se** *Med*, to get weak; to grow feeble; to waste away

deshecho, *adj*, *Med*, emaciated (*una persona*); weak (*una persona*), broken (*la salud*)

deshidratación, *f*, dehydration

deshidratado, *adj*, dehydrated

deshidratante, *adj*, dehydrant

deshidratar, to dehydrate

deshidrogenasa, dehydrogenase; ~ **láctica** lactic dehydrogenase

deshinchar, to deflate

deshipnotizar, to dehypnotize

deshonra, shame (*vergüenza*)

deshonrar, to shame (*quitar la honra*)

deshumanizante, *adj*, dehumanizing

deshumectante, *adj*, dehumidifier

deshumedecedor, *m*, *adj*, dehumidifier

deshumedecer, to dehumidify

deshumedecimiento, dehumidification

desilusión, *f*, disappointment (*decepción*); disillusion(ment)

desinfectante, *m*, *adj*, disinfectant

desinfectar, to disinfect

desinfestación, *f*, disinfestation

desinflar, to deflate

desintoxicación, *f*, drug withdrawal

desintoxicante, *adj*, detoxifying

desintoxicar, to detoxicate; to detoxify

desintubación, *f*, extubation

desintubar, to extubate

desjarretar, to hamstring (*cortar el tendón de la corva*)

deslizamiento   mandibular, mandibular glide

deslizar, to slip (*caerse*); ~**se** to slide (*sobre el agua*)

desmadejado, *adj*, lank (*desgarbado*)

desmadejamiento, lankiness (*flojedad del cuerpo*)

desmagnetizar, to demagnetize

desmantelar, to dismantle

desmasculinización, *f*, demasculinization

desmayarse, to black out; to faint

desmayo, blackout (*privación de sentido*); dismay; exanimation; faint; fainting spell

desmedro, *Med*, emaciation; thinness; weakness

desmejorado, quedar, to not look well

desmejorar, *Med*, to affect the health of; to weaken; ~**se** *Med*, to lose one's health; to waste away

desmembramiento, dismemberment

desmembrar, to amputate; to dismember; to divide

desmineralización, *f*, demineralization

desmoralización, *f*, demoralization

desmoralizador, *m*, *adj*, demoralizer; demoralizing

desmoralizante, *adj*, demoralizing

desmoralizar, to demoralize; ~**se** to become demoralized

desnaturalizado, *adj*, denatured

desnervar, to enervate

desnucleado, adj, denucleated
desnudarse, to strip naked (a sí mismo); to undress
desnudez, f, nudeness; nakedness
desnudo, adj, bare; naked (parte del cuerpo); nude; ~ de la cintura para arriba bare from the waist up; ~ de la cintura para abajo bare from the waist down
desnutrición, f, malnutrition; ~ húmeda kwashiorkor
desnutrido, adj, malnourished; fam, undernourished
desobediencia, disobedience; naughtiness
desobediente, adj, naughty (mal educado)
desocupado, adj, empty; void; idle
desocuparse, Arg, Chi, Ven, to give birth
desodorante, m, adj, deodorant; m, deodorizer
desodorizar, to deodorize
desolladura, abrasion (arañazo, herida)
desorden, m, disorder (confusión); litter (basura); mess (revoltijo); ~ nervioso m, nervous disorder
desordenar, to disturb (mover de sitio); to make a mess (una habitación)
desorganización, f, disorganization
desorientación, f, disorientation; ~ total total disorientation
desorientado, adj, confused/out of touch with reality
desoxidación, f, deoxidization
desoxiefedrina, desoxyephedrine
desoxirribonucleasa, deoxyribonuclease; desoxyribonuclease
desoxirribonucleico, adj, deoxyribonucleic; desoxyribonucleic
despachar, to send for; ~ (una receta) to fill (a prescription)
despacio, adv, slowly
despechar, Chi, Hond, PR, to wean
despecho, Chi, Hond, PR, weaning
despedazar, to mangle (destrozar)

despedir (i), to dismiss; to give off (un olor, gas, etc.); ~se (de) to say goodbye
despegamiento, detachment
despegar, to peel off (la pared, etc.)
despensa, Chicano, medicine cabinet
despercudido, adj, light-skinned (de tez clara)
desperdicios, wastes; waste products
despertador, m, alarm clock
despertar (ie), to arouse; to awaken (a alguien); to wake up; ~se to awaken o.s.; to wake o.s. up
despiadado, adj, merciless
despierto, adj, awake
despiojamiento, delousing
despiojar, to delouse
despistado, adj, absent-minded
desplazamiento, dislocation; displacement
desplazar, to displace; ~se to get around on one's own
desplomarse, to collapse
despojo, debris
despolarización, f, depolarization
despolarizar, to depolarize
desprender, to release (gas, etc.); ~se Med, to become detached (la retina); ~se de to separate from
desprendimiento, detachment; ~ de la placenta abruptio placentae; ~ de la retina detachment of retina; ~ prematuro de la placenta placenta abruptio
desproteinización, f, deproteinization
destacado, adj, outstanding; prominent (sobresaliente)
destacar, to stand out
destemplado, adj, Med, feverish; indisposed
destemplanza, Med, feverish condition; slight fever; indisposition; malaise
desteñir (i), to fade (el color al lavarse)

destetar, to wean
destete, *m*, weaning
destilación, *f*, distillation; filtration; ~ seca dry distillation
destilado, *adj*, distillate
destilar, to distil; to filter; *Med*, to ooze (*sangre*)
destino, fate (*suerte*)
destoxicación, *f*, detoxication; detoxification; ~ metabólica metabolic detoxication
destoxicar, to detoxicate
destoxificante, *adj*, detoxifying
destreza, skill
destripado, *slang*, hernia
destrozar, to ravage
destructibilidad, *f*, vulnerability
destructivo, *adj*, destructive
destruido, *adj*, destroyed
destruir, to destroy; to obliterate
desuso, disuse
desvanecerse, *Med*, to faint (away)
desvanecido, *adj*, *Med*, faint; giddy; dizzy; caer ~ to fall in a faint
desvanecimiento, dizziness; fainting spell; giddiness
desvariar, *Med*, to be delirious; ~ en su delirio to rave in one's delirium
desvarío, delirium; raving
desvelarse, to stay awake
desvelo, wakefulness
desventaja, disadvantage
desvergonzado, *adj*, immodest (*descarado*); impudent
desvergüenza, immodesty (*descaro*)
desvestirse (i), to undress
desviación, *f*, by-pass/bypass; deviation; shunt; ~ de la columna vertebral spinal curvature; ~ de la normalidad departure from normal; ~ del eje eléctrico axis deviation; ~ estándar standard deviation; ~ estrábica strabismic deviation; ~ hacia dentro de los dedos del pie toeing in; ~ hacia fuera de los dedos del pie toe-

ing out; ~ manifiesta strabismus; ~ media mean deviation; ~ primaria primary deviation; ~ secundaria secondary deviation
desviar, to deflect
desvirgamiento, defloration
desvitalización, *f*, devitalization
desvitalizado, *adj*, devitalized
desvitalizar, to devitalize
detección, *f*, detection; ~ temprana early detection
detectar, to detect
detención, *f*, arrest
detener la respiración, to hold one's breath
detergente, *m*, *adj*, detergent
deteriorante, *adj*, deteriorative
deteriorarse, to deteriorate (*desgastarse*)
deterioro, deterioration (*con el uso*)
determinación, *f*, determination; ~ del cariotipo karyotyping; ~ del grupo sanguíneo blood typing; ~ del sexo sex determination
determinante, *m*, *adj*, determinant
determinar, to gauge (*evaluar*)
devanarse de dolor, *Cu*, *Guat*, *Mex*, to double up with pain
devaneo, *Med*, delirium
devolver (ue), to return; to give back; to yield; *fam*, to barf *vulg* (*vomitar*); to throw up; to vomit; ~ la salud a alguien to restore s.o. to health; ~ la vista a alguien to restore s.o.'s sight
dexedrina, dexedrine/dexies/dextroamphetamine[2]; peaches[2]
dextrina, dextrin; starch sugar
dextrinasa, dextrinase
dextroanfetamina, dexedrine/dexies/dextroamphetamine[2]
dextrosa, dextrose; diabetic sugar; grape sugar
día, *m*, day
diabetes, *f*, *form*, diabetes; ~ albuminúrica chronic nephrosis; ~ alimentaria alimentary diabetes; ~ asociada con gota gouty

diabetes; ~ **carencial** hunger diabetes; ~ **cerebral** cerebral diabetes; ~ **con obesidad** fat diabetes; ~ **diastásica** enzymic diabetes; ~ **esteroide** steroid diabetes; ~ **gotosa** gouty diabetes; ~ **inocente** diabetes innocens; ~ **insípida** diabetes insipidus; ~ **lábil** brittle diabetes; ~ **lipógena** fat diabetes; ~ **mellitus** diabetes mellitus; ~ **pancreática** pancreatic diabetes; ~ **por punción** puncture diabetes; ~ **que guarda relación con enfermedad del páncreas** pancreatic diabetes; ~ **renal** renal diabetes; ~ **sacarina** diabetes mellitus; ~ **temporal** temporary diabetes; ~ **tóxica** toxic diabetes; ~ **verdadera** true diabetes

diabético, *m, adj*, diabetic

diabetis, *f*, diabetes

diablito, *slang*, rubber (*condón*)

diablos[1], devils[2]; red devils[2]; reds[2] (*barbitúricos , seconal*); LSD

diafisaria, *adj*, diaphysary

diáfisis, *f*, diaphysis

diaforesis, *f, form*, diaphoresis

diafragma, *m*, diaphragm *Anat*; diaphragm (*anticonceptivo*); ~ **anticonceptivo** diaphragm; ~ **contraceptivo** diaphragm

diagnosis, *f, inv*, diagnosis (*pl, diagnoses*); diagnostic (*ciencia*)

diagnosticador, -ra, *m/f*, diagnostician

diagnóstico, diagnosis (*pl, diagnoses*) (*de una enfermedad*); *m, adj*, diagnostic; ~ **biológico** biological diagnostic; ~ **bucal** oral diagnosis; ~ **clínico** clinical diagnostic; ~ **de laboratorio** laboratory diagnostic; ~ **de presunción** tentative diagnosis; ~ **de probabilidad** tentative diagnosis; ~ **diferencial** diagnostic workup; differential diagnostic; workup; ~ **directo**

direct diagnostic; ~ **equivocado** misdiagnosis; ~ **físico** physical diagnosis; ~ **histológico** tissue diagnosis; ~ **patológico** pathologic diagnostic; ~ **por exclusión** diagnostic by exclusion; ~ **roentgenológico** roentgen diagnostic; ~ **serológico** serum diagnostic; ~ **topográfico** topographic diagnostic

diagrama, *m*, chart; diagram

diálisis, *f, inv*, dialysis (*pl, dialyses*); ~ **peritoneal** peritoneal dialysis

dializado, *m, adj*, dialyzed

dializador, *m*, dialyzer

diámetro, diameter; ~ **de la pelvis** pelvic diameter; ~ **del cráneo** cranial diameter

diapasón, *m*, diapason; tuning fork

diapositiva, slide *Photo*; ~ **en color** color slide

diariamente, *adv*, diurnally

diario, *m*, newspaper; *adj*, daily

diarrea, diarrhea; loose bowels; ~ **del viajero** traveler's diarrhea; ~ **disenteriforme** dysenteric diarrhea; ~ **epidémica** epidemic diarrhea; ~ **estival** summer diarrhea; ~ **líquida** watery diarrhea; ~ **matinal** morning diarrhea

diastema, *m*, diastem *Dent*

diástole, *f*, diastole

diastólico, *adj*, diastolic

diatermia, diathermy; ~ **de onda corta** short wave diathermy; ~ **de onda ultracorta** ultrashort wave diathermy; ~ **médica** medical diathermy; ~ **quirúrgica** surgical diathermy

diazepam, *m*, diazepam

dibujo, design; drawing

dicipela, *Chicano*, erysipelas

diclorhidrato de quinina, quinine dihydrochloride

dictamen, *m*, advice

diente, *m*, jag (*borde dentado*);

tooth; ~ **anterior** anterior tooth; ~ **ausente** missing tooth; ~ **bucal** buccal tooth; ~ **caduco** deciduous tooth; ~ **canino** canine tooth (*colmillo*); cuspid; eyetooth; ~ **cariado** cavity *Dent*; ~ **cuspídeo** cuspid tooth; ~ **de ajo** *fam*, large misshapened tooth; ~ **de juicio** wisdom tooth; ~ **de leche** baby tooth; deciduous tooth; ~ **de resina acrílica** acrylic resin tooth; ~ **desvitalizado** devital tooth; ~ **en clavija** peg tooth; ~ **flojo** loose tooth; ~ **impactado** impacted tooth; ~ **incisivo** *form*, incisor tooth; ~ **incluido** impacted tooth; ~ **inferior** lower tooth; ~ **mamón** baby tooth; ~ **molar** molar tooth; ~ **moteado** mottled tooth; ~ **permanente** permanent tooth; ~ **picado** cavity *Dent*; ~ **podrido** caries; ~ **posterior** posterior tooth; ~ **postizo** artificial tooth; false tooth; ~ **premolar** bicuspid; ~ **que se mueve** loose tooth; ~ **relleno** filled tooth; ~ **retenido** unerupted tooth; impacted tooth; ~ **salido** buck tooth; ~ **saliente** buck tooth; ~ **saltón** buck tooth; ~ **superior** upper tooth; ~ **supernumerario** supernumerary tooth; ~ **temporal** deciduous tooth; temporary tooth; ~ **vital** vital tooth

dientes, *m*, teeth; ~ **blancos** white teeth; ~ **caducos** milk teeth; ~ **de leche** baby teeth; milk teeth; ~ **manchados** stained teeth; ~ **moteados** mottled teeth; ~ **parejos** even teeth; ~ **podridos** decayed teeth; ~ **separados** rake teeth; ~ **sin cúspides** cuspless teeth

dieta, diet; ~ **absoluta** absolute diet; ~ **alimenticia** nutritional diet; ~ **blanda** bland diet; ~ **de eliminación** elimination diet; ~ **de escaso residuo** low residue diet; ~ **de líquidos** liquid diet; ~ **de residuo ácido** acid-ash diet; ~ **de residuos alcalinos** alkaliash diet; ~ **desclorurada** saltfree diet; dechlorinated diet; ~ **diabética** diabetic diet; ~ **grasosa** diet rich in fat; ~ **hídrica** fluid diet; ~ **láctea** milk diet; ~ **ligera** light diet; ~ **que sigue las reglas dietéticas judías** kosher diet; ~ **rica en grasas** high fat diet; ~ **sin sal** salt-free diet

dietética, dietetics

dietético, dietician/dietitian; *adj*, dietary; dietetic

dietetista, *m/f*, dietician/dietitian

dietilamida del ácido lisérgico/ DAL, lysergic acid diethylamide/ LSD

dietilestilbestrol/DES, *m*, diethylstilbestrol/DES

dietista, *m/f*, dietician/dietitian

diez años de prisión[6], dime[2] *slang*

diez dólares[6], dime[2] *slang*

difenhidramina, diphenhydramine

diferencia pronunciada, marked difference

diferenciación, *f*, differentiation; ~ **correlativa** correlative differentiation; ~ **funcional** functional differentiation

difícil, *adj*, hard (*complicado*); sticky (*situación/persona*)

dificultad, *f*, difficulty; ~ **al respirar** dyspnea; ~ **al tragar** dysphagia; ~ **en** difficulty in; ~ **en diferenciar ciertos colores** color blindness

dificultar, to make difficult

dificultoso, *adj*, labored

difteria, diphtheria; ~ **cutánea** cutaneous diphtheria; ~ **de los terneros** calf diphtheria; ~ **faríngea** pharyngeal diphtheria; ~ **laríngea** laryngeal diphtheria; ~ **quirúrgica** surgical diphtheria

difunto, dead person; *m, adj*, deceased; *fam*, corpse; *adj*, late (*fallecido*)

difusión, *f*, diffusion; release (*del medicamento, luz, etc.*); ~ **lenta** slow release; ~ **periódica** timed release; ~ **prolongada** extended release; ~ **regulada** sustained release; timed release

difuso, *adj*, widespread

digerible, *adj*, digestible; digested

digerir (ie), to digest

digestibilidad, *f*, digestibility

digestible, *adj*, digestible

digestión, *f*, digestion; ~ **biliar** biliary digestion; ~ **difícil** maldigestion; ~ **gástrica** gastric digestion; ~ **intestinal** intestinal digestion; ~ **pancreática** pancreatic digestion; ~ **primaria** primary digestion; ~ **salival** salivary digestion; ~ **secundaria** secondary digestion

digestivo, *adj*, digestant; digestive

digitalina, digitalin; digitalis

digitalis, *f*, digitalis

dignidad, *f*, self-respect

digno de confianza, *adj*, safe (*que merece confianza*)

dilantina, dilantin

dilatación, *f*, dilation; enlargement; ~ **del corazón** dilation of the heart; ~ **del cuello de la matriz** dilation of the cervix; ~ **del estómago** dilation of the stomach; ~ **digital** digital dilation; ~ **y legrado** dilation and curettage/D & C; ~ **y raspado** dilation and curettage/D & C

dilatador, *m*, dilator

dilatar, to enlarge *Med*; ~**(se)** to dilate; ~ **las pupilas** to dilate the pupils

dilear[1], to traffic in drugs

dilema, *m*, quandary

diliar[1], to traffic in drugs

diligente, *adj*, diligent; hardworking

dilución, *f*, dilution

diluir, to dilute

diluvio, deluge

dinámica, dynamics

dinámico, *adj*, dynamic

dinero, money

dioptría, diopter

dióptrico, *adj*, dioptric

diosa verde[1], marijuana

dióxido, dioxide; ~ **de carbono** carbon dioxide

diplomado, *adj*, diplomate

diplopía, double vision; diplopia form

dirección, *f*, direction

directiva, management (*equipo de directores*)

directo, *adj*, straight

director, -ra, *m/f*, principal (*de una escuela, etc.*)

directriz, *f*, guideline (*dirección*)

dirigido hacia dentro, *adj*, varus

dirigir, to manage (*una empresa*)

disartria espasmódica, stuttering

discernir (ie), to discern

disco, disc; dish; disk; ~ **calcificado** calcified disc; calcified disk; ~ **de esmeril** emery disk; ~ **dental** dental disk; ~ **desplazado** slipped disc; slipped disk; ~ **herniador** herniated disk; ~ **intervertebral** intervertebral disk; ~ **intervertebral luxado** slipped disc/slipped disk; ~ **óptico** optic disc

discografía, diskography

discograma, *m*, diskogram

discreto, *adj*, closemouthed

discúlpeme, pardon me

discutible, *adj*, questionable

disecante, *adj*, dissecting

disecar, *Med*, to dissect

disección, *f*, dissection; ~ **cadavérica** cadaverous dissection; ~ **de una vena** venous cutdown; ~ **roma** blunt dissection; ~ **cortante** sharp dissection

diseminado, *adj*, disseminated

diseminar(se), to disseminate
disentería, dysentery; ~ **amebiana** amoebic dysentery; ~ **amibiana** amoebic dysentery; ~ **bacilar** bacillary dysentery
diseño de la dentadura, denture design
disfemia espasmódica, stuttering
disfiguración, *f,* disfigurement
disforme, *adj,* deformed (*feo*)
disfrutar con, to lap (*sacar provecho*); to enjoy (*poseer salud, herencia, etc.*)
disfunción, *f,* dysfunction; ~ **cardíaca** D.A.H./disordered action of the heart; ~ **dental** dental dysfunction
disgustado, *adj,* angry; upset
dislexia, dyslexia
dislocación, *f, form,* dislocation (*de un hueso*); luxation; sprain; ~ **compuesta** compound dislocation; ~ **congénita** congenital dislocation; ~ **iterativa** habitual dislocation; ~ **traumática** traumatic dislocation
dislocado, *adj,* dislocated; strained (*los huesos*)
dislocar, to disjoint; to strain (*espalda*); ~**(se)** to dislocate; ~ **el hombro** to dislocate one's shoulder; ~ **un hueso** to slip a bone
dismenorrea, difficult menstruation; dysmenorrhea; ~ **adquirida** acquired dysmenorrhea; ~ **inflamatoria** inflammatory dysmenorrhea; ~ **mecánica** mechanical dysmenorrhea; ~ **tubárica** tubal dysmenorrhea
disminución, *f,* decrease; ~ **de la tirantez** relaxation of tension
disminuir, to cut down (on); to decrease; to lessen; ~ **por roce** to erode; ~ **progresivamente** (*un tratamiento*) to taper; ~**(se)** to diminish; ~**se** to get smaller
disnea, *form,* dyspnea; breathlessness; labored respiration; respiratory distress; ~ **cardíaca** cardiac dyspnea; ~ **de esfuerzo** exertional dyspnea; ~ **paroxística** *form,* air hunger; paroxysmal dyspnea; ~ **renal** renal dyspnea
disolvente, *m, adj,* dissolvent
disolver (ue), to dissolve; to melt
disparates, *m, pl,* nonsense
dispareunia, dyspareunia; painful coitus
dispensación, *f,* dispensation
dispensar, to dispense
dispensario, clinic (*lugar donde se ofrece ayuda médica gratuita*); dispensary; surgery (*consultorio*); ~ **de empleados** employees' health service
dispénseme, pardon me
dispepsia, *form,* dyspepsia; indigestion; *fam,* constipation; ~ **ácida** acid dyspepsia; ~ **flatulenta** flatulent dyspepsia; ~ **gástrica** gastric dyspepsia; ~ **nerviosa** nervous dyspepsia; ~ **refleja** reflex dyspepsia; ~ **salival** salivary dyspepsia
dispersar, to disperse
displasia, dysplasia
disponible, *adj,* available; disposable
disposiciones negras, *f,* tarlike stools
dispositivo, device; ~ **de caucho** rubber-dam; ~ **intrauterino** intrauterine device/IUD
distal, *adj,* distal
distancia, distance; ~ **focal** focal distance; ~ **pupilar** pupillary distance
distender (ie), to distend (*la piel*); to expand; to strain (*un músculo*); to tear (*un músculo, un ligamento*)
distensión, *f,* distention; elongation; *Med,* strain; ~ **muscular** muscular strain
distobucal, *adj, Dent,* distobuccal

distobucooclusal, *adj*, *Dent*, disto-bucco-occlusal
distobucopulpar, *adj*, *Dent*, disto-buccopulpal
distocervical, *adj*, *Dent*, distocervical
distogingival, *adj*, *Dent*, distogingival
distolabial, *adj*, *Dent*, distolabial
distolabioincisivo, *adj*, *Dent*, distolabioincisal
distolingual, *adj*, *Dent*, distolingual
distolinguoclusal, *adj*, *Dent*, distolinguo-occlusal
distolinguoincisivo, *adj*, *Dent*, distolinguoincisal
distolinguopulpar, *adj*, *Dent*, distolinguopulpal
distooclusal, *adj*, *Dent*, disto-occlusal
distopulpar, *adj*, *Dent*, distopulpal
distopulpolabial, *adj*, *Dent*, distopulpolabial
distopulpolingual, *adj*, *Dent*, distopulpolingual
distorsión, *f*, distortion; *Anat*, torsion; twisting
distracción, *f*, distraction
distractibilidad, *f*, distractibility
distraído, *adj*, absent-minded
distribución, *f*, distribution; **~ de frecuencia** frequency distribution
distribuidor automático, *m*, vending machine
distribuir, to give out
distrofia, *f*, dystrophy; malnutrition; **~ muscular** muscular dystrophy; **~ muscular progresiva** progressive muscular dystrophy; **~ pulmonar** vanishing lung
disuadir a alguien de (+ *infinitive*), to restrain s.o. from (+ *gerund*)
disuria, dysuria
diteria, *fam*, diphtheria
DIU, *m*, IUD/intrauterine device
diuresis, *f*, diuresis (*pl*, *diureses*); **~ tubular** tubular diuresis

diurético, *m*, *adj*, diuretic; **~ cardíaco** cardiac diuretic; **~ directo** direct diuretic; **~ indirecto** indirect diuretic; **~ mecánico** mechanical diuretic; **~ salino** saline diuretic
diurno, *adj*, diurnal
divergencia, divergence; **~ vertical negativa** negative vertical divergence; **~ vertical positiva** positive vertical divergence
divergente, *adj*, divergent
diverticulitis, *f*, diverticulitis
divertículo, diverticulum (*pl*, *diverticula*)
divertido, *adj*, jolly (*entretenido*)
divertirse (ie), to amuse o.s.; to enjoy o.s.; to have a good time; to have fun
divieso, boil
divina[1], LSD
división, *f*, division (*sección*); **~ celular** cellular division; **~ celular (in)directa** (in)direct cell division; **~ de células** cellular division; **~ anormal de células** abnormal cellular division; **~ multiplicativa** multiplicative division
divorciado, *adj*, divorced; *m*, divorcee
divorciar, to divorce; **~se (de)** to get divorced (from)
divorcio, divorce
doblar, to bend; to double; to fold; to bend over; **~(se)** to flex; to overdose; **~se** to bend down; to bend over; to buckle (*rodillas*); to double up (*de dolor*)
doble, *adj*, double; **amputación a ~ colgajo** *f*, double flap amputation; **~ ciega** double blind; **~ enlace** *m*, double bond; **estudio ~ a ciegas** double-blind study; **tono ~** double murmur; **visión ~** *f*, double vision; **vista ~** double vision
doblez, *m*, bend; doubling; fold

(*pliegue*); cuff (*de los pantalones*); hem (*costura*); *f,* deceitfulness; insincerity

dócil, *adj,* docile; meek

doctor, -ra, *m/f,* doctor; physician; ~ **en medicina** *m/f,* medical doctor; ~ **en Medicina Veterinaria** Doctor of Veterinary Medicine/D.V.M.; ~ **en Quiropodia Quirúrgica** Doctor of Surgical Chiropody/D.S.C.

doctrina, doctrine

dolencia, ache; affection *Med;* ailment; disease; malady; sickness; *fam,* earache

doler (ue), to ache; to hurt; ~**le a uno** (+ *noun*)to be sore

doliente, *adj, Med,* aching; ill; *m/f, Med,* patient; sick person

dolor, *m,* ache pain; agony; distress; pain; sensitivity; sore; soreness; ~ **a la presión** tenderness; ~ **agudísimo** excruciating pain; ~ **agudo** sharp pain; ~ **al orinar** pain when urinating; dysuria; ~ **articular** joint pain; ~ **clavado** sharp pain; ~ **cólico** colicky pain; ~ **con ardor** burning pain; ~ **constante** constant pain; ~ **continuo** steady pain; ~ **corneal** keratalgia; ~ **de** (+ *parte del cuerpo*) (*part of body*) ache; ~ **de aire en el estómago** heartburn *fam*; ~ **de barriga** bellyache; ~ **de cabeza** headache; ~ **de cabeza anémico** anemic headache; ~ **de cabeza congestivo** congestive headache; ~ **de cabeza en grupos** cluster headache; ~ **de cabeza histamínico** histamine headache; ~ **de cabeza por punción** puncture headache; ~ **de cabeza por tensión** tension headache; ~ **de cabeza por tensión nerviosa** tension headache; ~ **de cabeza pulsátil** throbbing headache; ~ **de cabeza reflejo** reflex headache; ~ **de cabeza vascular** vascular

headache; ~ **de crecimiento** growing pain; ~ **de dientes** toothache; ~ **de espalda** backache; ~ **de estómago** stomach ache; ~ **de garganta** sore throat; ~ **de garganta por estreptococo** strep throat; ~ **de hijá** *fam,* menstrual cramp; ~ **de ijar**[5] *fam,* flank pain; ~ **de la regla** *fam,* menstrual cramp; ~ **de la vesícula** gallbladder attack; ~ **de la vesícula biliar** cholecystitis; ~ **de los dientes** odontalgia; ~ **de miembro fantasma** phantom limb pain; ~ **de muelas** toothache; ~ **de oído** earache; ~ **de oídos** sore ears; otalgia; ~ **de ojos** sore eyes; ~ **de panza** *fam,* abdominal cramp; ~ **de parto** labor pain; ~ **de pecho** pain in the chest; ~ **de pujos** bearing-down pain; ~ **de sentidos** *fam,* earache; ~ **de tripa** bellyache; ~ **de vientre** bellyache; ~ **del costado** flank pain; ~ **del crecimiento** growing pain; ~ **del período** menstrual cramp; ~ **dragante** dragging pain; ~ **en el riñón** nephralgia; ~ **errante** wandering pain; ~ **errático** wandering pain; ~ **espasmódico** cramp; ~ **expulsivo** bear down pain; expulsive pain; ~ **fantasma** ghost pain; ~ **fuerte** severe pain; ~ **fulgurante** shooting pain; ~ **intenso** intense pain; ~ **intenso en los huesos** osteocopic pain; ~ **intenso, profundo de la cabeza** encephalalgia; ~ **irradiado** radiating pain; ~ **lancinante** twinge; knifelike pain; ~ **leve** mild pain; ~ **localizado** localized pain; ~ **menstrual** menstrual cramp; ~ **migratorio** wandering pain; ~ **moderado** moderate pain; ~ **mordiente** gnawing pain; ~ **opresivo** pressure-like pain; dragging pain; ~ **penetrante** boring pain; ~ **por**

hambre hunger pain; ~ **poso-peratorio** postoperative pain; ~ **producido por aplicación de calor** thermalgesia; ~ **pungitivo** punching pain; ~ **punzante** twinge; ~ **que viene y se va** intermittent pain; ~ **quemante** burning pain; ~ **radicular** root pain; ~ **referido** referred pain; ~ **severo** severe pain; ~ **sordo** dull pain; ~ **subjetivo** subjective pain; ~ **tardío** delayed pain; ~ **terebrante** boring pain; dragging pain; ~ **torácico** thoracic pain; ~ **urente** scalding pain

dolores, throes *pl*; ~ **de estómago** abdominal cramp; ~ **de hambre** hunger pain; ~ **del alumbramiento** afterpains; ~ **del parto** throes of childbirth; ~ **de(l) parto** *fam*, contractions *Obst*; ~ **en el pecho** chest pains; ~ **falsos** false pain; ~ **intermenstruales** intermenstrual pain; ~ **premonitorios** premonitory pain

dolorido, *adj*, aching; painful (*resultado de un golpe*); sore; tender

dolorimiento, tenderness

dolorosamente, *adv*, *Med*, painfully

doloroso, *adj*, aching; afflictive; tender (*dolorido*); painful (*físicamente*)

domicilio, home; permanent address

dominancia, dominance; ~ **cerebral** cerebral dominance; ~ **lateral** lateral dominance; ~ **ocular** ocular dominance

dominante, *adj* dominant

dominar, to master; ~ **el inglés** to be fluent in English

dominio de sí mismo, self-control

dompear[1], to dump (*deshacerse de*); *Chicano*, to throw up; to vomit

dompedro[1], blue star[2]; flying saucers[2] (*semillas de dondiego*); morning glory seeds[2]

donado, *adj*, donor

donador, -ra, *m/f*, *adj*, donor; ~ **general** general donor; ~ **universal** universal donor

donante, *m/f*, blood donor; donor; ~ **de sangre** blood donor; ~ **universal** universal blood group donor; ~ **universal de sangre** general donor of blood

donar, to donate (*sangre*); to give

donatario, donee

doncellez, *f*, *Anat*, maidenhead; hymen

doña[4], untranslated female title; ~ **blanca**[1] cocaine; ~ **Juanita**[1] marijuana; ~ **Prudencia**[1] *slang*, rubber (*condón*)

doñajuanita[1], marijuana

dorado, *adj*, golden

dorar[1], to smoke marijuana

dormido, *adj*, numb

dormir (ue), to sleep; ~ **a alguien** to put s.o. to sleep; ~ **como un lirón** to sleep like a log; ~ **con alguien** to have sexual relations; ~ **demasiado** to oversleep; ~ **doce horas seguidas** to sleep around the clock; ~ **la mona** *fam*, to sleep it off; ~ **más de lo previsto** to oversleep; ~**se** to become numb; to go to sleep (*extremidad*); to fall asleep (*echar una cabezada*)

dormitar, to nap

dorsal, *adj*, dorsal

dorso, back (*de la mano*); ~ **de la mano** back of the hand; ~ **de la nariz** bridge of the nose

dos, *inv*, two; ~ **veces al día** *b.i.d./ bis in die/* twice a day

dosificación, *f*, dosage (*determinación*); titer/titre

dosis, *f*, *inv*, dose (*cantidad de medicina*); dosage; dosis; potion; shot ; ~ **curativa** curativa dosis; ~ **de mantenimiento** maintenance dose; ~ **de prueba** test dose; ~ **de refuerzo** booster dose; ~ **de sostén** maintenance dose; ~ **diaria** daily dose; ~ **dia-**

ria recomendada recommended dietary allowance; ~ **efectiva E.D.**/effective dose; ~ **efectiva mínima** minimum effective dose; ~ **eficaz** effective dose/ E.D.; ~ **excesiva**[1] hot shot[2] (*sobredosis que muchas veces es fatal*); overdose; ~ **fatal media** median lethal dose; ~ **inicial** loading dose; ~ **letal media** median lethal dose; ~ **letal mínima** L.F.D./least fatal dose; minimum lethal dose; ~ **máxima** maximum dose; ~ **media** average dose; ~ **mínima** minimum dose; ~ **mortal** lethal dosage; lethal dose; ~ **óptima** optimum dose; ~ **refuerzo** booster dose; ~ **tolerada máxima** maximum tolerated dose

dotar, to endow

dracma, *m*, *Pharm*, dram

Dramamina, *f*, Dramamine

drástico, *adj*, drastic

dren, *m*, drain; ~ **por contraabertura** stab wound drain; ~ **por transfixión** stab wound drain

drenaje, *m*, drain; drainage (*quirúrgico*); ~[1] *Chicano*, catheter; ~ **por aspiración** suction drainage; ~ **por irrigación** tidal drainage; ~ **por succión** suction drainage

drenante, *adj*, draining

drenar, to drain (*un absceso*)

drepanocitemia, sickle cell anemia; sickle cell disease; drepanocytemia

drepanocito, sickle cell; drepanocyte *form*

drepanocitosis, *f*, sickle cell anemia

droga, cribsheet; dope; drug (*droga narcótica*); medicine; ~ **alucinadora** drug hallucinogenic; hallucinogen; ~ **alucinante**[1] LSD; ~ **antagonista** antagonistic drug; ~ **antihistamínica** antihistamine; ~ **estupefaciente** narcotic;

~ **LSD** LSD; ~ **milagrosa** wonder drug; ~ **psicodélica** psychedelic; ~ **que produce hábito** habit-forming drug; ~ **somnífera** narcotic

drogadicción, *f*, addiction (*droga*); habit

drogadicto[1], drug addict; hype[2] (*un adicto que se da inyecciones subcutáneas*); junkie[2] (*adicto a narcóticos*); user[2]; ~ **a cola**[1] gluey[2]

drogado[1], *adj*, high on[2] (*drogas narcóticas*)

drogarse, to be on drugs

droguería, *SpAm*, drugstore

drosofila, drosophila

drugstore, *m*, *Chicano*, drugstore

ducha, douche; shower bath; shower; ~ **interna** douche; ~ **vaginal** douche

ducharse, to douche; to shower

duda, doubt

dudar, to doubt

duela, fluke; ~ **hepática** liver fluke; ~ **intestinal** intestinal fluke; ~ **pulmonar** lung fluke

dulce, *m*, candy (*un pedazo de dulces*); *m*, *adj*, sweet; ~**s** *pl*, candy; sweets; ~**s**[1] LSD

dulcificante, *m*, sweetener

duodenal, *adj*, duodenal

duodenitis, *f*, duodenitis

duodeno, duodenum

duplicación, *f*, doubling

duración, *f*, duration; length (*tiempo*); ~ **de vida** life span; ~ **del embarazo** length of pregnancy/LOP; ~ **larga de la vida** longevity

duradero, *adj*, chronic; durable; lasting

duramadre, *f*, dura mater; ~ **encefálica** endocardium

durante, during; ~ **24 horas** around the clock; ~ **todo el año** all the year round

durar, to last; to go on for; ~ **más (tiempo) que** to outlive

durazno, peach (tree)

dureza, lump; hardness; hard patch; ~ **permanente** permanent hardness; ~ **temporal** temporary hardness

duricia, callosity

durmiéndose[1], falling out[2] (*sobredosis de drogas narcóticas*); ~ **a medias**[1] falling out[2] (*sobredosis de drogas narcóticas o tranquilizantes*)

durmiente, *adj,* dormant

duro, *adj,* tough; hard (*consistencia*); stiff (*difícil de mover*); ~ **de oído** hard of hearing; dull of hearing; **estar** ~ *Mex, Ur,* to be drunk

---

[1] Este vocabulario es nuevo y todavía no se encuentra en el *Diccionario de la lengua española,* publicado por la Real Academia Española. Forma pate del argot o la lengua de la calle. Se supone que el género es obvio a menos que sea indicado.

[2] Forma parte del vocabulario inglés actual de los drogadictos.

[4] La palabra *doña* va seguida por el nombre de bautismo de una mujer casada o una viuda; no se traduce generalmente.

[5] *Mal de ijar* o *dolor de ijar* se aplica a cualquier dolor que pega a una mujer por el lado del vientre, de la barriga, o cintura. Puede ser causado per torcijones, apendicitis, infección, quiste o tumor en los ovarios o la matriz, o por infección del sistema urinario.

[6] El nombre viene del hecho de que originalmente el paquete de drogas tenía un valor de diez dólares.

ebrio, *adj*, drunk

eccema, *m/f*, [*Ú.m.c.m.*], eczema; ~, **asma y fiebre del heno** EAHF/eczema, asthma, and hay fever; ~ **del lactante** infantile eczema; ~ **escamoso** squamosum eczema; ~ **fisurado** crackled eczema; ~ **húmedo** moist eczema; ~ **infantil** infantile eczema; ~ **marginado** jock(ey) itch; ~ **seborreico** seborrheic eczema; seborrhea; ~ **seco** dry eczema; ~ **vacunado** eczema vaccination

echar, to give off; to impose; to throw; ~ **al bote** to bewitch; ~ **de menos** to miss (*a una persona*); ~ **dientes** to cut teeth; ~ **el bofe** *PR*, to pant with exhaustion; ~ **la cabeza hacia atrás** to lean one's head back; ~ **sal a** to salt (*adobar*); ~ **una carta en el correo** to mail a letter; ~ **una ojeada a** to look over (*mirar por encima*); ~ **una siesta** to take a nap; **~se a llorar** to burst into tears

eclampsia, eclampsia

eclipsado, *adj*, *fam*, *SpAm*, deformed

ecocardiografía, echocardiogram

ecocardiograma, *m*, echocardiogram

ecoencefalografía, echoencephalography

ecología, ecology

economía, economy

económicamente independiente, *adj*, self-supporting

ecosistema, *m*, ecosystem

ectodermo, ectoderm

ectopia, ectopia; ~ **testicular** ectopia of the testicles

ectópico, *adj*, ectopic

ectoplasma, *m*, ectoplasm

ecuación, *f*, equation; ~ **lineal** linear equation; ~ **química** chemical equation

ecuador, *m*, equator; ~ **de la célula** equator of the cell; ~ **del cristalino** equator of crystalline lens; ~ **del ojo** equator of the eyeball

eczema, *m/f*, [*Ú.m.c.m.*], eczema; (*Vea eccema.*)

edad, *f*, age; ~ **del chivateo** *Chicano*, awkward age; ~ **del pavo** awkward age; ~ **madura** middle age; ~ **mental** mental age; ~ **procreadora** childbearing age

edema, *m*, edema; tumefaction; ~ **angioneurótico** angioneurotic edema; ~ **cardíaco/cardiaco** cardiac edema; ~ **carencial** hunger edema; ~ **de hambre** famine edema; hunger edema; hunger swelling; ~ **pulmonar** pulmonary edema; ~ **agudo de pulmón** acute pulmonary edema

educación, *f*, education; training; ~ **higiénica** health education; ~ **para la salud** health education

educar, to educate; to train

EEG/electroencefalograma, *m*, EEG/electroencephalogram (*prueba de las ondas cerebrales*)

efectivo, cash; *adj*, effective

efecto, effect; ~ **acumulativo** cumulative effect; ~ **adverso** adverse effect; ~ **colateral** side effect; ~ **de sumación** additive effect; ~ **secundario** side effect; **~s tardíos** after-effects

efedrina, ephedrine

efélides, *f*, *pl*, *form*, ephelides *form*; freckles

efervescente, *adj*, effervescent

eficaz, *adj*, effective; efficient

eficiencia, efficiency

eficiente, *adj*, efficient
eflorescencia, *form*, efflorescence
efluxión, *f*, effluxion
ego, ego
egocéntrico, *adj*, egocentric; self-centered
ejecutivo, *adj*, executive
ejercer, to exercise (*autoridad, influencia*); to follow (*practicar una carrera*); ~ **presión sobre** to exert pressure on
ejercicio, exercise; ~ **activo** active exercise; ~ **activo contra resistencia** active resistive exercise; ~ **estático** static exercise; ~ **físico** physical exercise; ~ **físico moderado** moderate physical exercise; ~ **pasivo** passive exercise; ~ **respiratorio** breathing exercise; ~ **terapéutico** corrective exercise; ~**s físicos para adelgazar** reducing exercises; ~**s físicos para reducir peso** reducing exercises
el defecar, number two *euph*
el orinar, number one *euph*
el tiempo requerido para hacer algo, length of time required to do something
E.L.A./esclerosis lateral amiotrófica, *f*, A.L.S./amyotrophic lateral sclerosis
elástica, *f*, *adj*, elastic
elasticidad, *f*, elasticity; ~ **pulmonar** lung elasticity
elástico, *adj*, elastic
electivo, *adj*, elective
electricidad, *f*, electricity; ~ **dinámica** dynamic electricity; ~ **estática** static electricity; ~ **galvánica** galvanic electricity
eléctrico, *adj*, electric; electrical
electrificar, to electrify
electrista, *m/f*, electrician
electroanálisis, *m*, electroanalysis
electrobisturí, *m*, electrocautery
electrocardiografía, ECG/EKG/ electrocardiogram; electrocardiography

electrocardiógrafo, electrocardiograph
electrocardiograma, *m*, ECG /EKG /electrocardiogram; heart tracing; ~ **de esfuerzo** stress test; ~ **de esfuerzo con dipiridamol** dipyridamole stress test; ~ **de esfuerzo con talio** thallium stress test
electrocirugía, electrosurgery
electrocoagulación, *f*, electrocoagulation
electrocución, *f*, electrocution
electrocutar, to electrocute
electrochoque, *m*, electroshock
electrodiagnóstico, *m*, *adj*, electrodiagnostic
electrodiálisis, *f*, electrodialysis
electrodo, electrode; ~ **de aguja** needle electrode; ~ **despolarizante** depolarizing electrode; ~ **terapéutico** therapeutic electrode
electroencefalografía/EEG electroencephalography/EEG
electroencefalograma/EEG, *m*, brain-wave test; electroencephalogram/EEG
electroforesis, *f*, electrophoresis; ~ **en bloques de almidón** electrophoresis on starch block; ~ **en tira de papel** electrophoresis on paper strips
electroimán, *m*, electromagnet
electrólisis, *f*, electrolysis
electrolítico, *adj*, electrolytic
electrólito, electrolyte
electromagnético, *adj*, electromagnetic
electromagnetismo, electromagnetism
electromiografía/EMG, electromyography/EMG
electromiograma, *m*, electromyogram
electrón, *m*, electron
electrónica, electronics
electrónico, *adj*, electronic
electroshock, *m*, *Chicano*, electroshock

electroshockterapia, ECT (*terapia electroconvulsiva*); *Chicano*, EST (*terapia de electrochoque*)

electroterapia, electrotherapy; ~ por choque electroshock therapy

elefancía, elephantiasis

elefante blanco[1], LSD

elefantiasis, *f*, elephantiasis

elegante, *adj*, smart (*a la moda*)

elegible, *adj*, eligible

elegir (i), to choose; ~ (*una actividad*) to take up

elemento, element; ~ anatómico anatomic element; ~s constituyentes constituent elements; ~ electronegativo electronegative element ; ~ electropositivo electropositive element; ~ morfológico morphological element; ~ trazador tracer element

elevación, *f*, elevation; ridge

elevado, *adj*, elevated

elevador, *m*, elevator (*Dent: ascensor*)

elevar, to elevate (*alzar*); to raise

eliminación, *f*, elimination

eliminar, to defecate; to eliminate; to pass (*cálculos, parásitos, etc.*)

elixir, *m*, elixir

elongación, *f*, elongation; ~ quirúrgica de los nervios surgical elongation of nerves

emaciación, *f*, emaciation

emasculación, *f*, emasculation

embalsamamiento, embalming; embalmment

embalsamar, to embalm

embarazada, *adj*, pregnant

embarazar, to embarrass (*hacer pasar un apuro*); ~se to become pregnant

embarazo, pregnancy; ~ ectópico ectopic pregnancy; ~ en los tubos tubal pregnancy; ~ falso hysteric pregnancy; false pregnancy; pseudocyesis; ~ fuera de la matriz ectopic pregnancy; ~ histérico hysteria pregnancy; ~ incompleto incomplete preg-

nancy; ~ ovárico ovarian pregnancy; ~ tubárico tubal pregnancy

embarazoso, *adj*, embarrassing

embargo, *Med*, indigestion

embarsado[1], *adj*, high on[2] (*drogas narcóticas*)

embetunado[1], *adj*, high on[2] (*drogas narcóticas*)

embolectomía, embolectomy

embolia, embolism; ~ cerebral cerebral embolism; (cerebrovascular) stroke; ~ coronaria coronary embolism; ~ de la retina retinal embolism; ~ gaseosa air embolism; ~ linfática lymphogenous embolism; ~ pulmonar pulmonary embolism; ~ retrógrada retrograde embolism

embolio, cerebral vascular accident

embolismo, embolism

embollado[1], *adj*, high on[2] (*drogas narcóticas*)

embollarse[1], to get high[2]

émbolo, embolus (*pl, emboli*); piston/plunger of a syringe; ~ canceroso cancer embolus; ~ de aire air embolus; ~ de grasa fat embolus; ~ en silla de montar straddling embolus; ~ obturador obturating embolus

emborracharse, to be/get drunk

embotado, *adj*, dull (*sentido*); stiff (*Med: dormido*)

embotamiento, stiffness (*de las extremidades*)

embotar(se), to dull (*sentidos*); to stiffen (*extremidades*)

embriagado, *adj*, drunk; intoxicated

embriagar, to inebriate

embriago, *adj*, intoxicated

embriaguez, *f*, drunkenness; ebriety; inebriation; intoxication

embriocardia, embryocardia

embriología, embryology

embriólogo, embryologist

embrión, *m*, embryo

embrioterapia, embryotherapy
embriotomía, decapitation
embrujar, to hex
embudo, funnel
emergencia, emergency
emesis, *f, adj,* emesis
emético, *m, adj,* emetic; vomitive
EMG/electromiografía, EMG/ electromyography
EMG/electromiograma, *m,* EMG/ electromyogram
eminencia, eminence (*elevación de*); ~ **metatarsiana**, ball of the foot; ~ **tenar** ball of thumb
emisión (nocturna), *f,* (nocturnal) emission
emisor, *m,* sender; issuer; transmitter
emitir, to emit; to give off (*un sonido*)
emocional, *adj,* emotional
emocionar, to excite (*conmover*)
emoliente, *m, adj,* emollient
emolio, *Chicano,* (cerebrovascular) stroke
empacar, to pack *Med*
empacamiento en sábana fría/ mojada, wrapping in a cold/wet sheet
empachar(se), to get sick from overeating; *Med,* to give indigestion to; to make uncomfortable; ~**se** *Med,* to get/have indigestion; ~**se** *PR,* to get sick
empacho[4], *fam,* constipation; surfeit *ethn*
empalagoso, *adj,* sickly (*sabor*)
empancinar(se), *PR,* to eat too much
empañado, *adj,* blurred; blurry
empañarse to blur (*visión*)
empapar la gasa en un antiséptico, to soak gauze in antiseptic
empaque, *m, Chicano,* temporary filling
emparejar, to match
empastadura, filling *Dent*
empastar, to fill *Dent*; to do a filling; to fill a tooth

empaste, *m,* filling *Dent*; inlay; ~ **dental** dental filling; ~ **provisional** temporary filling; ~ **temporal** temporary filling
empatía, empathy
empedarse, *Mex, Ríopl,* to get drunk
empedido, *adj,* crippled
empeine, *m,* groin; instep (*del pie*); ringworm; tinea; *fam,* crotch
empelotado, *adj, Col, Chi, Cu, Mex,* naked
empeoramiento, deterioration (*condición del paciente*); worsening
empeorar, to go downhill; to make worse; to worsen; ~**(se)** to deteriorate (*condición del enfermo*); ~**se** to get worse
empezar (ie), to begin; to come on; to start; ~ **desde el principio** to start from scratch
empinarse, to bend over
empírico, *adj,* empiric
emplaste, *m,* dressing (*vendaje*)
emplasto, plaster *Med*; poultice; ~ **adhesivo** adhesive plaster; ~ **de mostaza** mustard plaster; ~ **frío** cold pack; ~ **para callos** corn plaster
empleador, -ra, *m/f,* employer
empleo, employment; exertion (*fuerza*); job; work
emplomadura, *Arg,* filling *Dent*
emplomar, *Arg,* to fill *Dent*
empolvado, *adj,* powdery
emponzoñar, to poison
empotrar, to embed/imbed
empujar, to push (*tocar; abrirse paso a codazos*); to thrust
empujón, *m,* jerk (*avance rápido que se da*); push (*impulso que se da con fuerza para mover o apartar*)
empuñar, *Chi,* to clench (*el puño*)
emulsificación, *f,* emulsification
emulsión, *f,* emulsion
emulsionar, to emulsify
emulsor, *m, adj,* emulsifier
en, *prep* in; on; ~ **aumento** grow-

ing; ~ **ayunas** fasting condition; on an empty stomach; ~ **broma** as a joke; ~ **carne viva** raw wound; ~ **casa** at home; ~ **caso de que** in case of; ~ **consideración a** in consideration of ; ~ **cuestión** under consideration; ~ **curso** in progress; ~ **diálisis** dialysis; ~ **el acto** outright (*de una vez*); ~ **el ambiente** *PR*, gay; ~ **el caso de que** in case of; ~ **el cuerpo vivo** in vivo; ~ **el marco de** within the framework of; ~ **embudo** funnel; ~ **estado** *fam*, pregnant; ~ **estado desesperado** past recovery; ~ **garra** claw; ~ **la movida** *PR*, busy; ~ **onda**[1] LSD; ~ **polvo** powdered; ~ **punto** prompt; ~ **realidad** in reality; ~ **seguida** immediately; right away; ~ **su sano juicio** in one's right mind; ~ **todas partes** everywhere; ~ **vacío** in a vacuum; ~ **voz alta** aloud

enajenación, *f*, absentmindedness; estrangement; ~ **mental** *Med*, mental derangement; insanity

enajenamiento, estrangement

enamoriscar[1], to smoke marijuana

enardecerse, *Med*, to become inflamed

enanismo, dwarfism; nanism

enano, dwarf; midget

encabezamiento, heading

encachorrarse, *Col*, to get angry

encajamiento (de la cabeza fetal), engagement *Obst*

encajar, to engage; to fit (in); to embed/imbed; to set (*un hueso*); ~**se** to go down in the birth canal

encalabrinar, *Med*, to make dizzy; to make giddy

encalamocarse, *Col, Ven*, to get drunk

encalatarse, *Perú*, to strip naked

encamado, *adj*, bedridden; **estar** ~ to be confined to bed

encamar, *CA, Mex*, to hospitalize; to take to the hospital

encandilarse, *Mex, PR*, to get mad; *Col, Perú, PR*, to be scared

encanecer, to go grey; to grey

encanecimiento, growing gray/grey

encanto, spell (*invocación mágica*)

encapsulación, *f*, encapsulation

encapsulado, *adj*, encapsulated

encaramar, *Col, CR*, to embarrass; ~**se** *Col, CR*, to get embarrassed

encargarse de, to take charge of

encargo, **estar de**, *Arg, RD, Ur*, to be pregnant

encarnar, *Med*, to heal (up)

encefalalgia, *form*, encephalalgia

encefalitis, *f*, brain fever; encephalitis; ~ **aguda diseminada** acute disseminated encephalitis; ~ **hemorrágica** hemorragic encephalitis; ~ **postinfectiva** post-vaccinalis encephalitis; ~ **purulenta** purulent encephalitis

encéfalo, *Anat*, encephalon

encefalografía, encephalography

encefalograma, *m*, encephalogram

encefalomielitis, *f*, encephalomyelitis

encefalopatía, encephalopathy

encendedor, *m*, cigarette lighter

encender (ie), to light (*prender*); to turn on; to warm up; ~**se (ie)** to flare up (*las pasiones; una llama*)

encerrado, *adj*, enclosed

enchinarse la piel, to get goose bumps

enchincharse, *Guat, Mex, Perú, PR*, to get infested with bugs

enchismarse, *PR*, to get mad

enchufe, *m*, electric socket; electrical plug

enchulao, *adj, PR*, infatuated

enchularse, *PR*, to become infatuated

encía, gingiva *Dent*; gum (*de la boca*); ~**s dolorosas** sore gums

encinta, *adj*, pregnant

enclavar, to imbed

enclenco, *adj, Col, PR*, weak; sickly

enclenque, *adj*, sickly (*enfermizo*); *m/f*, sickly person

encoger, to shrink (*ropa, etc.*); ~**(se) las rodillas** to pull up one's knees

encolerizar, to anger; ~**se** to flare up (*con furia*)

enconado, *adj, Med,* inflamed; sore

enconar, to irritate (*una herida*); ~**se** to fester

encono, *Cu, Mex,* inflammation; swelling

enconoso, *adj, Med,* sensitive

encontrar (ue), to find; ~**(se) (con)** to meet (*reunirse*); ~**se mal** to feel ill

encordio, swollen gland in groin

encorvamiento, droop (*de la espalda*)

encorvar (ue), to droop (*de la espalda*); ~**(se)** to flex; ~**se** to hunch one's back

encostración, *f,* incrustation

encubrir, to cover up (*esconder*)

encuentro, meeting

encuerar, *Chi, Cu, Mex,* to strip (naked); ~**se** *Chicano,* to undress

encuevao, *adj,* holed up in one's house

endaórtico, *adj,* endaortic

endarterectomía, endarterectomy

endarteria, endarterium

endeble, *adj, Med,* feeble; frail; weak

endémico, *adj,* endemic

endentecer, to cut teeth; to teethe

enderezar, to reduce a fracture; ~**los dientes** to straighten the teeth

endocardio, endocardium

endocarditis, *f,* endocarditis; ~ **bacteriana aguda** acute bacterial endocarditis; ~ **fetal** fetal endocarditis; ~ **infectiva** infective endocarditis; ~ **maligna** malignant endocarditis; ~ **séptica** septic endocarditis; ~ **ulcerativa** ulcerative endocarditis; ~ **ulcerosa** ulcerative endocarditis

endocráneo, endocranium

endocrino, *adj,* ductless *Anat;* endocrine

endocrinología, endocrinology

endocrinólogo, endocrinologist

endodermo, endoderm

endodoncia, *form,* root canal work

endodontista, *m/f,* endodontist

endodontitis, *f,* endodontitis

endometrio, endometrium

endometriosis, *f,* endometriosis

endometritis, *f,* endometritis

endomiocárdico, *adj,* endomyocardial

endoplasma, *m,* endoplasm

endorfina, endorphin

endoscopia, endoscopy; ~ **gástrica** gastroscopy

endoscopio, endoscope

endostetoscopio, endostethoscope

endotraqueal, *adj,* endotracheal

endrogado[1], *adj,* drugged

endrogar[1], to drug

endurecer, to harden

endurecimiento, hardening; induration; lump

eneldo, dill

enema, *m/f,* [*Ú.m.c.f.*] enema; ~ **alimenticia** nutrient enema; ~ **ciega** blind enema; ~ **de bario** barium enema; ~ **de contraste (doble)** (double) contrast enema; ~ **de limpieza** cleansing enema; ~ **de retención** retention enema; ~ **jabonosa** soapsuds enema; ~ **nutritiva** nutrient enema; ~ **opaca** barium enema

energía, energy; ~ **atómica** nuclear energy; ~ **cinética** kinetic energy/KE; ~ **nuclear** nuclear energy; ~ **química** chemical energy; ~ **radiante** radiant energy

enérgico, *adj,* alert; energetic; vigorous

enervación, *f,* enervation

enfadado, *adj,* angry

enfadao, *adj, PR,* angry (*más que irritado*)

enfadar, to anger; ~**se** to get angry; to get mad

enfatizar, to stress; *SpAm,* to emphasize

enferma, *euph*, menstruation

enfermar, to lay up; to make ill; ~se to fall sick; to get sick; to become sick; ~se *Chicano*, to be in labor

enfermedad, *f, form*, disease; affection *Med*; affliction *Med*; complaint; disorder (*afección*); illness; infirmity; malady; sickness; ~ **aguda** acute disease; acute illness; ~ **articular degenerativa** degenerative joint disease; ~ **benigna** ailment; mild disorder; ~ **cancerosa** malignant disease; ~ **cardíaca** heart disease; ~ **cardiovascular** cardiovascular disease; ~ **casera**[5] folk illness; ~ **celíaca** celiac disease; ~ **comunicable** communicable disease; ~ **contagiosa** contagious disease; contagious illness; ~ **crónica** chronic disease; chronic illness; ~ **crónica respiratoria** chronic respiratory disease; ~ **de almacenamiento de glucógeno** glycogen storage disease; ~ **de Alzheimer** Alzheimer's disease; ~ **de andancia** *Chicano*, disease that is "going around"; ~ **de carácter** disease of social pathology; ~ **de células falciformes** sickle cell disease; ~ **de Cooley** thalassemia major; ~ **de declaración obligatoria** notifiable disease; ~ **de Hodgkin** malignant granulomatosis; lymphogranulomatosis/ Hodgkin's disease; ~ **de Kaposi** Kaposi's disease; ~ **de lesiones mínimas** minimal change disease; ~ **de los buceadores** decompression sickness; ~ **de los buzos** *sg*, "the bends"; caisson disease; ~ **de los huesos** bone disease; ~ **de los riñones** kidney disease; ~ **de membrana hialina** hyaline membrane disease; ~ **de Ménière** Ménière's disease; ~ **de notificación** notifiable disease; ~ **de Parkinson** shaking palsy; Parkin-

son's disease; ~ **de San Valentín** epilepsy; ~ **de suero** serum sickness; ~ **de Tay-Sachs** (*idiocia amaurótica*) Tay-Sachs disease; ~ **de transmisión sexual** sexually transmitted disease/ STD; ~ **de Vicente** trench fever; ~ **del carácter** character disorder; ~ **del corazón** heart disease; heart problems; ~ **del hígado** liver complaint; ~ **del sueño** sleeping sickness; ~ **del tejido conjuntivo** connective tissue disease; ~ **emocional** mental disease; ~ **endañada** *Chicano, Mex*, disease due to an act of witchcraft; ~ **estival** summer complaint; ~ **fibroquística** fibrocystic disease; ~ **fibroquística del páncreas** fibrocystic disease of the pancreas; ~ **fibroquística ósea** fibrocystic disease of the bone; ~ **funcional** functional disease; ~ **genética** genetic disease; ~ **genitourinaria** genitourinary disease; ~ **glosopeda** foot-and-mouth disease; hoof-and-mouth disease; ~ **grave** serious illness; ~ **hemática** hemophilia; ~ **hereditaria** hereditary disease; ~ **infecciosa** infectious disease; ~ **inflamatoria pélvica** pelvic inflammatory disease/PID; ~ **intersticial pulmonar** interstitial lung disease; ~ **leve** minor illness; ~ **lunática** epilepsy; ~ **maligna** malignancy; ~ **matutina** morning sickness; morning nausea; ~ **mental** mental illness; mental disease; ~ **moral** disease of social pathology; character disorder; ~**es nerviosas** neurological disorder; ~ **obligatoria** reportable disease; ~ **oportunista infecciosa** opportunistic infectious disease; ~ **orgánica** organic illness (*mal*); ~ **pasada sexualmente** sexually transmitted disease/STD; ~ **por arañazo de gato** cat-scratch disease; ~ **por descompresión** "bends"; decompression sickness; ~ **primaria** primary disease; ~ **profesional** industrial disease; occupational disease; ~ **progresiva** progressive illness; ~ **pulmonar** pulmonary disease (*pulmón*); ~ **pulmonar obstructiva crónica/ EPOC** chronic obstructive pulmonary disease/ COPD; ~ **que anda** *Chicano*, disease that is "going around"; ~ **respiratoria** respiratory ailment; ~ **respiratoria crónica** chronic respiratory disease/ CRD; ~ **sanguínea** blood disease; ~ **tra(n)smisible** communicable disease; contagious illness; transmittable disease; ~ **tropical** tropical illness (*mal*); ~ **vascular periférica** peripheral vascular disease; ~ **venérea** venereal disease / VD; sexually transmitted disease/STD

enfermera, nurse (*para los enfermos*); ~ **anestesista** nurse-anesthetist; ~ **ambulante** visiting nurse; ~ **auxiliar** assistant nurse; ~ **de cargo** charge nurse; ~ **de día** day nurse; ~ **de guardia** nurse on duty; ~ **de hospital** hospital nurse; ~ **de noche** night nurse; ~ **de piso** ward nurse; ~ **de planta** ward nurse; ~ **de salud pública** public health nurse; ~ **de sección** charge nurse; ~ **diplomada** graduate nurse; registered nurse; ~ **domiciliaria** home nurse; ~ **escolar** school nurse; ~ **general** general duty nurse; ~ **graduada** graduate nurse; registered nurse; ~ **jefe/jefa** head nurse; ~ **mayor** head nurse; ~ **pediátrica** child's nurse; ~ **práctica** practical nurse; ~ **privada** private nurse; ~ **registrada** registered nurse; ~ **titulada** registered nurse/RN; ~ **visitadora** visiting nurse; ~ **visitante** visiting nurse; ~ **con título** registered nurse

enfermería, infirmary; nursing; ~ **especial** special nursing; general duty nursing

enfermero, male nurse; medical orderly; ~ **anestesista** nurse-anesthetist; ~ **ambulante** visiting nurse; ~ **asistente** nurse's aide; ~ **auxiliar** assistant nurse; ~ **con título** registered nurse; ~ **de cargo** charge nurse; ~ **de día** day nurse; ~ **de guardia** nurse on duty; ~ **de hospital** hospital nurse; ~ **de noche** night nurse; ~ **de piso** ward nurse; ~ **de planta** ward nurse; ~ **de salud pública** public health nurse; ~ **de sección** charge nurse; ~ **diplomado** graduate nurse; registered nurse; ~ **domiciliario** home nurse; ~ **escolar** school nurse; ~ **general** general duty nurse; ~ **graduado** graduate nurse; registered nurse; ~ **jefe** head nurse; ~ **mayor** head nurse; ~ **pediátrico** child's nurse; ~ **práctico** practical nurse; ~ **privado** private nurse; ~ **registrado** registered nurse/RN; ~ **titulado** registered nurse/RN; ~ **visitador** visiting nurse; ~ **visitante** visiting nurse

enfermizo, *adj*, ailing; feeble; unhealthy; infirm; sickly (*persona*)

enfermo, patient; ~ **hospitalizado** inpatient; *adj*, ill; sick

enfermoso, *adj*, *SpAm*, (*Vea enfermizo.*)

enfisema, *m*, emphysema; ~ **alveolar** alveolar emphysema; ~ **pulmonar** pulmonary emphysema; ~ **suplementario** compensatory emphysema; ~ **traumático** surgical emphysema

enflaquecer, to emaciate; ~**se** to become thin

enflaquecimiento, emaciation; weight loss

enfocar, to concentrate on; to shine a light on something; ~ **la vista** to focus

enfogonado, *adj*, angry

enfogonarse, *PR*, to get mad; (*Vea mad.*)

enfrentar(se) con, to confront; to face; ~**se a** to cope with

enfrente, *adv*, opposite; ~ **de** *prep*, opposite

enfriamiento, cooling

enfriar(se), to dull (*emociones*)

engañar, to delude

engaño, delusion

engarrotarse, *SpAm*, to get stiff; to go numb (*extremidad*)

engendrar, to cause; to engendrate; to father; to inseminate

engendro, abortion; deformed child

engerido, *adj*, *Col*, *Ven*, weak; sickly

engordar, to grow fat; to fatten

engranarse, *Arg*, to get angry

engrandecerse, to get larger

engrasar, to grease

engrifar[1], to administer marijuana to someone; ~**se**[1] to take marijuana

enguatado, padding *Surg*

engullir, to engorge; to gulp down

enjuagar, to rinse; to wipe (dry); ~ **las lágrimas a alguien** to wipe s.o.'s eyes; ~**se** to rinse out; ~ **la frente** to wipe one's brow; ~ **las lágrimas** to wipe one's eyes

enjuagatorio, mouth wash

enjuague, *m*, rinse

enjuañangarse, *PR*, to be exhausted

enjuto, *adj*, lean (*cara*)

enlace, *m*, bond; link; linkage

enlazamiento, *form*, bonding

enlazar, to link

enloquecer, to go mad; ~**(se)** to go crazy

enloquecido, *adj*, frenzied

enmarañarse, to get tied up in knots

enmarihuanar[1], to administer marijuana to someone; ~**se**[1] to take marijuana

enmascarado, *adj*, masked

enmascarar, to mask; to obscure

enmendar (ie), to emend

enmohecer(se), to rust; to mildew; to mold

enojadizo, *adj*, huffy

enojado, *adj*, angry; upset; mad (*enfadado*)

enojar, to anger; ~**se** to get angry; to get mad

enorme, *adj*, enormous

enquistado, *adj*, encysted

enredado, *adj*, tangled

enredar, to tangle

enriquecer, to enrich

enriquecido, *adj*, enriched

enrojecer, to redden; ~**se** to blush

enrojecido, *adj*, flushed

enrojecimiento, redness

enrollar, to roll

enroquecimiento, huskiness

ensalada, salad

ensalmar huesos, to set bones

ensalmo, *Med*, quack remedy; quack treatment

ensanchador, *m*, reamer

ensanchamiento, enlargement

ensanchar, to widen

ensayar, to taste (*probar*)

ensayo, trial; test; **tubo de ~** test tube

enseñar, to show (*mostrar*); to teach; ~ **los dientes** *fam*, to show one's teeth

ensimismarse, to become lost in thought

ensordecer, to deafen

ensordecimiento, deafness; deafening; ear-piercing (*sonido*); ear-shattering

ensuciar, to defecate; to dirty; to make a mess (*necesidades corporales*); ~**se** to get dirty

ensueño, daydream

entablazón, *f*, *Chicano*, constipation; stomach obstruction

entablillado, *adj*, in a splint

entablillar, to put in splints

enteco, *adj*, frail; sickly; weak

entender (ie), to understand
entendido, *m, adj, fam*, gay
enterectomía, enterectomy
enteritis, *f*, enteritis; **~ cicatrizante crónica** cicatrizing chronic enteritis
entero, *adj*, entire; whole; outright (*completa*)
enterología, enterology
enterólogo, *m, adj*, enterologist
enteropatía, enteropathy
entierro, funeral
entorpecer, to clog (*estorbar*); to numb
entorpecimiento, numbness
entorunarse[1], to get mad; *PR*, to become irritable
entrada, entrance; intake (*de aire*); mouth (*abertura*)
entrado en años, *adj*, advanced in years
entrañas, bowels; entrails; guts *fam*
entrar (en), to enter (*penetrar*); to go in (*caber*); **~ calores** to get the chills; **~le calores y fríos** *fam*, to have chills
entre comidas, in-between meals
entrega[1], drop[2]
entrenamiento, training (*deportes*)
entrenar(se), to train
entrepierna, crotch; **~s** crotch
entresijo, *fam*, genitals; groin
entrevista, interview
entripar, *Mex*, to soak; *Arg, Col, Ec*, to anger; to upset
entropía, entropy
entuerto, postpartum cramp; **~s** *pl*, afterpains
entumecer, to numb; **~(se)** to stiffen (*extremidades*); **~se** to bloat
entumecido, *adj*, numb; stiff (*Med: dormido*)
entumecimiento, numbness
entumido, *adj*, numb
enturbiamiento, cloudiness; fogging
entusiasmo, excitement (*ilusión*)
enucleación, *f*, enucleation
enuresis, *f*, bed-wetting

envaramiento, *Mex*, stiffness (*entumecimiento*)
envararse, *Mex*, to become stiff
envase, *m*, bottle; jar
envejecer, to age; **~(se)** to grow old
envejecido, *adj*, aged
envejecimiento, aging; old age
envenenamiento, poisoning; **~ de la sangre** *fam*, blood poisoning; **~ del plomo** lead poisoning; **~ plúmbico** lead poisoning; **~ por comestibles** food poisoning
envenenar, to poison; to pollute (*el aire*); **~(se)** to poison (*uno mismo*); **~se** to be poisoned
enviar, to refer (*un paciente*); to ship (*transportar*)
envidioso, *adj*, jealous
envinado, *adj, Arg*, drunk
envoltura, *fam*, bandage; envelope (*membrana limitante de algunos virus*)
envolver (ue), to roll; **~(se)** to wrap up
enyerbar[1], to smoke marijuana; **~se** *Guat, Mex*, to poison oneself
enyesadura, cast (*para inmovilizar una extremidad rota*); **~ para caminar** walking cast
enyesar, to put in a cast; to put in a plaster cast
enzima, enzyme; **~ bacteriana** bacterial enzyme; **~ coagulante** coagulating enzyme; **~ de unión** joining enzyme; **~ inorgánica** inorganic enzyme
eñangotao, *adj, PR*, squatting
eosinófilo, eosinophil
epazote, *m*, wormseed; Mexican tea; (*Vea té de epazote*); **~**[1] marijuana
epiblasto, epiblast
epicanto, epicanthus
epicardio, epicardium
epicarditis, *f*, epicarditis
epicondilalgia del húmero, tennis elbow
epicondilitis humeral, *f, form*, ten-

nis elbow; humeral epicondylitis *form*

epicóndilo, epicondyle
epidemia, epidemic; outbreak (*de una enfermedad*)
epidémico, *adj*, epidemic
epidemiología, epidemiology
epidemiólogo, epidemiologist
epidérmico, *adj*, epidermal
epidermis, *f*, epidermis
epidídimo, epididymis
epidural, *adj*, epidural
epífisis, *f*, epiphysis (*cabeza ósea*)
epigastrio, pit; ~ **del estómago** pit of stomach
epiglotis, *f*, epiglottis
epiglotitis, *f*, epiglottitis
epilepsia, *form*, falling sickness; epilepsy; ~ **abortiva** abortive epilepsy; ~ **autonómica diencefálica** autonomic diencephalic epilepsy
epiléptico, *m*, *adj*, epileptic
epinefrina, epinephrine
episiotomía, episiotomy
episodio, episode; event
epistaxis, *f*, *form*, nose bleeding; nosebleed; epistaxis *form*
epitelio, epithelium; ~ **celiado** ciliated epithelium; ~ **cilíndrico** columnar epithelium; ~ **escamoso** squamous epithelium; ~ **estratificado** stratified epithelium; ~ **falso** false epithelium
equilibración, *f*, equilibration; ~ **oclusal** occlusal equilibration
equilibrar, to balance; to equilibrate
equilibrio, balance (*físico, mental, etc.*); equilibrium; ~ **acidobásico** acid-base equilibrium; ~ **fisiológico** physiologic equilibrium; ~ **homeostático** homeostatic equilibrium; ~ **radioactivo** radioactive equilibrium
equimosis, *f*, ecchymosis
equiparar, to match
equipo, equipment; gear (*colección de instrumentos y aparatos es-*

peciales para un trabajo); outfit (*conjunto de cosas para uso particular*); team; ~ **de primeros auxilios** first aid kit; ~ **de técnicos** team of technicians; ~ **de urgencia** first aid kit; ~ **médico** medical team; medical unit; ~ **hipodérmico** artillery[2] (*término de las drogas*); gun[2] (*drogas*)
equivalente, *m*, equivalent
equivocación, *f*, misunderstanding
equivocarse (acerca de), to be mistaken (about)
erección, *f*, erection
eréctil, *adj*, erectile
erina, dissecting hook
erisipela, erysipelas; red fever; ~ **de la costa** coast erysipelas; ~ **lombarda** pellagra; ~ **médica** erysipelas idiopathic; ~ **migratoria** migrant erysipelas
eritema, *m*, erythema; ~ **de los pañales** baby rash; ~ **endémico** endemic erythema; ~ **infeccioso** infectiosum erythema; ~ **inflamatorio** inflammatory erythema; ~ **multiforme** multiform erythema; ~ **nudoso (sifilítico)** nodosum erythema (syphiliticum); ~ **solar** sun burn
eritroblasto, erythroblast; ~ **basófilo** basophilic erythroblast
eritroblastosis, *f*, erythroblastosis
eritrocito, *form*, erythrocyte (*glóbulo rojo*); red blood cell; red blood corpuscle; ~ **acrómico** achromic erythrocyte; ~ **inmaduro** immature erythrocyte
eritrodermia, erythrodermia
eritromicina, erythromycin
eritrosedimentación, *f*, erythrocyte sedimentation
erógeno, *adj*, erogenous
erosión, *f*, erosion; ~ **cervical** cervical erosion
erosionar(se), to erode
eroticismo, eroticism
erótico, *adj*, erotic
erotismo, erotism

erradicar, to eradicate

errante, *adj,* wandering

errático, *adj,* erratic

erróneo, *adj,* erroneous

error, *m,* error; mistake; slip (*equivocación*); ~ **de alineación** misalignment; ~ **de cálculo** miscalculation

eructación, *f,* belching

eructar, to belch; to burp

eructo, belch; burp; eructation *form;* ~ **acedo** burping (*amargo*)

erupción, *f,* efflorescence; eruption; outbreak (*de espinillas*); ~ **(cutánea)** rash; ~ **cutánea** impetigo; ~ **debida al calor** prickly heat; ~ **por medicamentos** drug eruption; ~ **vesicular** vesicular eruption

erutar, to belch; to burp

esbozo, design; drawing

escala, scale (*instrumento de medida*); ~ **centígrada** centigrade scale; ~ **de Apgar** Apgar score; ~ **de Celsius** Centigrade scale; ~ **de Fahrenheit** Fahrenheit scale; ~ **móvil** sliding scale

escaldadura, scald (*quemadura*); ~ (*en los bebés*) diaper rash

escaldar, to scald (*quemarse la piel*); ~**se la mano** to scald one's hand

escalera, stairway; ~ **de incendios** fire escape; ~ **mecánica** moving staircase; escalator; ~**s** stairs

escalofrío, chill; shiver (*con catarro*)

escalpelo, dissecting knife; scalpel

escama, flake (*de la piel*); scale (*Med; de la piel*); scale (*de pez, serpiente, etc.*)

escamar, to scale (*quitar las escamas*)

escamoso, *adj,* flaky

escán, *m, Chicano,* scan

escándalo, outrage (*atención pública*)

escandaloso, *adj,* outrageous (*que causa escándalo*)

escaparse, to escape

escape, *m,* escape (*de gas, vapor, etc.*); leak (*de gas*); release (*de gas, vapor*) (*steam*); ~ **ventricular** ventricular escape

escápula, shoulder blade; scapula

escarapelarse, *Mex, Perú,* to get gooseflesh; to tremble all over

escarbadientes, *m, inv,* toothpick

escarbar, to scratch (*una gallina, etc.*)

escarceo, *PR,* brawl

escarcha, frost

escariador, *m,* broach *Dent*

escarificación, *f,* scarification

escarpín, *m,* pump (*zapato*)

escasez, *f,* thinness (*de pelo*); shortage

escasifoyao, *adj, PR,* in bad condition

escasifoyarse, *PR,* to be exhausted

escaso, *adj,* meager; scanty; scarce

escatimar sus fuerzas, to save one's strength

escayola, calcium sulfate; cast (*para inmovilizar una extremidad rota*); plaster (*for an injury*)

escindir, to excise

esclera, sclera

esclerosis, *f,* sclerosis; ~ **diseminada** multiple sclerosis; ~ **en placa** multiple sclerosis; ~ **lateral amiotrófica/E.L.A.** amyotrophic lateral sclerosis/A.L.S.; ~ **múltiple** multiple sclerosis; ~ **pulmonar** pulmonary sclerosis

escleroso, *adj,* hard (*tejido*)

esclerótica, *Anat,* sclera; *adj,* sclerotic

escoba, broom

escobillón, *m,* cotton swab; swab

escocer (ue), to smart (*irritar*)

escoger, to choose

escoliosis, *f,* scoliosis; spinal curvature; ~ **postural** habit scoliosis

esconder, to conceal; ~**se** to hide

escondido, *adj,* occult

escopolamina, scopolamine

escorbuto, scurvy

escotadura, notch

escotoma, *m, form,* scotoma (*manchas enfrente de los ojos*)

escozor, *m*, itching; smarting pain; smarting (*sensación de una herida*)

escrachar(se), *PR*, to break (*dañar*)

escribir, to write; ~ **a máquina** to type; ~ **el español con fluidez** to write Spanish fluently

escritura, writing; ~ **como en un espejo** mirror writing; ~ **en espejo** mirror writing

escrófula, scrofula/scrophula

escroto, scrotum

escrúpulo, qualm (*remordimiento*); scruple

escrutar para detectar (+ *enfermedad*), to screen for (+ *illness*)

escrutinio, screening; ~ **multifásico** multiphasic screening

escuchar, to listen (to); ~**le los pulmones** to listen to one's lungs

escudo, shield (*IUD*); ~ **ocular** eye shield; eye-shield; ~ **para el pezón** nipple shield

escuela, school

escupidera, emesis basin

escupir, to cough up; to expectorate; to spit; ~ **en la taza** to spit in the bowl; ~ **sangre** to spit blood

escurribanda, *f*, *fam*, *Med*, diarrhea

escurrimiento, draining; dripping; ~ **de la nariz** rhinitis; ~ **posnasal** postnasal drip

esencia, essence; ~ **de eucalipto** eucalyptus oil; ~ **de menta** essence of peppermint; ~ **de trementina** turpentine

esencial, *adj*, essential

esofagoscopia, esophagoscopy

esfera, ball; sphere; ~ **de acción** scope (*terreno de acción*); ~ **de actividad** field of activity

esfigmomanometría, sphygmomanometry

esfigmomanómetro, blood pressure cuff; sphygmomanometer *form*

esfínter, *m*, sphincter; ~ **del cardias** cardiac sphinter; ~ **pilórico** pylori(c) sphincter

esforzarse (**ue**), to exert oneself; ~ **demasiado** to overdo

esfuerzo, effort; exertion (*empleo enérgico de la fuerza física contra alguna resistencia*); ~ **mental** mental strain; ~ **personal** self-help

esfumarse, to make oneself scarce; to vanish (*desaparecer*)

esgarrar, to cough up phlegm

esgolizarse, *PR*, to slip unexpectedly

esguabinao, *adj*, *PR*, apathetic

esguabinarse, *PR*, to be exhausted

esguanimao, *adj*, *PR*, in bad condition

esguince, *f*, sprain; ~ **vertebral** back strain

eslecharse, *vulg*, to climax (*sexualmente*); to come (*culminación sexual*); to reach sexual climax; *vulg*, *PR*, to ejaculate

eslembao, *adj*, *PR*, wearing adenoidal expression

eslembarse, *PR*, to be absent-minded; to be inattentive

esmalte, *m*, enamel; ~ **manchado** mottled enamel; ~ **moteado** mottled enamel; ~ **para las uñas** nail polish

esmamoniao, *adj*, *PR*, in bad condition (*cosas*); exhausted (*persona*)

esmamoniarse, *PR*, to be exhausted

esmayao, *adj*, extremely hungry; *PR*, starving

esmegma, *m*, smegma

esmonguillarse, *PR*, to be exhausted

esñemar(se), *PR*, to be sexually impotent

esofágico, *adj*, esophageal

esofagitis, *f*, esophagitis; ~ **péptica** peptic esophagitis; ~ **por reflujo** reflux esophagitis

esófago, esophagus; gullet

esofagología, esophagology

esofagoscopia, esophagoscopy

esofagoscopio, esophagoscope

esofagospasmo, esophagospasm

esoforia, internal/convergent strabismus

esotropía, internal/convergent strabismus

espabilar la borrachera, to sober up
espacio, length (*de tiempo*); space; ~ **de dentadura** denture space; ~ **epidural** epidural space; ~ **muerto** dead space; ~ **subgingival** gingival crevice
espalda, back (*de una persona*)
espaldarazo, slap (*en la espalda*)
espaldilla, shoulder blade (*omóplato*)
español, *m*, *adj*, Spanish; Spaniard
esparadrapo, adhesive strip; adhesive tape
esparcir, to spread out (*derramarse*)
esparlotear(se), *PR*, to be absent-minded
espárrago, asparagus
espaseao[1], *adj*, *Chicano*, *PR*, high on[2] (*drogas narcóticas*); ~[1] *adj*, *Chicano*, stoned on marijuana
espasmo, cramp; reflex jerk; jerk (*acción refleja*); spasm; ~ **bronquial** bronchial spasm; ~ **centelleante** lightning spasm; ~ **facial** facial spasm; ~ **masticatorio** lockjaw; ~ **muscular** twitching; ~ **por torsión** torsion spasm; ~**s respiratorios** breath holding
espasmódico, *adj*, spasmodic; spastic
espástico, *adj*, spasmodic; spastic
espatarrao, *adj*, sitting with the legs apart
espatarrarse, to open one's legs wide
especia, spice
especial, *adj*, special
especialista, *m/f*, specialist; ~ **en enfermedades de los ojos** ophthalmologist; ~ **en enfermedades venéreas** venereologist; ~ **en fracturas** orthopedist; ~ **en lentes** optometrist; ~ **en logopedia** speech pathologist; ~ **en ortopedia** orthopedist; ~ **en señoras** *fam*, gynecologist
especialización, *f*, specialization
especializado, *adj*, specialized

especializarse, to specialize
específico, *adj*, specific; *m*, *Med*, patent medicine; ~ **de grupo** group-specific
espécimen, *m*, specimen
espéculo, speculum
espejeras, *f*, *pl*, *Cu*, chafing
espejismo, mirage
espejo, mirror; ~ **de dentista** dental mirror; ~ **dental** dental mirror; ~ **frontal** head mirror; ~ **vaginal** vaginal speculum
espejuelos, *m*, *pl*, eyeglasses; *Cu*, glasses; spectacles
espera, wait; waiting
esperanza, hope; ~ **de vida** life expectancy
esperar, to expect; to hope (for); to wait (for)
esperma, semen; sperm
espermaticida, *m*, spermicide; ~ **vaginal** vaginal spermicide; vaginal spermaticide
espermatocele, *m*, spermatocele
espermatocito, spermatocyte
espermatogénesis, *f*, spermatogenesis
espermatozoide, *m*, sperm; spermatozoid; spermatozoon
espermiograma, *m*, spermiogram
espesar, to thicken; ~**se** to clog up (*condensar líquido*)
espeso, *adj*, thick (*consistencia*)
espesor, *m*, thickness (*dimensión*)
espesura, thickness (*consistencia*)
espetar la uña, *PR*, *fam*, to aggravate a problem
espicharse, *Cu*, *Mex*, to get thin; *Mex*, to feel ashamed; *Guat*, to get scared
espina, bone (*de un pez*); fish bone; thorn; ~ **bífida** spina bifida; ~ **dorsal** backbone; spinal column
espinaca, spinach
espinal, *adj*, spinal
espinazo, backbone; *fam*, back
espinilla, *Med*, blackhead (*debido al acné*); pimple; ~**s** *fam*, acne; *Anat*, shin; shinbone

espiración, *f*, expiration; exhalation
espiral, *m*, spiral (*IUD*); ~ **intra-uterino** intrauterine loop
espirar, to expire (*exhalar*)
espiritismo, spiritism
espiritista, *m/f*, spiritist
espíritu, *m*, spirit
espirógrafo, spirograph
espirograma, *m*, spirogram
espirometría, spirometry; ~ **bron-coscópica** bronchoscopic spiro-metry
espirómetro, spirometer
espiroscopio, spiroscope
esplenectomía, splenectomy
esplenorragia, splenorrhagia
espliego, lavender
esplín, *Chicano*, spleen
espolón, *m*, spur; ~ **calcáneo** cal-caneal spur
espolvorear, to dust (*polvos*)
espondilartritis, *f*, spondylarthritis
espondilosis, *f*, spondylosis
esponja, sponge; ~ **de gelatina** gel foam
esponjoso, *adj*, cancellous; spongy
espontáneo, *adj*, spontaneous
espora, spore
esporádico, *adj*, sporadic
esporoblasto, sporoblast
esporozoarios, sporozoa (*sg, sporo-zoon*) (*parásito*)
esposa, wife
esposo, husband
espray, *m*, *Chicano*, spray
espulgar, to delouse
espuma, foam; lather (*jabón*); ~ **vaginal** vaginal foam (*anticon-ceptivo*)
espumoso, *adj*, foamy; frothy
esputo, saliva; spit *Med*; sputum; ~ **de sangre** spit of blood; ~ **san-griento** blood in the sputum; ~ **sanguinolento** bloody sputum
esquelético, *adj*, skeletal
esqueleto, frame (*estatua*); frame-work *Dent*; skeleton
esquema, *m*, drawing

esquimosis de los párpados, *f*, *form*, black eye
esquinancia, quinsy (*garganta do-lorida*)
esquirla, bone splinter; splinter (*de un hueso*)
esquistasis, *f*, schistasis
esquistosoma, *m*, schistosoma (*pa-rásito*)
esquizofrenia, schizophrenia
esquizofrénico, *adj*, schizophrenic
esquizoide, *m/f*, *adj*, schizoid
esquizoidia, schizoidism
esquizoidismo, schizoidism
estabilidad de la dentadura, *f*, denture stability
estabilizar, to stabilize
estable, *adj*, stable
establecer, to lay down (*determinar*)
estacada, *SpAm*, wound; prick
estacar, *Ven*, to prick; to wound
estación, *f*, season of year; station; ~ **de ayuda** aid station; ~ **de descontaminación** decontami-nation station
estadística, statistics; ~**s demográ-ficas** vital statistics; ~**s médicas** medical statistics; ~**s vitales** vital statistics
estado, shape (*condición*); state; status; ~ **avanzado de gestación** advanced stage of pregnancy; ~ **civil** marital status; ~ **de ánimo** mood; state of mind; ~ **de an-siedad** state of anxiety; ~ **de choque** state of shock; ~ **de con-ciencia** consciousness; ~ **de de-presión** state of depression; ~ **de reposo** resting state; ~ **de salud** condition; state of health; ~ **general** condition; general condition; ~ **habitual** base-line/baseline (*examen físico o de comportamiento de un enfermo*); ~ **hipometabólico** hypometabolic state; ~ **interesante** *Chicano*, *euph*, pregnancy; ~ **mental** men-tal state; ~ **secundario** sec-

ondary stage; ~ **vegetativo persistente** persistent vegetative state

estafilocócico, *adj*, staphylococcal

estafilococo, staphylococcus (*pl, staphylococci*)

estampar, to stamp (*pegar*)

estampilla, *SpAm*, stamp

estancamiento, engorgement

estancia, stay

estándar, *m, adj*, standard

estandarización, *f*, standardization

estandarizar, to standardize

estante, *m*, shelf; stand

estar, to be; ~ **a dieta** to be on a diet; ~ **a millón**[1] to be higher than a kite[2]; to be stoned[2]; ~ **acostado boca arriba** *adj*, to be on one's back; ~ **afónico** *fam, adj*, to be hoarse; ~ **agobiado de trabajo** *adj*, to be up to the elbows in work; ~ **alterado** *fam, adj*, to be anxious; ~ **aquejado de** *adj*, to be afflicted with; ~ **archivado** *adj*, to be on file; ~ **atento** *adj*, to look out for (*prestar atención*); ~ **autorizado** *adj*, to be authorized; to be at liberty; ~ **borracho** *adj*, to have a jag on *slang*; ~ **cacarizo** *adj*, to have pockmarks; ~ **calado hasta los huesos** *adj*, to be drenched to the skin; ~ **caquis maquis** *euph*, to be dirty; ~ **chocho** *adj*, to be in one's dotage; ~ **cohibido** *adj*, to feel inhibited; ~ **como un guanime** *PR*, to be tired; ~ **como un paslote** *PR*, not to be alert; ~ **con alguien** to have sexual relations; ~ **con familia** to be expecting; ~ **conforme con el debido nivel** to be up to standard; ~ **congestionado** *adj*, to be congested; ~ **constipado** *adj*, to be congested; ~ **coronando** to crown; ~ **crudo**[1] *adj, Mex*, to have a hangover; ~ **de acuerdo** to be of the same opinion; ~ **de acuerdo (con)** to agree

(with); ~ **de carreritas** to have the trots (*diarrea*); ~ **de goma** *CA*, to be hungover; ~ **de mal humor** to grouch; ~ **de moda** to be in vogue; ~ **de parto** to be in labor; to lie in (*debido al parto*); ~ **de pie** to stand; ~ **de servicio** to be on duty; ~ **desesperado** *fam, adj*, to be anxious; ~ **desgonzado** *fam, adj*, to fatigue (*cansado*); ~ **desocupado** *adj*, to be at liberty (*libre*); ~ **desombligado** *adj*, to have an umbilical hernia; ~ **duro** *fam*, to have constipation; ~ **embarazada de ___ meses** to be ___ months pregnant; ~ **en boga** to be in vogue; ~ **en contacto con** to be exposed to; ~ **en desacuerdo con** to take issue with; to be at variance with; ~ **en el dique** *PR*, to give up alcohol; ~ **en el umbral de la vida** to be on the threshold of life; ~ **en la plantilla** to be on the staff; ~ **en las últimas** to be on one's last legs; ~ **en nada** *fam*, not to be alert; ~ **en un dilema** to be in a quandary; ~ **en un hilo** *PR*, to be on the verge of something; ~ **enamorado de** *adj*, to have a crush on; ~ **encamado** *adj*, to be on one's back (*estar enfermo*); ~ **enferma** *fam*, to menstruate; ~ **enojado** *adj*, to be in a huff; ~ **entripado** *fam*, to have constipation; ~ **expuesto a** *adj*, to be exposed to; ~ **fichao** *slang*, to be under surveillance under; ~ **incapacitado** *adj*, to be laid up; ~ **indispuesta** to menstruate; ~ **interesado en** *adj*, to be interested in; ~ **lleno de agujetas** *adj*, to be stiff all over; ~ **mala** to menstruate; ~ **mala de la garra** to menstruate; ~ **mala de la luna** to menstruate; ~ **mareado** to feel dizzy; ~ **más jalao que un timbre de guagua**[1] *PR*, to be higher than a kite[2]; ~ **mediagua** *slang*, to be/get drunk; ~ **muerto de hambre** *adj*, to be famished; ~ **muerto de miedo** *adj*, to be overcome by fear; ~ **nervioso** *adj*, to be anxious; ~ **obstruido** *adj*, to be congested; ~ **ocioso** *adj*, to idle (*estar libre*); ~ **pachucho** *adj*, *Spain*, to be under the weather; ~ **parado** *adj*, *SpAm*, to be standing (up); ~ **paralizado** *adj*, to be paralyzed; ~ **perdido por** *adj*, to have a crush on; ~ **poco dispuesto a** *adj*, to be loath to; ~ **por debajo del nivel correcto** to be below standard; ~ **postrado de dolor** *adj*, to be overcome by pain; ~ **predispuesto a favor de** *adj*, to be prejudiced in favor of; ~ **predispuesto contra** *adj*, to be prejudiced against; ~ **profundamente dormido** *adj*, to be sound asleep; ~ **recuperándose** to be on the road to recovery; ~ **rendido** *fam*, *adj*, to fatigue (*cansado*); ~ **repantigado en un sillón** *adj*, to slouch in a chair; ~ **ronco** *fam*, *adj*, to be hoarse; ~ **seguro** *adj*, to be sure; ~ **sentado con el cuerpo encorvado** to sit hunched up

estasis, *f*, stasis

estático, *adj*, static

estatura, frame (*altura*); height; stature

estearato de magnesio, magnesium stearate

estenosis, *f*, stricture; ~ **aórtica** aortic stenosis; ~ **esofágica** esophageal stenosis; ~ **mitral** mitral stenosis; ~ **pulmonar** pulmonary stenosis

estereopsia, *form*, depth perception; stereopsis

estéril, *adj*, barren; infertile; sterile

esterilidad, *f*, sterility; ~ **femenina** feminine sterility; ~ **masculina** masculine sterility; ~ **permanente** permanent sterility

esterilización, *f*, sterilization (*tipo de control de la natalidad*)

esterilizado, *adj*, sterile; sterilized

esterilizador, *m*, sterilizer

esterilizar, to sterilize; ~ **las botellas** to sterilize the bottles

esternón, *m*, breast bone/breastbone; sternum

esteroide, *m*, steroid

estertor, *m*, mucous rale; rale; rattling; ~ **agónico** death rattle; ~ **crujiente** rackling rale; ~ **de burbujas** bubbling rale; ~ **de chasquido** clicking rale; ~ **de la muerte** death rattle; ~ **de retorno** redux rale; ~ **húmedo** moist rale; ~ **seco** dry rale; ~ **sibilante** sibilant rale; whistling rale; ~ **traqueal** tracheal stertor

estertoroso, *adj*, stertorous

estético, *adj*, esthetic

estetoscopio, stethoscope; ~ **fetal** fetoscope

estigma, *m*, birthmark; stigma

estilete, *m*, probe; stylet

estimar, to esteem; to value

estimulante, *m*, amphetamines; mood elevator; pep pill; stimulant; *adj*, exciting

estimular, to stimulate

estímulo, stimulus

estíptico, *adj*, styptic; constipated

estiramiento, *form*, pulled muscle; stretching; ~ **de la piel** face lift; ~ **facial** face lift

estirar, to stretch; ~**le a alguien la piel de la cara** to have a face lift

estirón, *m*, growth spurt

estítico, *adj*, *fam*, *El Sal*, constipated

estival, *adj*, summer

estofa[1], *PR*, heroin

estofón, *m*, *PR*, bookworm

estomacal, *adj*, stomach

estómago, stomach; *fam*, abdomen; ~ **revuelto** upset stomach; ~ **sucio**[6] constipation; dyspepsia; *Chicano*, indigestion; ~ **suelto** diarrhea; ~ **vacío** hollow stomach

estomatitis, *f*, stomatitis
estomatología, dentistry; stomatology
estomatólogo, *adj*, stomatologist
estornudar, to sneeze
estornudo, sneeze
estrabismo, *form*, strabismus; ~ (convergente) cross-eye; ~ convergente internal strabismus; ~ divergente external strabismus; ~ externo external strabismus; ~ interno internal strabismus
estrabómetro, strabometer
estragado, *adj*, broken (*salud*)
estragao, *adj*, extremely hungry
estragos, *m*, *pl*, havoc
estrangulación, *f*, strangulation; ~ herniaria hernial strangulation
estrangular, to constrict (*una vena*)
estranguria, strangury
estrasijao, *adj*, extremely hungry; *adj*, *fam*, *PR*, undernourished
estratigrafía, scan
estrato, layer
estrechar, to constrict (*hacer estrecho*)
estrechez, *f*, narrowing; narrowness; ~ de miras narrow-mindedness; *Med*, stricture
estrecho, *adj*, close; narrow; ~ de cara narrow-faced; ~ de pecho narrow-breasted; narrow-chested; ~ medio de la pelvis midpelvic plane
estregar, to scrub (*con un cepillo*)
estrellita, *fam*, floater (*en el ojo*)
estremecerse, to quake (*temblar*); to shake with (*temor*)
estremecimiento, shiver (*de miedo*)
estrenuo, *adj*, strenuous
estreñido, *adj*, constipated
estreñimiento, constipation; ~ espasmódico spastic constipation
estreñir, to bind (*retrasar el curso del contenido intestinal*); ~se to become constipated
estreptobacilo, streptobacillus
estreptococia, *form*, strep throat

estreptococo, streptococcus; ~ leve mild streptococcus
estreptomicina, streptomycin
estrés, *m*, stress; ~ emocional *Chicano*, emotional stress; ~ personal personal stress
estriado, *adj*, striated
estriaciones cutáneas, *f*, skin striae
estrías, stretch marks; striae (*sg*, *stria*)
estribo, stapes; stirrup; stirrup bone
estricnina, strychnine
estricto, *adj*, strict
estrictura, stricture
estrillar, *Perú*, *Ríopl*, to get cross
estrillo, *Perú*, *Ríopl*, bad temper
estriol, *m*, estriol
estroc, *m*, *Chicano*, cerebral vascular accident; (cerebrovascular) stroke
estrógeno, estrogen
estroncio, strontium
estropajo, dishcloth; scouring pad
estropear, to maim; to spoil *Med*
estructura, framework; structure; ~s de soporte de la dentadura denture supporting structures
estruma, *m*, goiter
estuche, *m*, glass case; kit; ~ de disección dissecting set; ~[1] artillery[2] (*término de las drogas*); fit[2]; gun[2]
estudiante, *m/f*, student; ~ de medicina medical student
estudio, observation; study; ~ doble a ciegas double-blind study; ~ electrofisiológico electrophysiologic study
estudioso, *adj*, studious
estufa, warming crib; incubator
estufear[1], to sniff residue of powdered narcotics; to snort[2] (*sorber los restos de los narcóticos en polvo*)
estufiar[1], to sniff residue of powdered narcotics; to snort[2]
estupefaciente[1], *m*, dope[2]; drug[2] (*narcótico*); narcotic; *adj*, stupefaciente[2]

estupendo, *adj*, stupendous

estupidez, *f*, stupidity

estúpido, *adj*, dull (*intelectual-mente*); stupid

estupor, *m*, lethargy; stupor

estupro, rape

etanol, *m*, ethanol

etapa, stage; ~ inicial de la enfermedad initial stage of the illness

éter, *m*, ether; ~ anestésico anesthetic ether; ~ de metilo methyl ether; ~ etílico ethyl ether

ética, ethics; ~ médica medical ethics; ~ profesional professional ethics

ético, *adj*, ethical

etileno, ethylene

etilo, ethyl; ~ acético ethyl acetate; ~ bromhídrico ethyl bromide; ~ yodhídrico ethyl iodide; yoduro de ~ ethyl iodide

etiología, etiology

etiológico, *adj*, etiological

etiqueta, label

étnico, *adj*, ethnic

etnografía, ethnography

etnología, ethnology

eucalipto, eucalyptus

eucaliptol, *m*, eucalyptol

euforia, euphoria

eugenesia, eugenics

eugenol, *m*, eugenol *Dent*

eunuco, eunuch

eupareunia, normal coitus; vaginal coitus

eutanasia, euthanasia; mercy death/killing

evacuación, *f*, evacuation; bowel movement; stool; ~ del vientre bowel movement; feces

evacuar, to have a bowel movement; to evacuate; *Med*, to drain

evaluación, *f*, evaluation

evaluar, to evaluate

evaporación, *f*, evaporation

evaporarse, to evaporate

eversión, *f*, eversion

evidencia, evidence

evidente, *adj*, evident

evisceración, *f*, evisceration

evitar, to avoid; to save (*prevenir*); ~ inconvenientes to obviate

evolución, *f*, evolution

evolucionar, to evolve

exacerbación, *f*, exacerbation

exacto, *adj*, accurate

exageración, *f*, exaggeration

exagerado, *adj*, exaggerated

exagerar, to overdo

exaltación, *f*, exaltation

examen, (*pl*, exámenes) *m*, (lab) test; observation; ~ a simple vista naked eye examination; ~ bajo anestesia EUA/ exam under anesthesia; ~ con rayos x x-ray examination; ~ de (la) sangre blood test; ~ de capacidad mental mental test; ~ de conejo rabbit test; ~ de la lengua glossoscopy; ~ de la vista testing of vision; eye test; ~ de las huellas para la identificación de las personas dactyloscopy; ~ de leche milk testing; ~ de los senos breast examination; ~ de orina urinalysis; ~ físico physical examination; ~ ginecológico pelvic examination; pelvic; ~es hematológicos blood studies; ~ macroscópico gross examination; ~ médico medical exam; *Chicano*, medical examination; ~ médico minucioso thorough medical exam; ~ oftalmológico eye/ophthalmologic exam; ~ otorrinolaringológico ENT exam; ~ radiológico x-ray examination; ~ tacto rectal rectal examination; ~ vaginal para el cáncer Pap smear; ~ visual eye examination

examinación, *f*, examination

examinador, -ra, *m/f*, examiner; ~ médico medical examiner

examinar, to examine; to investigate (*evaluar*); to look at; to observe; to test; ~ con rayos x to x-ray (*en una pantalla fluorescente*)

exanguinotransfusión, *f*, exchange transfusion; exsanguinotransfusion

exánime, *adj*, lifeless

exantema, *m*, *form*, exanthem; rash; ~ **medicamentoso** drug rash; ~ **por calor** heat rash; ~ **vesicular** vesicular exanthem

excavación, *f*, excavation

excavador, *m*, excavator; ~ **dental** dental excavator

exceder, to exceed; ~ **en número** to outnumber

excelente, *adj*, excellent

excéntrico, *adj*, eccentric

excesivamente cuidadoso, *adj*, overcareful

excesivamente gordo, *adj*, overweight

excesivamente grueso, *adj*, overweight

excesivo, *adj*, excessive

exceso, excess; ~ **de cetonas en la orina** hyperketonuria; ~ **de confianza** overconfidence; ~ **de peso** overweight

excipiente, *m*, vehicle *Med*

excisión, *f*, excision; removal; ~ **de heridas** wound excision

excitabilidad, *f*, excitability

excitación, *f*, excitement; ~ **(directa) (indirecta)** (direct) (indirect) excitation; ~ **eléctrica** electric shock

excitante, *adj*, excitant; *adj*, *Med*, stimulating; *m*, *Med*, stimulant

excitar, to arouse (*sexualmente*)

excrecencia, growth (*tumor*); outgrowth (*algo que crece*)

excreción, *f*, ejection; excretion; ~ **urinaria** urinary output

excremento, bowel movement; excrement; excretion; feces; stool; ~ **aguado** mushy stool; ~ **suelto** diarrhea; loose bowels

excretar, to have a bowel movement

excusa, excuse

excusado, latrine; lavatory (*baño*); restroom; toilet

exhalación, *f*, exhalation

exhalar, to exhale; ~ **el último suspiro** to draw one's last breath

exhaustivo, *adj*, comprehensive

exhumación, *f*, disinterment; exhumation

exigente, *adj*, demanding

eximir, to exempt (*liberar*)

existencia, existence

existente, *adj*, actual (*en este momento*)

exitante[1], *m*, stimulant

éxito, success

exocrino, *adj*, exocrine

exodoncia, exodontics (*trata de la extracción de los dientes*)

exodontista, *m/f*, exodontist

exodontología, exodontology

exonerar el vientre, to have a bowel movement

exótico, *adj*, exotic

exotropía, external strabismus

expandir, to expand

expansor, *m*, expander; ~ **del plasma** plasma volume expander

expectación, *f*, expectation; ~ **de (la) vida** expectation of life

expectante, *adj*, expectant

expectativa de vida, life expectancy

expectoración, *f*, expectoration

expectorante, *m*, *adj*, expectorant

expectorar, *form*, to expectorate *form*; to cough up

expediente, *m*, dossier; file (*reporte*); record (*carpeta del enfermo*); ~ **del paciente** medical record (*del enfermo*)

experiencia, experience; ~ **mala en el uso de drogas** bad trip[2]; ~ **traumática** traumatic experience

experimentación, *f*, experimentation

experimentar, to experience

experimento, experiment

experto, *adj*, experienced; *m*, *adj*, expert

expirar, to expire (*morir*)

explicación, *f*, explanation

explicar, to explain

exploración, *f*, examination; exploration; ~ **nuclear** (nuclear) scan

explorador, *m*, explorer (*instrumento*); *adj*, exploratory *Surg*

explorar, to explore *Surg*; *Med*, to probe

exploratorio, *adj*, exploratory

explotación, *f*, rupture (*absceso*)

explotarse, to rupture (*un absceso: reventar*)

exponer, to expose

exposición, *f*, exposure

expresar, to express

expresión, *f*, expression

exprimir, to express (*estrujar*)

expulsar, to expel; ~ **aire** *form*, to breathe out

expulsión, *f*, ejection; expulsion; ~ **de la placenta** delivery of the placenta; ~ **de las secundinas** afterbirth

éxtasis, *f*, ecstasy

extender (ie), to prolong (*prolongar*); to spread limbs

extensión, *f*, extension; incidence (*de una enfermedad*); length (*de tiempo*); range (*de conocimiento, voz*); scale (*de un disastre, etc.*); ~ **de sangre** film of blood; blood smear

extenso, *adj*, extense; extensive

extenuación, *f*, abatement

exterior, *adj*, exterior; external; outer; *m*, exterior; outside

externo, *adj*, external; outer

extinto, *adj*, *Chi*, *Mex*, *Ríopl*, *euph*, deceased; dead

extintor de incendios, *m*, fire extinguisher

extirpación, *f*, extirpation; ~ **de la matriz** hysterectomy; ~ **de la pulpa** pulp extirpation

extirpar, to enucleate; to eradicate; to remove; to stamp out; *Med*, to remove surgically; ~ **un ganglio o ganglios** to deganglionate

extracción, *f*, extraction; ~ **con fórceps** forceps delivery; ~ **de nalgas** breech extraction; breech delivery; ~ **de várices** vein stripping; ~ **del nervio** root canal work

extracto, extract; ~ **alergénico** allergenic extract; ~ **animal** animal extract; ~ **compuesto** compound extract; ~ **de hígado** liver extract; ~ **de hígado para uso parenteral** parenteral liver extract; ~ **de paratiroides** parathyroid extract; ~ **de polen** pollen extract; ~ **de raíz orozuz (puro)** (pure) licorice root extract; ~ **de regaliz (puro)** (pure) licorice root extract; ~ **pancreático** pancreatic extract

extraer, to extract (*to remove, take out*); to pull out; to remove; to take out

extrañar, to miss (*una persona*); to surprise (*sorprender*)

extraño, *adj*, extraneous; quaint (*raro*); strange

extraordinario, *adj*, extraordinary

extrapolar, to extrapolate

extrarrápido, *adj*, quick-acting

extrasensorial, *adj*, extrasensory

extrasístole, *f*, anticipated systole; extrasystole; ~ **auricular** auricular extrasystole; ~ **auriculoventricular** auriculoventricular extrasystole; ~ **interpolada** interpolated extrasystole; ~ **nodal** nodal extrasystole; ~ **retrógrada** retrograde extrasystole; ~ **ventricular** ventricular escape; ventricular extrasystole

extrauterino, *adj*, extrauterine

extremidad, *f*, extremity; limb; ~**es frías** cold extremities; ~ **inferior/superior** lower/upper extremity

extremo, *adj*, extreme; ~ **distal** distal end *Dent*

extrínseco, *adj*, extrinsic

extrovertido, *m*, *adj*, extrovert; outgoing (*personalidad*)

extubación, *f,* extubation
extubar, to extubate
exuberante, *adj,* exuberant
exudado, *m,* exudate
exudar, to exude

eyaculación, *f,* ejection; **~ precoz** ejaculatio praecox; **~ prematura** ejaculatio praecox; **~ nocturna** nocturnal emission
eyacular, *form,* to ejaculate

---

[1] Este vocabulario es nuevo y todavía no se encuentra en el *Diccionario de la lengua española*, publicado por la Real Academia Española. Forma pate del argot o la lengua de la calle. Se supone que el género es obvio a menos que sea indicado.

[2] Forma parte del vocabulario inglés actual de los drogadictos.

[4] El verdadero nombre de esta enfermedad es *impacción*, Raras veces consiste en una verdadera obstrucción del intestino. Con más frecuencia otras dolencias producen señas nombradas *empacho*. Esto puede ser producido por una bola de lombrices o excremento duro, o por disentería con torcijones, o por una úlcera del estómago, o por la mala alimentación. Muchas personas consideran que cualquier malestar del estómago es *empacho*, especialmente si tienen gases o están "sofocadas." Echan la culpa al diablo o a una bruja. Acuden a curanderos que curan a estas personas poniendo ventosas, entre otras cosas, para "poder sacar una bola de pelo y espinas."

[5] Hay discusiones breves de muchas de las enfermedades caseras en esta obra bajo el nombre de la enfermedad específica. Para aún más discusión, hay que referir a *Conversational Spanish for Medical Personnel*, 2a edición, por Rochelle K. Kelz, New York: Delmar, 1982, págs. 386–396.

[6] Muchas personas de herencia hispana se preocupan del estómago sucio y piensan que es necesario limpiar el cuerpo. Toman un té medicinal como *té de epazote* (vea pág. 494) y un laxante. Estas personas opinan que una enfermedad que resulta de un estómago sucio es *empacho*.

F

fábrica, factory
facciones, *f*, features
facies, *m, inv*, facies
fácil, *adj*, easy; ~ **de engañar** easy (*crédulo*)
fácilmente, *adv*, easily
factor, *m*, factor; ~ **antihemofílico** antihemophilic factor/AHF; ~ **antihemorrágico** (*Vitamina K*) antihemorrhagic factor; ~ **de riesgo** risk factor; ~ **genético** genetic factor; ~ **madurador de eritrocitos** erythrocyte maturation factor; ~ **proteína animal** animal protein factor; ~ **Rh** Rh factor; ~ **Rhesus** Rh factor; ~ **tromboplástico del plasma** plasma thromboplastic factor; ~ **VIII de la coagulación de la sangre** (*factor antihemofílico A*) factor VIII, in the clotting of blood (*Antihemophilic factor A*); ~ **IX de la coagulación de la sangre** (*factor antihemofílico B*) factor IX, in the clotting of blood (*Antihemophilic factor B*)
facultad, *f*, faculty; school (*dentro de una universidad*); ~ **de enfermería** nursing school; ~ **de fusión** fusion faculty; ~ **de medicina** medical school; ~ **germinativa** germinative faculty
facultativa, midwife (*sin formación profesional*)
facultativo, physician; surgeon; *adj*, medical; **cuadro** ~ medical staff; **dictamen** ~ *m*, medical report; **parte** ~ *m*, medical bulletin
faja, band; belt; binder; girdle; ~ **abdominal** belly binder; swathing bandage; truss; ~ **médica** supporter; ~ **obstétrica** obstetric binder
fajar, to bandage

fajero, belly binder
fajita, belly binder; belly band
falange, *f*, phalanx
falda, skirt
fálico, *adj*, phallic
fallar, to fail
fallecer, to die; to expire (*morir*)
fallecido, *adj*, late (*difunto*); ~ **al llegar** *adj*, DOA/dead on arrival
fallecimiento, death; decease; demise
fallo, failure; ~ **cardíaco** cardiac arrest; ~ **del corazón** heart failure; ~ **múltiple de órganos** multiple organ failure
falo, phallus
falsear, to sprain
falseo, *Chicano*, sprain
falsificación, *f*, falsification
falso, false
falta, defect; lack; ~ **de(l) aire** air hunger; shortness of breath; ~ **de aliento** shortness of breath; ~ **de animación** lifelessness; ~ **de confianza** lack of confidence; ~ **de conocimiento** unconsciousness; ~ **de control** lack of control; ~ **de credibilidad** lack of credibility; ~ **de ejercicio** lack of exercise; ~ **de oxígeno** oxygen deficiency; ~ **de peso** underweight; ~ **de sensación** numbness; ~ **de uso** disuse
faltar, to lack; to miss (*cita*); to be missing; ~**le el aire** to be short of breath; ~**le la respiración** to be short of breath
fama, reputation
familia, family; ~ **degenerada** degenerate family; ~ **interracial** racially mixed family
familiar, *adj*, familial; *m*, family member; relative

fango, mud (*barro*)
fantasear, to dream
fañoso, hairlip
farfallota, *PR*, mumps
farfullar, to babble (*hablar de modo incoherente*)
farfullo, babble (*habla incoherente*)
faringe, *f*, pharynx
faringitis, *f*, pharyngitis
farmacéutico, druggist; pharmacist; *adj*, pharmaceutical
farmacia, pharmacy; *Chicano, Spain*, drugstore
fármaco, dope[1]; narcotic; drug (*medicamento*); ~ **no caducado** in date medication
farmacodependencia, (drug) addiction; (drug) dependence; (drug) dependency; habit
farmacodependiente, *form*, (drug) addict
farmacología, pharmacology
farmacólogo, pharmacologist
farol, *m*, light (*de la calle*)
farruto, *adj, Arg, Bol, Chi*, sickly (*enfermizo*)
fascia, fascia (*pl, fasciae*)
fascículo, bundle; tract *Anat*; ~ **acústico central** central tract of auditory nerve; ~ **muscular** muscle bundle; ~ **solitario** respiratory column; ~**s descendentes** descending tract
fase, *f*, phase; stage; ~ **del parto** stage of pregnancy; ~ **expulsiva** expulsive stage; ~ **placentaria** placental stage
fastidio, weariness
fatal, *adj*, fatal (*muy grave*)
fatiga, exhaustion; fatigue (*cansancio*); tiredness; weariness; *slang*, asthma; ~ **ocular** eyestrain; ~ **sin causa** unexplained fatigue
fatigar, to fatigue (*cansar*)
fauces, *f, pl*, fauces; gorge
favor, *m*, favor
febrífugo, *m, adj*, antipyretic
febril, *adj*, febrile

fecha, date (*calendario*); ~ **calculada de parto** E.D.C./expected date of confinement; ~ **de caducidad** expiration date; ~ **de nacimiento** date of birth; ~ **esperada del parto** E.D.D./expected date of delivery
fecundación, *f*, fertilization; ~ **del huevo** *f*, conception
fecundizar, to impregnate
fecundo, *adj*, fruitful
felación, *f*, fellatio (*felatorismo*)
felatorismo, fellatio (*felación*)
felicidad, *f*, happiness
feliz, *adj*, happy
femoral, *adj*, femoral
fémur, *m*, femur; thigh bone
fenicladina, angel dust[2] (*PCP*); phencyclidine; dust[2] (*cocaína, PCP*); PCP
fenilcetonuria, phenylketonuria/PKU
fenilquetonuria, phenylketonuria/PKU
fenobarbital, *m*, phenobarbital
fenómeno, phenomenon
feo, *adj*, nasty (*herida, corte*)
fermentación, *f*, fermentation
fermentar, hacer, to ferment
fermento, ferment; yeast
ferropenia, iron deficiency
fértil, *adj*, fertile
fertilización, *f*, fertilization
fertilizar, to impregnate
férula, splint; ~ **de yeso** plaster splint
fetichismo, fetishism
fetidez de aliento, *f*, foul breath
fétido, *adj*, evil-smelling; foul
feto, fetus
fetoscopio, fetoscope
fiambrera, takeout food eaten at home
fibra, fiber; strand; ~ **elástica** elastic fiber; yellow fiber; ~ **motriz** motor fiber; ~ **muscular** muscle fiber; ~ **nerviosa** nerve fiber
fibrilación, *f*, fibrillation; ~ **auricular** atrial fibrillation; auricular

fibrillation; ~ **ventricular** ventricular fibrillation

fibrina, fibril; fibrin

fibrinógeno, fibrinogen

fibrocístico, *adj*, fibrocystic

fibroide, *m, adj*, fibroid

fibroideo, *adj*, fibroid

fibroma, *m*, fibroma; fibrous tumor; **~s en el útero** polyps in the uterus

fibroquístico, *adj*, fibrocystic

fibrosis quística, *f*, cystic fibrosis

fíbula, fibula

fibular, *adj*, fibular

ficha médica, medical card

fichero, card index file

fideo, noodle

fiebre, *f*, fever; temperature; *fam, Mex*, hepatitis; ~ **abdominal** typhus fever; ~ **amarilla** black vomit; yellow fever; ~ **continua** continued fever; ~ **de Colorado** Colorado tick fever; ~ **de conejo** rabbit fever; ~ **de deshidratación** dehydration fever; ~ **de la sed** *fam*, dehydration fever; ~ **de las cotorras** parrot fever; ~ **de las Montañas Rocosas** Rocky Mountain fever; tick fever; ~ **de las trincheras** trench fever; ~ **de los campamentos** epidemic typhus; ~ **de los cinco días** trench fever; ~ **de los hospitales** hospital fever; ~ **de Malta** Malta fever; ~ **de origen desconocido** F.U.O./fever of undetermined origin; ~ **de tres días** German measles; rubella; ~ **de un día** *fam*, ephemeral fever; ~ **de(l) heno** hay fever; ~ **del Mediterráneo** Mediterranean fever; ~ **del valle** coccidiodomycosis; valley fever; ~ **efímera** ephemeral fever; ~ **entérica** enteric fever; ~ **escarlatina** scarlet fever; ~ **exantemática** exanthematous fever; ~ **fugaz** *fam*, ephemeral fever; ~ **ganglionar** acute infectious adenitis fever; ~ **glandular** glandular fever; ~ **in-**

termitente intermittent fever; relapsing fever; chills and fever; ~ **manchada** spotted fever; ~ **medicamentosa** drug fever; ~ **moderada** low-grade fever; ~ **neurogénica** neurogenic fever; ~ **ondulante** Malta fever; undulant fever; ~ **palúdica** malaria; malarial fever; ~ **paratífica** paratyphoid fever; ~ **paratifoidea** enteric fever; paratyphoid fever; ~ **por mordedura de rata** rat-bite fever; ~ **producida por infección** catheter fever; ~ **puerperal** childbed fever; ~ **punticular** spotted fever; ~ **purpúrea (de las Montañas Rocosas)** spotted fever; ~ **recurrente** relapsing fever; ~ **remitente** remittent fever; ~ **reumática** rheumatic fever; ~ **reumática (aguda)** (acute) articular rheumatism; ~ **roja** dengue fever; ~ **rompehuesos** breakbone fever; dengue; dengue fever; three-day fever; ~ **telúrica** paludism; ~ **térmica** heat apoplexy; heat stroke; thermic fever; ~ **tifoidea** enteric fever; typhoid fever; ~ **tra(n)smitida por garrapatas** Colorado tick fever; ~ **tropical** yellow fever

figura, figure

fijación, *f*, fixation; ~ **obsesiva** obsessive fixation

fijador, *m, adj*, fixative

fijar, to fix; to determine; **~se (en)** to notice; to pay attention; **~se en (+ infinitive)** to be intent on (+ *gerundio*); ~ **la hora de** to schedule (*citas, etc.*); ~ **la mirada** to stare

fila, line (*de gente esperando*)

filamento, filament; strand; thread

filamentoso, *adj*, threadlike

filerazo[1], fix[2] (*una inyección intravenosa de drogas*)

filerearse[1], to bang[2]; to fix[2] (*inyectar drogas*); to inject oneself with drugs; to hit up[2]

filero[1], nail[2] (*aguja para inyectar drogas narcóticas*); needle[2]; spike[2] (*una aguja hipodérmica*)
filete, *m*, crown of tooth
filmar, to film
filo, edge; ~ **cortante** cutting edge
filorazo, *Chicano*, knife wound
filtración, *f*, filtration
filtrado, filtrate; *adj*, filtered
filtrar, to filter; to filtrate
filtro, filter; ~ **intermitente de arena** intermittent sand filter; ~ **lento de arena** slow sand filter; ~ **percolador** percolating filter; ~ **por escurrimiento** trickling filter; ~ **solar** sunscreen
fin, *m*, end; goal; ~ **de semana** weekend
financiero, *adj*, financial
fingimiento, pretense (*simulación*); simulation
fingir, to make believe; to pretend (*simular*); ~**se** to pretend to be; ~**se enfermo** to malinger
firma, signature
firmar, to sign
firme, *adj*, hard (*músculo*)
física, physics
físicamente, *adv*, physically
fisicista, *m/f*, physicist
físico, build; *adj*, physical
fisicoculturista, *m/f*, bodybuilder
fisiología, physiology
fisiológico, *adj*, physiological
fisiólogo, physiologist
fisión, *f*, fission; ~ **binaria** binary fission; ~ **nuclear** nuclear fission
fisioterapeuta, *m/f*, physiotherapist
fisioterapia, physical therapy; physiotherapy
fisioterapista, *m/f*, physiotherapist
fístula, fistula; ~ **ciega** blind fistula; ~ **congénita de la oreja** ear pit; ~ **rectovaginal** rectovaginal fistula; ~ **urinaria** urinary fistula
fisura, crack (*astilla*); fissure; hairline fracture; ~ **auricular** auricular fissure
fitoca[1], marijuana

flac(c)idez, *f*, flabbiness; limpness
flác(c)ido, *adj*, flabby; flaccid; floppy; lax (*carne*); limp
flaco, *adj*, emaciated; gaunt; thin; lank (*seco*); lean (*persona*); skinny; slender
flacura, lankiness (*delgadez*)
flagelación, *f*, flagellation
flagelados, flagellate protozoa
flanela, flannel
flaquear, to sag (*esfuerzos*); ~**le las piernas a alguien** to quake at the knees
flaqueza, thinness (*delgadez de una persona*)
flato, flatus
flatulencia, flatulence
flauta[1], marijuana
flebitis, *f*, phlebitis; thrombophlebitis
flebografía, phlebography; venogram; venography
flebograma, *m*, phlebogram; venogram
flebotomista, *m/f*, phlebotomist
flebótomo, sandfly fever; three-day fever
flema, mucus; phlegm; sputum
flemón, *m*, abscess; boil; ~ **(dentario)** gumboil
flexible, *adj*, flexible; limber (*una cosa*)
flexión, *f*, flexion
flexura, back; bend; curve; fold; ~ **de la pierna** back of the knee; bend of the knee; ~ **del brazo** bend of the arm
flictena, blister
flojera, *fam*, fatigue (*cansancio*)
flojo, *adj*, flabby; floppy (*flácido*); lax (*entrañas*); lax (*no estirado*); mild (*comida, bebida*); slack (*inactivo*)
flor, *f*, flower; ~ **de Juana**[1] marijuana; ~ **de la vida** prime
flores blancas, *fam*, white discharge
florido, *adj*, florid; full-blown (*refiriendo al síntoma*)

flotante, *adj*, floating
fluctuación, *f*, fluctuation; vacillation
fluctuar, to fluctuate; to vacillate
fluido, *m*, *adj*, fluid
fluir, to flow; to stream (*líquido*)
flujo, discharge (*fluido*); efflux; flow; lochia; ~ **blanco** white discharge; ~ **de sangre** bleeding; ~ **de sangre por la vagina inesperadamente** breakthrough bleeding; ~ **menstrual** menstrual flow; ~ **plasmático renal** renal plasma flow; ~ **plasmático renal efectivo** ERPF/effective renal plasma flow; ~ **purulento** pus; ~ **retrógrado** backflow; reflux; ~ **retrógrado pielovenoso** pyelovenous backflow; ~ **sanguíneo** *form*, blood flow; ~ **sanguíneo renal** renal blood flow; ~ **vaginal** vaginal discharge; ~ **vaginal blancuzco** leukorrhea
flúor, *m*, fluorine
fluoración, *f*, fluoridation
fluorescente, *adj*, fluorescent
fluoridación, *f*, fluoridation
fluoroscopia, fluoroscopy
fluoroscopio, fluoroscope
fluorosis dental, *f*, mottled enamel
fluoruro, fluoride
flúter, *m*, flutter *Card*
flux, *m*, *Ven*, *Carib*, suit
fobia, phobia
foco, focus (*pl*, *foci*); ~ **de la infección** focus of infection
fofo, *adj*, limp (*blando*)
fogajes, *m*, *PR*, hot flashes (*de la menopausia*)
foliculitis, *f*, folliculitis
folículo, follicle; ~ **de De Graaf** grafian follicle; ~ **ovárico** ovarian follicle; ~ **piloso** hair follicle
folleto, booklet; pamphlet
fomentación, *f*, fomentation
fomento, foment; ~**s de agua caliente** hot wet compress
fondillo, *Cu*, buttock

fondo, fundus; ~**s públicos** public funds; ~ **del ojo** eyeground; ~ **oscuro** dark field
fondongo, *slang*, buttock
fonendoscopio, stethoscope
foniatría, speech therapy
fontanela, fontanelle; ~ **caída** *ethn*, fallen fontanel
foramen, *m*, foramen
fórceps, *m*, forceps *Obst*
forense, *adj*, forensic
forma, form (*apariencia*, *condición*); shape; ~ **de los parásitos en heces** form of parasite in feces; ~ **de masaje en dirección de la corriente venosa** effleurage; ~ **facial** face form *Dent*; ~ **oclusal** occlusal form
formación, *f*, formation; training (*educación*); ~ **obrera** workers' training; ~ **profesional** professional training; vocational training
formaldehido, formaldehyde
formar, to form; to fashion; ~ **capas** to layer; ~ **costra** to cake; ~ **un enlace con** to bond; ~**se ampollas** to blister
fórmula, formula; ~ **dental** dental formula; ~ **empírica** empirical formula; ~ **hemática** blood formula; differential blood count; ~ **leucocitaria** differential leukocyte count; ~ **química** chemical formula
formulario, form (*documento*)
fornicar, *form*, to fornicate
fornido, *adj*, able-bodied
fórnix, *m*, fornix
forro, jacket (*de un disco, libro, etc.*); lining; *vulg*, *Arg*, condom; rubber (*anticonceptivo*)
fortalecer, to build up (*dar fortaleza*); to fortify
fortificante, *adj*, fortifying
fortificar, to fortify
fortuito, *adj*, chance; fortuitous
forúnculo, *var*, boil; ~ **oriental** Yemen ulcer

forzado, *adj*, sickly (*sonrisa*); strained (*risa, voz*)

forzar (ue), to force; to strain (*risa, voz*)

fosa, fossa (*pl, fossae*); recess *Anat*; socket (*glena*); ~ **cubital** bend of the elbow; ~ **lumbar** loin; ~ **nasal** nasal cavity; nostril; ~ **pequeña** fovea

fosfato, phosphate

fósforo, match; phosphorus

fosita, fovea

fotografía, photography

fotosensible, *adj*, photosensitive

fototerapia, light therapy

fóvea, *form*, fovea; ~ **central** fovea centralis; ~ **centralis** macula lutea

fracasar, to fail

fracaso, failure

fractura, break *Ortho*; fracture; rupture (*hueso*); ~ **abierta** compound fracture; open fracture; ~ **cerrada** closed fracture; ~ **completa** complete fracture; ~ **complicada** compound fracture; complicated fracture; ~ **compuesta** compound fracture; ~ **con hundimiento** depressed fracture; ~ **con impacto** impacted fracture; ~ **conminuta** comminuted fracture; ~ **del cráneo** skull fracture; ~ **desviada** depressed fracture; ~ **empotrada** impacted fracture; ~ **en mariposa** butterfly fracture; ~ **en ojal** buttonhole fracture; ~ **en rama verde** green stick fracture; ~ **en tallo verde** green stick fracture; ~ **espiral** spiral fracture; ~ **espiroidea** spiral fracture; ~ **espontánea** spontaneous fracture; ~ **impactada** impacted fracture; ~ **incompleta** incomplete fracture; ~ **lineal** linear fracture; ~ **maleolar** ankle fracture; ~ **mayor** serious fracture; ~ **múltiple** multiple fracture; ~ **oblicua** oblique fractura; ~ **patológica** pathologic fracture; ~ **perforante** perforating fracture; ~ **por arrancamiento** avulsion fracture; ~ **por compresión** compression fracture; ~ **por esfuerzo** stress fracture; ~ **por torsión** torsion fracture; ~ **simple** simple fracture; ~ **supracondílea** supracondylar fracture; ~ **transcondílea** transcondylar fracture; ~ **y luxación** dislocation fracture

fracturar(se), to break *Ortho*; to fracture

frágil, *adj*, brittle; delicate; fragile; frail

fragilidad, *f*, fragility; ~ **de la sangre** fragility of the blood; ~ **de los huesos** hereditary fragility of bone

fragmentación, *f*, fragmentation; ~ **del miocardio** fragmentation of myocardium

fragmento, fragment; ~s **óseos** bone fragments

frajo[1], jive stick[2] (*cigarrillo de mariguana*); joint[2] (*cigarrillo de mariguana*); marijuana; ~ **de seda**[1] jive stick[2] (*cigarrillo de mariguana*)[1]; marijuana cigarette

frambesia, yaws

frambuesa, raspberry

francamente, *adv*, outright

franco, *adj*, outright (*directo*)

franja, fringe

frasco, bottle (*para píldoras*); flask; jar; vial

frazada, blanket

frecuencia, frequency; rate; ~ **audible** audio frequency; ~ **cardíaca** H.R./heart rate; ~ **del pulso** pulse rate; ~ **respiratoria** respiratory rate

frecuente, *adj*, frequent

frecuentemente, *adv*, frequently; often

fregar, to scrub (*quirúrgicamente*)

freír (i), to fry

frenesí, *m*, frenzy

frenético, *adj*, frantic; frenetic
frénico, *adj*, phrenic
frenillo, frenum (*de la lengua*)
frenillos, bands *Dent*; braces *Dent*
frenos, bands (*aparato para los dientes*); braces *Dent*
frente, *f*, brow; forehead; ~ **a** *prep*, opposite
fresa, strawberry; bur *Dent*; drill *Dent*; ~ **dental** dental drill
fresada, blanket
fresco, *adj*, cool; fresh
fricción, *f*, friction; rub
frigidez, *f*, frigidity
frígido, *adj*, frigid
frío, *adj*, cold (*temperatura*); *m*, *slang*, *Mex*, mucus; *m*, *SpAm*, malaria; ~ **de la matriz** female sterility; ~ **en la matriz** cold in the womb (*una causa de la esterilidad*); frigidity
frito, *adj*, fried
friza, *PR*, *DR*, blanket
frontal, *adj*, frontal
frotación, *f*, rub
frotar, to grate; to rub; ~**se** to rub
frotis, *m*, smear; ~ **de Papanicolaou** Pap smear; ~ **sanguíneo** blood smear
fructosa, fructose
fruncir el ceño, to frown
frustración, *f*, frustration
fruta, fruit; ~ **cítrica** citrus fruit
fuego, fire; light (*llama*); *fam*, fever blister; ~**s** *pl*, *fam*, herpes; ~ **de San Antonio** St. Anthony's fire; erysipela; ~ **en la boca** cold sore; ~ **en los labios** cold sore
fuente, *f*, source; fountain; *fam*, bag of waters; ~ **de agua potable** drinking fountain; ~ **de energía** source of energy; ~ **luminosa** light source; ~ **para beber** drinking fountain
fuera de, *prep*, outside of; ~ **de lugar**

out of place; ~ **del alcance de niños** out of reach of children
fuerte, *adj*, great (*dolor*); high (*fiebre*); husky; severe; strong (*olor*, *bebida*); tough; vivid (*impresión*)
fuerza, force; strength; ~ **catabólica** catabolic force; ~ **de cara** cheek (*audacia*); chutzpah; ~ **de puños** elbow grease; ~ **de voluntad** willpower; ~ **extra** extra strength; ~ **interior** inner strength; ~ **radical** reserve force; ~ **vital** life force; vital force
fuga, leak (*de gas o un líquido*)
fugaz, *adj*, fleeting; fugitive
fumar, to smoke; ~ **menos** to cut down on smoking
fumigación, *f*, fumigation
fumigar, to fumigate
función, *f*, function; ~**es vitales** vital functions
funcional, functional
funcionamiento, performance; ~ **defectuoso** malfunction
funcionar en vacío, to idle (*motor*, *máquina*)
funda, large shopping bag; *PR*, bag of marijuana; bag of grass; ~ **de almohada** pillowcase; ~ **de gafas** glass case
fundamental, *adj*, essential
fundillo, *Mex*, anus; buttock
funduscopio, funduscope
funeraria, funeral home
fungicida, *m*, *adj*, fungicide
furioso, *adj*, livid; mad (*enojado*)
furor, *m*, furor; fury; rage
furúnculo, *form*, boil; furuncle; *fam*, abscess
fusión, *f*, fusion; ~ **de las imágenes dobles** binocular fusion; ~ **espinal** spinal fusion
futuro, *m*, *adj*, future

---

[1] Este vocabulario es nuevo y todavía no se encuentra en el *Diccionario de la lengua española*, publicado por la Real Academia Española. Forma parte del argot o la lengua de la calle. Se supone que el género es obvio a menos que sea indicado.
[2] Forma parte del vocabulario inglés actual de los drogadictos.

G

gacho, *adj*, drooping (*oreja*)

gafas, *f*, *pl*, eyeglasses; glasses; spectacles; ~ **ahumadas** dark glasses; ~ **de sol** sun glasses/sunglasses

galería[1], (shooting) gallery[2] (*lugar para picarse con drogas o ingerirlas*)

galillo, *fam*, uvula; *PR*, voice box

gallazo[1], fix[2] (*una inyección intravenosa de drogas*)

galleta, cracker; cracker[2] (*Drug: para animales, mezclada con LSD*); ~ **blanca** soda cracker

gallo, crack (*de la voz*)

galón, *m*, gallon

galvánico, *adj*, galvanic

galvanizar, to electroplate

galvanoplastia, electroplating

gama, range (*de frecuencias, colores, etc.*)

gamaglobulina, gamma globulin

gameto, gamete

gammagrama, *m*, scan (*nuclear*)

ganancia, gain

ganar, to gain

ganas, *f*, *pl*, itch; desire; ~ **de comer** appetite; **tener** ~ **de** (+ *infinitive*), to feel like (+ *gerundio*)

gancho, clasp *Dent*; clothes hanger; hanger; hook (*ayuda para sostener o levantar una carga*); ~ **continuo** continuous clasp *Dent*

ganchudo, *adj*, hooked (*encorvado*)

ganga, *PR*, *Chicano*, gang (*pandilla*); ~[1] marijuana

ganglio, bubo; ganglion; node (*ganglio linfático*); ~**s basales** basal ganglia; ~ **cardíaco** cardiac ganglion; ~ **cervical inferior** inferior cervical ganglion; ~ **cervical medio** middle cervical ganglion; ~ **cervical superior** superior cervical ganglion; ~ **ciliar** ciliary ganglion; ~ **com-**

puesto palmar compound palmar ganglion; ~ **diafragmático** diaphragmaticum ganglion; ~ **esfenopalatino** sphenopalatine ganglion; ~ **espiral** spiral ganglion; ~ **esplácnico** splanchnic ganglion; ~ **estrellado** stellate ganglion; ~ **frénico** phrenic ganglion; ~ **geniculado** facial ganglion; ~ **inferior del vago** inferior vagus ganglion; ~ **lenticular** lenticular ganglion; ~ **linfático** lymph node; ~ **mesentérico superior** superior mesenteric ganglion; ~ **ótico** otic ganglion; ~ **petroso** petrous ganglion; ~ **submandibular** submandibular ganglion; ~ **superior del vago** superior ganglion of the vagus; ~ **trigémino** trigeminal ganglion; ~ **yugular** jugular ganglion

ganglioglioma, *m*, ganglioglioma

gangrena, gangrene; ~ **diabética** diabetic gangrene; ~ **espontánea** spontaneous gangrene; ~ **gaseosa** gas gangrene; ~ **hospitalaria** hospital gangrene; ~ **húmeda** moist gangrene; ~ **infecciosa** hot gangrene; ~ **por decúbito** bed sore; ~ **seca** dry gangrene; ~ **senil** senile gangrene

gangrenoso, *adj*, gangrenous

ganja[1], marijuana

garantizar, to guarantee

garañón, *m*, *Mex*, *slang*, stud *slang*

garfio, hook (*gancho*)

garganta, throat; ~ **inflamada** sore throat

gargao, sputum

gárgara, gargle; ~**s** gargling

gargarismo, gargle (*líquido*)

gargarizar, to gargle

garrapata, chigger flea; tick (*in-*

secto); ~ **americana del perro** American dog tick; ~ **de las costas del Pacífico** Pacific coast tick; ~ **de las Montañas Rocosas** Rocky Mountain tick; ~ **de los bovinos** cattle tick

garrote, *m*, garrot

garrotillo, croup; diphtheria; inflammation of the throat

garza, *PR*, tall woman with skinny legs

gas, *m*, gas; ~ **asfixiante** poison gas; ~ **de hulla** coal gas; ~ **de los pantanos** marsh gas; ~ **exhilarante** *m*, *slang*, gas (*óxido nitroso*); ~ **hilarante** *m*, *slang*, gas (*óxido nitroso*); laughing gas; ~ **inerte** inert gas; ~ **lacrimógeno** tear gas; ~ **natural** natural gas; ~ **oleificante** ethylene sewer gas; ~ **tóxico** poison gas; ~**es arteriales** arterial blood gas

gasa, gauze; ~ **absorbente** absorbent gauze; ~ **absorbente estéril** sterile absorbent gauze; ~ **absorbible** absorbable gauze; ~ **antiséptica** antiseptic gauze

gaseosa de jengibre, ginger ale

gasita con alcohol, alcohol pad

gasolina, gasoline

gasometría, arterial blood gas

gastado, *adj*, worn out

gastar menos en cigarrillos, to cut down on smoking

gasto, cost; expense; output; ~ **cardíaco** cardiac output; ~ **energético** energy output; ~ **urinario** urinary output; ~**s de mantenimiento** living expenses

gastralgia, heartburn

gástrico, *adj*, gastric

gastritis, *f*, gastritis

gastroduodenal, *adj*, gastroduodenal

gastroenteritis, *f*, gastroenteritis; ~ **hemorrágica** hemorrhagic gastroenteritis; ~ **infecciosa aguda** acute infectious gastroenteritis

gastroenterología, gastroenterology

gastroenterólogo, gastroenterologist

gastrointestinal, *adj*, GI/gastrointestinal

gastrología, gastrology

gastrorrea, gastrorrhea

gastroscopia, gastroscopy

gastroscopio, gastroscope

gatear, to crawl

gatillo, dental forceps; forceps *Dent*

gatito, kitten

gato[1], heroin

gaveta, drawer

gavos[1], marijuana

gaznate, *m*, gullet; windpipe; *fam*, trachea

gel, *m*, gel

gelatina, gelatin; ~ **anticonceptiva** contraceptive jelly; ~ **medicinal** medicinal gelatin

gelatinificar, to gelatinize

gelatinoso, *adj*, gelatinous

gelfoam, gelfoam

gélido, *adj*, icy

gemelo, twin; ~**s fraternos** fraternal twins; ~**s idénticos** identical twins; ~**s que no se parecen** fraternal twins

gemido, groan (*quejido*); moan (*lamento*)

gemir (i), to groan (*lamentarse*); to moan (*quejarse*)

gen, *m*, gene; ~ **dominante** dominant gene; ~ **ligado al sexo** sex-linked gene; ~ **recesivo** recessive gene

generación, *f*, generation; ~ **alternante** alternate generation; ~ **espontánea** spontaneous generation

general, *adj*, systemic

generalizar, to generalize

generar, to generate

genérico, *adj*, generic

género, gender; kind

generoso, *adj*, rich (*vino*)

genética, genetics
genético, *adj*, genetic
genetista, *m/f*, geneticist
genio, genius
genital, *adj*, genital
genitales, *m, pl*, genitalia; private parts
genitourinario, *adj*, G.U./genitourinary
geomedicina, geomedicine
gerencia de servicios médicos, management of health services
geriatra, *m/f*, geriatrician
geriatría, geriatrics; ~ **dental** dental geriatrics
geriátrico, *adj*, geriatric
germen, *m*, germ; ~ **de trigo** wheat germ
germicida, *adj*, germicidal; *m, adj*, germicide
germinación, *f*, germination
gerodoncia, gerodontics *Dent*
gerodontista, *m/f*, gerodontist *Dent*
gerontología, gerontology
gerontólogo, gerontologist
gestación, *f*, childbearing; gestation
gestacional, *adj*, gestational
gesto, gesture
giardia, giardia
gigante, *m, adj*, giant
gillette, *m, CA*, razorblade
gimnasia, gymnastics; ~ **ocular** ocular gymnastics; ~ **vocal** vocal gymnastics
ginebra, gin
ginecología, gynecology
ginecológico, *adj*, gynecologic; gynecological
ginecólogo, gynecologist
ginger ale, *m*, ginger ale
gingiva, gingiva *Dent*; ~ **alveolar** alveolar gingiva; ~ **bucal** buccal gingiva; ~ **labial** labial gingiva; ~ **lingual** lingual gingiva
gingival, *adj*, gingival *Dent*
gingivitis, *f*, gingivitis; ~ **marginal supurativa** suppurative marginal gingivitis; ~ **ulcerosa necrosante**

aguda acute necrotizing ulcerative gingivitis
gingivolabial, *adj*, gingivolabial *Dent*
gira[1], *PR*, trip on drugs
gis[1], LSD
glacial, *adj*, glacial
glacis[1], *m*, cocaine
glande, *m*, glans (*pene*)
glándula, gland; ~ **accesoria** accessory gland; ~ **adrenal** adrenal gland; ~ **bucal** buccal gland; ~ **carotídea** carotid gland; ~ **carótidea** carotid gland; ~ **de Cowper** Cowper's gland; ~ **de la próstata** prostate gland; ~ **de secreción interna** ductless gland; ~**s de secreción interna** endocrine system; ~ **duodenal** duodenal gland; ~ **endocrina** ductless gland; endocrine gland; ~ **excretora** excretory gland; ~ **excretoria** excretory gland; ~ **inflamada** sore gland; ~ **intestinal** intestinal gland; ~ **lagrimal** lacrimal gland; tear gland; ~ **linfática** lymph gland; ~ **mamaria** mammary gland; ~ **nasal** nasal gland; ~ **paratiroide** parathyroid gland; ~ **paratiroides** parathyroid gland; ~ **parótida** parotid gland; ~ **parotídea** parotid gland; ~ **pineal** pineal gland; ~ **pituitaria** pituitary; pituitary gland; ~ **prostática** prostate gland; ~ **salival** salivary gland; ~ **sebácea** sebaceous gland; ~ **sublingual** sublingual gland; ~ **submandibular** submandibular gland; ~ **submaxilar** submaxillary gland; ~ **sudorípara** sweat gland; ~ **suprarrenal** adrenal gland; ~ **timo** thymus gland; ~ **tiroide** thyroid gland; ~ **tiroidea** thyroid gland; ~ **tiroides** thyroid gland
glandular, *adj*, glandular
glaucoma, *m*, glaucoma
glicemia, *form*, blood sugar
glicerina, glycerine

glicerol, *m*, glycerine; glycerol
glicina, glycine
glicógeno, glycogen
glicol, *m*, glycol
globito, *slang*, rubber (*profiláctico*)
globo, globe; light bulb; sphere; ~ **del ojo** eyeball; ~ **ocular** ball of eye; eyeball; ~[1] *slang*, barbiturate; balloon[2] (*de heroína*)
globulina, globulin; ~ **gamma** gamma globulin
globulino, plaque
glóbulo, blood cell; corpuscle; ~ **blanco** white blood cell; white blood corpuscle; ~ **blanco de la sangre** leukocyte; white blood cell; ~ **rojo** erythrocyte; red blood cell; red blood corpuscle
glosopeda, foot and mouth disease
glotis, *f*, glottis
glucagón, *m*, glucagon
glucatonia, glucatonia
glucemia, *form*, blood sugar; ~ **en ayunas** fasting blood sugar
glucocinético, *adj*, glucokinetic
glucogenasa, glycogenase
glucógeno, glycogen; ~ **hepático** hepatic glycogen; ~ **tisular** tissue glycogen
glucólisis, *f*, glycolysis
glucometabólico, *adj*, glycometabolic
gluconato de calcio, calcium gluconate
glucoproteína, *m/f*, glycoprotein
glucosa, dextrose; glucose; grape sugar; ~ **en ayunas** fasting glucose; **prueba de tolerancia a la** ~ glucose tolerance test
glucósido, glucoside; glycoside; ~ **cardíaco** cardiac glycoside
glucosina, glucosin
glucosuria, glycosuria; ~ **adrenalínica** epinephrine glycosuria; ~ **alimentaria** alimentary glycosuria; ~ **digestiva** digestive glycosuria; ~ **emocional** emotional glycosuria; ~ **hipofisaria** pituitary glycosuria; ~ **no diabética** non-diabetic glycosuria; ~ **renal** renal glycosuria; ~ **tóxica** toxic glycosuria

glufo[1], glue sniffer[2]; ~[1] *adj*, high from glue sniffing
glutamato monosódico, monosodium glutamate/MSG
glutamina, glutamine
glúteo, buttock; gluteal region
glutina, glutin
GNO/garganta, nariz, y oídos, ENT/ear, nose, and throat
gobierno, government
golden[1], marijuana
golosinas, *f*, *pl*, sweets
golpe, *m*, beat; blow; crack; sock (*puñetazo*); stroke (*pegada*); *fam*, concussion; trauma; ~ **de calor** heat apoplexy; heat stroke; ~ **de sol** sun stroke; ~ **en la nuca** whiplash; ~ **torácico** *m*, precordial thump; ~[1] heroin
golpear, to beat (*dar con el puño*); to hit (*pegar*); to knock (*dar un golpe*); to slap (*abofetear*); ~ **ligeramente** to dab; ~**se** to hit oneself
golpeteo, tap
golpiza, assault; beating
goma, elastic band; bubblegum; glue; gum; *slang*, condom; rubber (*contraceptivo*); ~[1] *slang*, opium; heroin
gomitar, *fam*, to throw up; to vomit
gónada, gonad
gonadal, *adj*, gonadal
gonadocinético, *adj*, gonadokinetic
gonadotropina, gonadotropin; ~ **coriónica** chorionic gonadotropin; ~ **coriónica humana** human chorionic gonadotropin/HCG; ~ **hipofisaria** pituitary gonadotropin
gongolí, *m*, *PR*, (*syn para gongulén*) insect (*tipo de insecto*)
gongulén, *m*, *PR*, (*syn para gongolí*) insect (*tipo de insecto*)
gonococo, gonococcus (*pl*, *gonococci*)

gonorrea, clap *vulg*, (*enfermedad venérea*); gonorrhea
gonorreico, *adj*, gonorrheal
gordo, *adj*, fat (*obeso*)
gordura, fat (*obesidad*); obesity
gorgotear, to gurgle
gorgoteo, gurgling
gorra[1], cap[2] (*cápsula*); ~[1] heroin capsule; ~s **amarillas**[1] nebbis[2]
gorro, cap (*que cubre la cabeza*); ~ **cervical** cervical cap (*contraceptivo*)
gota, drip; drop *Med* (*de sangre, sudor, agua, etc.*); gout; *slang*, gonorrhea; ~ **a gota** drip by drip; ~ **a gota intravenosa** drip intravenous; ~ **articular** articular gout (*ataca a las articulaciones*); ~ **asténica** chronic rheumatism; ~ **coral** epilepsy; ~ **de los pobres** poor man's gout; ~s **de polio** oral vaccine (*vacuna de Sabin*); ~ **latente** masked gout; ~ **metastática** misplaced gout; ~s **nasales** nose drops; ~s **oftalmológicas** eye drops; ~s **óticas** ear drops; ~ **para la tos** cough drop; ~s **para polio** Sabin's oral polio vaccine; ~ **retrógrada** misplaced gout; ~ **retropulsa** misplaced gout; retrocedent gout
goteador, *m*, eyedropper (*un cuentagotas*)
gotear, to dribble (*caer gota a gota*); to drip; to drop (*echar gota a gota*)
goteo, drip (*caída de gotas*); ~ **nasal** nasal drip
gotera, leak (*en un techo*)
gotero, drip apparatus; ~ (*para los ojos*) *SpAm*, eyedropper (*cuentagotas*)
gotita, droplet
gotoso, *adj*, gouty
grabar, to record (*en cintas, discos*)
gracias, thank you
gracioso, *adj*, funny
gradiente, *m*, gradient; ~ **auriculoventricular** atrioventricular gradient; ~ **mitral** mitral

gradient; ~ **ventricular** ventricular gradient
grado, degree; ~ **de toxicidad** toxicity rating; ~ **de validez** validity
graduado, *adj*, graduate; *adj*, graduated
gradual, *adj*, gradual
graduar, to calibrate (*termómetro*)
gráfica, chart; graph
gráfico, graph; *adj*, vivid (*descripción*); ~ **de la temperatura** temperature chart
grafito, graphite
grafospasmo, graphospasm (*calambres de escritor*)
gragea, sugar-coated pill
gramnegativo, *adj*, gram-negative
gramo, gram; ~[1] packet of heroin
grampositivo, *adj*, gram-positive
gran mal, *m*, grand mal; major epilepsy
grande, *adj*, big; large
granizo, cataract
grano, grain; skin lesion; pustule; sore (*llaga*); open skin wound; wheal; whitehead; chancre; venereal lesion; *fam*, abscess; ~s *pl*, *fam*, hives; ~ **de la cara** pimple; ~ **enterrado** boil; furuncle
granuja, *slang*, measles
granulación, *f*, granulation
granular, *adj*, grainy; granular
gránulo, granule; ~ **basófilo** basophil granule; ~ **eosinófilo** eosinophil granule; ~ **neutrófilo** neutrophil granule
granulocito, granulocyte
granulocitosis, *f*, granulocytosis
granuloma, *m*, granuloma; ~ **benigno de tiroides** benign granuloma of thyroid; ~ **infeccioso** infectious granuloma; ~ **lipoideo** lipoid granuloma; ~ **ulcerativo de los genitales** ulcerating granuloma of the pudenda
granulomatosis, *f*, granulomatosis; ~ **lipoide** lipoid granulomatosis; ~ **maligna** malignant granulomatosis

granulomatoso, *adj*, granulomatous
grapa, clip; staple
grapadora, stapler
grasa, fat (*cuerpo graso*); grease
(*materia grasienta*); ~ **en las venas** fat in the veins; *fam*, cholesterol; **~s de animal** animal fats; **~s saturadas** saturated fats; **~s**[1] LSD
grasiento, *adj*, oily
grasoso, *adj*, fatty; greasy
grass[1], marijuana
gratificación, *f*, gratification
gratis, *adj*, free (*que no cuesta nada*)
grave, *adj*, acute (*critical*); grave; seriously ill; nasty (*accidente*); serious (*enfermedad, herida, situación*); earnest
gravedad, *f*, gravity; ~ **específica** specific gravity
grávida, *adj*, gravida; pregnant
gravidez, *f*, gestation; gravidity; pregnancy
gravídico, *adj*, gravidic
GRD/grupo relacionado diagnósticamente, *m*, DRG/ diagnostically related group
greña, shock of hair; **~s** *fam*, hair
griefo[1], marijuana
grieta, crack (*fisura*); fissure; split (*en la piel*); ~ **del pezón** nipple crack; cracked nipple; **~s en el paladar** cleft palate; **~s radiales** radial cracks
grifa[1], Acapulco gold[2] (*mariguana*); marijuana
grifear[1], to smoke marijuana
grifo[1], Afro; Acapulco gold[2] (*mariguana*); marijuana; marijuana user
grilla[1], marijuana
gripa, flu; grippe; influenza
gripe, *f*, flu; grippe; influenza; ~ **asiática** Asiatic flu
gris, *adj*, gray/grey
gritar, to cry (*de dolor, sorpresa, etc.*); to scream; to yell; ~ **de dolor** to scream with pain

grito, cry (*de dolor, sorpresa, etc.*); scream; yell; ~ **de dolor** cry of pain
grosero, *adj*, gross (*descortés; vulgar*); rough (*carácter, lenguaje*)
grosor, *m*, thickness (*dimensión; volumen*)
gruesa, *f*, gross (*doce docenas*); *adj*, *fam*, pregnant
grueso, *adj*, coarse; fat (*obeso*); gross (*espeso*); thick (*dimensión*)
gruñido, grunt (*sonido*)
gruñir, to gnarl; to groan (*refunfuñar*); to growl (*un perro*)
grupo, group; unit; plant; set; ~ **dental** dentist's operating equipment; ~ **ejecutivo** executive group; ~ **médico** medical group; ~ **sanguíneo** blood group; blood type *form*
guábara, *PR*, freshwater shrimp
guacho, *adj*, *esp. Chi, Perú, Ríopl*, homeless (*persona*); orphaned; *Chi, Perú, Ríopl*, abandoned child; homeless child; illegitimate child
guagua, *m/f*, *Chi, Ec, Perú*, baby (*infante*); *Bol, Arg, Ur, PR*, kid; *f*, *PR*, bus
guaguana, *slang*, scabies
guama, *Col, Ven*, calamity; disaster; misfortune
guante, *m*, glove; **~s de goma** *pl*, rubber gloves; **~s estériles** sterile gloves
guantón, *m*, *SpAm*, blow; hit; slap
guapo, *adj*, handsome
guarapear(se), *RD*, to drink; to get drunk
guardar, to hold (*tener*); to keep; to save (*reservar para más tarde*); to store; ~ **cama** to stay in bed; to keep to one's bed; to be laid up
guardería, day care center; nursery; ~ **infantil** day-care center; day nursery; nursery
guardia nocturna, night watch
guardián, guardian

guares, *m*, *pl*, twins
guargüero, *SpAm*, throat; throttle *Anat*
guari, *m*, *Chi*, throat; throttle *Anat*
guasana, gnat
guata, padding *Surg*; wad; *Arg*, *Chi*, *Perú*, belly; stomach; paunch; **echar ~** to get fat
guato[1], marijuana
guatón, *adj*, *Arg*, *Chi*, *Perú*, fat; paunchy; pot-bellied
guayaba, *SpAm*, guava; *Ec*, ankle; **~s** *CR*, (protruding) eyes
guayabo, *Col*, grief; sorrow; *Col*, *fam*, hangover
guayacol, *m*, guaiacol
guayao, *adj*, *PR*, intoxicated
guayar(se)[1], to get drunk; to get zonked; **~(se)** *PR*, to tie one on (*emborracharse*)
gubia, gouge
güegüecho, *CA*, *Mex*, goiter; *adj*, *CA*, *Mex*, suffering from a goiter
güelegüele, *m/f*, *PR*, idler

güelepega[1], *PR*, glue sniffer[2]
güera[1], marijuana
güero, *adj*, *Mex*, *CA*, blond; fair (*tez*)
guerra nuclear, nuclear war
gueto, *PR*, *Chicano*, ghetto
guía, guidance; guide
guijón, *m*, cavity *Dent*
guillao, *adj*, *PR*, stingy
güina, *Mex*, chigger flea
guineo, *PR*, banana
guiño, eye-wink; winking
guisado, stew
guisante, *m*, pea
gurbia, *PR*, switchblade knife
gusano, maggot; worm; **~ tableado** solium (*tenia*)
gustarle a uno, to like (*caerle bien*)
gustativo, *adj*, taste
gustatorio, *adj*, gustatory
gustillo, aftertaste
gusto, taste; *slang*, scabies
gutapercha, gutta-percha
gutural, *adj*, throaty

[1] Este vocabulario es nuevo y todavía no se encuentra en el *Diccionario de la lengua española*, publicado por la Real Academia Española. Forma parte del argot o la lengua de la calle. Se supone que el género es obvio a menos que sea indicado.
[2] Forma parte del vocabulario inglés actual de los drogadictos.

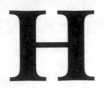

H

H[1], *f,* heroin

haba, bean

habanita[1], marijuana

haber, to have *aux;* **~ perdido el juicio** to be out of one's mind; **~se picado** *adj,* to be in a huff

hábil, *adj,* experienced

habilidad, *f,* management (*destreza*)

hábito, (drug) addiction; habit

habituación, *f,* habit

habituamiento a las drogas, drug addiction

hablar, to speak; **~ con voz gangosa** to nasalize; **~ inglés con soltura** to be fluent in English; **~ español con soltura** to speak Spanish fluently; **~ por señas** to sign (*para los sordos*); **~ un español bueno** to speak fluent Spanish

habón, *m,* wheal

hacer, to do; to make; to pack (*una maleta, etc.*); **~se** (+ *noun of profession*) to become (*alguna profesión*); **~(se)a la glu(fa)**[1] to sniff glue[2]; **~se abortar** have an abortion; **~ adelgazar** to reduce (*peso*); **~ agua** *Chicano,* to urinate; **~ bajar por fuerza** to bear down; **~ buche** *fam,* to demonstrate annoyance; **~ buches (de sal)** *fam,* to gargle; **~ caca** *slang, juv,* to have a bowel movement; *vulg,* to move the bowels; **~ calentamiento** to warm up (*antes de hacer ejercicios*); **~ calor** to be hot (*clima*); **~ caso omiso de** to deliberately pass over; to fail to mention; to override; **~ certificación** to warrant's vote to make a date; **~ cola** to queue up; **~ correr líquido** to run (*un líquido*); **~ cosquillas** to tickle; **~ daño** to damage; to hurt (*doler*);

to injure; **~se daño** to harm oneself; to get hurt; **~ del baño** *Mex, fam,* to have a bowel movement; **~se demasiado grande para** to outgrow (*la ropa*); **~ ejercicio** to work out; **~ ejercicios (moderado)(con)** to exercise (moderately)(*el cuerpo*); **~ errores** to make mistakes; **~ eructar** to burp (*un bebé*); **~ esfuerzos** to exert oneself; **~ esfuerzos para respirar** to gasp for air; **~ frente con** to cope with; **~ frío** to be cold (*clima*); **~ gárgaras** to gargle; **~ hervir** to boil (*agua*); **~ madurar un absceso** to draw an abscess; **~ más ancho** to widen; **~se más grande** to get larger; **~se moretones** to bruise; **~ olvidar** to outlive (*sobrevivir*); **~ padecer hambre** to famish; **~ (la) pipi/pipí** *slang, juv,* to pee *slang;* to urinate; **~ popó** *slang, juv,* to have a bowel movement; **~ práctica de clínica** to walk the wards; **~ preguntas** to ask (*preguntar*); **~ provecho** to be beneficial; **~ prueba(s) cruzada(s)** to cross match; **~ pupú** *slang, juv,* to have a bowel movement; **~ que uno vuelva bruscamente a la realidad** to jolt someone back to reality; **~ una receta** to fill a prescription; **~ rechinar (los dientes)** to grind (one's teeth); **~ ruido** to make noise; **~ salir** to push out; **~ saltar las lágrimas a uno** to make s.o. cry, **~ sangrar** to draw blood; to let bleed; **~ testamento** to make one's will; **~ turno** to make an appointment; **~ un análisis** to do an analysis; **~ un diagnóstico** to diagnose; **~ un error** to miscalculate; **~ un** esfuerzo excesivo to overexert oneself; ~ un frotis to take a swab; ~ un mal to hex; ~ un puño to make a fist; ~se un seguro to take out insurance; ~ una infusión de to infuse; ~ una intervención quirúrgica to operate; ~ una mueca to grimace; ~ una pregunta to question; ~ una punción to tap; ~ una respiración profunda to take a deep breath; ~ una sangría to let bleed; ~ una transfusión to give a transfusion; to transfuse; ~ visitas to make rounds

hacia (a)dentro, *adv*, inward
hachich, *m*, hash/hashish[2]
hachis, *m*, hash/hashish[2]
halitosis, *f*, halitosis
hallar, to find
hallazgo, finding; ~ de laboratorio laboratory finding
halógeno, *m*, *adj*, halogen
halotano, halothane
halterio, dumbbell
hambre, *f*, famine; hunger; ~ hormónica hormone hunger
hambreado, *SpAm*, (*Vea hambriento.*)
hambriento, *adj*, hungry; ravenous
hambruna, *Arg*, *Col*, ravenous hunger; **tener ~** *Arg*, *Col*, to be ravenously hungry
hambrusia, *Mex*, *PR*, ravenous hunger; **tener ~** *Mex*, *PR*, to be ravenously hungry
hamburguesa, hamburger
harina, flour
haschich, *m*, hash/hashish[2]
hashi[1], marijuana
haz, *m*, knot (*de nervios*); ~ ascendente ascending tract; ~ central del timo central tract of thymus; ~ electrónico electron beam; *f*, *Anat*, face
hebilla, buckle
heces, *f*, *pl*, stool; ~ alquitranadas tarlike stools; ~ biliosas spinach stool; ~ depigmentadas clay-col-

ored stools; ~ espumosas spluttery stool; ~ fecales bowel movement; feces; ~ jabonosas soapy stool; ~ sanguinolentas bloody stool

hechicería, bewitchment; witchcraft
hechizar, to cast a spell on
hecho, *adj*, made
hedor, *m*, stink
helado, ice cream; *adj*, iced; icy
heladura, frostbite
helar (ie), to freeze
helena[1], heroin
helio, helium
hélix, *m*, helix
helminto, helminth
hemangioma, *m*, hemangioma; ~ capilar capillary hemangioma; ~ cavernoso cavernous hemangioma
hemático, *adj*, hematic
hematíe, *m*, erythrocyte; red blood cell
hematimetría, blood count
hematoblasto, hematoblast; plaque
hematócrito, hematocrit; red cell mass
hematofilia, hemophilia
hematología, hematology
hematólogo, hematologist
hematoma, *m*, hematoma; ~ aneurismático aneurysmal hematoma; ~ dural dural hematoma; ~ pélvico pelvic hematoma; ~ periorbitario black eye; ~ subdural subdural hematoma
hematuria, hematuria
hembra, female
hemeralopia, *form*, day blindness
hemicránea, migraine
hemiplejía, hemiplegia
hemisferio, hemisphere; ~ cerebral cerebral hemisphere; ~ dominante dominant hemisphere
hemocultivo, blood culture
hemodiálisis, *f*, hemodialysis
hemofilia, hemophilia; ~ esporádica sporadic hemophilia; ~ hereditaria hereditary hemophilia

hemofílico, bleeder; hemophiliac; *adj*, hemophiliac; *adj*, hemophilic
hemoglobina, hemoglobin; ~ **inactiva** inactive hemoglobin; ~ **oxigenada** oxidized hemoglobin; ~ **reducida** reduced hemoglobin
hemograma, *m*, differential count
hemólisis, *f*, hemolysis
hemolítico, *adj*, hemolytic
hemorrafilia, hemophilia
hemorragia, bleeding; exanguination; hemorrhage; hemorrhaging; ~ **arterial** arterial hemorrhage; ~ **cerebral** brain stroke; cerebral hemorrhage; ~ **de disrupción** *fam*, breakthrough bleeding; ~ **detrás de la córnea** hyphemia; ~ **espontánea** essential hemorrhage; spontaneous hemorrhage; ~ **externa** external hemorrhage; ~ **funcional** functional bleeding; ~ **inesperada** breakthrough bleeding; ~ **inevitable** unavoidable hemorrhage; ~ **interna** internal bleeding; internal hemorrhage; ~ **masiva** massive hemorrhage; ~ **nasal** *form*, bloody nose; nose bleed/nosebleed; ~ **oculta** occult bleeding; concealed hemorrhage; ~ **primaria** primary hemorrhage; ~ **puerperal** postpartum hemorrhage; ~ **pulmonar** pulmonary hemorrhage; ~ **recurrente** recurring hemorrhage; ~ **renal** renal hemorrhage; ~ **secundaria** secondary hemorrhage; ~ **subaracnoidea** subarachnoid hemorrhage; ~ **uterina** flooding; ~ **vascular** (cerebrovascular) stroke; ~ **venosa** venous hemorrhage
hemorrágico, *adj*, hemorrhagic
hemorroidal, *adj*, hemorrhoidal
hemorroide(s), *f*, hemorrhoids; piles

hemostático, *m*, *adj*, hemostatic
hemóstato, *m*, *adj*, hemostat
hendidura, *form*, cleft; crevice; groove; ~ **auricular** auricular groove; ~ **de la nuca** nuchal groove; ~ **del obturador** obturator groove; ~ **del olfatorio** olfactory groove; ~ **infraorbital** infra-orbital groove; ~ **meníngea** meningeal groove; ~ **milohioidea** mylohyoid groove; ~ **nasal** nasal groove; ~ **neural** neural ridge; ~ **occipital** occipital groove; ~ **palatina** cleft palate; ~ **peroneal** peroneal groove; ~ **poplítea** popliteal groove; ~ **sigmoidea** sigmoid groove
heparina, heparin
heparinizar, to heparinize
hepático, *adj*, hepatic; liver
hepatitis, *f*, hepatitis; ~ **infecciosa** infectious hepatitis; ~ **por transfusión** transfusion hepatitis; ~ **viral** viral hepatitis
herbáceo, *adj*, herbaceous
herbario, *adj*, herbal
herbicida, *m*, herbicide
herbolario, herbalist
heredado, *adj*, inherited
hereditario, *adj*, hereditary; inherited
herencia, heredity; inheritance; ~ **cruzada** sex-linked inheritance; ~ **ligada al sexo** sex-linked inheritance
herida, cut (*llaga*); hurt; injury; wound; ~ **abierta** open wound; ~ **anfractuosa** ragged wound; ~ **de bala** bullet/gunshot wound; ~ **incisa** incised wound; ~ **lacerada** lacerated wound; ~ **mortal** death wound; lethal wound; ~ **penetrante** puncture wound; ~ **por bala** gunshot wound; ~ **por punción** puncture wound; ~ **punzante** puncture wound; ~ **superficial** flesh wound; ~

supurante suppurating wound; wound oozing pus

herido, *adj*, injured

herir (ie), to hit; to hurt; to injure; to stick (*con cuchillo, puñal, etc.*); to tear (*los tejidos*); to wound

hermana, sibling; sister

hermanastra, stepsister

hermanastro, stepbrother

hermano, brother; sibling; ~ **carnal** blood brother

herméticamente cerrado, airtight

hermético, *adj*, airtight; gastight

hernia, hernia; rupture; ~ **abdominal** abdominal hernia; ~ **adquirida** acquired hernia; ~ **cística** cystic hernia; ~ **congénita** congenital hernia; ~ **congénita del ombligo** omphalocele; ~ **crural** femoral hernia; crural hernia; ~ **del ombligo** umbilical hernia; ~ **discal** disk protrusion; ~ **enquistada** encysted hernia; ~ **epigástrica** epigastric hernia; ~ **estrangulada** strangulating hernia; ~ **femoral** femoral hernia; ~ **hiatal** hiatal hernia; hiatus hernia; ~ **inguinal** inguinal hernia; ~ **inguinal directa** direct hernia; ~ **inguinal externa** indirect hernia; ~ **inguinal indirecta** indirect hernia; ~ **inguinal interna** direct hernia; ~ **inguinal oblicua** indirect hernia; ~ **intermuscular** intermuscular hernia; ~ **intersticial** interstitial hernia; ~ **oculta** concealed hernia; ~ **por deslizamiento** sliding hernia; ~ **retrógrada** retrograde hernia; ~ **umbilical** umbilical hernia; ~ **vesical** hernia of the bladder

heroica[1], heroin

heroína, boy[2] *slang*; H[2] *slang*; heroin; junk[2] *vulg*

herpe(s), *m/f*, [*Ú.m.c.m.*], herpes; *m/f*, [*Ú.m.c.m.*], *pl*, shingles; ~(s)[4] **facial** herpes facialis; ~(s)[4] **febril** fever blister; herpes febrilis; ~(s)[4] **genital** genital herpes; herpes genitalis; ~(s)[4] **labial** fever blister; ~s[4] **labial** cold sore; ~(s)[4] **menstrual** herpes menstrualis; ~(s)[4] **simple** herpes simplex; ~(s)[4] **zoster** herpes zoster

herpético, *adj*, herpetic

herramienta[1], artillery[2] (*término de las drogas*); gun[2]

herre[1], *f*, artillery (*término de las drogas*); gun[2]

herrumbre, *f*, rust (*en metal*)

hervedera, *PR*, heartburn

hervido, *adj*, boiled

hervir (ie), to boil (*agua*); ~ **a fuego lento** to simmer; ~ **las botellas** to boil the bottles

heterosexual, *m/f*, *adj*, heterosexual

heticarse, *PR*, *RD*, to contract tuberculosis

hetiquencia, *PR*, tuberculosis

hiatal, *adj*, hiatal

hiato, hiatus; ~ **superior del esófago** esophagus thoracic inlet

hibernante, *adj*, hibernating

híbrido, *m*, *adj*, hybrid

hidátide, *f*, hydatid

hidratante, *adj*, moisturizing

hidrocarburo, hydrocarbon

hidrocefalia, hydrocephaly

hidrocéfalo, hydrocephalus; ~ **adquirido** acute hydrocephalus; ~ **agudo** acute hydrocephalus; ~ **comunicante** communicating hydrocephalus

hidrocele, *m/f*, [*Ú.m.c.m.*] hydrocele; ~ **cervical** cervical hydrocele; ~ **congénito** congenital hydrocele; ~ **enquistado** encysted hydrocele

hidrocloruro, hydrogen chloride

hidrocortisona, hydrocortisone

hidrodinámica, hydrodynamics (*ciencia*)

hidrodinámico, *adj*, hydrodynamic

hidroelectricidad, *f*, hydroelectricity

hidroeléctrico, *adj*, hydroelectric
hidrofobia, hydrophobia; rabies
hidrófobo, *m/f*, *adj*, hydrophobic
hidrogenar, to hydrogenate
hidrogenión, *m*, hydrogen ion
hidrógeno, hydrogen; ~ **pesado** double weight hydrogen
hidrólisis, *f*, hydrolysis
hidromasaje, *m*, hydromassage
hidrómetro, hydrometer
hidropesía, dropsy *Med*; ~ **anémica aguda** acute anemic dropsy; ~ **cardíaca** cardiac dropsy; ~ **cutánea** cutaneous dropsy
hidrópico, *adj*, dropsical
hidrosálpinx, tubal dropsy
hidróxido de sodio, sodium hydroxide
hidruro, hydride
hiedra, ivy; ~ **venenosa** poison ivy
hiel, *f*, bile; gall
hielo, ice; ~ **seco** dry ice
hierba, grass; herb; weed; ~[1] marijuana
hierbabuena, mint
hierbajo, weed
hierro, iron (*metal*); iron vitamin; needle (*una aguja hipodérmica*); ~ **utilizable** available iron; ~s forceps; ~[1] nail[2] (*aguja para una inyección de drogas*)
hifemia, hyphemia
hígado, liver; ~ **adiposo** fatty liver
higiene, *f*, hygiene; ~ **bucal** oral hygiene; ~ **corporal** body hygiene; ~ **mental** mental hygiene; ~ **personal** personal hygiene
higiénico, *adj*, hygienic; sanitary
higienista, *m/f*, *adj*, hygienist; ~ **dental** dental hygienist
higienizar, *SpAm*, to clean up; ~se *Arg*, to wash; to bathe
hijastro, stepson
hijastra, stepdaughter
hijo, son; ~s offspring; ~ **de leche** foster child
hilachas blancas, white spots
hilao, *slang*, *PR*, chewing tobacco

hilas, *f*, *pl*, lint
hilo, thread; ~ **dental** dental floss
himen, *m*, hymen
hincada, *Col*, *Cu*, *Perú*, *PR*, *Ven*, thrust; *Perú*, *PR*, sharp rheumatic pain
hincadura de alfiler, pinprick
hincarse, to kneel
hinchado, *adj*, bloated; distended; swelling; swollen
hinchar, to blow up (*con la boca*); to distend (*el vientre*); to inflate (*o con la boca o con una bomba*); to pump up (*con una bomba*); to swell (*el vientre, el cuerpo, la piel*); *fig*, to irritate (*irritar*); ~(se) to bloat; ~se to balloon (*inflarse*); to swell up (*el cuerpo y la piel*)
hinchazón, *f*, bump; edema; distension; lump; swelling; tumefaction; *fam*, abscess
hipar, to hiccough/hiccup
hipear, *Mex*, (*Vea hipar.*)
hiperacidez, *f*, hyperacidity
hiperactividad, *f*, hyperactivity
hiperactivo, *adj*, hyperactive
hiperbárico, *adj*, hyperbaric
hipercetonuria, *form*, hyperketonuria
hiperflexión, *f*, hyperflexion
hiperglucemia, hyperglycemia
hiperlipidemia, hyperlipidemia
hipermetabolismo, hypermetabolism
hipermétrope, *m*, *adj*, farsighted (person)
hipermetropía, farsightedness; presbyopia
hiperope, *m*, *adj*, farsighted (person)
hiperopía, farsightedness; presbyopia
hiperopsia, farsightedness; presbyopia
hiperparatiroideo, *adj*, hyperparathyroid
hiperparatiroidismo, hypeparathyroidism
hiperparotidia, hyperparotidism

hiperparotidismo, hyperparotidism
hiperpiesia, *form,* hyperpiesia
hiperplasia, hyperplasia
hiperqueratosis, *f,* hyperkeratosis
hipersensibilidad, *f,* hypersensibility
hipersensible, *adj,* hypersensitive
hipertensión, *f,* hyperpiesia; hypertension/HPN (*presión arterial alta*); ~ **arterial** high blood pressure; hypertension; ~ **benigna** benign hypertension; ~ **esencial** essential hypertension; ~ **maligna** malignant hypertension; ~ **pálida** pale hypertension; ~ **paroxística** paroxysmal hypertension; ~ **portal** portal hypertension; ~ **pulmonar** pulmonary hypertension; ~ **renal** renal hypertension; ~ **vascular** vascular hypertension
hipertenso, *adj,* hypertensive
hipertermia, hyperthermia
hipertérmico, *adj,* hyperthermal
hipertiroideo, *adj,* hyperthyroid
hipertiroidismo, hyperthyroidism; ~ **enmascarado** masked hyperthyroidism; ~ **oculto** masked hyperthyroidism
hipertonía, hypertonia
hipertónico, *adj,* hypertonic
hipertrofia, hypertrophy; ~ **compensadora** compensatory hypertrophy; ~ **complementaria** complementary hypertrophy; ~ **de adaptación** adaptive hypertrophy; ~ **prostática benigna** benign prostatic hypertrophy; ~ **simulada** simulated hypertrophy
hipertrófico, *adj,* hypertrophic
hiperventilación, *f,* hyperventilation
hipiar, *Mex,* (*Vea hipar.*)
hipnosis, *f,* hypnosis
hipnótico, *m, adj,* hypnotic
hipnotismo, hypnosis; hypnotism
hipnotista, *m/f,* hypnotist

hipnotizador, -ra, *m/f,* hypnotist; *adj,* hypnotizing
hipnotizar, to hypnotize; to mesmerize
hipo, hiccough/hiccup
hipoactividad, *f,* hypoactivity
hipoalergénico, *adj,* hypoallergenic
hipoclorito de sodio, sodium hypochlorite (*blanqueo*)
hipocondría, hypochondria
hipocondríaco/hipocondriaco, *m, adj,* hypochondriac
hipocóndrico, *m, adj,* hypochondriac
hipocrático, *adj,* hippocratic
hipodérmico, *adj,* hypodermic
hipodermis, *f,* hypodermis
hipogástrico, *adj,* hypogastric
hipogenético, *adj,* hypogenetic
hipoglicemia, hypoglycemia
hipoglicémico, *adj,* hypoglycemic
hipoglotis, *f,* hypoglottis
hipoglucemia, hypoglycemia
hipoglucémico, *adj,* hypoglycemic
hipometabolismo, hypometabolism
hipoparatiroidia, hypoparathyroidism
hipoparatiroidismo, hypoparathyroidism
hipostasis, *f,* sediment; hypostasis *form*
hipotensión arterial, *f,* low blood pressure; hypotension (*presión arterial baja*)
hipotiroideo, *adj,* hypothyroid
hipotiroidismo, hypothyroidism
hipotónico, *adj,* floppy
hipoxia, hypoxia
hipóxico, *adj,* hypoxic
hipsus, *m,* hiccough/hiccup
hirsutismo, hairiness
hirsuto, *adj,* hairy
hirviendo, *adj,* boiling; scalding
hirviente, *adj,* boiling; scalding; ebullient
hisopillo, cotton swab
hisopo de algodón, cotton swab
histamina, histamine

histerectomía, hysterectomy; ~ **abdominal** abdominal hysterectomy; ~ **cesárea** cesarean hysterectomy; ~ **radical** radical hysterectomy; ~ **subtotal** subtotal hysterectomy; ~ **vaginal** vaginal hysterectomy

histeria, hysteria; hysterics; ~ **de ansiedad** anxiety hysteria

histérico, *adj*, hysteric; hysterical

histerismo, hysteria; hysterics

histidina, histidine

histología, histology

histólogo, histologist

historia, history/Hx; ~ **clínica** case history; medical history; record (*historial médico*); ~ **de la actual enfermedad** history of present illness/HPI; ~ **de la familia** family history; ~ **familiar** family history

historial, *m*, case history; ~ **médico** record (*hoja clínica del paciente*)

hito, goal

hocico, muzzle; ~ **de tenca** mouth-of-the-womb

hogar, *m*, home; ~ **adoptivo** foster home; ~ **de ancianos** nursing home; ~ **de convalecencia** convalescent home

hoja, blade (*de un cuchillo*); ~ **clínica** chart; medical form; medical history; ~ **de afeitar** razorblade; ~**s de eucalipto** eucalyptus leaves; ~**s de poleo** pennyroyal leaves; ~**es de yerbabuena** mint leaves; ~ **verde**[1] marijuana

hojuela, scale (*escama*)

holgazán, *adj*, lazy (*ocio*)

holgazanear, to idle (*gandulear*)

hombre, *m*, man

hombrera, shoulder strap

hombro, shoulder (*persona*); ~ **doloroso de los golfistas** golfer's arm

hombruno, *adj*, mannish

homeópata, *m/f*, homeopathist; *adj*, homeopathic

homeopatía, homeopathy

homicidio, homicide

homosexual, *m/f*, *adj*, homosexual; *m*, *adj*, queer *slang*

hondo, *adj*, deep; profound; heartfelt; **con ~ pesar** with heartfelt sorrow; with deep regret

hongo, fungus (*pl*, *fungi*); mushroom; ~**s del pie** athlete's foot; ~**s**[1] magic mushrooms[2]; psilocybin

honorarios médicos, doctor's fee

hora, hour; ~**s de consulta** office hours; ~**s de oficina** office hours; ~ **de verano** daylight-saving time; ~**s de visita** visiting hours; ~**s extraordinarias** *pl*, overtime

horario, schedule; timetable

horizontal, *adj*, flat

horma, last (*de un zapato*)

hormiga, ant; ~**s** *Med*, itch; pins and needles

hormiguear, to tingle

hormigueo, prickling pain; tingle; tingling; tingling sensation

hormiguilla brava, *PR*, insect (*tipo de*)

hormón, *m*, hormone

hormona, hormone; ~ **adrenocorticotrópica** adrenocorticotropic hormone/ACTH; ~ **adrenotrópica** adrenotropic hormone/ATH; ~ **condrotrópica** chondrotropic hormone; ~ **de(l) crecimiento** chondrotropic hormone; growth hormone/GH; ~ **estimulante de las células intersticiales** interstitial cell stimulating hormone/ICSH; ~ **estimulante del folículo** follicle-stimulating hormone/FSH; ~ **estimulante del tiroides** thyroid-stimulating hormone/ TSH; ~ **folicular** follicle hormone; ~ **folículo-estimulante** follicle stimulating hormone/FSH; ~ **foliculoes-**

timulante follicle stimulating hormone/FSH; **~ liberadora de gonadotropinas** gonadotropin-releasing hormone/GnRH; **~ luteinizante** luteinizing hormone/LH; lutein-stimulating hormone/LSH; **~ masculina** male hormone; **~ ovárica** ovarian hormone; **~ paratiroidea** parathyroid hormone/PTH; **~ tiroidea** thyroid hormone

hormonal, *adj*, hormonal

horneado, *adj*, baked

horno, oven

horquilla, hairpin

horrible, *adj*, hideous

hospicio, hospital for the poor; orphanage; hospice; **~ para ancianos** nursing home

hospital, *m*, hospital; **~ comunitario** community hospital; **~ de la comunidad** community hospital; **~ del condado** county hospital; **~ para veteranos** Veteran's Administration hospital; **~ privado** private hospital; **~ (p)siquiátrico**[5] mental hospital; **~ público** public hospital

hospitalización, *f*, hospitalization

hospitalizado, *adj*, hospitalized

hoy, today

hoyito, hole (*meato*)

hoyo, *Carib, Ríopl,* dimple; **~ de la nariz** *fam,* nostril

hoyuelo, dimple

Ht/hipermetropía total, Ht/total hypermetropia

huaco, *adj, SpAm,* toothless

huato[1], marijuana

hueco, gap (*cavidad*); hole; hollow; spare time (*tiempo libre*); *adj,* deep (*voz*); empty (*vacío*); hollow (*sonido*); spongy (*esponjoso*); **~ axilar** armpit

huella, mark (*señal*); print (*del dedo, pie, etc.*); *fam,* fingerprint; **~ dactilar** fingerprint; **~ digital** fingerprint

huérfano, orphan

huesecillo, ossicle

huesillo, ossicle

hueso, bone; pit (*de una fruta*); *fam, CA, Mex,* joint; **~s** *fam,* vertebra (*pl, vertebrae*); **~ alveolar** alveolar bone; **~ coxal** hip bone; **~ de la cadera** hip bone; **~ de la rodilla** kneecap (*rótula*); **~ del cuello** *fam,* collar bone/clavicle; **~ del pecho** breastbone; **~s del tarso** tarsal bone; **~ ilíaco** hip bone; ilium; **~ malar** cheek bone/cheekbone; jugal bone; **~s metatarsianos** metatarsal bones; **~ occipital** occipital bone; **~ parietal** parietal bone; **~ quebrado** *fam,* fracture; **~ supernumerario** accessory bone; **~ temporal** temple; **~ timpánico** tympanic bone

huésped, *m*, host

huesudo, *adj, fam,* big-boned

huevecillo, small egg (*de un parásito*)

huevo, egg; *fam,* ovum (*pl, ova*); **~ duro** hard-boiled egg; **~ frito** fried egg; **~ pasado por agua** soft-boiled egg; **~ revuelto** scrambled egg; **~s** *m, pl, vulg,* testicle; **~s** *pl, vulg, common* balls *slang*

hule, *m, slang,* condom (*anticonceptivo*); rubber *slang,* (*anticonceptivo*)

humanizado, *adj*, humanized

humano, *m, adj,* human

humectación, *f*, humidification

humectador, *m*, humidifier

humedad, *f*, dampness; humidity; moisture; **~ absoluta** absolute humidity; **~ relativa** relative humidity

humedecedor, *m, adj,* humidifier

humedecer, to dampen; to humidify; to moisten; to moisturize; to wet

humedecido, *adj*, humidified

humedecimiento, humidification
húmedo, *adj*, damp; humid; moist; wet; ~ **y con mucho calor** *adj*, sticky (*clima*)
húmero, humerus
humilde, *adj*, humble
humo, fumes; smoke
humor, *m*, humor *Anat*; mood; ~ **acuoso** aqueous humor; ~ **cristalino** crystalline humor; ~ **vítreo** vitreous humor
hundido, *adj*, broken down; depressed; hollow (*ojos, pecho, mejillas*); lank (*mejillas*)
huso, spindle; ~ **olfatorio** olfactory bundle; ~**s musculares** muscle spindles
huyente, *adj*, receding (*frente*)

---

[1] Este vocabulario es nuevo y todavía no se encuentra en el *Diccionario de la lengua española*, publicado por la Real Academia Española. Forma parte del argot o la lengua de la calle. Se supone que el género es obvio a menos que sea indicado.
[2] Forma parte del vocabulario inglés actual de los drogadictos.
[4] Se usa la palabra *herpes* muchas veces como palabra plural pero con adjetivo singular.
[5] Hoy es aceptable deletrear las palabras que antes se escribían con *psi-* en español (o *psy-* en inglés) sin la *p* que es consonante silenciosa en este caso.

I

ibuprofén, *m*, ibuprofen
ictericia, *form*, jaundice; ~ **infecciosa aguda** acute febrile jaundice; infectious jaundice; ~ **obstructiva** obstructive jaundice; ~ **por suero homólogo** homologous serum jaundice; ~ **toxémica** toxic jaundice; ~ **urobilínica** urobilin jaundice
ictérico, *adj*, jaundiced
ictiol, *m*, ichthyol
idea, hunch (*presentimiento*); idea; ~ **compulsiva** compulsive idea; ~ **de referencia** referential idea; ~ **dominante** dominant idea; ~ **fija** fixed idea
ideal, *m, adj*, ideal
idéntico, *adj*, identical
identidad, *f*, identity
identificación, *f*, identification
identificar, to identify; to recognize; ~**se con** to identify with
idiocia mongólica, Down's syndrome
idioma, *m*, idiom; language
idiopatía, idiopathy
idiosincrasia, idiosyncrasy
idiosincrásico, *adj*, idiosyncratic
idiota, *m/f*, idiot
idiotez, *f*, idiocy
idioventricular, *adj*, idioventricular
ido, *adj, SpAm*, absent-minded
iglesia, church
ignorancia, ignorance; ~ **crasa** gross ignorance
ignorar, to be unaware of; to be ignorant of; to not know; *Chicano*, to ignore
ijada, flank; loin; *Med*, pain in the side; stitch
ijar, *m*, flank; loin (*del hombre*)
ilegalidad, *f*, illegality
ilegitimidad, *f*, illegitimacy
ilegítimo, *adj*, illegitimate

ileítis, *f*, ileitis
íleo, ileus
íleon, *m*, ileum
ilíaco, *adj*, iliac
ilion, *m*, ilium
iluminación, *f*, illumination
iluminarse, to light up
ilusión, *f*, delusion; illusion
imagen, (*pl*, *imágenes*) *f*, frame (*en televisión, películas*); image; ~ **acústica** acoustic image; ~ **en espejo** mirror image; ~**es hechas por resonancia magnética** *pl*, magnetic resonance imaging /MRI; ~ **invertida** inverted image; ~**es por resonancia magnética** *pl*, magnetic resonance imaging /MRI; ~ **mental** visualization; ~ **sensorial** sensory image
imaginar, to daydream; to visualize; ~**se** to imagine
imaginario, *adj*, imaginary
imán, *m*, magnet; ~ **en herradura** horseshoe magnet
imbécil, *m/f, adj*, imbecile; *Med*, feeble-minded
impacción, *f*, impaction
impaciente, *adj*, impatient
impactado, *adj*, impacted
impacto, impaction
impalpable, *adj*, impalpable
impar, *adj*, odd; uneven; unpaired
impedimento, handicap; impediment; obstruction; ~ **en el aprendizaje** learning disability
impedir (**i**), to impede; to prevent; to prohibit (*prohibir*)
imperdible, *m*, safety pin
imperfección, *f*, defect
imperfecto, *adj*, imperfect
impericia, inexperience; malpractice
imperioso, *adj*, imperative (*urgente*)

impermeable, *m*, raincoat; *slang*, rubber (*condón*)
impertinente, *adj*, impertinent
impervio, *adj*, impervious
impétigo, impetigo
ímpetu, *m*, impetus (*fuerza*)
impetuoso, *adj*, rash (*persona*)
implantación, *f*, implant
implantar(**se**), to implant
implementación, *f*, implementation
implementar, to implement
implicar, to imply
implícito, *adj*, implicit
imponer, to impose; *Mex*, to accustom
importancia, importance
importante, *adj*, important
imposibilitado, *adj*, *Med*, crippled; disabled
imposibilitar, to make impossible
impotencia, impotence
impotente, *adj*, impotent
impredecible, *adj*, *CA*, *Mex*, *PR*, not predictable
impredictible, *adj*, unpredictable
impregnar, to impregnate
impresión, *f*, impression; ~ **digital** fingerprint
imprevisible, *adj*, not predictable
imprimir, to stamp (*una marca*)
improbable, *adj*, improbable
impronosticable, *adj*, not predictable
improvisado, *adj*, scratch
imprudente, *adj*, imprudent
impudente, *adj*, impudent
impúdico, *adj*, immodest (*sin pudor*)
impudor, *m*, immodesty (*falta de pudor*)
impulsar, to impel; to pump (*sangre*)
impulsivo, *adj*, impulsive
impulso, drive (*energía*); impulse; prompting; ~ **nervioso** nervous impulse; ~ **sexual** sex drive
impureza, impurity
inactivado, *adj*, dead (*inerte*)
inactivar, to inactivate; to kill

inactividad, *f*, disuse; inactivity
inactivo, *adj*, dormant; inactive
inadaptación, *f*, maladjustment
inadaptado, *adj*, maladjusted
inadecuación, *f*, inadequacy (*insuficiencia*); unsuitability (*impropiedad*)
inadecuado, *adj*, inadequate; inappropriate; unsuitable
inanición, *f*, starvation; inanition
inanimado, *adj*, inanimate
inapropiado, *adj*, inappropriate
inarticulado, *adj*, inarticulate
incachable, *adj*, *SpAm*, useless
incandescencia, glow
incapacidad, *f*, disability *Med*; handicap; impairment; incapacity; ~ **de trabajo** *Mex*, work excuse; ~ **financiera** inability to pay; ~ **física** physical disability; ~ **mental** mental disability
incapacitado, *adj*, disabled; handicapped
incapacitante, *adj*, incapacitating
incapacitar, to cripple; ~ (**para**) to disable (*legalmente*)
incapaz, *adj*, incapable
incarceración, *f*, incarceration
incendio, fire
incesante, *adj*, never-ceasing
incesto, incest
incidencia, incidence
incidente, *m*, incident
incisión, *f*, incision; wound; ~ **en el riñón** nephrotomy
incisivo, front tooth; incisor; ~ **central** central incisor; ~ **lateral** lateral incisor; ~ *adj*, incisive
inclinación, *f*, droop (*de la cabeza*); inclination; ~ **de la pelvis** inclination of the pelvis
inclinado, *adj*, drooping (*cabeza*)
inclinar, to droop (*cabeza*); ~(**se**) to lean; ~**se** to bend down; to bend over; to lean forward; ~**se hacia atrás** to bend back
incluir, to embody; to include; to rule in
incluso, *adv*, even

incoherencia, incoherence
incoherente, *adj*, incoherent
incomodidad, *f*, discomfort (*falta de comodidad*)
incómodo, *adj*, bothersome; uncomfortable
incompatibilidad, *f*, incompatibility; ~ **fisiológica** physiologic incompatibility; ~ **química** chemical incompatibility; ~ **terapéutica** therapeutic incompatibility
incompatible, *adj*, incompatible
incompetencia, incompetence
incompetente, *adj*, incompetent
incomprensible, *adj*, incomprehensible
inconsciencia, unconsciousness
inconsciente, *adj*, unconscious
incontinencia, incontinence; ~ **de esfuerzo** stress incontinence; ~ **fecal** fecal incontinence; ~ **por rebosamiento** overflow incontinence; ~ **urinaria** urinary incontinence; ~ **urinaria durante el día** day-dribbling
incontinente, *adj*, incontinent
inconveniente, *m*, liability (*desventaja*); objection (*dificultad*)
incordio, bubo; swollen gland in groin
incorporar, ~ **(a/con/en)** embody (in); to incorporate (in, into); ~ **a uno** to help s.o. to sit up (*en la cama*); to make s.o. sit up; ~**se** to sit up; ~**se en la cama** to sit up in bed
incorrecto, *adj*, inaccurate (*inexacto*)
increíble, *adj*, incredible
incrúspido, *adj*, *Col*, *Mex*, *Nic*, awkward; clumsy
incrustación, *f*, inlay
incrustar, to encrust; to incrust
incubadora, incubator; warming crib
incumbencia, scope (*obligación de una persona*)
incurable, *adj*, incurable

indagación, *f*, inquest; inquiry
indagar, to probe
indección, *f*, *Chicano*, injection
indecente, *adj*, gross (*muy malo*)
indecisión, *f*, indecisiveness
indemne, *adj*, safe (*seguro*)
independiente, *adj*, self-reliant
indicación, *f*, gauge (*muestra*); indication
indicador, *m*, gauge; indicator
indicar, to indicate; to point to; ~ **con la mano** to motion
índice, *m*, index finger; level; rate; ~ **de alcohol en la sangre** alcohol level in the blood; ~ **de enfermedad** sickness rate; ~ **de morbilidad** morbidity rate; ~ **de mortalidad** death rate; fatality rate; mortality rate; ~ **de mortinatalidad** stillbirth rate; ~ **de natalidad** birth rate; ~ **de sedimentación** sedimentation rate; ~ **de yodo** iodine number; ~ **metabólico** metabolic rate; ~ **pélvico** pelvic index; ~[1] marijuana
indicio, sign; trace *Med*; ~ **revelador** telltale sign
indiferente, *adj*, apathetic
indigestión, *f*, dyspepsia; indigestion; ~ **ácida** acid indigestion; ~ **gástrica** gastric indigestion; ~ **grasa** fat indigestion; ~ **nerviosa** nervous indigestion
indignidad, *f*, outrage (*afrenta*)
indique, *S*/*signa*/mark
indispensable, *adj*, imperative (*necesario*)
indisponer, *Med*, to make ill; to upset; ~**se** *Med*, to become ill
indisposición, *f*, *Med*, ailment; malaise
indispuesto, *adj*, *Med*, indisposed; a little ill; **sentirse** ~ *Med*, to feel a little ill
individual, *adj*, individual
individuo, individual
índole, *f*, nature
indolente, *adj*, indolent; lazy

indoloro, *adj*, painless (*físicamente*)
indometacina, indomethacin
indulgencia, leniency
indulgente, *adj*, lenient
indurado, *adj*, hard
inercia, inertia
inerte, *adj*, dead (*falto de vivacidad, etc.*)
inervación, *f*, innervation; nerve supply
inespecífico, *adj*, nonspecific
inestabilidad, *f*, instability
inestable, *adj*, unstable; shaky (*situación, etc.*); unsteady
inexacto, *adj*, inaccurate (*impreciso*)
infancia, childhood; infancy
infante, *m/f*, infant
infantil, *adj*, baby; babyish (*aniñado*)
infarto, heart attack; infarct; infarction; ~ **anémico** anemic infarct; ~ **cardíaco/cardiaco** myocardial infarction/MI; ~ **del corazón** heart attack; ~ **del miocardio** myocardial infarction/MI; ~ **embólico** embolic infarct; ~ **esplénico** splenic infarction; ~ **hemorrágico** hemorrhagic infarct; ~ **intestinal** intestinal infarction; ~ **miocardía-co/miocardiaco** myocardial infarction/MI; ~ **miocárdico** myocardial infarct/MI; ~ **pulmonar** pulmonary infarction; ~ **renal** renal infarction
infección, *f*, infection; *fam*, sepsis; ~ **aerógena** air-borne infection; ~ **de hongos** fungus infection; ~ **de la bolsa de lágrimas** dacryocystitis; ~ **de la sangre** *euph*, syphilis; ~ **de la vejiga** cystitis; ~ **de los oídos** ear infection; ~ **de los riñones** kidney infection; ~ **de serpigo** athlete's foot; ~ **del tracto urinario** urinary tract infection; ~ **directa** contact infection; ~ **en la sangre** *fam*, septicemia; ~ **estafilocócica** staphylococcal infection; ~ **focal** focal infection; ~ **pélvica** pelvic inflammatory disease

/PID; ~ **por candida** yeast infection; ~ **respiratoria viral** VRI/viral respiratory infection; ~ **secundaria** secondary infection; ~ **vaginal causada por una clase de hongos** yeast infection; ~ **viral** viral infection; ~ **de las vías respiratorias (superiores)** (upper) respiratory tract infection /URI
infeccioso, *adj*, infectious
infectado, *adj*, infected
infectar, to infect; ~**se (de)** to become infected (with)
infecundidad, *f*, sterility
infecundo, *adj*, barren; childless; sterile
infeliz, *adj*, unhappy
inferior, *adj*, inferior; lower (*físicamente*)
infértil, *adj*, infertile
infestación, *f*, infestation
infestar, to infest
infiltrado, *m*, *adj*, infiltrate
inflado (del estómago), *adj*, bloated
inflamable, *adj*, flammable
inflamación, *f*, inflammation; soreness; ~ **aguda** acute inflammation; ~ **crónica** chronic inflammation; ~ **de la córnea y la conjuntiva** keratoconjunctivitis; ~ **de la médula del hueso** osteomyelitis; ~ **de la mucosa uterina** endometritis; ~ **de la pulpa dental** endodontitis; ~ **de la rodilla** housemaid knee; ~ **de los bofes** *Chicano*, pleurisy; ~ **de los ojos** ophthalmia (*inflamación de los ojos*); ~ **de los pulmones** bronchitis; ~ **de riñones y vejiga urinaria** nephrocystitis; ~ **del hígado** hepatitis; ~ **productiva** productive inflammation
inflamado, *adj*, angry *Med*; inflamed; sore (*doloroso*)
inflamar, *Med*, to inflame; ~**se** to become inflamed
inflamatorio, *adj*, inflammatory

inflar(se), to puff out; to swell

inflexible, *adj*, hard (*reglas*); inflexible

inflexión de las rodillas, *f*, knee-bend(ing)

influenza, flu; influenza; ~ **asiática** Asiatic flu

información, *f*, information; ~ **confidencial** privileged information

informar, to inform (*comunicar*)

informe, *m*, report

infrarrojo, *adj*, infrared

infructuoso, *adj*, unsuccessful

infusión, *f*, infusion; ~ **salina** saline infusion

infuso, infusion

ingeniería, engineering; ~ **dental** dental engineering; ~ **genética** genetic engineering

ingeniero, engineer

ingenuidad, *f*, naiveté

ingenuo, *adj*, naive

ingerido, *adj*, *Col*, *Mex*, *Ven*, ill

ingerir (**ie**), to ingest; ~[1] to take (drugs); ~ **narcóticos**[1] to scoff[2] *slang*

ingestión, *f*, ingestion; intake; ~ **calórica** caloric intake; ~ **de líquidos** fluid intake

ingle, *f*, groin; inguinal region

ingrediente, *m*, ingredient

ingresado en una institución, *adj*, institutionalized

ingresar (**en**), to admit (*al hospital*); ~ **cadáver** to be dead on arrival (*al hospital*); ~**se** to be admitted (*al hospital*)

ingreso, admission (*al hospital*); intake; ~**s** income; admitting; ~**s accesorios** fringe benefits

ingurgitado, *adj*, engorged

inhabilidad, *f*, disability; incompetence

inhalación, *f*, inhalation; ~ **de humo** smoke inhalation

inhalador, *m*, *adj*, *Med*, inhaler; ~ (*dispositivo*)[1] inhaler

inhalante, *m*, inhalant

inhalar, to breathe in; to inhale (air); ~ **cola**[1] to inhale glue[2]; to sniff glue[2]

inherente, *adj*, inherent

inhibición, *f*, inhibition

inhibidor, *m*, inhibitor

inhibirse, to feel inhibited

inhumación, *f*, interment

inhumano, *adj*, inhuman; *adj*, *Chi*, dirty; disgusting

iniciar, to initiate; to start

ininflamable, *adj*, nonflammable

injerir (**ie**), to ingest; ~[1] to take (drugs); ~ **narcóticos**[1] to scoff[2] *slang*,

injertar, to graft; to implant

injerto, graft (*la piel*); implant; *Perú*, mestizo with Chinese blood ; ~ **animal** animal graft; ~ **autoepidérmico** autodermic graft; ~ **autógeno** autoplastic graft; ~ **autoplástico** autoplastic graft; ~ **cutáneo** full-thickness graft; ~ **cutáneo parcial** split-skin graft; ~ **de espesor parcial** split-skin graft; ~ **dermoepidérmico** full-thickness graft; ~ **en malla** mesh-graft; ~ **epidérmico de la piel del mismo paciente** autodermic graft; ~ **laminar** split-skin graft; ~ **libre** free graft; ~ **óseo** bone graft; ~ **tiroideo** thyroid graft; ~ **tomado del cuerpo del propio paciente** autoplastic graft; ~ **tubular** tube graft; tunnel graft

injuriar, to abuse; to harm; to injure

inmaculado, *adj*, immaculate

inmaduro, *adj*, immature

inmediatamente, *adv*, immediately; *stat/ statim*

inmediato, *adj*, immediate; prompt

inmersión, *f*, immersion

inmigrante, *m/f*, immigrant

inmigrar, to immigrate

inminente, *adj*, imminent; impending

inmoderado, *adj*, self-indulgent

inmodestia, immodesty (*falta de modestia*)

inmodesto, *adj*, immodest (*no humilde*)

inmóvil, *adj*, immobile; motionless; still (*que no se mueve*)

inmovilidad, *f*, immobility

inmovilización, *f*, immobilization

inmovilizar, to immobilize

inmune, *adj*, immune

inmunidad, *f*, immunity; ~ **activa** active immunity; ~ **adquirida** acquired immunity; ~ **antibacteriana** antibacterial immunity; ~ **artificial** artificial immunity; ~ **congénita** congenital immunity; ~ **específica** specific immunity; ~ **pasiva** passive immunity; ~ **placentaria** intrauterine immunity; ~ **racial** species immunity

inmunización, *f*, immunization; vaccine; ~ **masiva** mass immunization

inmunizar, to immunize

inmunocarácter, *m*, immunocharacter

inmunocompetente, *adj*, immunocompetent

inmunodeficiencia, immunodeficiency

inmunodeprimido, *adj*, immunodepressed

inmunogenética, immunogenetics

inmunología, immunology

inmunológico, *adj*, immune; immunologic/immunological

inmunólogo, immunologist

inmunosupresión, *f*, immunosuppression

inmunosupresor, *m*, immunosuppressant

inmunoterapia, immunotherapy

inmunotoxina, immunotoxin

inmunotransfusión, *f*, immunotransfusion

innato, *adj*, inborn; inbred

inocente, *adj*, *euph*, mentally retarded; *adj*, *Mex*, deformed

inoculación, *f*, inoculation; vaccination; ~ **protectora** protective inoculation

inocular, to inoculate (*contra* against; *de* with)

inocuo, *adj*, harmless

inodoro, toilet; ~ **portátil** commode; *adj*, odorless

inofensivo, *adj*, harmless; inoffensive

inoperable, *adj*, inoperable

inorgánico, *adj*, inorganic

inquieto, *adj*, uneasy; upset; restless

inquietud, *f*, anxiety

inquilinismo, tenancy

inquilino, tenant

insaciable, *adj*, voracious

insanable, *adj*, incurable

insania, insanity

insecticida, *m*, *adj*, insecticide

insecto, bug

inseguridad, *f*, insecurity

inseguro, *adj*, insecure

inseminación, *f*, insemination; ~ **artificial** artificial insemination

insensato, *adj*, mad (*imprudente*)

insensibilidad, *f*, *Med*, insensibility; unconsciousness

insensibilización, *f*, insensibility; unconsciousness

insensibilizador, *m*, *adj*, *Med*, anesthetic

insensibilizar, *Med*, to anesthetize

insensible, *adj*, impervious (*a las emociones*); *adj*, *Med*, insensible; unconscious; numb (*extremidades*)

insertar, to insert

insidioso, *adj*, insidious

insignificante, *adj*, negligible

insípido, *adj*, tasteless

insolación, *f*, heat apoplexy; heat stroke; sun stroke/sunstroke

insomnio, insomnia; vigilance *Med*

inspección, *f*, inspection

inspiración, *f*, *Med*, inhalation

inspirar, to inhale; *form*, to breathe in

instalaciones de laboratorio, *f*, laboratory facilities

instalar aire acondicionado en, to air-condition

instintivo, *adj*, instinctive

instinto, drive (*energía, impulso*); instinct; ~ **de rebaño** herd instinct

institución, *f*, institution

instrucción, *f*, instruction; **instrucciones** directions; ~ **higiénica** health education

instructivo, package insert

instrumento, apparatus; ~ **afilado** sharp-edged instrument; **~s de exploración** examining instruments

insuficiencia, failure (*órgano*); inadequacy; incompetence; insufficiency; ~ **aórtica** aortic insufficiency; ~ **cardíaca/cardiaca** cardiac insufficiency; heart failure; ~ **cardíaca anterógrada** forward heart failure; ~ **cardíaca congestiva** congestive heart failure; ~ **cardíaca retrógrada** backward heart failure; ~ **cardíaca ventricular derecha** right ventricular heart failure; ~ **cardíaca ventricular izquierda** left ventricular heart failure; ~ **circulatoria aguda** acute circulatory insufficiency; ~ **coronaria** coronary insufficiency; ~ **de la válvula mitral** mitral valve insufficiency; ~ **de las válvulas cardíacas** incompetence of the cardiac valves; ~ **hepática** liver failure; hepatic insufficiency; ~ **mitral** mitral insufficiency; ~ **pancreática** pancreatic insufficiency; ~ **placentaria** placental insufficiency; ~ **pulmonar** pulmonary insufficiency; ~ **renal** kidney failure; renal failure; renal insufficiency; ~ **respiratoria** respiratory failure; ~ **vascular** vascular insufficiency; ~ **venosa** venous insufficiency

insuficiente, *adj*, insufficient

insuflación, *f*, insufflation; ~ **endotimpánica** tubal insufflation; ~ **tubárica** tubal insufflation

insulina, insulin

insulinasa, insulinase

insulínico, *adj*, insulin

insulinoshockterapia, insulin shock therapy

insultar, to offend

insulto, insult; *Chicano, Mex, Nic,* indigestion; *Arg, Ven,* fainting fit

inteligencia, intelligence; mind

inteligente, *adj*, able-minded; intelligent; smart

inteligible, *adj*, intelligible

intención, *f*, intention

intencional, *adj*, intentional

intensidad, *f*, rate; ~ **de crecimiento** growth rate; ~ **del metabolismo basal** basal metabolic rate/BMR; metabolic rate; ~ **del ruido** noise level; ~ **eléctrica** electric intensity

intensificar, to intensify

intenso, *adj*, vivid (*color*); intense

interacción, *f*, interaction

intercambiable, *adj*, exchangeable

intercambio, exchange; ~ **de gases** exchange of gases; ~ **de iones** ion exchange; ~ **iónico** ion exchange; ~ **materno-fetal** maternal-fetal exchange; ~ **respiratorio** respiratory exchange

intercostal, *adj*, intercostal

interdependencia, interdependence

interés, *m*, interest

interesado, *adj*, interested

interesar, to interest

interfase, *f*, interface

interferencia, interference; ~ **cuspídea** cuspal interference; ~ **viral** viral interference

interferir (**ie**), to interfere

interferón, *m*, interferon

interino, *adj*, acting (*provisional*)

interior, *m, adj*, inside; inner

interiorizar, *SpAm*, to look into

interlocutor, -ra, *m/f*, speaker

intermediario, *m, adj*, intermediary; intermediate

intermitente, *adj*, intermittent; spasmodic

internado, internship; *adj*, hospitalized; institutionalized

internamente, *adv*, internally

internar, to hospitalize; to house; to put in a home (*a un anciano*); ~ (en) to admit (to) (*un hospital*); to commit (to) (*un manicomio*); to confine (in) (*un hospital*); ~se to be admitted (*al hospital*)

internista, *m/f*, internist

interno, intern; ~ del hospital intern; *adj*, internal; medial; por vía interna internally

interóseo, *adj*, interosseous

interpretación, *f*, interpretation

interpretar, to interpret

intérprete, *m/f*, interpreter; translator

interrumpido, *adj*, interrupted

interrumpir, to interrupt

interrupción de coito, *f*, coitus interruptus

interruptor, *m*, interrupter; switch *Elect*

intersticial, *adj*, interstitial

intersticialoma, *m*, interstitialoma

intervalo, gap (*espacio*); interval (*tiempo*); ~ auscultatorio auscultatory gap

intervención, *f*, interference; intervention; *Med*, operation; ~ (p)siquiátrica[4] psychiatric intervention; ~ quirúrgica operation; surgical intervention

intervenir, to intervene (en; in); *Med*, to operate on

intestinal, *adj*, intestinal

intestino, intestine; ~s *pl*, entrails; guts *fam*; ~ ciego blind gut; cecum (*pl, ceca*); ~ delgado small bowel; small intestine; ~ grueso large bowel; large intestine; ~ inferior bowel; ~ mayor colon; large intestine; ~ medio midgut

intimidad, *f*, intimacy

intimidar, to intimidate

íntimo, *adj*, intimate

intolerancia, intolerance

intoxicación, *f*, intoxication; poisoning; ~ alimenticia food poisoning; ~ botulínica botulism poisoning; ~ con alimentos food poisoning; ~ de la sangre *fam*, blood poisoning; ~ de orín uremia; ~ del embarazo toxemia of pregnancy; ~ palúdica paludism; ~ por estafilococos staphylococcal poisoning; ~ por monóxido de carbono carbon monoxide poisoning; ~ por salmonellas salmonella poisoning; ~ saturnina lead poisoning

intoxicado, *adj*, drunk

intoxicante, *m*, intoxicant; poison

intoxicar, to poison

intracapsular, *adj*, intracapsular

intradérmico, intradermal

intradermorreacción, *f*, intradermoreaction

intranquilizar, to make uneasy; to worry; ~se to be anxious; to get worried

intranquilo, *adj*, anxious; uneasy; worried

intratable, *adj*, inoperable

intravascular, *adj*, intravascular

intravenoso, *adj*, intravenous

intrínseco, *adj*, intrinsic

introducir, to insert; to introduce (*algo en*)

introvertido, *m, adj*, introvert; *adj*, introverted

intubación, *f*, intubation

intubar, to intubate

intususcepción, *f*, intussusception

inundación, *f*, deluge; flooding

invadir, to invade

invaginación, *f*, invagination; ~ intestinal intestinal invagination; ~ uterina uterine invagination

invalidez, *f*, disability

inválido, *m, adj*, cripple; invalid; *adj*, disabled; weak; maimed

invasibilidad, *f*, invasiveness

invasión, *f*, invasion

invasor, *adj*, invasive

inventariar, to schedule (*inscribir*)
inventario, schedule (*documento legal*)
inversión, *f*, reversal; ~ **del sexo** sex reversal
invertebrado, *m, adj*, invertebrate
investigación, *f*, research
investigador, **-ra**, *m/f*, investigator; researcher
investigar, to investigate
invisible, *adj*, invisible; *m, Arg*, hairpin; *m, Mex*, hairnet
involuntariamente, *adv*, involuntarily
involuntario, *adj*, involuntary
inyección, *f*, jab *fam* (*de una aguja*); injection; shot; ~ **de penicilina** penicillin injection; ~ **de prueba** challenge injection; ~ **de refuerzo** booster shot; ~ **endovenosa** intravenous injection; ~ **epidural** epidural injection; **hacerse** ~ to give oneself an injection; ~ **hipodérmica** hypodermic injection; ~ **intracardíaca** intracardiac injection; ~ **intracutánea** intracutaneous injection; ~ **intradérmica** intradermic injection; ~ **intramuscular** intramuscular injection; ~ **intravenosa** intravenous injection; **ponerse** ~ to give oneself an injection; ~ **preparante** preparatory injection; ~ **secundaria** booster shot; ~ **sensibilizante** exciting injection; ~ **subcutánea** subcutaneous injection
inyectable, *adj*, injectable
inyectado, *adj*, injected; **ojos ~s (en sangre)** bloodshot eyes
inyectar, to give a shot; ~ **drogas directamente en la vena principal del brazo** to mainline[2]; ~ **narcóticos** to skin[2] *slang*; ~**(se)** to inject (oneself); ~**se** to inject oneself with drugs
ion/ión, *m*, ion; ~ **negativo** *m*, negative ion
ionización, *f*, ionization

ionizante, *adj*, ionizing
ionizar, to ionize
iontoforesis, *f*, iontophoresis
ir, to go; *Med*, to be; to get along; ~**se** to go away (*salir*); ~ **a comer jobos** *fam*, to play hooky; ~ **al baño** to go to the bathroom; ~ **al sobre** *PR*, to go to bed/to hit the sack; ~ **en auxilio de** to go to the aid of; to go to the rescue of; ~ **en contra de** to go against; ~ **más despacio** to slow down (*al caminar, etc.*); ~ **para viejo** to be getting elderly; ~ **y venir** to come and go
iridectomía, iridectomy
iris, *m*, iris (*del ojo*)
irradiación, *f*, irradiation
irradiar, to eradiate; to irradiate
irregular, *adj*, irregular; spasmodic; uneven
irresponsable, *adj*, irresponsible
irreversible, *adj*, irreversible
irrigación, *f*, douche; irrigation; lavage
irrigador, *m*, irrigator
irrigar, to irrigate
irritabilidad, *f*, irritability; ~ **nerviosa** nervous irritability; ~ **vesical** irritability of the bladder
irritable, *adj*, irritable
irritación, *f*, annoyance (*estado*); irritation
irritador, *adj*, irritating
irritante, *adj*, irritant; irritating
irritar, to anger; to irritate (*órgano, piel*); to inflame; ~**se** to become irritated
iscuria, ischuria
isla, island; ~**s de Langerhans** islands of Langerhans
islote, *m*, islet; ~**s de Langerhans** islands of Langerhans; islets of Langerhans
isómero, isomer
isométrico, *adj*, isometric
isoprenalina, isoprenaline; isoproterenol
isoproterenol, *m*, isoproterenol

isotónico, *adj*, isotonic

isotópico, *adj*, isotopic

isótopo, isotope; ~ **estable** stable isotope; ~ **indicador** tracer; ~ **radiactivo** radioactive isotope; radioisotope; radioactive tracer

isquemia, ischemia; ~ **cerebral transitoria** transient ischemic attack/TIA

isquémico, *adj*, ischemic

isquiático, *adj*, ischiatic

isquiocavernoso, *adj*, ischiocavernous

isquiocoxígeo, *adj*, ischiococcygeus

isquiofemoral, *adj*, ischiofemoral

isquion, *m*, ischium

istantino, *fam*, anus

istmo, isthmus; ~ **de la trompa de Eustaquio** isthmus of the Eustachian tube

izquierda, left hand; left side; left-hand side; **estar a la** ~ to be on the left of; **seguir** (**i**) **por la** ~ to keep (to the) left

izquierdo, *adj*, left; left-hand; left-handed

---

[1] Este vocabulario es nuevo y todavía no se encuentra en el *Diccionario de la lengua española*, publicado por la Real Academia Española. Forma parte del argot o la lengua de la calle. Se supone que el género es obvio a menos que sea indicado.

[2] Forma parte del vocabulario inglés actual de los drogadictos.

[4] Hoy es aceptable deletrear las palabras que antes se escribían con *psi-* en español (o *psy-* en inglés) sin la *p* que es consonante silenciosa en este caso.

J

jaba, *PR*, a piece of soap
jabón, *m*, soap; ~ **blando** green soap; soft soap; ~ **germicida** germicidal soap
jabonadura, lather (*jabón*)
jacket[1], *m*, a fix of heroin (*un filerazo*)
jadeante, *adj*, breathless; panting
jadear, to gasp; to pant
jadeo, gasp (*dificultad en respirar*)
jaipa[1], mainliner[2]
jaipo, *slang*, hypodermic needle used to inject drugs; ~[1] mainliner[2]
jalá[1], *PR*, hit of marijuana; toke of marijuana or hashish
jalaita[1], *PR*, hit of marijuana; toke of marijuana or hashish
jalao, *adj*, intoxicated
jalar, to pull; ~**se** *PR*, to leave (*irse*)
jalea, jelly; ~ **anticoncepcional** contraceptive jelly; ~ **cardíaca** cardiac jelly; ~ **glicerinada** glycerin jelly; ~ **vaginal** vaginal jelly (*control de la natalidad*)
jaleo, *PR*, indigestion; stomach upset; upset stomach
jamás, *adv*, ever
jamón, *m*, ham; *PR*, bachelor
jamona, *PR*, spinster
jane, *adj*, *Hond*, harelip
janguear, *Chicano*, to hang around
jani[1], marijuana
jaqueca, headache; migraine
jarabe, *m*, syrup (*medicación*); ~ **de cereza** cherry syrup; ~ **de ipeca** syrup of ipecac; ~ **de ipecacuana** syrup of ipecac; ~ **de regaliz** licorice syrup; ~ **para la tos** cough syrup
jarra, jar; pitcher
jefa/jefe, *f/m*, boss; employer; ~ **de enfermeras** head nurse; nursing supervisor; ~ **de turno** charge nurse; ~ **de la casa** head of household; ~ **de la familia** head of household

Jefferson[1], marijuana
jején, *m*, *CA*, *SpAm*, gnat; sandfly; *Mex*, a great number
jender(se), *PR*, to tie one on (*emborracharse*)
jendío, *adj*, *PR*, (severely) intoxicated
jengibre, *m*, ginger
jerga, jargon
jeringa, hypodermic needle; syringe; ~ **con aguja hueca** hollow needle syringe; ~ **con cilindro de cristal** glass cylinder syringe; ~ **de lavativa** enema syringe; ~ **desechable** disposable syringe; ~ **esterilizada** sterile syringe
jeringuilla, syringe; ~ **descartable** disposable syringe; ~ **hipodérmica** hypodermic syringe; ~[1] nail[2] (*aguja para picarse*); needle[2]; spike[2] (*una jeringa hipodérmica*)
jey fiver, *m/f*, *Chicano*, hay fever
jijene, *m*, sandfly
jimagua, *m/f*, *Cu*, twin
jincarse, to bang; ~[1] to fix[2] (*picarse o filerearse*); to inject oneself with drugs; to hit up[2]
jinquetaza, *PR*, blow (*golpe con el puño*)
jiotes, *f*, *fam*, tinea corporis
jiribilla, *PR*, hyperactive child
jiricua, *slang*, vitiligo
jodido, *adj*, in poor health
jofaina, basin (*lavabo*); washbowl/washbasin
joroba, hump; humpback (*giba*); hunch (*corcova*)
jorobado, humpback; hunchback

(*persona*);   *adj*,   humpbacked; hunchbacked

jorobar, to annoy; to harass; **~se** to get cross; to get fed up (*hartarse*)

joven, *m/f*, young person; ~ (*de 13 a 19 años*) teenager

joyanco, hole in the ground

joyas, jewelry

Juana[1], Acapulco gold[2]; marijuana

juanetazo, *PR, fam*, straight shot of alcoholic drink

juanete, *m*, bunion

Juanita[1], Acapulco gold[2]; marijuana

jubilado, senior citizen; *adj*, retired (*que no trabaja*)

jugar (ue), to play

jugo, juice; ~ **de arándano** cranberry juice; ~ **de china** *PR*, orange juice; ~ **de ciruela pasa** prune juice; ~ **de fruta** fruit juice; ~ **de limón** lemon juice; ~

de naranja orange juice; ~ **de tomate** tomato juice; ~ **de toronja** grapefruit juice; ~ **digestivo** enzyme; ~ **gástrico** gastric juice; ~ **intestinal** intestinal juice; **~s pancreáticos** pancreatic juices

jugoso, *adj*, juicy

juicio, mind (*inteligencia*); sanity (*cordura*); senses *Med* (*sensatez*)

jumazo, *PR*, cigar

junta, board; ~ **administrativa** administrative counsel

juntar, to join; **~se** to have intercourse

juntura, *Anat*, joint; ~ **serrátil** serrated suture (*articulación fija*)

juramento, oath; ~ **hipocrático** Hippocratic Oath

justo, *adj*, fair (*imparcial*)

juvenil, *adj*, juvenile; youthful

juventud, *f*, youth

juyir(se), *PR*, to be afraid

---

[1] Este vocabulario es nuevo y todavía no se encuentra en el *Diccionario de la lengua española*, publicado por la Real Academia Española. Forma parte del argot o la lengua de la calle. Se supone que el género es obvio a menos que sea indicado.

[2] Forma parte del vocabulario inglés actual de los drogadictos.

kefir, *m,* kefir
keroseno, kerosene
kikear[1], *Chicano,* to clear up; to kick the habit
kilocaloría, kilocalorie
kilogramo, kilogram
kilolitro, kiloliter
kilómetro, kilometer
kilovatio, kilowatt

kilovatio-hora, *m,* kilowatt-hour
kleenex, *m,* facial tissues; Kleenex
knife[1], *m,* cocaine
kotex, *m,* sanitary napkin; sanitary pad
Kris Kras[1], marijuana
kwashiorkor, *m,* malnutrition; kwashiorkor

---

[1] Este vocabulario es nuevo y todavía no se encuentra en el *Diccionario de la lengua española,* publicado por la Real Academia Española. Forma parte del argot o la lengua de la calle. Se supone que el género es obvio a menos que sea indicado.

L

la cosa[1], heroin
la duna[1], heroin
la otra cosa[1], any narcotic substitute
la parte de atrás de, the back of
la salud[1], LSD
la semana pasada, last week
la verde[1], marijuana
la voluntad de vivir, will to live
la posición de un diente en relación a la lengua y el carrillo, buccolingual relationship
laberintitis, *f*, labyrinthitis
laberinto, labyrinth; ~ membranoso membranous labyrinth
laberintosis, *f*, labyrinthosis
labial, *adj*, labial
labihendido, harelip
labilidad del humor, *f*, lability; emotional instability
labio, labium (*pl*, *labia*); lip; ~ cucho *Chicano*, harelip; ~ hendido cleft lip; ~ inferior lower lip; ~ leporino cleft lip; harelip; ~s mayores labia majora; ~s menores labia minora; ~ superior upper lip
labioalveolar, *adj*, labio-alveolar
labiodental, *adj*, labiodental
labiolectura, lip reading
labor, *m*, task; *f*, labor
laboratorio, laboratory; ~ clínico clinical laboratory; ~ médico medical laboratory; ~ de Investigación de Enfermedades Venéreas VDRL/Venereal Disease Research Laboratory
laboratorista, *m/f*, laboratory technician
laceración, *f*, laceration; wound
lacerado, *adj*, lacerated
lacerar, to lacerate; to tear (*desgarrar*)

lacio, *adj*, lank (*pelo*)
lacra, *Med*, mark; scar; trace; *SpAm*, sore; ulcer
lacrar, *Med*, to infect; to injure the health of; to strike (with a disease)
lacrimal, *adj*, lachrymal
lactación, *f*, lactation
lactagogo, lactagogue
lactancia, lactation; nursing; ~ artificial bottle feeding; ~ maternal breast feeding; ~ natural breast feeding
lactante, *m/f*, baby (*infante*); infant; suckling; ~ azul *m/f*, blue baby; *adj*, nursing; mujer ~ *f*, nursing mother
lactar, to lactate; to nurse
lactasa, lactase
lactato, lactate
lácteo, *adj*, dairy; lacteal; milk; milky
lactodensímetro, lactodensimeter
lactosa, lactose (*se usa para cortar la heroína*)
LAD/lipoproteína de alta densidad, HDL/high density lipoprotein
ladilla, crab louse; parasitic cyst
lado, side; ~ derecho inferior right lower side; ~ derecho superior right upper side; ~ izquierdo inferior left lower side; ~ izquierdo superior left upper side
ladrar, to yelp
ladrido, barking
ladrilla, brick; ~[1] brick (*por lo común un kilo de mariguana u otra droga narcótica*)
lágrima, tear (*de llorar*); teardrop; ~s de cocodrilo crocodile tears
lagrimal, *adj*, lachrymal

lagrimear, to shed tears (*una persona*); to water (*los ojos*)
laguna, lacuna; ~ **auditiva** tone gap; ~ **de absorción** absorption lacuna; ~ **mental** blackout (*un fallo de memoria*); ~ **sanguínea** blood lacuna
lamer, to lick
lámina, lamina
laminectomía, laminectomy
laminografía, scan
lámpara, lamp; light (*luz*); ~ **de arco** arc lamp; ~ **de cuarzo** quartz lamp; ~ **de rayos ultravioletas** ultraviolet lamp; ~ **de techo** overhead light; ~ **de vapores de mercurio** mercury vapor lamp; ~ **solar** sunlamp
lamparón, *m, Med*, scrofula
lamprea, *Med*, sore; ulcer
lancinante, *adj*, nagging (*dolor*)
langosta, lobster
languidecer, to languish
languidez, *f*, languidness
lanolina, lanolin
lanzar gritos de dolor, to scream with pain
lapa, leech (*persona pegajosa*)
laparoscopia, laparoscopy
laparotomía, laparotomy
lápiz, *m*, pencil
lapso, lapse
larga duración, *f*, longstanding
laríngeo, *adj*, laryngeal
laringoscopia, laryngoscopy
largo, length; *adj*, long
larguirucho, *adj*, lank (*alto y delgado*)
laringe, *f*, larynx
laringectomía, laryngectomy
laríngeo, *adj*, laryngeal
laringitis, *f*, laryngitis
laringoscopia, laryngoscopy
laringoscopio, laryngoscope
larva, maggot; larva
lascadura, *Mex*, abrasion; sore
láser, *m*, laser
lástima, pity; shame; **llorar ~s** to moan and groan; to feel sorry for oneself

lastimada, *Mex*, (*Vea lastimadura*.)
lastimado, *adj*, sore (*herido por un golpe*)
lastimadura, bruise; hurt; injury; sore; sprain; wound
lastimar, to hurt (*hacer daño*); to injure (*herir*); ~**se** to get hurt; to wound
lastimoso, *adj*, sorry (*condición*)
lata, can (*envase*)
latente, *adj*, dormant; latent
látex, *m*, latex
latido, beat (*corazón, pulso*); stroke (*latido del corazón*); throb (*del corazón*); hunger pang; pain, twinge; throbbing (*de una herida*); *Chicano*, palpitation; spasm; ~ **arterial** arterial beat; ~ **cardíaco/cardiaco** heartbeat; ~ **del corazón** heartbeat; ~ **del corazón fetal** fetal heart tone; ~ **ectópico** ectopic beat; ~ **epigástrico** epigastric throbbing; ~ **irregular** irregular heartbeat (*arritmia*); ~ **normal del corazón** normal heartbeat; ~ **prematuro** anticipated systole; premature beat
latigazo, whiplash
latir, to beat (*corazón*); to palpitate; to throb (*corazón, pulso*); ~ **a ritmo acelerado** to race (*corazón, pulso, etc.*); ~ **irregularmente** to flutter (*pulso*); ~ **violentamente** to pound (*corazón*)
lauca, *Chi*, baldness; loss of hair
laucadura, *Chi*, baldness
lauco, *adj*, *Chi*, bald
lavable, *adj*, washable
lavabo, lavatory (*lavamanos*); washbowl/washbasin
lavacara, *Col, Ec*, washbasin
lavado, enema; lavage (*del estómago, etc.*); purge; washing out (*del estómago*); ~ **broncoalveolar** bronchoalveolar lavage; ~ **bucal** mouth wash; ~ **de la sangre** systemic lavage; *fam*, blood lavage; ~ **gástrico** gastric lavage;

~ **interno** douche; ~ **intestinal**
intestinal lavage; ~ **peritoneal**
peritoneal lavage; ~ **pleural**
pleural lavage; ~ **vaginal** douche
lavador, *m*, *Arg*, *Para*, washbasin
lavaje, *m*, *Med*, enema
lavamanos, *m*, *inv*, lavatory (*lavabo*)
lavandería, laundry (*lugar*)
lavaojos, *m*, *inv*, eye cup
lavaplatos, *m/f*, *inv*, [*Ú.m.c.m.*],
dishwasher
lavar, to bathe (*una herida*); to
scrub (*quirúrgicamente*); to wash;
~ (**y planchar**) to launder; **~se** to
wash oneself
lavativa, *fam*, enema
lavativo, purge
lavatorio, lavatory (*lavamanos*)
laxante, *m*, laxative
laxativo, *m*, *adj*, laxative
laxo, *adj*, easy (*moral*, *costumbre*);
lax (*disciplina*)
lazariento, *adj*, *Arg*, *Mex*, *Nic*, leprous
lazarín, *m*, leprosy
lazarino, leper
lazo, loop (*IUD*)
**LBD/lipoproteína de baja densi-
dad**, LDL low density lipoprotein
LEC/líquido extracelular, ECF/
extracellular fluid
lección, *f*, lesson
leche, *f*, milk; *vulg*, semen; ~ **agria**
sour milk; ~ **baja en grasa** low
fat milk; ~ **bronca** *Mex*, raw
milk; ~ **con chocolate** chocolate milk; ~ **condensada** condensed milk; ~ **de cabra** goat's
milk; ~ **de magnesia** milk of
magnesia; ~ **de vaca** cow's milk;
~ **descremada** skim(med) milk;
~ **desnatada** skim(med) milk; ~
en polvo powdered milk; ~ **entera** whole milk; ~ **esterilizada**
sterilized milk; ~ **evaporada**
evaporated milk; ~ **evaporizada**
evaporated milk; ~ **fortificada**
fortified milk; ~ **fresca de vaca**

fresh milk; ~ **homogeneizada**
homogenized milk; ~ **humana
exprimida** EBM/expressed
breast milk; ~ **materna** breast
milk; mother's breast milk; ~
pasteurizada pasteurized milk;
~ **sin procesar** raw milk
lecho, bed (*fig. mortuario, etc.*); ~
capilar bed capillary; ~ **de la
uña** nail bed; ~ **de muerte**
death bed; ~ **mortuorio** death
bed; ~ **ungueal** nail bed
lechoso, *adj*, milky
lechuga, lettuce
lecitina, lecithin
lectura, reading
**LED/lupus eritematoso disemi-
nado**, *m*, LED/lupus erythematosus disseminata
leer, to read
legaña, gum (*de los ojos*); rheum
legítimo, *adj*, legitimate
lego, *adj*, lay
legra, curette
legrado, *fam*, curettage; D & C
legumbre, *f*, legume; vegetable
leishmaniasis, *f*, leishmaniasis
lejano, *adj*, dim (*distante*); far away
lejía, lye
lengua, tongue; ~ **cubierta** coated
tongue; ~ **depapilada** bald
tongue; ~ **desatada** loose
tongue; ~ **materna** native
tongue; ~ **negra peluda** black
hairy tongue; ~ **pastosa** morning tongue; ~ **quemante** burning tongue; ~ **saburral** coated
tongue; encrusted tongue;
furred/furry tongue; ~ **sucia**
coated tongue; ~ **tostada** baked
tongue; ~ **vellosa** hairy tongue
lenguado, sole (*pescado*)
lenguaje, *m*, idiom; speech; ~
cercenado slurred speech; ~
titubeante clipped speech
lenguazo[1], heroin
lente[4], *m/f*, [*Ú.m.c.m.*], lens; **~s** *m*,
pl, eyeglasses; eyewear; **~s** *m*, *pl*,
Mex, glasses; spectacles; ~ **bifo-**

cal bifocal lens; ~ **cóncava** concave lens; ~ **convexa** convex lens; ~ **correctivo** corrective lens; ~ **de aumento** magnifying lens; ~ **de catarata** cataract lens; ~ **de contacto** contact lens; ~ **de contacto blando** soft contact lens; ~ **de contacto duro** hard contact lens; ~ **poroso** gas permeable contact lens; ~**s suaves** soft lenses; ~ **intraocular** lens implantation; ~ **pequeño** lenticula; ~**s protectores** protective eyewear; ~ **tórica** toric lens; ~ **trifocal** trifocal lens

lenteja, lentil
lentilla, *Spain*, contact lens
lentitud, *f*, slowing
lento, *adj*, lingering (*muerte*); slow
leñazo, blow (*garrotazo, etc.*)
leñito[1], jive stick[2] (*cigarrillo de mariguana*); marijuana cigarette
leño[1], jive stick[2], joint (*cigarrillo de mariguana*); marijuana cigarette
lepra, Hansen's disease; leprosy; *fam*, eczema; ~ **italiana** pellagra
leproso, leper
leptomeninges, *f*, leptomeninges
leptospirosis, *f*, leptospirosis
lerdo, *adj*, backward; dull (*torpe*)
lerenes, *m, pl, vulg*, balls; testicle
lesbiana, *f, adj*, lesbian
lesbianismo, lesbianism
lesbismo, lesbianism
lesión, *f*, damage; injury; lesion; sore; ~ **de latigazo** whiplash; ~ **degenerativa** degenerative lesion; ~ **estructural** structural lesion; ~ **expansiva** expanding lesion; ~ **macroscópica** gross lesion; ~ **microscópica** minute lesion; ~ **precancerosa** precancerous lesion; ~ **primaria** primary lesion; ~ **sistematizada** systemic lesion; ~ **total** total lesion; ~ **tóxica** toxic lesion; ~ **vascular** vascular lesion
lesionar, to damage; to hurt (*herir*); to injure; ~**se** to be injured

letal, *adj*, lethal *Med*
letalidad, *f*, deadliness
letargia, lethargy
letárgico, *adj*, deathlike; lethargic
letargo, lethargy
letra inclinada hacia la izquierda, backhand (*escritura*)
leucanemia, leukanemia
leucemia, leukemia; ~ **aguda** acute leukemia; ~ **aplástica** aplastic leukemia; ~ **basófila** basophilic leukemia; ~ **de células indiferenciadas** undifferentiated cell leukemia; ~ **de células plasmáticas** plasma-cell leukemia; ~ **granulocítica** granulocytic leukemia; ~ **hepática** hepatic leukemia; ~ **linfática** lymphatic leukemia; ~ **linfoblástica** lymphoblastic leukemia; ~ **linfocítica (aguda)** (acute) lymphocytic leukemia; ~ **linfógena** lymphogenous leukemia; ~ **linfoide (crónica)** (chronic) lymphoid leukemia; ~ **mieloblástica** myeloblastic leukemia; ~ **mielocítica** myelocytic leukemia; ~ **mielógena (crónica)** (chronic) myelogenous leukemia; ~ **mieloide (crónica)** (chronic) myeloid leukemia; ~ **transitoria** temporary leukemia
leucémico, *adj*, leukemic
leucemoide, *adj*, leukemoid
leucoblasto, leukoblast; ~ **granular** granular leukoblast
leucocito, leukocyte; white blood cells; white blood corpuscle; ~ **acidófilo** acidophil leukocyte; ~ **agranulocito** agranular leukocyte; ~ **basófilo** basophil leukocyte; ~ **granuloso** granular leukocyte; ~ **linfoide** lymphoid leukocyte; ~ **neutrófilo** neutrophil leukocyte; ~**s nucleados** nucleated leukocytes; ~ **polimorfonuclear** polymorphonuclear leukocyte; ~ **sin gránulos** lymphoid leukocyte

leucocitosis, *f*, leukocytosis
leucoplaquia, leukoplakia
leucoplasia, leukoplasia
leucorrea, leukorrhea; ~ **periódica** periodic leukorrhea
levadura, yeast; ~ (**en polvo**) baking powder; ~ **de cerveza** Brewer's yeast
levantamiento, lift
levantar, to hold up (*alzar*); to lift; to raise; to lift up (*recoger*); to turn (*trastornar*); ~ **ampollas en** to blister; ~ **el cadáver** to remove the corpse; ~ **la cabeza hacia arriba** to raise one's head; ~**se** to get up; to raise oneself (*ponerse de pie*); to stand up
leve, *adj*, easy (*castigo, etc.*); light (*enfermedad*); light (*no grave*); mild; minor (*insignificante*); slight
ley, *f*, law; ~, **reflejo, signo, síndrome de Babinski** *m*, Babinski's law, reflex, sign, syndrome
libido, libido; ~ **bisexual** bisexual libido
libra, pound (*peso, moneda*)
libre, *adj*, promiscuous (*sexualmente*); ~ **albedrío** free will; ~ **de gérmenes** *adj*, germ free; ~ **de polvo** *adj*, dust-free; ~ **de servicio** off duty
licencia, license
licenciado, *Mex*, lawyer
licor, *m*, liquor
licuar, to liquefy
licuefacer, to liquefy
lidocaína, lidocaine
liendre, *f*, nit
liga, tourniquet
ligado, *adj*, bound; linked; ~ **al cromosoma X** *adj*, X-linked
ligadura, bond; ligation; ligature; tourniquet; ~ (**de**) **los tubos** tubal ligation; ~ **de trompas** tubal ligation
ligamenta, ligamentum; ~ **accesoria plantaria** ligamenta acceso-

ria plantaria; ~ **flava** flava ligamenta
ligamento, ligament; ~ **accesorio** accessory ligament; ~**s anchos de los párpados** orbital septum; ~ **arterial** arteriosum ligamentum; ~ **cervical posterior** nuchae ligamentum; ~ **gastropancreático** gastropancreatic fold; ~ **transverso de la pelvis** floor of the pelvis; ~**s plantares accesorios de las articulaciones metatarsofalángicas** ligamenta accesoria plantaria; ~ **redondo** teres ligamentum; ~**s transversos de las articulaciones metatarsofalángicas** ligamenta accesoria plantaria
ligar, to attach; to ligate; to tie together; ~ **los tubos de Falopio** to tie the tubes; ~ **los tubos uterinos** to tie the tubes; ~ **trompas** to tie the tubes
ligazón de tubos, *f*, tubal ligation
ligeramente, *adv*, lightly; mildly; slightly
ligero, *adj*, light (*color, peso*); mild; ~ **estrabismo** cast; slight squint (*ligera bizquera*)
lima, file (*herramienta*); lime (*fruta*); ~ **para las uñas** nail file
limaduras, filings
limar, to file down; to polish; to smooth
limbo, limbus
limitación, *f*, limitation; ~ **de la natalidad** birth control
limitado, *adj*, limited
limitante, *adj*, limiting
limitarse a, to keep to (*restringirse a*)
límite, *m*, limit; ~**s** range; ~ **de asimilación** assimilation limit; ~ **de saturación** saturation limit
limo, mud (*légamo del río*)
limoso, *adj*, muddy
limpiador de agua a presión, *m*, waterpick
limpiar, to clean; to wipe (clean);

~ (**mariguana**)[1] to manicure[2] (*limpiar y preparar la mariguana para liar cigarrillos*); ~ **el pico** *PR*, to kill; ~**se** to clean oneself; to wipe oneself (*después de una evacuación intestinal*)

limpieza, cleaning *Dent*; cleanliness

limpio, *adj*, clean; pure

limpión, *m*, wipe

linaje, *m*, lineage

linaza, linseed

lindano, lindane

línea, line; ~ **abdominal** abdominal line; ~ **capilar** hairline; ~ **curva** curved line; ~ **de absorción** absorption line; ~**s de fuerza magnética** magnetic lines of force; ~ **de hendidura** cleavage lines; ~ **de oclusión** line of occlusion; ~ **de puntos** dotted line; ~ **de referencia** base-line; ~ **discontinua** dashed line; ~ **mamilar** nipple line; ~ **media** midline; ~ **oblicua** oblique line; ~ **primitiva** primitive streak; ~ **visual** line of sight

lineal, *adj*, lineal

linfa, lymph

linfático, *adj*, lymphatic

linfoblasto, lymphoblast

linfocito, lymphocyte

linfogranuloma venéreo, *m*, lymphogranuloma venereum/LGV

linfogranulomatosis, *f*, lymphogranulomatosis/Hodgkin's disease

linfoide, *adj*, lymphoid

linfoma, *m*, lymphoma

lingual, *adj*, lingual

linimento, liniment

lío, mess (*embrollo*); pack (*paquete*)

lipectomía, lipectomy

lipemia, lipemia

lipidemia, lipidemia

lípido, lipid

lipoide, *m*, lipoid

lipoideo, *adj*, lipoid

lipoma, *m*, lipoma

lipón, *adj*, *Ven*, pot-bellied

lipoproteína, lipoprotein; ~ **de alta densidad**/LAD high density lipoprotein/HDL; ~ **de baja densidad**/LBD low density lipoprotein/LDL

liposarcoma, *m*, liposarcoma

liposoluble, *adj*, liposoluble

liposucción, *f*, liposuction

lipotimia, fainting spell

liquen, *m*, lichen; ~ **plano** lichen planus

liquidar una cuenta, to settle an account

líquido, *m*, *adj*, fluid; liquid; ~[1] angel dust (*PCP*); dust (*cocaína*, *PCP*); PCP; ~ **amniótico** amniotic fluid; ~ **cefalorraquídeo**/LCR cerebrospinal fluid/CSF; ~ **cerebrospinal**/LCS cerebrospinal fluid/CSF; ~ **en el escroto** *fam*, hydrocele; ~ **filtrado** filtrate; ~ **pleural** pleural fluid; ~ **seminal** seminal fluid; ~ **sinovial** synovial liquid

lisiado, *adj*, crippled; lame; maimed; injured

lisiar, to cripple (*tullir*); to maim (*un miembro*); to injure (*herir*)

lisina, lysine

liso, *adj*, even (*suave, sin asperezas*); smooth

lista, list; ~ **de accidentados** casualty/casualties list; ~ **de colorantes** table of stains; ~ **de espera** waiting list; ~ **de hígado** (*liquid*) liver extract; ~ **de intercambios** exchange list

listerina, *fam*, mouthwash

listo, *adj*, ready; able-minded; smart (*inteligente*); *adj*, *fam*, available

litio, lithium

litotomía, lithotomy

litotripsia, lithotripsy

litro, liter

llaga, fester; sore (*úlcera*); wound; ~ **de cama** bed sore/bedsore; ~

de fiebre fever blister; ~ **por decúbito** bed sore/bedsore; ~ **ulcerosa** canker; canker sore

llama, flame; **~s capilares** capillary flames

llamada telefónica, telephone call

llamar, to call; ~ **al médico** to send for the doctor; ~ **por bíper**[1] to page (*usando un aparato portátil*); ~ **por teléfono** to telephone; ~ **por vocina**[1] to page (*por altavoz*); **~se** to be called; to be named

llamaradas, hot flashes

llanto, cry (*con lágrimas*); wailing

llave, *f*, key (*para cerradura*); ~ **dental** tooth key *Dent*

llegar, to arrive; to come; to reach; ~ **hasta el extremo de** to go to the length of; ~ **tarde** to be late (*una persona*)

llenar, to fill; ~ (**una receta**) to fill (*a prescription*); ~ **un formulario** to fill out a form; ~ **una planilla** to fill out a form

lleno, *adj*, full; ~ **de alegría** *adj*, overjoyed; ~ **de costras** *adj*, scabby; ~ **de moretones** black and blue

llevado por el aire, *adj*, airborne

llevar, to carry; to wear; ~ **a cabo** to carry out; to go through with; ~ **en camilla** to carry on stretcher; ~ **retraso** to be late (*un tren, avión, etc.*); **~se un chasco** to be let down

llorar, to cry (*con lágrimas*); to weep; ~ **hasta dormirse** to cry oneself to sleep; ~ **la muerte de** to mourn for

lloroso, *adj*, weeping

lluvia, rain; ~ **de estrellas**[1] LSD; ~ **radiactiva** fallout

lo contrario, opposite

lo demás, *slang*, placenta

lo más pronto posible, as soon as possible

lo mismo, the same thing

lo siento, excuse me (pardon)

lobanillo, wen

lobar, *adj*, lobar

lobectomía, lobectomy; ~ **completa** complete lobectomy; ~ **izquierda anterior** left lower lobectomy; ~ **parcial** partial lobectomy

lobotomía, lobotomy

lobulillo, lobule

lóbulo, ear lobe; lobe; ~ **fusiforme** occipitotemporal convolution; ~ **occipital** occipital lobe; ~ **parietal** parietal lobe; ~ **pequeño** lobule; ~ **terminal** endlobe

local, *adj*, local

localización, *f*, localization; ~ **electiva** selective localization

localizador, *m*, locator

localizar, to localize; to locate (*buscar y encontrar*)

loción, *f*, lotion; ~ **bronceadora** suntan lotion; ~ **contra los insectos** insect repellent; ~ **de calamina** calamine lotion; ~ **para el sol** suntan lotion

loco, *adj*, crazy; insane; lunatic; mad; nut (*enfermo mental*); **~**[1] *adj*, high on[2] (*drogas narcóticas*)

locote[1,] *adj*, high on[2] (*drogas narcóticas*)

lóculo, loculus

locura, craziness; insanity; madness; ~ **de doble forma** manic-depressive insanity; ~ **maníaco-depresiva** manic-depressive insanity

lodo, mud

logafasia, logaphasia

logopatólogo, speech pathologist

logoterapia, speech therapy

lombriz, *f*, worm (*parásito*); ~ **chiquita afilada** threadworms; ~ **de gancho** uncinaria (*anquilostoma*); ~ **de látigo** trichocephalus; ~ **grande redonda** ascaris (*ascáride*); ~ **solitaria** tapeworm

lomo, shoulder (*animal*); loin; *fam*, back

longevidad, *f*, life span; longevity
longitud, *f*, length; ~ **de onda** wavelength; ~ **vértex-rabadilla** crown-rump length; ~ **vértex-talón** crown-heel length
longitudinal, *adj*, longitudinal
longitudinalmente, *adv*, lengthwise
loquillo, *adj*, crazy
loquios, lochia
lora, *Col, Ec, PR, Ven*, open wound; serious wound
loro, *Chi*, bedpan
lovastatina, lovastatin
LSD[1], acid[2] (*LSD*); (green) barrels/(the) beast[2]
lubricante, *m, adj*, lubricant
lubricar, to lubricate
lubricativo, *adj*, lubricant
lucas[1], Acapulco gold[2] (*mariguana*); marijuana
lucha, fight
luchar, to fight
lucidez, *f*, lucidity; sanity (*en sano juicio*)
lúcido, *adj*, lucid
lúes, *f*, lues; syphilis
lugar, *m*, place (*posición; sitio*); spot (*paraje*); ~ **de nacimiento** birthplace; ~ **donde se deja o se esconde una droga** drop[2]
lumbago, low back pain; lumbago; ~ **isquémico** ischemic lumbago
lumboartrosis, *f*, lumboarthrosis
lumbodorsal, *adj*, lumbodorsal
lumbosacro, *adj*, lumbosacral

lumbricida, *m, adj*, lumbricide
lumpectomía, lumpectomy
luna, *Chicano*, menstruation
lunar, *m*, beauty mark; birthmark; blemish mole; nevus (*pl, nevi*)
lunático, *m, adj*, lunatic
lupa, magnifying glass; magnifying lens
lupia, wen; cyst; *m/f, Hond*, quack doctor
lupo, loop; birth control
luposo, lupous
lupus, *m*, lupus; ~ **eritematoso discoide** discoid lupus erythematosus; ~ **eritematoso generalizado** disseminatus lupus erythematosus; systemic lupus erythematosus
luquete, *m, Chi*, bald spot (*en la cabeza*)
lustroso, *adj*, glossy
lútea, macula lutea
luteína, lutein
lúteo, *adj*, luteal
luto, mourning
luxación, *f*, dislocation; luxation
luz, *f*, light; light (*lámpara*); **baño de ~** light bath; ~ **brillante** glare (*luz deslumbrante*); ~ **del día** daylight; ~ **del sol** sunlight; ~ **deslumbrante** glare (*luz brillante*); ~ **difusa** diffused light; **golpe de ~** light stroke; ~ **neón** neon light; ~ **polarizada** polarized light

---

[1] Este vocabulario es nuevo y todavía no se encuentra en el *Diccionario de la lengua española*, publicado por la Real Academia Española. Forma parte del argot o la lengua de la calle. Se supone que el género es obvio a menos que sea indicado.
[2] Forma parte del vocabulario inglés actual de los drogadictos.
[4] Cuando se refiere a *gafas/spectacles*, la palabra suele ser masculina—*los lentes*. Cuando se refiere a *lentes refringentes/refractive lenses*, la palabra suele ser femenina—*las lentes*.

M

macanazo, blow (*por la porra de un policía*)

macerar, to macerate

machacar, to crush (*moler*); to nag (*molestar con insistencia*); to pound (*en un mortero*)

macho, *m*, *adj*, male

machucar, to crush (*dedo, pie, etc.*); to mash (*aplastar*)

macis, *f*, mace

macoña[1], marijuana

macrobiótico, *adj*, macrobiotic

macrocefalia, macrocephalia

macrocito, macrocyte

macrocosmo, macrocosm

macrodoncia, macrodontia

macrófago, macrophage

macroscópico, *adj*, macroscopic

mácula, macula; ~ **densa** macula densa

maculosa de las Montañas Rocosas, Rocky Mountain fever

madera, wood

madrastra, stepmother

madre, *f*, mother; ~ **adoptiva** foster mother; ~[1] dope pusher; peddler[2] (*persona que proporciona drogas*)

madurar, to come to a head (*un absceso*); to grow up; to mature

madurez, *f*, maturity

maduro, *adj*, mature; ripe (*fruta; absceso*)

mafú[1], *m*, (*uncommon*) hashish; ~[1] marijuana

mafufa[1], marijuana

magnesia, magnesia

magnesio, magnesium

magnético, *adj*, magnetic

magnetismo, magnetism

magnetizar, to magnetize

magnificación, *f*, magnification

magrez, *f*, thinness (*de una persona*); weight loss

magro, *adj*, lean (*carne*)

magullado, *adj*, bruised

magulladura, bruise (*contusión*); contusion

magullamiento, bruise

maíz, *m*, corn (*comida*)

majadero, *PR*, badly behaved child

maje, *m*, *PR*, (*syn: mime/noseeums*); insect (*tipo de insecto*); (*Vea mime.*); *m*, *PR*, gnat

mal, *m*, affliction *Med*; disease; harm; illness; malady; malaise; sickness; ~ **caduco** epilepsy; ~ **comicial** epilepsy; ~ **de arco** *slang*, tetanus; ~ **de bubas** *slang*, syphilis; ~ **de Down** Down's syndrome; ~ **de garganta** sore throat; ~ **de garganta por estreptococo** strep throat; ~ **de Hansen** leprosy; ~ **de hiel** cholecystitis; gallbladder disease; ~ **de ijar**[6] flank pain; ~ **de la rosa** pellagra; ~ **de las encías** pyorrhea; ~ **de los aviadores** air sickness; ~ **de madre** morning sickness; ~ **de mar** seasickness; ~ **de monja** housemaid knee; ~ **de oídos** sore ears; ~ **de ojo** hex (*maleficio*); *fam*, conjunctivitis; pinkeye; ~ **de orín** urinary problem; *slang*, gonorrhea; ~ **de pintas** psoriasis; ~ **de pinto** spotted sickness; ~ **de riñón** kidney disease; ~ **de San Guido** chorea; ~ **de San Juan** epilepsy; ~ **de San Lázaro** leprosy; ~ **de San Pedro** epilepsy; ~ **de San Vito** chorea; ~ **de sol** pellagra; ~ **del apendis** *fam*, appendicitis; ~ **del corazón** heart disease; *fam*, heart attack; ~ **del pecho** asthma; ~ **francés** *slang*, syphilis; ~ **intelectual** epilepsy; ~ **napolitano** syphilis; ~ **puesto** hex (*maleficio*); **mal**[7]/**malo**/**mala** *adj*, bad; ~ **adaptado** *adj*, misfit; ~ **aire** *m*, bad air; ~ **aliento** bad breath; halitosis; ~ **asistido** *adj*, *fam*, malnourished; ~ **criado** *adj*, misbehaved; ~ **educado** *adj*, impolite; ~ **informado** *adj*, misinformed; ~ **juicio** bad judgment; ~ **nutrido** *adj*, malnourished; ~ **ojo** evil eye; ~ **olor corporal** *m*, body odor; ~ **parto** miscarriage; ~ **sabor de boca** *m*, aftertaste; ~ **ventilado** *adj*, close (*ventilación de un cuarto*); stuffy (*ventilación*); ~ **viaje** *m*, bad trip²; **mala alimentación** *f*, malnutrition; **mala alimentación mojada** kwashiorkor; **mala alimentación seca** marasmus; **mala conducta** naughtiness (*mal comportamiento*); **mala digestión** *f*, indigestion; **mala salud** *f*, ill health; sickliness; **mala voluntad** *f*, prejudice (*hostilidad*); *adv*, badly; ill

malabsorción, *f*, malabsorption
malaria, malaria; blackwater fever; marsh fever; ~ **perniciosa** pernicious malaria
malariología, malariology
malarioterapia, malariotherapy
maleficio, hex (*mal de ojo*); spell (*sortilegio*)
maléolo, ankle; malleolus
malestar, *m*, ailment; discomfort (*sensación de indisposición*); distress (*dolor*); indisposition; malaise; ~ **postalcohólico** hangover; ~**es de la mañana** morning nausea; ~**es de la vesícula biliar** gallbladder disorder
maleta, suitcase
maletín, *m*, doctor's bag; ~ **médico** doctor's bag
malformación, *f*, malformation; ~ **congénita** congenital malformation
malformativo, *adj*, misformed
malfuncionamiento, malfunction
malfuncionar, to malfunction
malgastar, to waste

malhumorado, *adj*, bad-tempered (*de vez en cuando*); grouchy (*de mal humor*)
malicia, malice
malicioso, *adj*, evil-minded; malicious
malignidad, *f*, malignancy
maligno, *adj*, malignant
malintencionado, *adj*, evil-minded
malla, mesh
malnutrición, *f*, malnutrition
malo, *adj*, bad; ill; naughty (*bad*); sick (*Vea mal/malo/mala.*); ~ **para la salud** bad for one's health
maloclusión, *f*, malocclusion
maloja¹, *PR*, marijuana
maloliente, *adj*, evil-smelling
malparto, abortion; miscarriage
malposición mandibular, *f*, jaw malposition
malpraxis, *f*, malpractice; malpraxis
maltasa, maltase
maltosa, malt sugar; maltose
maltratar, to abuse
maltrato, abuse; ~ **de los niños** child abuse
maluso, misuse
mama, breast; mamma; mammary gland; ~ **supernumeraria** supernumerary mamma
mamá, mom; mother
mamadera, breast pump; nipple (*de un biberón*); nursing bottle; *SpAm*, baby bottle
mamar, to breast feed; to nurse (*una crianza*); to suck
mamífero, *m*, *adj*, mammalian
mamila, nipple (*de un hombre*)
mamilar, *adj*, mammillary
mamografía, mammogram; mammography
mamograma, *m*, mammogram
mamón, *m*, *Chicano*, pacifier
mamoplastia, mammoplasty
mampostial, *m*, *PR*, candy (*hecho de coco y melaza*)
manar, to stream (*sangre*)
manazo, *Ríopl*, slap (*golpe con la mano*)

mancha, blemish; mole; spot; stain (*mancilla*); dab; macula; **~s blancas en la uña** leuconychia; **~s de color amarillo** xanthoma; **~s de flujo vaginal sanguinolento** vaginal spotting; **~ de la preñez** chloasma; facial discoloration; mask of pregnancy; **~ de lágrima** tearstain; **~ de sangre** bloodstain; **~s de sangre** spotting; **~ del embarazo** chloasma; facial discoloration; mask of pregnancy; **~s frente a los ojos** scotoma (*una zona visual insensible a la luz en la retina*); **~s hepáticas** liver spots; **~s oscuras en la piel** skin blotches; **~ volante** floater (*en el ojo*)

manchado, spotting; **~ del pulmón** *Mex*, *fam*, tuberculosis; *adj*, soiled (*sucio*); stained; **~ de sangre** *adj*, bloodstained

manchar, to stain

manco, *adj*, crippled (*hand*); maimed; one-armed; one-handed; one-armed person (*del brazo*); one-handed person (*de la mano*); cripple

mandar, to order *Med*; to send

mandíbula, jaw (*de personas*); jawbone; lower jaw; mandible; **~ crujiente** crackling jaw; **~ rota** broken jaw

mandibular, *adj*, mandibular

manejar, to drive; to handle

manejo, management (*de personas, de herramientas, etc.*)

manera, manner; way

manga, sleeve

manganeso, manganese

mangar, to catch someone doing something illegal or forbidden

mango, handgrip (*de una raqueta, un palo*); handle; neck (*de un instrumento o cuchillo*); shaft

mangonear, *PR*, to goof off

manguera, air duct; ventilation shaft; hose (*una manga de riego*); tube

manguito, cuff; **~ de presión sanguínea** blood pressure cuff; **~ rotador del hombro** rotator cuff of the shoulder

maní, *m*, peanut; **~**[1] marijuana

manía, madness; mania; **~ aguda alucinatoria** acute hallucinatory mania; **~ danzante** dancing mania; **~ depresiva** manic depression; **~ histérica** hysterical mania; **~ puerperal** puerperal mania

maníaco, *adj*, mad (*loco*); maniac; **~-depresivo** *adj*, manic-depressive

maniamelancolía, manic-depressive insanity

manicomio, insane asylum; hospital for the insane; madhouse

manicura, manicure

manidiestro, *adj*, right handed

manifestación, *f*, manifestation

manifestar (ie), to manifest

manifiesto, *adj*, evident; obvious

maniobra, maneuver/manoeuver

manipulación, *f*, manipulation

mano, *f*, hand; **~ en garra** claw hand; **~ segura** steady hand; **~ zampa** clubhand

manso, *adj*, meek

manta, blanket

manteca, fat (*grasa*); lard (*del cerdo*); **~ de cacahuete** peanut butter; **~ de cacao** cocoa butter; **~**[1] bad heroin; heroin

mantecado, ice cream

mantener, to feed (*alimentar*); to keep; to maintain; to raise (*una familia*); to support (*hacer provisión para; sostener*); **~ con vida** to keep alive; **~ en vida** to keep alive; **~se a distancia de** to stand clear of

mantengo, hand-out; *fam*, government subsidy

mantenido, *adj*, supported

mantenimiento, maintaining; maintenance

mantequilla, butter

mantillas, swaddling clothes

manual, *m, adj,* manual

manzana, apple; *Mex,* Adam's apple

mañana, morning; tomorrow; ~ **por la mañana** tomorrow morning

mapache, *m,* raccoon

maquillaje, *m,* makeup

maquillar, to apply makeup (*aplicar productos de maquillaje*); ~**se** to put on makeup

máquina, machine; ~ **de afeitar** safety razor; ~ **de cortar** slicer; ~ **ultrasónica** ultrasonic machine

maquinilla de afeitar, safety razor

maquinilla de seguridad, safety razor

marasmo, consumption; marasmus (*mala alimentación*)

maravilloso, *adj,* marvelous

marca, make (*fabricación*); mark (*signo; huella; cicatriz; picadura*); score (*resultado*); ~ **de nacimiento** birthmark

marcado, *adj,* marked

marcador de paso, *m,* pacemaker

marcador de ritmo, *m,* pacemaker

marcapaso(s), (cardiac) pacemaker

marcar, to label; to mark (*ropa*); to record (*un termómetro, etc.*)

marcas, landmarks; ~[1] tracks[2] (*cicatrices y traques causados por el uso de agujas hipodérmicas*)

marcha, gait; ~ **antálgica** antalgic gait; ~ **de ánade** waddle; ~ **diagnóstica** diagnostic approach; workup; ~ **espasmódica** spastic gait; ~ **paralítica** paralytic gait; ~ **sobre los talones** heel walking; ~ **torpe** clumsiness of gait; ~ **zafia** clumsiness of gait

marchito, *adj,* withering

marco, frame (*de un cuadro, una puerta, una ventana*)

mareado, *adj,* airsick; seasick; dizzy; giddy; light-headed (*de alcohol*)

marear, *Med,* to make s.o. feel sick; to make s.o. feel dizzy; to make s.o. seasick; ~**se**, *Med,* to feel sick (*tener nauseas*); to become dizzy (*estar aturdido*); to be/feel/get seasick; to feel giddy; to feel faint

mareo, dizziness; giddiness; motion sickness; seasickness; *fam,* fainting spell; ~ **en un vehículo** carsickness ~**en viaje aéreo** air sickness

marfil, *m,* ivory

margarina, margarine

Margarita[1], marijuana

margen, *m,* edge; margin; *f,* range; ~ **de error** range of error

mari[1], marijuana

María Juanita[1], marijuana

María[1], marijuana

Mariana[1], marijuana

maricocaimorfi[1], user of marijuana/cocaine/morphine

maricón, *m, adj,* queer *slang*

marido, husband

marifinga[1], marijuana

mariguana[1, 4], Acapulco gold[2] (*mariguana*); marijuana

mariguano[1], doper[2]; marijuana user

marihuana[1, 4], marijuana; tea[2]; weed[2]

marihuanar[1], to administer marijuana to someone

marihuano[1], marijuana user

marijuana[1, 4], marijuana

marijuano[1], marijuana user

marinola[1], marijuana

mariola[1], marijuana

mariólogo, malariologist

mariposa, *vulg,* gay male

mariscos, *m, pl,* shellfish

marital, *adj,* marital

marizazo[1], cocaine

mármol, *m,* marble

marquita[1], marijuana

marrayo, *PR,* candy (*hecho de coco y melaza*)

marrón, *adj,* maroon

martillo, hammer (*del oído medio*); malleus; hammer; ~ **neumático** air hammer

Mary Jane[1], marijuana
Mary Popins[1], marijuana
más, *adj*, *adv*, more; ~ **caliente** warmer; ~ **despacio** more slowly; ~ **gráfico** *adj*, clearer; ~ **o menos** more or less; ~ **tarde** *adj*, later
masa, mass
masaje, *m*, massage; ~ **auditivo** auditory massage; ~ **cardíaco/cardiaco externo** external cardiac massage; ~ **electrovibratorio** electrovibratory massage; ~ **facial** facial
mascar, to chew
máscara, mask; ~ **antigás** gas mask; ~ **de oxígeno** oxygen mask; ~ **del embarazo** mask of pregnancy; ~ **equimótica** ecchymotic mask; ~ **gravídica** mask of pregnancy; ~ **mortuoria** death mask
mascarilla, mask; ~ **de oxígeno** oxygen mask; ~ **mortuoria** death mask
mascaura, wad of chewing gum; *slang*, *PR*, wad of chewing tobacco
masculino, *adj*, male; masculine
mascullamiento, mumbling
mascullar, to mumble
masivo, *adj*, massive
masoquismo, masochism; *adj*, masochistic
masoquista, *m/f*, masochist; *adj*, masochistic
mastectomía, mastectomy; ~ **radical** radical mastectomy
masticar, to chew; to masticate
mastitis, *f*, mastitis; ~ **cística** cystic mastitis; ~ **flemonosa** gathered breast; ~ **por estasis** caked breast
mastocito, mastocyte
mastoidectomía, mastoidectomy
mastoideo, *adj*, mastoid
mastoides, *f*, *adj*, mastoid
mastoiditis, *f*, mastoiditis
masturbación, *f*, masturbation
masturbar(se), to masturbate
matadero, bad hospital
matar, to kill; ~ **a alguien a puña-**ladas to stab s.o. to death; ~**le el nervio a alguien** to remove the nerve *Dent*
matasanos, *m*, *inv*, quack; ~ **avaricioso**[5] hungry croaker
matayerbas, *m*, *inv*, herbicide
mate, *adj*, dull (*sonidos*)
materia, matter (*substancia*); pus *Med*; ~ **blanca** white matter; ~ **cerebral** brain matter; ~ **fecal** bowel movement; excrement; feces; ~ **gris** grey matter; *fam*, cerebral cortex; ~ **radioactiva** radioactive material
material, *m*, *adj*, material; ~ **áspero inabsorbible** roughage; ~ **de base** base material *Dent*; ~ **dental** dental material; ~ **negro**[1] opium; ~**es restauradores** restorative materials; *f*, matter (*substancia*)
maternal, *adj*, maternal
maternidad, *f*, maternity
matidez, *f*, dullness (*sonido*)
matiz, *m*, hue (*shade*)
matojo, weed
matrimonial, *adj*, marital
matrimonio, marriage
matriz, *f*, matrix; uterus; womb; ~ **de la uña** nail bed
maxilar, *m*, jawbone; maxilla; upper jaw; ~ **inferior** lower jaw; lower jawbone; ~ **superior** upper jaw; upper jawbone; *adj*, maxillar; maxillary
maxilofacial, *adj*, maxillofacial
maxilofaríngeo, *adj*, mandibulopharyngeal; maxillopharyngeal
maxilolabial, *adj*, maxillolabial
maxilomalar, *adj*, jugomaxillary
mayonesa, mayonnaise
mayor, *adj*, older
mayoría, majority
mazorca, *sg*, *slang*, teeth
meadera, *Chicano*, frequent urinating
mear, to urinate
meato, meatus
mecánico, mechanic; *adj*, mechanical

mecanismo, mechanism; ~ **de defensa** defense mechanism; ~ **de escape** escape mechanism

mechero, cigarette lighter; jet (*boquilla de los aparatos de alumbrado*)

mechón, *m*, bunch (*de pelo*)

mecos, *m*, *pl*, *vulg*, semen; ~ *m*, *slang*, sperm

media, stocking; ~**s** hose (*stocking*); ~ **compresiva** surgical stocking; ~**s compresivas** leggings (*para después de la cirugía*); ~ **elástica** elastic stocking; ~**s pantalón** panty hose; ~**s para várices** stockings for varicose veins

mediador, -ra, *m/f*, mediator

mediano, *adj*, median; medium

medianoche, *f*, midnight

mediar, to mediate

medicación, *f*, medication; ~ **conservadora** conservative medication; ~ **derivativa** substitutive medication; ~ **tiroides** thyroid pill

Medicaid, *m*, Medicaid

medicamento, drug; medicament; medication; medicine; remedy; ~ **que produce hábito** habit-forming drug; ~**s sicativos** exsiccant drugs

medicar, to medicate

Medicare, *m*, Medicare

medicina, drug; medicament; medication; medicine; remedy; stuff (*medicine*); medicine; ~ **clínica** clinical medicine; ~ **colonial** tropical medicine; ~ **comunal** community medicine; ~ **de la botica** patent medicine; ~ **de la farmacia** patent medicine; ~ **deportiva** sports medicine; ~ **ecológica** environmental medicine; ~ **experimental** experimental medicine; ~ **familiar** family practice; family medicine; ~ **forense** forensic medicine; ~ **geriátrica** geriatric medicine; ~ **homeopática** homeopathic medicine; ~ **interna** internal medicine; ~ **legal** forensic medicine;

medical jurisprudence; ~ **nuclear** nuclear medicine; ~ **ocupacional** occupational medicine; ~ **operatoria** operative medicine; ~ **para dolor** analgesia; ~ **patentada** patent medicine; ~ **preventiva** preventive medicine; ~ **(p)sicosomática**[8] psychosomatic medicine; ~ **registrada** patent medicine; ~ **socializada** socialized medicine; ~ **tropical** tropical medicine; ~ **veterinaria** veterinary medicine

medicinal, *adj*, medicated

medicinar, to dose; to medicate

médico, doctor; M.D.; medical doctor; physician; *adj*, medical; medicine; ~ **a cardo** attending physician; ~ **a cargo** attending physician; ~ **adscrito/médica adscrita** attending physician; ~**asistente** attending physician; ~ **consultor/médica consultora** consulting physician; medical consultant; ~ **de apelación** consulting physician; medical consultant; ~ **de atendencia** attending physician; ~ **de cabecera** attending physician; family doctor; family physician; ~ **de consulta** medical consultant; ~ **de cuidado general** primary care physician; ~ **de guardia** physician on call; ~ **de hospital** house physician; resident physician; ~ **de la familia** family doctor; family physician; ~ **forense** coroner; forensic physician; medical examiner; ~ **general** general/GP practitioner; ~ **interno/médica interna** house surgeon; intern; ~ **practicante** intern; ~ **privado/médica privada** private doctor; ~ **que emite informes** (**para una compañía de seguros**) medical examiner; ~ **recomendante** referring physician; ~ **residente** house/resident physician; ~ **rural** country doctor

medicolegal, *adj*, medicolegal
medida, dose; measure; measurement; ~ **extraordinaria** extraordinary measure; ~ **preventiva** preventive measure; precautionary measure; ~ **de seguridad** safety measure
medio, medium; *m*, *adj*, middle; *adj*, half; ~ **aclarante** clearing medium; ~ **de contraste** contrast medium; ~ **de cultivo** culture medium; ~ **de restricción** restraining device; ~ **dormido** *adj*, half asleep; ~ **nutritivo** nutrient medium; ~ **sordo** hard of hearing; ~**s visuales** visual aids
mediodía, *m*, noon
medir (**i**), to gauge; to measure
meditar, to meditate
medroso, *adj*, afraid; fearful
médula, marrow; ~ **del hueso** bone marrow; ~ **espinal** spinal cord; medulla dorsalis; medulla spinalis; ~ **oblonga(da)** medulla oblongata; ~ **ósea** bone marrow; medulla ossium; ~ **suprarrenal** medulla suprarenal
medusa, jellyfish
megadosis, *f*, *inv*, megadose
megalocito, megalocyte
megalomanía, megalomania
megavitamina, megavitamin
mejilla, cheek
mejor, *adj*, better
Mejoral, *m*, *Mex*, aspirin
Mejoralito, *Mex*, children's aspirin
mejorar, to improve; to progress *Med*; ~(**se**) to get better; to improve
melancolía, melancholia; ~ **agitada** agitated melancholia
melancólico, *adj*, gloomy; melancholy
melanina, melanin
melanoma, *m*, melanoma; ~ **maligno** malignant melanoma
melisa, balm

mella, gap *Dent*; jag (*de una rotura*); ~ **dentaria** gap in the teeth
mellado, *adj*, gap-toothed *Dent*; jagged
mellar, to jag; to lose one's teeth
mellizo, twin
melocotón, *m*, peach
membrana, membrane; ~ **de la placenta** placental membrane; ~ **hialina** hyaline membrane; ~ **mucosa** mucous membrane; ~ **perineal** perineal; ~ **permeable** permeable membrane; ~ **semipermeable** semipermeable membrane; ~ **serosa** serous membrane; ~ **sinovial** synovial membrane; ~ **timpánica** tympanic membrane; ~ **vitelina** yolk sac
memoria, memory; mind; ~ **auditiva** ear memory; ~ **inmediata** short-term memory; ~ **reciente** short-term memory; ~ **remota** long-term memory
memorizar, to memorize
menarca, menarche
menarquia/menarquía, menarche
menárquico, *adj*, menarchal
mención, *f*, mention
mencionar, to mention
menear(se), to jiggle; to sway
meníngeo, *adj*, meningeal
meninges, *f*, *pl*, meninges
meningitis, *f*, meningitis; ~ **aséptica** (**aguda**) (acute) aseptic meningitis; ~ **cerebral** cerebral meningitis; ~ **cerebrospinal** cerebrospinal meningitis; ~ **espinal** spinal meningitis; ~ **linfocítica** lymphocytic meningitis; ~ **tuberculosa** tubercular meningitis
meningococo, meningococcus
menisco, cartilage; meniscus
menjurje, *m*, stuff (*medicina*)
menopausia, change of life; menopause
menopáusico, *adj*, menopausal

menor, *m/f*, *adj*, minor (*edad, tamaño*)
menorragia, menorrhagia
menorralgia, menorrhalgia
menos, *adj*, *adv*, less
mensaje, *m*, message
menstruación, *f*, (*general term*) menses; menstrual period; menstruation; ~ **dolorosa** dysmenorrhea; menorrhalgia
menstrual, *adj*, menstrual
menstruar, to menstruate
menstruo, *sg*, menses
mensualmente, *adv*, monthly
mensuraciones, vital statistics (*de una mujer*)
mental, *adj*, mental
mentalidad, *f*, mentality
mente, *f*, mind; ~ **consciente** conscious mind
mentir (**ie**), to lie (*no decir la verdad*)
mentira, lie; ~ **piadosa** white lie
mentiroso, *adj*, liar
mentol, *m*, menthol
mentolato, *Chicano*, mentholatum
mentón, *m*, chin; mentum
menú, *m*, menu
menudo, *adj*, minor (*insignificante*)
meñique, *m*, little finger
mercurio, mercury
mercurocromo, Mercurochrome
meridiano, meridian; ~ **de la córnea** meridian of the cornea; ~ **del ojo** meridian of the eye
merienda, snack
mertiolato, Merthiolate
mes, *m*, menstruation; month
mesa, table; ~ **basculante** tilt-table; ~ **de cirugía** operating table; ~ **de exámenes** examining table; ~ **de exploración** examining table; ~ **de operaciones** operating table; ~ **de reconocimientos** (**médicos**) examining table; ~ **del parto** delivery table
mescalina[1], mescaline
mesencéfalo, midbrain

mesentérico, *adj*, mesenteric
mesenterio, mesentery
mesenteritis, *f*, mesenteritis
meserole[1], marijuana
mesial, *adj*, *Dent*, mesial
mesiobucal, *adj*, *Dent*, mesiobuccal
mesiobucooclusal, *adj*, *Dent*, mesiobucco-occlusal
mesiobucopulpar, *adj*, *Dent*, mesiobuccopulpal
mesiocervical, *adj*, *Dent*, mesiocervical
mesioclusal, *adj*, *Dent*, mesio-occlusal
mesioclusodistal, *adj*, *Dent*, M.O.D./ mesio-occlusodistal
mesiogingival, *adj*, *Dent*, mesiogingival
mesioincisivo, *adj*, *Dent*, mesio-incisal
mesiolabial, *adj*, *Dent*, mesiolabial
mesiolingual, *adj*, *Dent*, mesiolingual
mesiolinguoclusal, *adj*, *Dent*, mesiolinguo-occlusal
mesmerismo, hypnotism
mesocardio, mesocardium
mesodermo, mesoderm
mesogastrio, mesogastrium
meta, goal
metabólico, *adj*, metabolic
metabolismo, metabolism; ~ **basal** basal metabolism; ~ **constructivo** constructive metabolism; anabolism; ~ **destructivo** destructive metabolism; catabolism; ~ **en reposo** resting metabolism; ~ **endógeno** endogenous metabolism; ~ **exógeno** exogenous metabolism
metabolito, metabolite
metacarpiano, *adj*, metacarpal
metacarpo, metacarpus
metaciclina, metacycline
metadona, methadone
metafase, *f*, metaphase
metáfisis, *f*, metaphysis
metal, *m*, metal; ~ **alcalino** alkali metal

metalergia, metallergy
metamorfosis, *f*, metamorphosis
metampicilina, metampicillin
metano, marsh gas; methane *Chem*
metanol, *m*, methanol
metarcarpiano, *m*, *adj*, metacarpal
metástasis, *f*, metastasis
metastatizar, to metastasize
metatarsalgia, metatarsalgia; Morton's disease
metatarsiano, *adj*, metatarsal
metatarso, metatarsus
metazoos, metazoos; parasite louse; metazoa
meteorismo, meteorism
meter, to insert ; ~**se en un lío** to get into a mess
meticuloso, *adj*, meticulous
metilo, methyl
metílico, *adj*, methyl
metódico, *adj*, orderly
método, method; *Sig/ signetur*/directions; technique; ~ **anticonceptivo** birth control method; ~**s anticonceptivos para no tener niños** birth control methods; ~ **curativo** cure; ~ **de Billing** Billing's method; ~ **de(l) ritmo** rhythm method; ~ **de succión con ventosa** suction cup method; ~ **de tratamiento de las heridas** air dressing; ~ **ortóptico** orthoptic training; ~ **para creatinina** method for creatinine; ~ **que corrige la oblicuidad de los ejes visuales** orthoptic training; ~**s de laboratorio para prótesis dental** dental prosthetic laboratory procedures
metodología, methodology
métrico, *adj*, metric
metro, meter
metrodinia, metrodynia
metrosalpingitis, *f*, metrosalpingitis
mezcla, medley; mixture; to mix (*varios ingredientes*); to stir
mezquino, *Mex*, wart
mialgia, myalgia

miasma, *m*, miasma
miastenia grave, *f*, myasthenia gravis
miatrofia, myatrophy
mica[1], LSD
micción, *f*, miction; micturition; urination; voiding; ~ **al reírse** giggle micturition
micosis, *f*, mycosis
microbacteria, microbacterium
microbiano, *adj*, microbial
microbio, germ; microbe; bug *slang*
microbiología, microbiology
microcirugía, microsurgery
microficha, microfiche
microfilme, *m*, microfilm
microgramo, microgram
micrón, *m*, micron
microonda, microwave
microorganismo, microorganism
microscopia, microscopy
microscopio, microscope; ~ **binocular** binocular microscope; ~ **compuesto** compound microscope; ~ **de fase** phase difference microscope; ~ **electrónico** electron microscope; ~ **fluorescencia** fluorescence microscope
microsección, *f*, microsection
micrótomo, microtome
miedo, fear
miedoso, *adj*, afraid; fearful
miel, *f*, honey
mielastenia, myelasthenia
mielina, myelin
mielinado, *adj*, myelinated
mielinización, *f*, myelinization
mielitis, *f*, myelitis
mielocito, myelocyte
mielograma, *m*, myelogram
mieloide, *adj*, myeloid
mieloma múltiple, *m*, multiple myeloma
miembro, limb; penis; member; ~ **artificial** artificial limb; prosthesis; ~ **de la familia** family member; ~ **fantasma** phantom limb; ~ **viril** viril member *Anat*; ~ **del Colegio**

Norteamericano de Odontólogos F.A.C.D./Fellow of the American College of Dentists; ~ **del Colegio Norteamericano de Médicos** F.A.C.P./Fellow of the American College of Physicians; ~ **del Colegio Norteamericano de Cirujanos** F.A.C.S./Fellow of the American College of Surgeons

miércoles, *m*, *sg*, *euph*, bowel movement; excretion; feces

mierda, *vulg*, bowel movement; feces; shit

migración, *f*, migration

migraña, migraine headache; migraine

migratorio, *adj*, wandering

milagro, miracle

milagroso, *adj*, miraculous

mildeu, *m*, mildew (*en la vid*)

mildiu, *m*, mildew (*en la vid*)

miligramo, milligram

mililitro, ml/milliliter

milimetro, mm/millimeter

milque, *f*, *Chicano*, milk

mimar, to indulge; ~ **con exceso** to overindulge (*a un niño*)

mime[9], *m*, *PR*, gnat (*tipo de insecto*)

mineral, *m*, mineral

mínimo, minimum

ministro, minister

minucioso, *adj*, close (*detallado*); minute; thorough

mioatrofia/miatrofia, myatrophy

miocardia, miocardia/myocardia

miocárdico, *adj*, myocardial

miocardio, myocardium

miocardiopatía, myocardiopathy

miocarditis, *f*, myocarditis

mioceptor, *m*, myoceptor

miodinia, myalgia

miofibrilla, muscle rod; myofibrilla

miope, *m/f*, *adj*, myopic; *adj*, nearsighted; shortsighted

miopía, myopia; nearsightedness; ~ **progresiva** progressive myopia

miópico, *adj*, myopic

miorrelajante, *m*, muscle relaxant

miosclerosis, *f*, myosclerosis

miosis, *f*, myosis

miquear, *Chicano*, to goof off

mirada feroz, glare (*mirada airada*)

mirar, to look (at); ~ **hacia abajo** to look down (*bajar los ojos*); ~ **hacia arriba** to look up; ~ **hacia atrás** to look back

misa, Mass

misantropía, misanthropy

misántropo, *m*, misanthrope; *adj*, misanthropic

misericordia, mercy

misericordioso, *adj*, merciful

misoginia, misogyny

misógino, misogynist; *adj*, misogynous

mitad, *f*, half

mitigar, to alleviate; to ease; to mitigate

mitín popular, *m*, *Chicano*, mass meeting

mitocondria, mitochondria

mitosis, *f*, mitosis

mitral, *adj*, mitral

mixto, *adj*, mixed

mixtura, mixture

mocedad, *f*, youth

moco, mucus

mocosidad, *f*, mucus; phlegm

moda, mode; vogue

modelo, model; paradigm; *adj*, *inv*, model; ~ (**dental**) cast *Dent*; ~ **de diagnóstico** diagnostic cast; ~ **padrón** master cast

moderación, *f*, moderation

moderado, *adj*, moderate; temporate

moderar la marcha, to slow down *Auto*

moderno, *adj*, modern

modesto, *adj*, modest

modificación, *f*, adjustment; change; modification; ~ **de la conducta** behavior modification; ~**es químicas** chemical changes

modificar, to modify

modo, manner; mode; way; ~ **de empleo** instructions for use; ~

de ser makeup (*carácter*); **~ de vivir** life style; way of life /living

modorra, drowsiness

moho, mildew; mold (*hongos*); rust (*del hierro*)

moisés, *m*, *fam*, bassinet

mojado, *adj*, damp; wet

mojar, to moisten; to wet; **~se** to get wet

mola, mole; **~ carnosa** fleshy mole; **~ cística** cystic mole; **~ maligna** invasive mole

molar, *m*, molar; **~ impactado** impacted molar

molde, *m*, die (*instrumento que sirve para estampar o para dar forma a algo*); mold (*pieza en la que se hace en hueco una figura en sólido*)

molécula, molecule

moler (**ue**), to grind; to pound (*machacar*)

molestar, to anger (*enfadar*); to bother; to disturb (*incomodar*); to irritate (*irritar*); to mind (*importarle*); to object to; to trouble (*un dolor*)

molestia, annoyance (*una cosa*); discomfort (*un dolor físico, incomodidad*) disturbance (*inconveniente*); nuisance (*fastidio*)

molesto, *adj*, disturbing (*fastidioso*); irksome; irritating (*irritante*); upset

molido, *adj*, *fam*, aching all over *fig*

mollera, crown of the head; fontanelle; **~ caída**[10] *ethn*, fallen fontanel

mollero, *fam*, biceps

momentáneo, *adj*, fleeting

momento, moment

momia, mummy

momificación, *f*, mummification

mompes, *m*, *pl*, *Chicano*, mumps

mondadientes, *m*, *inv*, toothpick

monga, *PR*, bad cold; influenza; viral infection; (*Vea infección.*)

mongolismo, Down's syndrome; mongolism

mongoloide, *adj*, mongoloid

Monilia, Monilia

moniliasis, *f*, moniliasis

monitor, *m*, monitor; **~ cardíaco** cardiac monitor; pacemaker; **~ cardíaco fetal** fetal heart monitor; **~ cardíaco portátil** Holter monitor

monitoreo, monitoring

monitoría, monitoring; **~ cardíaca** cardiac monitoring; **~ de la presión arterial** blood pressure monitoring; **~ del corazón fetal** fetal heart monitoring; **~ electrónica** electronic monitoring

monitorizar, to monitor

monja, nun

mono, *adj*, cute

monoblasto, monoblast

monocítico, *adj*, monocytic

monocitos, nucleated leukocytes; monocytes

monocular, *adj*, one-eyed

mononucleosis, *f*, mononucleosis; **~ aguda** infectious mononucleosis; **~ infecciosa** infectious mononucleosis

monóxido de carbono, carbon monoxide

monstruo verde[1], marijuana

montaje, *m*, mounting

monte[1], Acapulco gold[2] (*mariguana*); marijuana

monto, total charge/cost

montura, frame (*de gafas*)

moqueadera, *Chicano*, nasal drip

moquear, to have a runny nose; to sniffle

moquera, *fam*, mucus; nasal drip; phlegm

mora[1], marijuana

morado, *adj*, purple; *adj*, *fam*, cyanotic

moral, *f*, morale; *adj*, moral

moraleja, moral

morbilia, measles; morbilli

morboso, *adj*, morbid

mordedura, bite (*animal*; *herida*); **~ de culebra** snake bite; **~ de escorpión** scorpion bite; **~ de ratones**

rat bite; ~ **de serpiente** snake bite; ~ **humana** human bite

morder (**ue**), to bite (*animales*); ~ **a dentelladas** to bite *Dent*; ~ (**los dientes**) to clench (teeth); **~se los labios/las uñas/la lengua** to bite one's lips/nails/tongue

mordida, bite (*animal*); ~ **de gato** cat bite; ~ **de perro** dog bite

mordisco, bite *Dent*; dental impression

moreno, black (*persona*); *SpAm*, mulatto; *adj*, brunette; *adj*, dark (*la tez*); dark skinned; swarthy; tanned; dark haired

morete, *m*, *Mex*, *Hond*, bruise

moreteado, *adj*, black and blue; *adj*, *Chicano*, bruised (*en todas partes*)

moretón, *m*, bruise (*equimosis*); contusion

morfi[1], morphine

morfina, morphine

morfiniento[1], user of morphine

morfinomanía[1], drug habit; morphinomania[2]

morfinómano[1], (drug) addict; junkie[2] (*un drogadicto*)

morfogénesis, *f*, morphogenesis

morfología, morphology

morgue, *f*, *Chicano*, morgue

moribundo, *adj*, dying

morir (**ue**), to die; to expire; ~ **apuñalado** *adj*, to be stabbed to death; ~ **de muerte natural** to die a natural death; **~se de cáncer** to die of cancer; **~se de frío** to freeze to death; **~se de hambre** to starve to death; **~se de miedo** to be scared to death

mormación, *f*, *Chicano*, nasal obstruction

morragia, *Chicano*, hemorrhage

mortal, *adj*, fatal (*accidente*); lethal; mortal

mortalidad, *f*, death rate; mortality; ~ **actual anual** annual actual mortality; ~ **de una enfermedad** case fatality rate; ~ **perinatal** perinatal mortality

mortificarse, *Mex*, *CA*, *Ven*, to be embarrassed

mortinatalidad, *f*, natimortality

mortinato, dead-born; stillbirth; *adj*, stillborn

mosalbete, *m/f*, headstrong teenager

mosca, fly (*insecto*); ~ **volante** floater (*en el ojo*)

mosquito, mosquito

mostacho, moustache

mostaza, mustard; ~[1] marijuana

mostrar (**ue**), to show; ~ **los dientes** to show one's teeth; **~se activo** (**un medicamento**) to work

mota[1], Acapulco gold[2] (*mariguana*); marijuana

mote, *m*, nickname

moteado, *adj*, mottling

motear[1], to blow weed[2] (*fumar mariguana*); to smoke marijuana

motiado[1], *adj*, high on[2] (*mariguana; elevado a mil*)

motiar[1], to blow weed[2] (*fumar mariguana*); to smoke marijuana

moto[1], doper[2]; marijuana user; *slang*, *Mex*, infantum tetanus

motorizar[1], to smoke marijuana

motricidad, *f*, motor functions

mover (**ue**), to move; ~ **a tirones** to jerk (*a trompicones*); ~ **el vientre** to have a bowel movement

móvil, *adj*, mobile; movable; sliding (*escala*)

movilidad, *f*, mobility

movilización, *f*, mobilization

movilizar, to mobilize

movimiento, motion; movement; ~ **asociado** associated movement; ~ **automático** automatic movement; ~ **de la pierna** leg movement; ~ **de vaivén** to and fro movement; ~ **espontáneo** spontaneous movement; ~ **fetal** fetal movement; ~ **mandibular** jaw movement; ~ **mandibular funcional** functional mandibular movement; ~ **ocular rápido** rapid eye movement/REM; ~ **reflejo** reflex movement; ~ **vi-**

bratorio vibrating movement;
~s pasivos passive movements
mozusuelo, *Mex*, infantum tetanus
mucamo, orderly
muchacho, boy
muchacha, girl
muchas veces, *adv*, often
mucílago, mucilage
mucoide, *adj*, mucoid
mucosa, mucous membrane; mucosa
mucosidad, *f*, mucosity; ~ teñida de sangre bloody show
mucoso, *adj*, mucous
mudar, to break (*la voz*); to change; to molt; to move
mudez, *f*, dumbness *Med*; voicelessness; muteness; silence
mudo, *adj*, dumb (*sin poder hablar*); mute; ~ de nacimiento born dumb
mueca, grimace (*de dolor, etc.*)
muela, molar; back tooth; ~ cordal wisdom tooth; ~ de(l) juicio wisdom tooth; third molar
muérdago, mistletoe
muermo, glanders
muerte, *f*, death; fate (*suerte*); ~ aparente apparent death; ~ de familiares death in the family; ~ fetal fetal death; ~ súbita en la cuna crib death; (*Vea syndrome, sudden infant death/SIDS*); ~ súbita del lactante crib death; ~ súbita infantil crib death; ~ violenta casualty
muerto, *m, adj*, dead (*sin vida*); deceased; *fam*, corpse
muestra, gauge (*indicación*); sample; specimen; sign; ~ de excremento stool specimen; ~ de fatiga sign of fatigue; ~ de heces fecales stool specimen; ~ de la orina urine specimen; ~ de orina recogida a mitad de la micción midstream specimen; ~ de sangre blood sample; bloody show

muestreo al azar, random sample/sampling (*estadística*)
muestreo de la vellosidad coriónica, chorionic villi sampling/CVS
mufla, flask *Dent*
muguet, *m/f*, [*Ú.m.c.m.*] fungus—moniliasis; thrush
mujer, *f*, woman; ~ preñada gravida
mujercitas[1], psilocybin
mula[1], runner[2] (*portador de drogas*)
muleta, crutch
multicelular, *adj*, multicellular
multifuncional, *adj*, multifunctional
multípara, multipara
multiparidad, *f*, multiparity
multíparo, *adj*, multiparous
múltiple, *adj*, multiple
multiplicación, *f*, multiplication
mundo, world
muñeca, wrist; doll (*un juguete*)
muñón, *m*, stump (*en una amputación*)
murciélago, bat
mureler[1], LSD
murmullo, heart murmur; humming; murmur (*término general*); murmur (*de la voz, etc.*); ~ aórtico aortic murmur; ~ venoso humming-top murmur; ~ vesicular vesicular murmur
muscular, *adj*, muscular
musculatura, musculature
músculo, muscle; ~ antagonista antagonistic muscle; ~ cardíaco cardiac muscle; ~s del jarrete hamstring muscles; ~ deltoide deltoid muscle; ~ dérmico cutaneous muscle; ~s dorsales muscles of the back; ~ esquelético skeletal muscle; ~ estriado striated muscle; ~s flácidos flabby muscles; ~ flexor flexor muscle; ~ involuntario involuntary muscle; ~ liso smooth muscle; ~s oculares ocular muscles; ~s posteriores del muslo hamstring muscles; ~ transverso transverse muscle; ~

visceral visceral muscle; ~ **voluntario** voluntary muscle
musculoesquelético, *adj*, musculoskeletal
muslo, thigh
mutación, *f*, mutation
mutágeno, mutagen

mutante, *m*, *adj*, mutant
mutilación, *f*, mutilation
mutilar, to deface; to maim; to mutilate
mutismo, voicelessness; mutism
muy alto, *adj*, high up

---

[1] Este vocabulario es nuevo y todavía no se encuentra en el *Diccionario de la lengua española*, publicado por la Real Academia Española. Forma parte del argot o la lengua de la calle. Se supone que el género es obvio a menos que sea indicado.

[2] Forma parte del vocabulario inglés actual de los drogadictos.

[4] Sigo la forma del *Diccionario de la lengua española*, RAE, vigésima primera edición, 1992 que prefiere la *g*. La Academia acepta las variaciones que usan *h* y la lengua de la calle usa variaciones con *j*.

[5] Es un médico que escribe recetas para drogas narcóticas.

[6] *Mal de ijar* o *dolor de ijar* se aplica a cualquier dolor que pega a una mujer por el lado del vientre, de la barriga, o cintura. Puede ser causado por torcijones, apendicitis, infección, quiste o tumor en los ovarios o la matriz, o por infección del sistema urinario.

[7] Se usa esa forma cortada de *malo* antes de sustantivos masculinos singulares.

[8] Hoy es aceptable deletrear las palabras que antes se escribían con *psi-* en español (o *psi-* en inglés) sin la *p* que es consonante silenciosa en este caso.

[9] Un jején chiquitito encontrado en áreas húmedas cerca de la playa cuya picadura dura entre un par de horas y un par de días según la sensibilidad de su víctima.

[10] Esta enfermeded también se llama *caída de la mollera*. Vea la nota que aparece en página 328 acerca de sus causas y su tratamiento.

N

nacer, to be born

nacido, *adj*, born; *m*, tumor; *Carib, fam*, boil; **~s** *m, pl, fam*, abscess; **~ antes de la llegada** b.b.a./born before arrival; **~ muerto** *adj*, dead-born; still-born; **~ vivo** *adj*, liveborn

nacimiento, birth (*parto*); **~ con vida** live birth; **~ múltiple** multiple birth; **~ prematuro** birth premature; **~ tardío** post-term birth

nacionalidad, *f*, nationality

nada, nothing; **~ por (la) boca** NPO/*nihil per os*/nothing by mouth

nadar, to swim

nadie, no one; nobody

nafta, naphtha

naftol, *m*, naphthol

nalga, buttock; **~s** *fam*, bottom (*trasero*); hams *fam*; **~s** butt *vulg*

nanismo, nanism

napalm, *m*, napalm

naqueado, *adj, Chicano*, unconscious

naranja, orange (*fruta*); **~s**[1] amphetamines

narcisismo, ego libido; narcissism

narcisista, *adj*, narcissistic

narco, narcos[2]; narcs[2]; member of police narcotics squad[2]

narcoanálisis, *m, inv*, narcoanalysis

narcohipnosis, *f*, narcohypnosis

narcolepsia, narcolepsy; sleep apnea

narcoléptico, *adj, m*, narcoleptic

narcomanía, drug addiction

narcosis, *f*, narcosis; general anesthesia

narcótico, *m, adj*, drug (*droga*); merchandise[2] *slang*; narcotic; soporific; *sg*, knockout drops[2]; *vulg*, dope[2]

narcotraficante[1], *m/f*, dope pusher[2]; peddler[2] (*vendedor de drogas*)

nariz, *f*, nose; **~ ganchuda** hook(ed) nose; **~ tapada** stopped-up nose; stuffed nose; stuffed-up nose; **~ tupida** stuffed nose; stuffed-up nose

nasal, *adj*, nasal

nasociliar, *adj*, nasociliary

nasogástrico, *adj*, nasogastric

natal, natal

natalidad, *f*, birthrate; **~ dirigida** planned parenthood

natimuerto, stillbirth

nativo, *adj*, native

natural, *adj*, easy (*manera*); natural

naturaleza, nature; **~ de la enfermedad** nature of the illness; **~ humana** human nature

naturalista, *m/f*, naturopath

náusea, nausea; **~s** *pl*, queasiness (*bascas*); **~s del embarazo** morning sickness; **~ sin vomitar** dry heaves

nauseabundo, *adj*, sickening; sickly (*olor*)

nausear, to retch

navaja de afeitar, razor

navajazo, stab (*golpe con un cuchillo*)

navajita, razorblade

nave[1], LSD

nayotas, *pl, slang, Chicano*, nose

nebulización, nebulization

nebulizador, *m*, nebulizer

necesario, *adj*, compulsory; essential; necessary

necesidad, *f*, necessity; need; **~s calóricas** caloric needs; **~s energéticas** energetic needs; **~ urgente** compelling urge

necesitado, *adj*, down[2]; hurting[2] (*en necesidad de drogas*)

necesitar, to need

necrobiosis, *f*, necrobiosis; **~ lipóidica de los diabéticos** necrobiosis lipoidica diabeticorum

necrofilia, necrophilia
necrofobia, necrophobia
necrólisis epidérmica tóxica, scalded skin syndrome
necrología, necrology
necrosar, to necrotize
necrosis, *f*, necrosis; ~ aséptica aseptic necrosis; ~ avascular avascular necrosis; ~ colicuativa colliquative necrosis; ~ de coagulación coagulative necrosis; ~ de tejido adiposo fat necrosis; ~ embólica embolic necrosis; ~ grasa fat necrosis; ~ húmeda moist necrosis; ~ por decúbito decubital necrosis; ~ seca dry necrosis
necrótico, *adj*, necrotic
nefralgia, nephralgia
nefrectomía, nephrectomy
nefrítico, *adj*, nephritic
nefritis, *f*, nephritis; ~ aguda intersticial acute interstitial nephritis; ~ bacteriana bacterial nephritis; ~ crónica chronic nephritis; ~ embólica embolic nephritis; ~ focal focal nephritis; ~ intersticial crónica chronic interstitial nephritis; ~ supurada suppurative nephritis
nefrocalcinosis, *f*, nephrocalcinosis
nefrocistitis, *f*, nephrocystitis
nefrograma, *m*, nephrogram
nefrólisis, *f*, nephrolysis
nefrolito, nephrolith *form*; kidney stone
nefrología, nephrology
nefrólogo, nephrologist
nefroma, nephroma
nefromegalia, enlarged kidney
nefropatía, nephropathy
nefroptosis, *f*, nephroptosis
nefrosclerosis/nefroesclerosis, *f*, nephrosclerosis
nefrosis, *f*, nephrosis; ~ aguda acute nephrosis; ~ crónica chronic nephrosis
nefrótico, *adj*, nephrotic
nefrotomía, nephrotomy

negación, *f*, denial
negar (ie), to deny; ~ con la cabeza to shake one's head; ~se a dar su consentimiento to withhold one's consent
negativismo, negativism
negativo, *m*, *adj*, negative
negligencia, neglect; negligence; ~ médica malpractice
negligente, *adj*, negligent
negro, *adj*, black (*color*); negroid; black (*persona*); ~ de humo lamp black
nematelminto, nemathelminth; roundworm
nematocida, *m*, *adj*, nematocide
nematodo, eel worm; nematode
nena, baby (*infante*); infant
nene, *m*, baby (*infante*); infant
neófito, *m*, *adj*, neophyte
neoformación, *f*, tumor; neoformation
neomicina, neomycin
neón, *m*, neon
neonatal, *adj*, neonatal
neonato, *adj*, newborn; neonate
neonatología, neonatology
neonatólogo, neonatologist
neoplasia, malignant disease; neoplasia
neoplasma, *m*, tumor; neoplasm
neoplástico, *adj*, neoplastic
nervio, nerve; ~s *fam*, anxiety; ~ acústico nerve deafness; ~ aplastado pinched nerve; ~ atrapado pinched nerve; ~ ciático sciatic nerve; ~ comprimido entrapped nerve; ~ craneal cranial nerve; ~ dental dental nerve; ~ hipogloso twelfth nerve; ~ motor motor nerve; ~ neumogástrico vagus; ~ oculomotor third nerve; ~ olfatorio olfactory nerve; ~ óptico optic nerve; ~ parasimpático parasympathetic nerve; ~ pellizcado pinched nerve; ~ sensorial sensory nerve; ~ simpático sympathetic nerve; ~ vago *form*; vagus

nerviosidad, *f*, nervousness
nerviosismo, jitteriness; nervousness
nervioso, *adj*, anxious; nervous
neumatosis, *f*, pneumatosis
neumaturia, pneumaturia
neumococemia, pneumococcemia
neumococo, pneumococcus
neumógrafo, pneumograph
neumólogo, lung specialist; pulmonologist
neumonectomía, pneumonectomy
neumonía, pneumonia; ~ por aspiración aspiration pneumonia
neumonitis, *f*, pneumonitis; pneumonia
neumopatía, lung disease
neumotórax, *m*, pneumothorax
neural, *adj*, neural
neuralgia, neuralgia; ~ cardíaca cardiac neuralgia; ~ degenerativa degenerative neuralgia; ~ del trigémino trigeminal neuralgia; ~ facial face-ache
neurastenia, nervous breakdown; neurasthenia
neurasténico, *adj*, neurasthenic
neuritis, *f*, neuritis; ~ alcohólica alcoholic neuritis; ~ degenerativa degenerative neuritis; ~ diabética diabetic neuritis; ~ palúdica malarial neuritis; ~ traumática traumatic neuritis
neuroanatomía, neuroanatomy
neuroblasto, neuroblast
neuroblastoma, *m*, neuroblastoma
neurocirugía, neurosurgery
neurocirujano, neurosurgeon
neuroendocrinología, neuroendocrinology
neurofarmacología, neuropharmacology
neurofibroma, *m*, neurofibroma
neurofisiología, neurophysiology
neuroléptico, *adj*, neuroleptic
neurología, neurology
neurológico, *adj*, neurologic; neurological
neurólogo, neurologist

neuroma, *m*, neuroma; ~ de amputación amputation neuroma; ~ mielínico myelinic neuroma
neuromuscular, *adj*, neuromuscular
neurona, neuron; ~s nerve cells; ~ aferente afferent neuron; ~ eferente efferent neuron; ~ motora motor neuron; ~ motora inferior lower motor neuron; ~ motora periférica peripheral motor neuron; ~ motora superior upper motor neuron; ~s posganglionares postganglionic neurons; ~s preganglionares preganglionic neurons; ~ sensorial periférica peripheral sensory neuron
neurooftalmología, neuro-ophthalmology
neuropatía, neuropathy
neuropatología, neuropathology
neuro(p)siquiatra[5], *m/f*, neuropsychiatrist
neurosífilis, *f*, neurosyphillis; ~ meningovascular meningovascular neurosyphillis
neurosis, *f*, neurosis; ~ de ansiedad anxiety neurosis; ~ de asociación association neurosis; ~ de indemnización compensation neurosis; ~ obsesivo-compulsiva obsessive-compulsive neurosis; ~ profesional occupational neurosis
neurosquelético, *adj*, neuroskeletal
neurosqueleto, neuroskeleton
neurótico, *adj*, neurotic
neurovascular, *adj*, neurovascular
neutralización, *f*, neutralization
neutralizar, to neutralize
neutro, *adj*, neuter; neutral
neutrófilo, neutrophil; ~ en banda rod neutrophil; ~ filamentoso filamented neutrophil; ~ polimorfonuclear polymorpho-nuclear neutrophil
nevar (ie), to snow
nevera, ice box; refrigerator

nevo, mole (*lunar*); nevus (*mancha en la piel*); ~ **anémico** anemicus nevus; ~ **cavernoso** cavernosus nevus; strawberry nevus; ~ **intermedio** junction nevus; ~ **intradérmico** common mole; ~ **pigmentario** pigmented mole; pigmentosus nevus; ~ **piloso** hairy mole; ~ **vascular** vascularis nevus

NGB/numeración de glóbulos blancos, *f,* WBC/white blood count

NGR/numeración de glóbulos rojos, *f,* RBC/red blood count

niacina, niacin

nice[1], cocaine

nicho, recess (*cavidad pequeña*)

nicotina, nicotine

nictalopia/nictalopía, *form,* night blindness; nyctalopia

nicturia, nycturia

nido, nest

niebla, fog

nieto, grandson

nieve, *f,* snow; sherbet; ~ **carbónica** dry ice; *Mex,* ice cream; ~[1] big C[2] (*cocaína*); candy[2] (*cocaína*); cocaine; coke[2], gin[2]; girl[2]; happy dust[2]; heroin

nigua, chigger flea; chigoe; jigger

nilón, *m,* nylon

ninfómana, nymphomaniac

ninfomanía, nymphomania

ninguno, *pron, adj,* none

niña, girl; ~ **del ojo** pupil of the eye

niñera, baby nurse; nurse (*ama de cría*)

niñez, *f,* childhood

niño[4], child; kid; ~ **rojo** *fam, Costa de Oro,* kwashiorkor; ~**s**[1] psilocybin

nistagmo, nystagmus; ~ **amaurótico** amblyopic nystagmus; ~ **rotatorio** eye rolling

nitrato, nitrate; ~ **de plata** silver nitrate; ~ **de potasio** potassium nitrate

nitrificante, *adj,* nitrifying

nitrito, nitrite

nitro(glicerina), nitro(glycerin)

nitrobenceno, nitrobenzene

nitrógeno, nitrogen; ~ **líquido** liquid nitrogen; ~ **total** total nitrogen

nitroso, nitrous

nivel, *m,* level; ~ **de colesterol** cholesterol count; ~ **de vida** standard of living; ~ **habitual** base-line/baseline (*valor del laboratorio*); ~ **líquido** fluid level

no, no (*en respuestas*); not (*delante de un verbo*); ~ **absorbible** *adj,* nonabsorbable; ~ **adherente** *adj,* nonadherent; ~ **bajar la regla** to miss a period; ~ **dar resultado** to have no effect; ~ **disyunción** *f,* nondisjunction; ~ **doler (ue) ni una uña** *PR,* to be in perfect health; to be in perfect shape; ~ **estar de servicio** to be off duty; ~ **imponible** *adj,* nontaxable; ~ **infeccioso** *adj,* noninfectious; ~ **inflamable** *adj,* nonflammable; ~ **invasor** *adj,* noninvasive; ~ **mostrar (ue) interés alguno en** to be apathetic towards; ~ **parar la pata** *PR,* to be away from home a lot; ~ **pegar ojo en toda la noche** to not have a wink of sleep all night; ~ **permanente** *adj,* deciduous; ~ **picante** *adj,* bland (*comida*); ~ **sentarle (ie) bien a uno** to disagree with one; ~ **sentir (ie) nada** to feel nothing; ~ **soporta peso** NWB/non-weight bearing; ~ **tener pelos en la lengua** not to mince one's words; to be outspoken; ~ **tener razón** *f,* to be wrong; ~ **tratado** *adj,* untreated

noche, *f,* night

noción, *f,* awareness; idea

nocivo, *adj,* bad; deleterious; detrimental; harmful; noxious; ~ **para la salud** bad for one's health

nocturno, *adj,* nocturnal

nodo, node *Card;* ~ **atrioventricular** atrioventricular node; ~ **au-**

riculoventricular auriculoventricular node; ~ **sinoauricular** sinoatrial node

nodriza, baby nurse; wet nurse

nodular, *adj*, nodular

nódulo, node (*nodo*); nodule; ~ **de los cantantes** singers' node; ~ **linfático** lymph node; ~ **vocal** singers' node; ~**s de color amarillo** xanthoma

nombre, *m*, name (*de bautismo*); ~ **común** common name; ~ **de soltera** maiden name

nomenclatura, nomenclature; ~ **binaria** binomial nomenclature

noradrenalina, norepinephrine

norepinefrina, norepinephrine

norma, norm

normal, *adj*, normal

norsa, *Chicano*, nurse (*para los enfermos*)

norte, *m*, north

nose[1], cocaine

nosocomio, *Chicano*, hospital

nostalgia, homesickness; nostalgia

nota[1], *f*, high on[2] (*drogas narcóticas*)

notable, *adj*, marked

notar, to notice; to observe

noticias, news

notificar, to notify

notoriedad, *f*, notoriety

novia, fiancée

novio, fiancé

novocaína, novocaine

nube, *f*, film (*en la córnea del ojo*); nebula; opacity (*del ojo*); ~ **en el ojo** *fam*, cataract

nuca, back of the neck; nape (*del cuello*); neck (*parte posterior del cuello*); ~ **tiesa** *fam*, stiff neck

nuclear, *adj*, nuclear; **colorante ~**, *m*, nuclear stain

núcleo, core; nucleus; ~ **ambiguo** large cell nucleus; ~ **coloreado** nuclear stain

nucléolo, nucleolus

nucleótido, nucleotide

nudillo, knuckle

nudo, knot; node (*general*); ~ **de cirujano** surgeons' knot; ~ **doble** double knot; ~ **en la garganta** gulp (*de ansiedad*); ~ **linfático** *fam*, lymph node

nuevo, *adj*, new

nuez, *f*, nut (*comestible*); ~ **de Adán** Adam's apple; ~ **de la garganta** *fam*, Adam's apple

nuligrávida, nulligravida

nulípara, *f*, *adj*, nonparous; nulliparous

nulo, *adj*, null

numeración de glóbulos blancos, *f*, WBC/white blood count

número, number; ~ **atómico** atomic number; ~ (*de zapatos, guantes*) size

nunca, *adv*, never; not ever

nutricio, nutrient; *adj*, nutritious

nutrición, *f*, nourishment; nutriment; nutrition; ~ **defectuosa** malnutrition; ~ **parenteral total** total parenteral nutrition

nutricional, *adj*, nutritional

nutrimento, nutriment

nutriólogo, nutritionist

nutrir, to nourish

nutritivo, *adj*, nourishing; nutritional; nutritious; *m*, nutrient

---

[1] Este vocabulario es nuevo y todavía no se encuentra en el *Diccionario de la lengua española*, publicado por la Real Academia Española. Forma parte del argot o la lengua de la calle. Se supone que el género es obvio a menos que sea indicado.

[4] Muchas variantes existen para este sustantivo. Hay la influencia de los muchos dialectos indios de todas partes.

[5] Hoy es aceptable deletrear las palabras que antes se escribían con *psi-* en español (o *psy-* en inglés) sin la *p* que es consonante silenciosa en este caso.

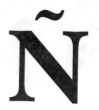

ñácara, *CA*, ulcer; *CA*, sore

ñame, *m*, yam

ñangado, *adj*, *Cu*, knock-kneed; bow-legged

ñango, *adj*, *slang*, stupid; *adj*, *PR*, idiotic; *adj*, *Mex*, weak; feeble; *Chi*, short-legged; *Arg*, *Ur*, clumsy

ñangotao, *adj*, *slang*, submissive

ñangotarse, *Col*, *PR*, to squat; to crouch down

ñangue, *adj*, *PR*, idiotic

ñanguería, *slang*, stupidity

ñaño, *Col*, *Perú*, child

ñata, *SpAm*, nose; *Peru*, death

ñeques, *m*, *Ec*, fists

ñisca, *CA*, *Col*, excrement

ñoca, *Col*, crack; fissure

ñoco, *PR*, *fam*, amputee; *adj*, *Col*, *PR*, *SD*, *Ven*, one-handed; missing a finger; *PR*, *fam*, amputee

ñola, *Col*, *Guat*, excrement; *Guat*, *Hond*, ulcer; sore

ñoño, cuddling

ñusca, *Col*, *Ec*, excrement

ñutir, to grunt

o[4], or
obedecer, to obey
obediencia, obedience
obediente, *adj*, obedient
obesidad, *f*, obesity
obeso, *adj*, fat; obese
obituario, obituary
objeción, *f*, objection
objetar, to object
objetivo, goal; objective
objeto, object
oblicuo, *adj*, oblique
obligación, *f*, obligation
obligado, *adj*, compulsory; obliged
obligar, to obligate; ~ **a guardar cama** to lay up (*tener que guardar cama*)
obligatorio, *adj*, obligatory
obnubilación, *f*, obnubilation
obradera, *Col, Guat, Pan*, diarrhea
obrar[5], to work; *Mex, CA, fam,* to have a bowel movement; to move the bowels; ~ **con sangre** to have dysentery
obscenidad, lewdness
obsceno, *adj*, lewd
observación, *f*, follow-up; observation; ~ **continuada** monitoring; ~ **médica** case report
observador, -ra, *m/f, adj*, observant; observer
observar, to notice; to observe
obsesión, *f*, obsession; ~ **con el fuego** pyromania
obsesivo-compulsivo, *adj*, obsessive-compulsive
obstaculizar, to hinder; to interfere
obstáculo, bar; obstacle
obstetra, *m/f*, obstetrician
obstetricia, midwifery; obstetrics
obstétrico, obstetrician; *adj*, obstetric; obstetrical
obstrucción, *f*, block (*bloqueo*); blockage; obstruction; *SpAm,* interference; ~ **de la tripa** bowel obstruction; ~ **intestinal** intestinal obstruction
obstructivo, *adj*, obstructive
obstruir, to block (*Anat: cerrar; Dent: estorbar*); to hinder; to obstruct; ~ **el nervio** to block the nerve
obtener, to get; to obtain
obturación, *f*, inlay; obturation; ~ **dentaria** dental obturation
obturador, *m, adj*, obturator
obturar, *form,* to fill *Dent;* to obturate
obtuso, *adj*, blunt; obtuse
obvio, *adj*, obvious
occipital, *m, adj*, occipital
occipucio, occiput
ocio, leisure; **ratos de** ~ leisure time
ocitócico, *adj*, oxytocics
ocitocina, oxytocin
ocluir, to occlude; ~**se** to occlude *Dent*
oclusal, *adj*, occlusal
oclusante, *adj*, occluding
oclusión, *f*, occlusion; ~ **anormal** abnormal occlusion; ~ **balanceada mecánicamente** mechanically balanced occlusion; ~ **borde a borde** edge-to-edge occlusion; ~ **bucal** buccal occlusion; ~ **de la mufla** flask closure; ~ **de los dientes** contact of teeth; ~ **de prueba de la mufla** trial flask closure; ~ **distal** distal occlusion; ~ **intestinal** intestinal occlusion; ~ **labial** labial occlusion; ~ **lingual** lingual occlusion
oclusivo, *adj*, occlusive
ocronosis, *f*, ochronosis
octano, octane
ocular, *m*, eyepiece; *m, adj*, ocular

oculectomía, ocular enucleation

oculista, *m/f*, oculist

ocultar, to conceal; to hold back (*la verdad*)

oculto, *adj*, latent (*escondido*); occult

ocupación, *f*, occupation

ocupacional, *adj*, occupational

ocupado, *adj*, busy (*persona*); occupied; **estar ocupada** to be pregnant (*para mujeres*)

ocupar, to occupy; **~se de** to look after

ocurrir, to happen; to occur

odiar, to hate

odio, hate

odontalgia, toothache

odontología, *form*, dentistry; odontology; **~ operatoria** operative dentistry; **~ preventiva** preventive dentistry; **~ prostética** prosthetic dentistry; **~ quirúrgica** dental surgery

odontólogo, dental surgeon; dentist; odontologist

odontonecrosis, *f*, tooth decay

odontopediatra, *m/f*, pediatric dentist

odontoplerosis, *f*, dental filling

odontoscopio, dental mirror; odontoscope

ofender, to offend

ofensa, offense

oferta, offer

oficial, *m, adj*, official

oficina, office

oficio, occupation

ofrecer, to offer

ofrecimiento, offer

oftalmía, ophthalmia (*inflamación del ojo*); **~ contagiosa** conjunctivitis; pinkeye

oftálmico, *adj*, ophthalmic

oftalmología, ophthalmology

oftalmólogo, ophthalmologist

oftalmoplejía, ophthalmoplegia

oftalmoscopia, ophthalmoscopy; retinoscopy

oftalmoscopio, ophthalmoscope

oído, ear (*órgano de oír*); hearing; **~ externo** external ear; outer ear; **~ interno** inner ear; labyrinth; **~ medio** middle ear

oír, to hear; **~ por casualidad** to overhear; **~ voces** to hear voices; *m*, hearing

ojeada, glance

ojera, circle under the eye; eye cup; **~s** eye shield

ojeroso, *adj*, hollow-eyed (*causado por enfermedad o fatiga*); haggard

ojete, *m*, *slang*, anus; arse *slang* (*ano*)

ojituerto, *adj*, squint-eyed; cross-eyed

ojo, eye; **~ amoratado** black eye; **~s capotudos** *Chicano*, bulging eyes; **~ de pescado** *fam*, plantar wart; **~ de vidrio** glass eye; **~ derecho** *o.d./oculus dexter/*right eye; **~ excitante** exciting eye; **~s fatigados** eyestrain; **~ inyectado de sangre** bloodshot eye; **~ izquierdo** *o.l./oculus laevus/*left eye; **~s llorosos** watery eyes; **~ monocromático** monochromatic eye; **~ morado** black eye; **~s, oídos, nariz y garganta** EENT/eyes, ears, nose and throat; **~s saltones** bulging eyes; **~ simpatizante** sympathizing eye; **~ tricromático** trichromatic eye

ojotes, *m*, *pl*, *CA, Col*, bulging eyes

ola, wave

oleadas de calor, flushes

oleólico, medicinal oil

oleoso, *adj*, oily

oler (ue), to smell; **~ cola**[1] to be flashing[6]; **~ mal** to smell nasty

olfativo, *adj*, olfactory

olfato, smell; *adj*, olfactory

olfatorio, *adj*, olfactory

oligoelemento, trace element

oliva, olive

olla, *slang*, *Chicano*, buttock

olor, *m*, odor; smell

olvidadizo, *adj*, absent-minded; forgetful

olvidar, to forget; **~se (de)** to forget

ombligo, belly button; navel; umbilicus; **~ salido** *slang*, umbilical hernia

ombligón, *m, slang,* umbilical hernia

ombliguero, belly binder

omisión, *f,* failure

omitir, to omit

omóplato, shoulder blade; scapula

O.M.S./organización para el mantenimiento de la salud, *f,* H.M.O./health maintenance organization

onanismo, onanism

oncocercosis/oncocerciasis, *f, form,* onchocerciasis; river blindness

oncógeno, *adj,* oncogenic; oncogenous

oncología, oncology

oncólogo, oncologist

oncoterapia, oncotherapy

onda, wave; **~ cerebral** brain wave; **~s sonoras** sound waves

onfalocele, *m,* omphalocele

onicofagia, onychophagia; nail biting

onicosis, *f,* onychosis

oniquia, onychia

onza, ounce; **~ líquida** fluid ounce

ooforectomía, oophorectomy

oogénesis, *f,* oogenesis

opa, *adj, Bol, Perú, Ríopl,* deaf and dumb

opacidad, *f,* cloudiness; haziness; opacity; **~ corneal** corneal opacity

opaco, *adj,* dull (*color*); opaque

opción, *f,* choice; option

operable, *adj,* operable

operación, *f,* operation; **~ cesárea** caesarean section; **~ de derivación** by-pass operation; **~ en dos tiempos** two-stage operation; **~ facial de estética** face lift

operar, to operate; **~ con éxito a un paciente** to bring a patient through; **~se (de)** to have an operation (on/for)

operativo, *adj,* operative

opiáceo, *m, adj,* opiate

opiado, opiate

opiato, opiate

opinión, *f,* opinion

opio, opium; **~ granulado** granulated opium; **~ pulverizado** powdered opium

opiomanía[1], opium addiction

opiómano[1], opium addict

oponer, to oppose

oportunidad, *f,* opportunity

oportunista, *m/f, adj,* opportunist; *adj,* opportunistic

oportuno, *adj,* well-timed

oposición, *f,* opposition

opoterapia, opotherapy; organotherapy

OPP/organización de proveedor preferido, *f,* PPO/preferred provider organization

opresión, *f, Med,* difficulty in breathing; tightness of the chest; **sentir (ie) ~** to find it difficult to breathe

opresivo, *adj,* crushing (*dolor*); oppressive

oprimir, to constrict (*comprimir*); to oppress

óptica, optics

óptico, optician; *adj,* optic; optical

optometría, optometry

optometrista, *m/f,* optometrist

opuesto, *adj,* opposite

oral, *adj,* oral

orange[1], LSD

órbita, eye socket; orbit; socket (*del ojo*)

orden, *(pl, órdenes) f,* order (*autorización*); regulations; **~ escrita** written order; **~es médicas** doctor's orders; *m,* order (*armonía; categoría*)

ordenado, *adj,* orderly

ordenar, to order

ordeñar, to milk

ordeño, milking

orear, to air (*colgar para secar*)

oreja, ear; external ear; outer ear

orejón, *m, Col,* goiter
orejudo, *adj,* big-eared
orgánico, *adj,* organic
organigrama, *m,* flowchart
organismo, organism; system
organización, *f,* organization; ~ **del mantenimiento de la salud** *f,* H.M.O./health maintenance organization; ~ **para el mantenimiento de la salud** *f,* H.M.O./ health maintenance organization
organizador, -ra, *m/f,* organizer
organizar, to organize
órgano, organ; ~ **absorbente** absorbent organ; ~ **de choque** organ of shock; **~s de los sentidos** sense organs; ~ **errante** wandering organ; **~s genitales** genitals; ~ **sensorio** sense organ; **~s vitales** vital organs
orgasmo, orgasm; ~ **sexual** sexual climax
orgullo, pride
orgulloso, *adj,* proud
orientación, *f,* orientation
orientado hacia el centro, *adj,* mesial
oriental, *adj,* oriental
orificación, *f,* inlay
orificar, to fill with gold
orificio, hole; orifice; ~ **de aeración** air vent
origen, *m,* origin
original, *adj,* original
orín, *m,* rust (*en hierro*); urine; **orines** *pl,* urine
orina, urine; ~ **de la mitad de la micción** midstream jet of urine
orinal, *m,* bedpan; urinal
orinar, to micturate; to urinate; to void; ~ **demasiado** *m,* polyuria; ~ **muy de seguido** *m,* frequent urinating; **~se** to urinate (involuntarily)
oriundo, *adj,* native born; *m,* native
oriza, acute catarrhal rhinitis
oro, gold; ~ **verde**[1] marijuana
orquidectomía, orchidectomy; orchiectomy

orquiectomía, orchidectomy; orchiectomy
orquiotomía, orchiotomy
orquitis, *f,* orchitis
ortodoncia, orthodontia; orthodontics
ortodoncista, *m/f, adj,* orthodontist; orthodontic
ortodóntico, *adj,* orthodontic
ortodontista, *m/f, adj,* orthodontist
ortopedia, orthopedics
ortopédico, orthopedist; ~ **dental** orthodontist; *adj,* orthopedic
ortopedista, *m/f, adj,* orthopedist
ortóptica, orthoptics
ortóptico, *adj,* orthoptic
ortoptista, *m/f,* orthoptist
ortoptoscopio, orthoptoscope
ortoscópico, *adj,* orthoscopic
ortoscopio, orthoscope
oruga, caterpillar
orzuelo, sty
oscilación, *f,* oscillation
oscilador, *m,* oscillator
oscilar, to oscillate; to swing (*vacilar*)
oscilógrafo, oscillograph
osciloscopio, oscilloscope
oscurecer, to grow dark
oscuro, *adj,* dark; dim (*sin brillo*)
óseo, *adj,* bone; bony; osseous
osículo, ossicle
osificación, *f,* ossification
osificar, to ossify
osteítis, *f,* osteitis; ~ **fibroquística** fibrosa cystica osteitis
osteoartritis, *f,* osteoarthritis; chronic rheumatism
osteoblasto, osteoblast
osteofito, osteophyte
osteogénesis, *f,* osteogenesis; ~ **imperfecta** brittle bones; osteogenesis imperfecta
osteogénico, *adj,* osteogenic
osteología, osteology
osteoma, *m,* osteoma
osteomielitis, *f,* osteomyelitis
osteonecrosis, *f,* osteonecrosis
osteópata, *m/f,* osteopath/D.O.

osteopatía, osteopathy
osteopático, *adj*, osteopathic
osteoporosis, *f*, osteoporosis; ~ **adiposa** adipose osteoporosis
osteosarcoma, *m*, osteosarcoma
osteosclerosis, *f*, osteosclerosis
osteosis, *f*, osteosis
osteotomía, osteotomy
ostra, oyster
otalgia, otalgia
ótico, *adj*, otic
otitis, *f*, otitis; ~ **externa** otitis externa; ~ **interna** labyrinthitis; otitis interna; ~ **media** otitis media; ~ **media aguda** acute ear
otoconio, ear dust
otofaríngeo, *adj*, otopharyngeal
otófono, hearing aid
otología, otology
otólogo, otologist
otorrea, otorrhea
otorrinolaringología, otolaryngology; otorhinolaryngology
otorrinolaringólogo, ENT/ear, nose and throat specialist; otolaryngologist; otorhinolaryngologist
otosalpinge, *m*, otosalpinx
otosclerosis, *f*, otosclerosis
otoscopia, otoscopy
otoscopio, eartrumpet; otoscope
otro, *adj*, other
oval, *m*, *adj*, oval
ovárico, *adj*, ovarian

ovariectomía, ovariectomy
ovario, *adj*, ovarian; ovary; ~ **poliquístico** polycystic ovary
ovariotomía, ovariotomy
oviducto, oviduct; ~**s de los mamíferos** Fallopian tubes
ovogénesis, *f*, oogenesis; ovogenesis
ovulación, *f*, ovulation; ~ **amenstrual** ovulation
ovular, to ovulate
óvulo, egg; ovum (*pl*, *ova*); ~**s** *pl*, vaginal suppositories
ovulogénesis, *f*, ovulogenesis
oxidación, *f*, oxidation
oxidar, to oxidize; to oxygenate; ~**(se)** to rust
oxidasa, oxidase
óxido, oxide; ~ **de carbono** carbon monoxyde; ~ **de cinc** zinc oxide; ~ **nitroso** gas *Chem*; nitrous oxide
oxigenación, *f*, oxygenation
oxigenado, *adj*, oxygenate
oxigenador, *m*, oxygenator
oxigenar, to oxygenize; to ventilate (*sangre*); to oxygenate
oxígeno, oxygen
oxigenoterapia, oxygen treatment
oxitocia, oxytocia
oxitócico, *adj*, oxytocic
oxitocina, oxytocin
oxiuro, pinworm; threadworms
ozono, ozone

---

[1] Este vocabulario es nuevo y todavía no se encuentra en el *Diccionario de la lengua española*, publicado por la Real Academia Española. Forma parte del argot o la lengua de la calle. Se supone que el género es obvio a menos que sea indicado.
[4] Antes de palabras que empiezan con *o* o con *ho*, la *o* cambia a la *u*.
[5] Este verbo también significa *evacuar*.
[6] Es la reacción eufórica inicial que tiene una persona al picarse con drogas narcóticas intravenosas.

P

PABA/ácido para-aminobenzoico, PABA/para-aminobenzoic acid

pabellón, *m*, ward; **~ externo de la oreja** *Anat*, external ear

pábulo, pabulum

pacha, *Chicano, CA*, baby bottle

pachaco, *adj, CA*, weak; feeble

pachangiar, *fam*, to have a good time

paciencia, patience

paciencioso, *adj, Chi, Ec*, patient

paciente, *m/f, adj*, patient; **~ ambulante** outpatient; **~ ambulatorio** ambulatory patient; outpatient; **~ con buen estado general** good risk patient; **~ con escaso riesgo** good risk patient; **~ de consulta externa** outpatient; **~ en fase terminal** terminally ill patient; **~ externo** outpatient

padecer, to withstand; **~ (de)** to suffer (from)

padecimiento, ailment; illness; sickness; suffering

padrastro, stepfather; *Med*, hangnail of finger

padre, *m*, father; **~s** *m, pl*, parents

padrino, godfather

pagado con anticipación, *adj*, prepaid

pagar, to pay (for); **~ al contado** to pay (in) cash; **~ por adelantado** to pay in advance; **cuenta a ~** outstanding account; unpaid bill

página, page

pago, payment

pagua, *Chi*, hernia

paguacha, *Anat*, hump; *Anat, fam*, head

país, *m*, country (*nación*)

paja, straw

pájaro, bird; homosexual

pajón, *Mex*, (*pelo*) straight

pala, shovel; *PR*, (**fig: buenas relaciones con gente que lo tiene todo**) influence

palabra, power of speech; faculty of speech; word; **perder (ie) la ~** to lose one's power of speech

paladar, *m*, palate; roof of mouth; **~ blando** soft palate; **~ duro** hard palate; bony palate; **~ hendido** cleft palate; **~ membranoso** soft palate; **~ óseo** hard palate; bony palate; **~ partido** cleft palate

palanca, lever

palangana, basin (*jofaina*); *Mex* washbowl/washbasin

palatino, *adj, Anat*, palatal

palatosquisis, *f*, cleft palate

paleta, bedpan; *fam*, tongue depressor; *Anat*, shoulder blade

paletero, *Ec*, tuberculosis

paletilla, *Anat*, shoulder blade (*omóplato*)

paliar, to alleviate

paliativo, *m, adj*, palliative

palidecer, to fade (*descolorarse*); to turn pale

palidez, *f*, pallor

pálido, *adj*, pale; sickly (*apariencia*)

palidoso, *adj, Perú*, pale; sickly (*apariencia*)

palillo de dientes, toothpick

paliquear, to chat

paliza, beating

palma, palm (*árbol; de la mano*); *PR*, tall person; **~ de la mano** palm; palm of the hand

palmada, slap (*golpe con la palma de la mano*)

palmar, *adj*, palmar

palmotearse las rodillas, to slap one's knees

palo, stick (*vara, pedazo de madera, etc.*); *fam*, straight shot of alcoholic drink; *slang*, (*prick*) penis

paloma, pigeon
palomitas de maíz, *f, pl,* popcorn
palpación, *f,* feeling (*método exploratorio donde se aplica los dedos o la mano sobre las partes externas del cuerpo*); palpation
palpar, to feel (for) (*tocar*); to palpate
palpitación, *f,* beat (*corazón*); fast heartbeat; flutter; heartbeat; palpitation; tachycardia; throb; ~ **cardíaca/cardiaca** heart palpitation; ~ **irregular** irregular heartbeat (*arritmia*); ~ **lenta** slow heartbeat; ~ **rápida** rapid heartbeat (*taquicardia*); ~ **rítmica** rhythmical heartbeat
palpitante, *adj,* throbbing (*corazón*)
palpitar, to beat (*corazón*); to flutter; to palpitate; to pound
palúdico, *adj, Med,* malarial
paludismo, fever; malaria; marsh fever; paludism; ~ **autóctono** autochthonous malaria
paludología, malariology
paludólogo, malariologist
pan, *m,* bread
pana, *Chi,* liver
panacea, cure-all
panadizo, felon
páncreas, *m,* pancreas
pancreático, *adj,* pancreatic
pancreatina, pancreatin
pancreatitis, *f,* pancreatitis
pancreocimina, pancreozymin
pandilla, gang (*callejera*)
panetela[1], marijuana
panículo adiposo subcutáneo, subcutaneous panniculus adiposus
pantaletas, *Mex,* panty/panties
pantalla, screen; (lamp)shade (*una lámpara*); *PR,* earring (*que no cuelga del lóbulo*); ~ **de plomo** lead screen
pantalón/pantalones, *m,* [*Ú.m.e.p.*], pants; slacks; trousers; *sg, Ec, Perú,* man; male

pantaloncillos, shorts (*calzoncillos*); men's underpants
pantimedias, panty hose
pantorrilla, calf (*pl, calves*) (*parte de la pierna*)
pantufla, slipper
panza, *fam,* abdomen; belly; paunch; *Chicano,* stomach; ~ **peligrosa** *slang,* appendicitis; bowel obstruction; peritonitis
panzazo, *Arg, Para, Perú,* blow to the stomach/belly
panzón, panzona, *adj,* potbellied; **panzona** *vulg,* pregnant
panzudo, *adj,* paunchy; potbellied
pañal, *m,* diaper; ~ **de tela** cloth diaper; ~ **desechable** disposable diaper
pañalitis, *f,* diaper rash
paño, chloasma (*descoloración facial, marca de embarazo*) *Med;* diaper; ~ (**caliente**) (hot) pack; ~ **de lavarse** washcloth; ~ **higiénico** sanitary napkin; sanitary towel; **~s en los ojos** eyepads
pañuelo, handkerchief; ~ **de papel** facial tissue; Kleenex; tissue (*papel*); **~s faciales** facial tissues
papa, *SpAm,* potato
papá, *m,* father
papada, double chin
papagayo, parrot; *Perú,* chamberpot; **enfermedad de los ~s** *f,* parrot fever
Papanicolaou, *m,* Pap smear; **test de ~** *m,* Pap smear
papaya, *SpAm,* papaya
papel, *m,* paper; ~ **de baño** toilet paper; toilet tissue; ~ **de excusado** toilet paper; ~ **de tornasol** litmus paper; ~ **higiénico** toilet paper; ~ **sanitario** toilet paper *CA;* **~**[1] heroin; LSD
papelera, waste basket
papelito[1], heroin
paper[1], LSD
paperas, mumps

papila, papilla; ~ **gustativa** taste-bud; ~ **interdentaria** gingival septum

papiloma, *m*, papilloma; **virus del** ~ **humano** *m*, human papilloma virus

papilomavirus humano/virus del papiloma humano, *m*, human papilloma virus/HPV

papo, *Med*, goiter

papudo, *adj*, double-chinned

papujo, *adj*, *Mex*, sickly; anemic; swollen

pápula, wheal; papule

paque de drogas[1], *m*, dime bag[2,4] (*un paquete de heroína, cocaína, o mariguana*)

paquete, *m*, bag; package; pack; ~[1] bindle[2] (*cantidad de mariguana y narcóticos*); ~ **de vendas** first aid packet

paquimeninge, *f*, pachymeninx

paquimeningitis, *f*, pachymeningitis

par, *m*, couple; pair; *f*, *pl*, placenta *sg*; *adj*, even (*número*)

para, *prep*, for; toward; in regard to; in order to; ~ **abajo** down; downward; downwards; ~ **arriba** up; upward; upwards; ~ **estar seguro** (in order) to be sure; ~ **uso externo** not to be taken internally

para-aminosalicílico, ácido/PAS, para-aminosalicylic acid/PAS

paracentesis, *f*, paracentesis

paracinesia, parakinesia

paradentio, paradentium

paradentitis, *f*, paradentitis

paradentosis, *f*, paradentosis

parado, estar, *adj*, *SpAm*, to be standing (up)

parafasia, paraphasia

parafina, paraffin

paraguas, *m*, *inv*, umbrella; *slang*, rubber (*condón*); *Col*, *Cu*, *Mex*, fungus

parálisis, *f*, palsy; paralysis; (cerebrovascular) stroke; ~ **agitante** Parkinson's disease; shaking palsy (*enfermedad de Parkinson*); ~ **ascendente aguda** acute ascending paralysis; ~ **bilateral** diplegia; ~ **bulbar crónica progresiva** Duchenne's paralysis; ~ **cerebral** cerebral palsy; cerebral paralysis; ~ **de la mitad inferior del cuerpo** paraplegia; ~ **de un lado del cuerpo** hemiplegia; ~ **facial** Bell's palsy; ~ **infantil** infantile paralysis; polio(myelitis); ~ **obstétrica** obstetrical paralysis; ~ **periódica familiar** familial periodic paralysis; ~ **progresiva** creeping paralysis

paralítico, *adj*, paralyzed; paralytic

paralización, *f*, numbness; palsy; paralysis

paralizar, to paralyze

paramédico, paramedic

parametrio, parametrium

parámetro, parameter; ~**s vitales** vital parameters

paranoia, paranoia

paranoico, *m*, *adj*, paranoid

parapareunia, extravaginal coitus

paraplasia, paraplasm

paraplejía, paraplegia; ~ **alcohólica** alcoholic paraplegia; ~ **espástica infantil** congenital spastic paraplegia

parapléjico, *adj*, paraplegic

para(p)sicología[6], parapsychology

parar(se), to stand up; to stop

parasimpático, *adj*, parasympathetic

parasitario, *adj*, parasitic

parasitismo, parasitism

parásito, parasite; *adj*, parasitic

parasitología, parasitology

parasitosis, *f*, parasite infestation

paratifoidea, *f*, paratyphoid

paratifoideo, *adj*, paratyphoid

paratifus, *f*, paratyphoid fever

paratiroidectomía, parathyroidectomy

paratiroides, *f*, *adj*, parathyroid

parche, *m*, dressing (*tirita*); patch;

~ **mucosa** mucous patch; ~**s para callos** corn plaster

parchecito, Bandaid

parcho, *Ven* (*Vea parche.*)

parcial, *adj*, partial

parcialmente sordo, hard of hearing

pardo, *adj*, brown

parecer, *m*, advice

parecer, to seem; ~ **enfermo** *adj*, to look ill

pared, *f*, wall; ~ **de los vasos sanguíneos** wall of the blood vessels; ~ **torácica** chest wall; ~ **vascular** vessel wall/V.W.; ~**es del sistema digestivo** walls of the digestive system

paregórico, paregoric

pareja, partner; other one (of a pair)

parénquima, *m*, parenchyma

parenteral, *adj*, parenteral; **vía** ~ parenteral route

parentesco, relation; relationship

paresia, paresis

pariente, relative; ~ **cercano** close relative; ~ **más cercano** next of kin; ~**s** *m*, *pl*, kin

parietal, *adj*, parietal

parir, to give birth; to deliver; *esp. Carib, fam*, to bear (*un niño*); *PR*, to vomit

paro, arrest; ~ **cardíaco** cardiac arrest; cardiac standstill; heart failure; ~ **del corazón** heart failure; ~ **respiratorio** respiratory arrest

paroniquia, paronychia

parorquidia, parorchidium

parótida, mumps; parotid; ~**s** *pl*, mumps

parotídeo, parotid

parotiditis, *f*, mumps

paroxismo, fit; paroxysm

paroxístico, *adj*, paroxysmal

parpadear, to blink; to flutter (*párpados*)

parpadeo, blink; eyelid winking; flutter (*de párpados*)

párpado, eyelid; ~ **superior** upper eyelid; **restregarse los** ~**s** to rub one's eyes

parque de niños, *m*, play pen

parte, *f*, part; ~ **artificial** prosthesis; ~ **baja de la espalda** lower back; ~ **del cuerpo** body part; ~**s** *pl*, *slang*, genitals; private parts; ~**s ocultas** *slang*, genitals; pubic region; ~**s privadas** *slang*, genitals; private parts; ~**s pudendas** genitals; privates *slang*

partear, *Obst*, to deliver

partenogénesis, *f*, parthenogenesis

partera, midwife (*con licencia, diplomada*)

participación, *f*, participation

participar, to participate

partícula flotante, floater (*en el ojo*)

particular, *adj*, particular; private

partida, certificate; ~ **de bautismo** baptismal certificate; ~ **de defunción** certificate of death; death certificate; ~ **de matrimonio** marriage certificate; ~ **de nacimiento** birth certificate

partido, *adj*, chapped; split; *adj*, *PR*, effeminate

partidura, fissure

partir, to split (*dividir*); ~ **en rajas** to slice (*rebanadas, etc.*); ~**se** to chap; ~**se unos dientes** to knock out some teeth; ~(**se**) *Cu*, to break *Ortho*

parto, birth (*nacimiento*); childbirth; delivery; labor; ~ **abdominal** abdominal delivery; ~ **artificial** artificial delivery; ~ **cesáreo** caesarean delivery; ~ **complicado** complicated labor; ~ **con fórceps** forceps assisted delivery; ~ **de nalgas** breech delivery; ~ **espontáneo** spontaneous labor; spontaneous delivery; ~ **falso** false labor pains; ~ **forzado** forced delivery; ~ **indoloro** natural childbirth; ~ **inducido** induced labor; ~ **inmaturo** immature labor; ~ **instrumental** instrumental labor; ~ **malogrado** miscarriage; ~ **muerto** stillbirth; ~ **múltiple** multiple childbirth; multiple birth; multiple labor; ~ **natural** natural birth; natural childbirth; ~ **podálico** podalic labor; ~ **por operación** caesarean delivery; ~ **prematuro** early birth; premature childbirth; premature delivery; premature labor; ~ **prematuro habitual** habitual premature labor; ~ **prolongado** delayed delivery; extended labor; prolonged labor; ~ **provocado** induced delivery; ~ **seco** dry labor; **asistir un ~** to deliver a baby; **estar de ~** to be in labor; **tener un ~ difícil** to have a difficult labor

parturición, *f*, parturition

parturienta, *f*, woman in labor; woman who has just given birth

pasa, raisin

pasado mañana, day after tomorrow

pasajero, *adj*, fleeting

pasar, to get over (*curarse de una enfermedad*; to give (*un catarro a alguien*); to endure; to go through (*dolor físico, desgracias, etc.*); to make (*una llamada; una visita*); to suffer; to happen; to pass; to wear off; ~ **gas** to pass gas; ~ **la mano sobre la superficie de** to rub; ~ **la noche** to stay overnight; ~ **por** to be considered; to enter; to go (through) (*atravesar*); to pass over; to go through (*sufrir una operación*); ~ **por alto** to leave out; to skip; to forget about; ~ **revista** to list; to review (*problemas*); ~ **vergüenza** to be embarrassed; ~ **visita** to call; to make a call; to pay a visit; ~**se** to get over

pasatiempo, hobby; pastime

pase, *m*, pass; ~ **del cuerpo** bowel movement; feces; ~[1] a fix of heroin[2] (*un filerazo que viene de aspirar heroína*); a hit of cocaine

or heroin[2]; a hit of marijuana[2]; *PR*, toke of marijuana or hashish

pasillo, hall; hallway; passage (*corredor*)

pasivo, *adj*, passive; ~**-agresivo** passive-aggressive

pasmado, *adj*, *SpAm*; ~ (*herida*) infected; unhealthy; ~ (*una persona*) unhealthy looking

pasmar, to stun

pasmazón, *m*, *Med*: *CA*, *Mex*, *PR*, lockjaw; tetanus; chill

pasmo, *Med*, lockjaw; tetanus; chill; *SpAm*, fever; inflammation; ~[5] *ethn*, infection; ~ **del parto** childbed fever; ~ **seco** lockjaw; tetanus

paso, step; ~ **de tortuga** slow walk; ~ **del tiempo** passage of time; ~ **regular** steady pace

pasoso, *adj*, *Chi*, perspiring; sweaty; *Ec*, contagious; *adj*, *Col*, *Chi*, *Guat*, *Perú*, *Ven*, absorbent

paspa, cracked skin; *Bol*, *Ec*, *Perú*, chapped skin

paspadura, cracked skin; *Ríopl*, chapped skin

pasparse, to crack (*piel*); *SpAm*, to chap

pasta, paste; ~ **de dientes** toothpaste; ~ **dentífrica** toothpaste; ~[1] heroin; ~**s** pasta (*sg, tallarines, etc.*)

pastel, *m*, pastry; pie

pasteurización, *f*, pasteurization

pasteurizar, to pasteurize

pastilla, lozenge; pill (*sólida*); tablet; ~ (*anticonceptiva*) birth control pill; contraceptive pill; ~ **de chupar** lozenge; ~ **para chupar** troche; ~ **para la tos** cough drop; cough lozenge; ~ **para no tener niños** birth control pill

pasto[1], marijuana

pastor, -ra, *m*, minister

pastoso, *adj*, doughy

pastura[1], marijuana

patacón, *m*, *Chi*, bruise; welt

patada, kick
pataletas, temper tantrum
patas de gallo, crow's feet
patata, potato
patela, patella
patelar, *adj*, patellar
patelectomía, patellectomy
patente, *m, Cu*, patent medicine
paternidad, *f*, fatherhood
patético, *adj*, pathetic
paticaliente, *adj, PR*, carefree
patidifuso, *adj, PR*, confused
patillas, whiskers
patizambo, *adj*, bandy-legged; pigeon-toed
pato, *slang*, bedpan
patogenia, pathogeny
patógeno, pathogen
patojo, *adj*, lame; *SpAm*, having deformed legs/feet; *CA, Col, Guat*, child; kid
patología, pathology; ~ **clínica** clinical pathology
patológico, *adj*, morbid; pathological
patólogo, pathologist
patrón, patrona, *m/f*, employer
pausa, break (*interrupción*); pause; wait; ~**s apnéicas** breath holding
pauta, guideline (*modelo*)
pava, *Chi, Mex*, chamber pot
pavico, *Chicano*, diaper
payuelas, *f, pl*, chickenpox
paz, *f*, peace
PCP, angel dust^2/PCP; dust^2 (*cocaína, PCP*); phencyclidine
pebete, -a, *m/f, Ríopl*, child
pecas, freckles
pecho, breast; *fam*, chest; thorax; ~**s pesados** heaviness in breasts
pechugón, *adj, Arg, Mex, PR*, big bosomed
pechuguera, *Bol, Col, Mex*, hoarseness; bronchitis; chest trouble
pecotra, *Chi, Anat*, bump; swelling
pectina, pectin; vegetable jelly
pectoral, *adj*, pectoral
peculiaridad, *f*, quirk (*rareza*)
pedacito, chip; ~**s de hielo** ice chips

pedazo, piece
pederse, *slang*, to fart *slang*,
pediatra/pedíatra, *m/f*, pediatrician
pediatría, pediatrics
pediátrico, *adj*, pediatric
pediculosis, *f*, pediculosis (*infestación*)
pedicura, pedicure
pedicuro, chiropodist
pedir (**i**), to ask (for); to request; ~ **permiso** to ask permission
pedo, *slang*, fart *slang*; flatus; gas (*aire*)
pedodoncia, pedodontia
pedodontista, *m/f*, pedodontist
pega, *Chi*, infectious period (*de enfermedad*)
pegadizo, *adj, Med*, contagious; catching; infectious
pegajoso, *adj*, sticky (*viscoso*); adhesive; *Med*, infectious; *Med*, catching
pegamento, glue; gum (*para pegar*)
pegar, to beat (*físicamente*); to hit (*golpear*); to knock; to give (*infectar*); to infect with; to pass on (*una enfermedad*); to glue; to stick (*adherir*); ~ **un salto** to leap up; ~ **un tortazo a uno** to slap someone on the face; ~**le a uno** to get a disease; to catch a disease; ~**se** to become stuck; ~**se** *Med*, to be catching; ~**se** *slang*, to cling (*ropa*)
pegoste, *m, CA, Col, Mex, Ven*, sticking plaster
peinarse, to comb one's hair
peine, *m*, comb; ~ **espeso** fine-toothed comb
peineta, *PR*, row of widely spaced teeth
peje grande^1, *m, PR*, *big cheese* in a dope ring^2
pejigar, to harass; *PR*, to irritate (*molestar*)
pelada, *SpAm*, haircut; *Chi, Ríopl*, bald head; **la ~** *Chi, Cu, Ec*, death

pelado, *Bol, Col, Pan*, child; kid; baby

peladura, peeling; ~ **química** chemical peeling

pelagra, pellagra

pelapatatas, *m, inv*, potato peeler

pelar, to peel (*fruta, patatas*); to shell (*habas, mariscos, etc.*); ~**se** to lose one's hair; to get one's hair cut; **pelársela** to pull back foreskin of penis

peldaño, stair (*de una escalera*)

película, film; ~ **de sangre fijada** fixed blood film

peligro, danger; hazard; risk; ~ **de aborto** danger of miscarriage; ~ **de contaminación** risk of contamination

peligroso, *adj*, dangerous; hazardous

pelirrojo, *adj*, red-haired

pelirubio, *adj*, fair-haired

pelitos, *m, pl, Chicano*, pubic hair

pellejo, flap of the skin

pellín, *m, Chicano*, buttock

pelo, hair; ~ **axilar** hircus; underarm hair; ~ **crespo** curly hair; ~ **de la axila** hircus; underarm hair; ~ **grifo** *Chicano*, kinky hair; ~ **liso** straight hair; ~ **pasudo** kinky hair; ~ **púbico** pubic hair; ~ **quebrado** wavy hair; ~ **rizado** curly hair

pelón, pelona, *m/f, SpAm*, child; kid; baby; **el ~** *Guat, Mex*, death

pelota, bump; ~**s** *pl, vulg*, testicle

pelú, *adj*, hairy; in need of a haircut; *adj, PR*, complicated

peluca, wig

peludo, *adj*, hairy; **agarrarse un ~** *Arg, Ur*, to get drunk

peluquearse, *SpAm*, to have a haircut

peluza, *Mex*, rubella

pelviano, *adj*, pelvic

pélvico, *adj*, pelvic

pelvimetría, pelvimetry

pelvímetro, pelvimeter

pelvis, *f*, pelvis; ~ **renal** renal pelvis

pena, ache; distress (*dolor*); grief; pity; sore; worry

penar, to agonize

penca, leaf (*de un cacto*); **agarrar una ~** *SpAm*, to get drunk

pendejos, *fam, slang, Arg*, pubic hair

pendenciero, *adj*, quarrelsome (*con tendencia a pelear*)

pendiente, *m*, earring (*que cuelga del lóbulo*); *adj*, outstanding (*sin hacer*); pending

penduloso, *adj*, pendulous

pene, *m, form*, penis

penetración, *f*, penetration

penetrante, *adj*, penetrating; deep (*una herida*)

penetrar, to penetrate; to pierce; ~ **en** to enter (*entrar en*)

penicilina, penicillin

penicilinorresistencia, penicillinresistance

penoso, *adj*, distressing (*doloroso*); painful (*difícil*)

pensar (**ie**), to believe; to think; ~ (+ *infinitive*) to intend to

pentotal, *m*, pentothal; ~ **de sodio** sodium pentothal; ~ **sódico** sodium pentothal

peña, *Ec, Guat, PR*, deaf person

peor, *adj, adv*, worse

pepas[1] *slang*, amphetamines

pepe, *m, Guat, Hond*, nursing bottle

pepenado, *CA, Mex*, orphan

pepinillo, pickle

pepita verde[1], marijuana

pepsicola[1], cocaine

pepsina, pepsin

péptico, *adj*, peptic

péptido, peptide

peptona, peptone

pequeñez del corazón, *f*, microcardia

pequeño, *adj*, little (*talla*); small; ~ **abultamiento** nodule; **pequeña amplificación** *f*, low magnification; ~ **mal** petit mal; **pequeña úlcera en la boca** canker sore

pera, bulb syringe; pear; ~ **de goma** rubber bulb; rubber suction ball

percepción, *f*, cognition; perception; ~ **de la profundidad** depth perception (*estereopsia*); ~ **extrasensorial** extrasensory perception/ESP

perceptible, *adj*, detectable; noticeable

percha, hanger (*ropa*); hook (*para colgar ropa*)

perchero, hanger (*colgador de la ropa*)

percibir, to perceive

percusión *f*, percussion

perder (**ie**), to grow out of (*una costumbre*); to lose (*no ganar*); to miss (*no hacer caso de*); to miss (*una oportunidad*); ~ **con la edad** to outgrow (*una costumbre, etc.*); ~ **el conocimiento** to black out; to lapse into unconsciousness; to lose consciousness; ~ **el juicio** to lose one's sanity; ~ **la conciencia** to lose consciousness; ~ **la razón** to lose one's sanity; ~ **peso** to lose weight; ~ **sangre** to menstruate; ~ **la voz** to lose one's voice

pérdida, loss; ~**s blancas** *fam*, leukorrhea; ~ **de apetito** loss of appetite; ~ **de conocimiento** loss of consciousness; unconsciousness; ~ **de equilibrio** loss of balance; ~ **de la tonicidad muscular** loss of muscle tone; ~ **de la voz** obmutescence; ~ **de memoria** loss of memory; memory loss; ~ **de peso** loss of weight; weight loss; ~ **de sangre** loss of blood; ~ **de sangre de poca intensidad** bleeding; ~ **de(l) sueño** loss of sleep; insomnia; ~**s fetales** fetal wastage; ~**s rojas** metrorrhagia; ~**s seminales** spermatorrhea

perdido, *adj*, missing

perdón, excuse me; pardon

perdonar, to pardon; **perdóneme** pardon me

perdurar, to last a long time

perejil, *m*, parsley

perezoso, *adj*, lazy; *m*, *Cu*, safety pin

perfeccionar, to improve

perfeccionista, *m/f*, perfectionist

perfectamente, *adv*, perfectly

perfecto, *adj*, perfect

perfil, *m*, profile (*of face*); ~ **facial** *m*, facial profile

perfilar, to outline; ~**se** *SpAm*, to get slim

perforación, *f*, perforation

perforado, *adj*, ruptured

perforador, *m*, drill

perforadora, punch (*para hacer agujeros en el papel*)

perforar, to drill; to perforate; to pierce; to punch (*el papel*)

perfume, *m*, perfume

perfusión, *f*, perfusion

perica, **agarrar una**, *Col*, *Ec*, *Pan*, to get drunk

pericárdico, *adj*, pericardial

pericardio, heart sac; pericardium

pericardiocentesis, *f*, pericardiocentesis

pericarditis, *f*, pericarditis; ~ **adhesiva** adhesive pericarditis; ~ **con derrame** pericarditis with effusion; ~ **constrictiva** constrictive pericarditis; ~ **hemorrágica** hemorrhagic pericarditis

pericazo[1], cocaine; ~ heroin

pericistitis, *f*, pericystitis

perico[1], *Cu*, *PR*, cocaine; ~[1] *Cu*, big C[2] (*cocaína*); candy[2] (*cocaína*)

pericondrio, perichondrium

pericote, *m*, *Arg*, *Perú*, child

pericráneo, scalp

periférico, *adj*, peripheral

perilla, bulb syringe; lobe (*de oreja*); *fam*, *Mex*, sty

perimetrio, perimetrium

perímetro, circumference; perimeter; ~ **cefálico** head circumference; ~ **de caderas** hip measurement

periné, *m*, perineum

perineal, *adj*, perineal; **desgarros** ~**es** perineal lacerations

perineo, perineum
periódico, newspaper; *adj*, periodical
período, period; period (*menstruación*); *fam*, menstruation; ~ **agónico** death struggle; ~ **de alumbramiento** third stage in birth process; ~ **de cuarentena** quarantine period; ~ **de dilatación** first stage in birth process; ~ **de incubación** incubation period; ~ **de latencia** lag; ~ **de rezago** lag period; ~ **de seguridad** safe period; ~ **del parto** stage of pregnancy; ~ **menstrual** menstrual period; ~ **puerperal** lying-in period; ~ **reproductivo** child-bearing period
periodoncia, periodontia; periodontics
periodontal, *adj*, periodontal
periodontio, periodontium
periodontista, *m/f*, periodontist
periodontitis, *f*, periodontitis; ~ **apical** apical periodontitis
periodonto, periodontium
periodontología, periodontology
periodontosis, *f*, periodontosis
perioniquia, perionychia
perioniquio, perionychium
periostio, periosteum
peristáltico, *adj*, peristaltic
peristaltismo, peristalsis
perito, *m*, *adj*, expert
peritoneal, *adj*, peritoneal
peritoneo, peritoneum
peritonitis, *f*, peritonitis; ~ **aguda** acute peritonitis; ~ **crónica adhesiva** chronic adhesive peritonitis; ~ **por perforación** perforative peritonitis
perjudicial, *adj*, detrimental
perlático, *adj*, paralytic; palsied
perleche, *f*, oral lesion
perlesía, paralysis; palsy
permanecer impasible, *fam*, not to move a muscle
permanente, *f*, *adj*, indwelling; permanent

permanganato de potasio, potassium permanganate
permiso, authorization; license; permission; permit; ~ **de convalencia** sick leave
permitir, to allow; to permit
pernear, to shake one's legs; to kick one's legs
perniabierto, *adj*, bow-legged
pernicioso, *adj*, deleterious; noxious; pernicious
peroné, *m*, calf bone; fibula
peroneal, *adj*, fibular; peroneal
peroneo, peroneum; *adj*, fibular
peróxido, peroxide; ~ **de benzoílc** benzoyl peroxide; ~ **de hidró geno** *form*, hydrogen peroxide; ~ **de sodio** sodium peroxide
perpetuar, to perpetuate
perro, dog; *Col*, drowsiness
perseguir (**i**), to pursue
perseveración, *f*, perseveration
persiana, shade (*enrollable*)
persistencia, persistence
persistente, *adj*, lingering (*olor*); nagging (*constante*); persistent; remaining
persistir, (**en** + *infinitive*) to persist (in + *gerundio*)
persona, person; ~ **anormal** psycho; ~ **muerta** deceased (individual)
personal, *m*, personnel; staff; *adj*, personal; ~ **del quirófano** (operating) theater staff; ~ **médico** house staff; medical personnel; ~ **sanitario auxiliar** nursing staff
personalidad, *f*, personality; ~ **antisocial** antisocial personality; ~ **esquizoide** schizoid personality; ~ **limítrofe** borderline personality; ~ **múltiple** multiple personality; ~ **obsesivo-compulsiva** obsessive-compulsive personality; ~ **paranoide** paranoid personality; ~ **pasivo-agresiva** passive-aggressive personality; ~ **(p)sicopática**[6] psychopathic personality
perspectiva, outlook

perspicaz, *adj*, keen
perspiración, *f*, transpiration; perspiration
perturbación, *f*, *Med*, upset; disturbance; mental disorder
perturbado, *adj*, upset; mentally unbalanced; *m*, mentally unbalanced person
perturbar, to disturb (*Med: la mente; el organismo*); to perturb (*mentalmente*); to unsettle; to upset
perversión, *f*, perversion; ~ **sexual** sexual perversion
pervertido sexual, sexual pervert
pesa, (*para balanzas; deportes*) weight; dumbbell
pesadez, *f*, heaviness (*del estómago, cabeza*); pigheadedness (*terquedad*); ~ **pélvica** bearing down; *fam*, fatigue (*cansancio*)
pesadilla, nightmare
pesado, *adj*, heavy
pesadumbre, *f*, grief
pesar, to weigh; ~ **más que** to outweigh
pesario, pessary; ~ **de diafragma** diaphragm pessary; ~ **oclusivo** occlusive pessary
pescado, fish (*comida*)
pescar, to fish; *Col*, *Ríopl*, to doze; ~ **una monga** *PR*, to catch a cold
pescozudo, *adj*, thick-necked
pescuezo, neck (*de un animal*)
pesimismo, pessimism; ~ **terapéutico** therapeutic pessimism
peso, weight; ~ **al nacer** birthweight; weight at birth; ~ **al nacimiento** birthweight; weight at birth; ~ **bruto** gross weight; ~ **corporal** body weight; ~ **de baño** bathroom scale; ~ **de nacimiento** birthweight; weight at birth; ~ **de nacimiento bajo** low birth weight; ~ **del cuerpo humano** human body weight; ~ **en seco** dry weight; ~ **escaso** underweight; ~ **específico** specific gravity; ~**s y medidas** weights and measures

pesquisa, inquest
pestaña, eyelash; lash
peste, *f*, plague (*enfermedad*); epidemic; *Perú*, *PR*, bubonic plague; *Chi*, smallpox; *Ríopl*, (any) infectious disease; ~ **blanca** tuberculosis; ~ **bubónica** bubonic plague; ~ **cristal** *fam*, chicken pox
pesticida, *m*, pesticide
pestilencia, pestilence
petaca, cigar case; *CA*, *Anat*, hump; ~**s** *Mex*, *Anat*, buttocks; big breasts
petacón, **petacona**, *adj*, *Mex*, *Perú*, *Ríopl*, short; plump; *Col*, lazy; potbellied
petacudo, *adj*, *Guat*, hunchbacked
petardo[1], *adj*, (*menos común*) high on[2] (*drogas narcóticas*)
petate[1], *m*, marijuana; ~ **del soldado**[1] marijuana
petequia, petechia (*pl*, *petechiae*)
petequial, *adj*, petechial
petición, *f*, request
petrificación, *f*, petrifaction
petróleo, petroleum
peyote, *m*, peyote; *fam*, mescaline
pez, *m*, fish (*en el agua*)
pezón, *m*, nipple (*del pecho femenino*); ~ **enlechado** caked breast; engorged nipple
pezonera, nipple shield; *Arg*, nursing bottle
P.G./práctica de un grupo, *f*, group practice/G.P.; **P.G./practicante general** *m/f*, G.P./general practitioner
pH, *m*, pH
piache, *m*, *Ven*, quack doctor
piamadre, *f*, pia mater
pibe, **piba**, *m/f*, *Bol*, *Chi*, *Ríopl*, child; kid
picada, bite/sting (*insecto*)
picado de viruelas, *adj*, pockmarked; variolous
picadura, bite/sting (*insecto*); mark (*de viruelas*); pit (*señal en la piel de viruelas, etc.*); stick (*de

una aguja, un insecto); sting; fam, cavity *Dent*; ~ **de abeja** bee sting; ~ **de alacrán** scorpion sting; ~ **de araña** spider bite/sting; ~ **de avispa** wasp sting; ~ **de avispón** hornet sting; ~ **de garrapata** tick sting; ~ **de hormiga** ant sting; ~ **de insecto** insect bite; ~ **de moscardón** botfly sting; ~ **de mosquito** mosquito sting; ~ **de nigua** chigoe/jigger/sandflea sting; ~ **de pulga** flea sting; ~ **de ubar** *fam*, black widow spider sting; ~ **de viuda negra** black widow spider sting

picante, *adj*, hot (*con especias*); spicy (*comida*); biting/sharp (*respuesta*); itchy

picao, *adj*, *PR*, intoxicated (*ligeramente*)

picar, to bite (*araña, pulga, serpiente*)/to sting (*abeja, avispa*); to itch (*escocer*); to mark (*viruelas*); to mince (*carne*); to stick (*agujerear*); to sting (*una herida*); to smart; ~**se** to go off in a huff; ~[1] to bang[2]; to fix[2] (*inyectarse con drogas*); to hit up[2]; to inject oneself with drugs

picarazado, *adj*, *Cu*, *PR*, pockmarked

picardía, naughtiness (*travesura*)

pícaro, *adj*, naughty (*niño travieso*)

picazón, *f*, itch (*sensación*); prickly heat; *m*, tingle; *m*, *fam*, itching

picor, *m*, ticklish itch; itch (*sensación*); itching

picoso, *adj*, pockmarked

picotada, bite; sting

picotazo, bite; sting

pie, *m*, foot; ~ **contrahecho** talipes; tibia varus; ~ **de atleta** athlete's foot; ~ **hueco** high arched foot; ~ **plano** flat foot; ~ **talo** talipes; ~ **zambo** clubfoot; talipes; *m*, *Arg*, kyllosis; ~ **zopo** talipes

piedra, stone; ~**s en el vesículo** biliary stones; ~ **en la vejiga** gall-stone; ~ **en la yel** *Chicano*, gall-stone; ~ **en los riñones** kidney stone; ~ **infernal** silver nitrate; ~ **nefrítica** kidney stone; ~ **pómez** pumice stone

piedrita de la luna[1], LSD

piel, *f*, fur (*de animal con pelo largo*)/leather (*cuero*); peel (*de las frutas*); skin; *fam*, complexion; ~ **agrietada** cracked skin; ~ **amarilla** jaundice; ~ **azulada** *fam*, cyanosis; ~ **de gallina** gooseflesh; ~ **de la cabeza** scalp; ~ **de oveja** sheepskin; ~ **flácida** loose skin; ~ **laxa** loose skin; ~ **marmórea** marbled skin; ~ **roja** chafing; ~ **viscosa** clammy skin

pielitis, *f*, pyelitis

pielocistitis, *f*, pyelocystitis

pielografía, pyelography

pielograma, *m*, pyelogram; ~ **excretorio** excretory pyelogram; ~ **intravenoso** intravenous pyelogram/IVP

pielonefritis, *f*, pyelonephritis

piemia, pyemia; septicemia

pierna, leg; *fam*, thigh; ~ **de pájaro** bird-leg; ~ **en paréntesis** bow-leg

pieza, part; piece; ~ **bucal** mouth-piece

pigmentación, *f*, pigmentation; ~ **extrínseca** extraneous pigmentation; ~ **palúdica** malarial pigmentation

pigmentario, *adj*, pigmentary

pigmento, pigment; ~**s biliares** bile pigments; ~ **purpúrico visual** visual purple

pija, *slang*, *Arg*, penis

pijamas, *f*, *pl*, pajamas

pila eléctrica, galvanic element

píldora, pill (*sólida*); ~ **anticonceptiva** birth control pill; oral contraceptive; ~ **de anticoncepción** birth control pill; ~ **diurética** diuretic; ~ **para control de embarazo** birth control pill; ~ **para dormir** sleeping pill; ~ **somnífera** sleeping pill

pildorear(se)[1], to ingest narcotic pills

pildoriar(se)[1], to ingest narcotic pills

pildoriento[1], user of pills[2]

píldoro[1], pill freak[2]; pill head[2]; pill popper[2]; *adj*, high on pills[2]

pilinga, *vulg*, penis

pillido, *Mex*, souffle

pilórico, *adj*, pyloric

píloro, pylorus

piloso, *adj*, hairy

piloto, pilot light

pilucho, *adj*, *Chi*, naked (from the waist down)

pimienta, pepper; ~ **negra** black pepper

pimiento, bell pepper; ~ **morrón** sweet pepper

pimpo, *adj*, gorged

pinchar, to inject; to jab (*con una aguja*); to prick; to stick; ~**le a uno** *Med*, *fam*, to give s.o. an injection

pinchazo, jab (*puñalada*); jab *fam*, (*de una aguja*); prick; stick (*de una aguja*)

pincho, thorn

pineal, *adj*, pineal

pingar, *vulg*, *PR*, to screw

pinguas[1], *pl*, narcotic pill

pinta, pint; spotted sickness

pintar, to paint

pinto, *adj*, very dark-skinned, lacking negroid features; ~ (*complexion*) blotchy

pintura, paint; ~ **con plomo** lead-based paint; ~ **de labios** lipstick

pinza, clamp; ~ **de cejas** tweezers; ~ **de garfios** hooked-forceps; ~**s** dental forceps; forceps (*quirúrgicas*); nippers; pliers; tongs; tweezers; ~**s de curación** dressing forceps; ~**s de dientes finos** fine-toothed forceps; ~**s de disección** dissecting forceps; ~**s de sutura** suture forceps; ~**s de torsión** torsion forceps; ~**s den-tadas** toothed forceps; ~**s hemostáticas** hemostatic forceps; hemostat; ~**s quirúrgicas** surgical forceps

pinzamiento del espacio discal, disc/disk space narrowing

pinzar, to clamp

piña, pineapple

piocha, beard; *fam*, chin

piojería, pediculosis (*infestación*)

piojo, louse (*pl*, *lice*) (*insecto*); ~ **de la cabeza** head louse; ~ **del cuerpo** body louse

piojoso, *adj*, scruffy (*apariencia descuidada*)

piorrea, pyorrhea

pipa, pipe (*para fumar*)

piperacina, piperazine

piperawitt, *m/f*, piperazine

piperidol, *m*, piperazine

pipeta, pipette

pipi/pipí, *m*, *fam*, number one *euph*; pee; urine

pique, *m*, *SpAm*, chigoe (*nigua*)

piquete, *m*, bite/sting (*insecto*); sting (*pinchazo*); small hole (*agujero*); ~ **de insecto** insect bite; sting (*de un insecto*); *f*, *Mex*, puncture *Med*; *m*, *Mex*, prick; stick (*de una aguja*); ~[1] *m*, heroin; injection (*de una substancia narcótica*)

piquiña, *PR*, aversion; itch (*sensación*)

piragua, cone of crushed ice with syrup

piridoxina, vitamin B_6

piriforme, *adj*, pear-shaped

pirinola, *Mex*, child

piripi, *adj*, jolly (*un poco borracho*)

pirosis, *f*, heartburn

pis, *m*, *fam*, pee

pisada, step

pisa-lengua, tongue depressor

pisalengua, tongue depressor

pisar, to tread

piscoiro *Chi*, child

piscolabis, *m*, *inv*, snack

piso, floor (*de un edificio*); story (*planta*); ~ **de maternidad** maternity floor; ~ **ginecológico** gynecological floor
pisotear, to tread
pisporra, *CA*, wart
pisporr(i)a, *Chicano*, lump on head
pisto, *adj*, drunk
pistola, gun
pit[1], LSD
pitillera, cigarette case
pitillo, *m*, *fam*, cigarette; ~[1] marijuana
pítima, drunken fit
pito, *slang*, penis; ~[1] jive stick[2] (*cigarrillo de mariguana*); joint[2]; marijuana
pitocín, *m*, pitocin
pitocina, pitocin
pitongo, *adj*, *Chi*, drunk
pitra, *Chi*, rash
pituita, *PR*, hay fever
pituitaria, *f*, pituitary
pituitario, *adj*, pituitary
piuria, pyuria
PIV/pielograma intravenoso, *m*, IVP/intravenous pyelogram
piyamas, *f*, *pl*, pajamas
pizca, speck (*una partícula*)
placa, film (*rayos x*); plate *Dent*, *Med* (*rayos x*);*SpAm*, skin blemish; ~ **bacteriana** plaque *Dent*; ~ **base** baseplate *Dent*; ~ **de Petri** Petri dish; ~ **de revelado rápido** rapid-developing film; ~ **terminal** end-plate; ~**s** denture plates
placebo, placebo
placenta, *form*, afterbirth; placenta; ~ **en herradura** horseshoe placenta; ~ **previa** placenta previa
placentario, *adj*, placental
placentografía, placentography
plaga, plague (*infortunio*)
plaguicida, *m*, pesticide
plan, *m*, plan (*esquema; propósito*); project; *Med*, regime; course of treatment; **estar a** ~ to be on a

course of treatment; ~ **de inmunización pediátrica** pediatric immunization schedule; ~ **de trabajo** work schedule
plancha, iron (*instrumento para planchar ropa*); *Dent*, dental plate
planchar, to iron; to press
planificación, *f*, planning; ~ **de la familia** family planning; ~ **familiar** family planning
planigrafía, scan
plano, *m*, *adj*, flat; ~ **de oclusión** occlusal plane; ~**s de clivaje** excisional planes
planovegus, *m*, flat foot
planta del pie, sole of the foot
plantar[1], to stash[2] (*esconder un suministro de drogas*)
plantear el problema (de), to raise the issue (of)
plantilla, insole (*para los zapatos*)
plaqueta, blood disk; blood platelet; plaque; platelet; ~ **sanguínea** nucleated leukocytes; blood platelet
plasma, *m*, plasma; ~ **sanguíneo** blood plasma
plasmaféresis, *f*, plasmapheresis
plasta, *vulg*, *PR*, impotent person
plástico, *adj*, artificial; *m*, *adj*, plastic
plastocito, plaque
plata, silver
platanillo, *fam*, calf (*pl*, *calves*) (*parte de la pierna*)
platelminto, flatworm
platillo, saucer
platina, slide (*de un microscopio*)
plato, dish; plate (*vajilla*)
pleito, lawsuit; suit (*legal*)
plenitud epigástrica, *f*, epigastric fullness
pleura, pleura (*pl*, *pleurae*)
pleuresía, pleurisy
pleuritis, *f*, pleurisy
plexo, plexus
pley, *m*, *Chicano*, game
pliegue, *m*, fold; furrow; ~ **cutáneo** skin fold; ~ **genital** genital

fold; ~ **neural** neural fold; ~ **umbilical lateral** lateral umbilical fold

plomazo, *CA, Mex,* bullet wound

plomo, lead

pluma, feather; pen (*para escribir*); ~ **estilográfica** fountain pen

plumafuente, *f, SpAm,* fountain pen

plumbismo, lead poisoning

plumero, *PR,* effeminate male; effeminate guy

plumilla, insect (*tipo de*)

plurípara, pluripara

población, *f,* population

pobre, *adj,* impecunious; poor

pobreza, misery (*miseria*)

poca sangre, *f, fam,* anemia

pocas veces, *adv,* seldom

pochola[1], marijuana

pocilga, pen (*para los cerdos*)

pocillo, small cup of coffee

pócima, brew; draught

poción, *f,* draft; draught; potion

poco, small (*cantidad*); ~ **atento** *adj,* inattentive; *m, adj, adv,* little (*cantidad*)

pod[1], marijuana

podagra, gout

poder, *m,* power; ~ **legal** power of attorney/POA

poder (**ue**), to be able

poderoso, *adj,* potent (*un veneno*)

podiatra/podíatra, *m/f,* chiropodist; podiatrist

podiatría, podiatry; chiropody

podiatrista, *m/f,* podiatrist; chiropodist

podólogo, chiropodist

podrido, *adj,* bad (*estropeado*); decayed; putrid; rotten; spoiled

polaridad, *f,* electric polarity

polen, *m,* pollen

policía, *f,* police (*cuerpo*); policewoman; *m,* policeman

polisaturado, *adj,* polysaturated

polilla, ringworm; tinea

polillo[1], marijuana

polimorfos, nucleated leukocytes— polymorphs

polio(mielitis), *f,* infantile paralysis; polio(myelitis)

pólipo, polyp; ~ **carnoso** fleshy polyp; ~ **hemorrágico** bleeding polyp; ~ **nasal** nasal polyp; **~s en el útero** polyps in the uterus

poliquístico, *adj,* polycystic

poliuria, polyuria

polivacuna, polyvalent vaccine

polivalente, *adj,* multifunctional

póliza, policy (*seguro*); ~ **de seguros** insurance policy; ~ **de seguros de cuidado dental** dental insurance policy; ~ **de seguros de salud** health insurance policy; ~ **de seguros de vida** life insurance policy; ~ **de seguros sobre la vida** life insurance policy

polla, *vulg,* penis

pollera, baby walker; *Ríopl,* skirt

pollo, *Chicano,* sputum

polución, *f,* pollution

polvito[1], cocaine

polvo, ~ (**de la tierra**) dust; ~ (*medicina; química*) powder; **~s** *pl,* talcum powder; powder (*cosmético*); **~**[1] angel dust[2] (*PCP*); cocaine; dust[2] (*cocaína, PCP*); heroin; PCP; ~ **amargo**[1] heroin; ~ **blanco**[1] heroin; ~ **de azufre** sulfur powder; ~ **de la casa** house dust; ~ **facial** facial powder; ~ **para los pies** foot powder

polvoriento, *adj,* powdery

polvoroso, *adj,* powdery

pomada, ointment; pomade; salve; unguent; ~ **de bacitracina** bacitratin ointment; ~ **de calamina** calamine ointment; ~ **de óxido de cinc** zinc oxide ointment; ~ **oftálmica de penicilina** penicillin eye ointment

pomo, bottle (*para las pastillas*); door knob; **~**[1] ampoule/ampule

pómulo, cheekbone; malar bone

ponche, *m,* punch (*una bebida*)

ponchera, *CA, Col, Mex, Ven,* washbowl/washbasin

ponderar, to ponder

poner, to give (*administrar*); to insert; to place; ~ **a dieta** to put on a diet; ~ **a la defensiva** to put on the defensive; ~ **a prueba** to test; ~ **de relieve** to emphasize; ~ **en cabestrillo** to put in a sling; ~ **en cuarentena** to put in quarantine; ~ **en movimiento** to put into action; ~ **en peligro** to endanger; to hazard; ~ **en práctica** to put into action; ~ **en yeso** to put in a cast; ~ **las medicinas fuera del alcance de los niños** to keep medicines away from children; ~ **los ojos en blanco** to roll one's eyes back; ~ **nervioso** *adj*, to excite (*irritar*); ~ **pleito** to sue; ~ **sangre** *fam*, to transfuse; to give a transfusion; ~ **tenso** *adj*, to tense (*los músculos*); ~ **una carga excesiva (a)** to overcharge *Elect*; ~ **una inyección** to give an injection; ~ **una mascarilla a** to mask; ~**(se) en marcha** to start (*una máquina*); ~**se** to insert; ~**se (+ adj) (Vea high.)** to be high²; ~**se (+ adj de estado emocional/mental)** to become/turn (+ *adj*); ~**se (+ sustantivo)** to put on (*ropa*); ~**se al tanto**¹ to get in the groove; ~**se alto** *fam, adj*, to be/get drunk; ~**se azul** to turn blue; ~**se chinito** *adj*, to get goose bumps; ~**se de cuclillas** to squat; ~**se de lado** to turn on one's side; ~**se de luto** to go into mourning; ~**se de pie** to stand up; ~**se dormido** *adj*, to turn numb; ~**se enfermo** *adj*, to be taken ill; ~**se furioso** *adj*, to get mad; ~**se histérico** *adj*, to go into hysterics; ~**se más grande** to get bigger; ~**se rojo** *adj*, to blush; ~**se rojo de ira** *adj*, to flush with anger; ~**se tenso** *adj*, to tense up; ~**se tieso** *adj*, to turn stiff
ponzoña, poison; venom
ponzoñoso, *adj*, poison (*serpiente, etc.*); poisonous

poporo, *Col, Ven*, bump; swelling
popular, *adj*, lay
por, per; ~ **(su) propia voluntad** of (*uno mismo*) own free will; ~ **cabeza** per capita; ~ **dentro** within; ~ **día** daily; per diem; ~ **ejemplo** e.g.; for example; ~ **el año** per anum; ~ **favor** please; ~ **inhalación** by inhalation; ~ **la noche** at night; during the night; ~ **la semana** per week; ~ **mes** per month; ~ **meses** *adv* monthly; ~ **minuto** per minute; ~ **precaución** just in case; ~ **si acaso** just in case; ~ **su bien** for your benefit; ~ **su propio bien** for your own good; ~ **una noche** overnight; ~ **vapor** by inhalation; ~ **vía bucal** *adv*, orally
porcelana, porcelain
porcentaje, *m*, percentage
porcino, *Med*, bump; swelling
porción, *f*, portion
poro, pore
pororó, *Ríopl*, popcorn
poroto, *Chi*, child
porquería, filth; mess (*algo que no vale*)
porra, *vulg*, head of penis
porrazo, sock (*golpe*)
porrigo, ringworm of the scalp
portaagujas, *m, inv*, needle holder
portador, -ra, *m/f*, agent (*causal*); ~ **activo** active carrier; ~ **de enfermedad** carrier (*de una enfermedad*); ~ **de microbios** carrier (*de una enfermedad*); ~**ra hemofílica** *f*, hemophiliac carrier
portalápiz, *m*, pencil holder; *slang*, rubber (*condón*)
portalentes, *m*, frame (*gafas*)
portaobjetivo (*del microscopio*), nosepiece
portaobjetos, *m, inv*, microscope slide; slide (*de un microscopio*)
portar, to carry; ~**se** to behave; ~**se mal** to misbehave
portátil, *adj*, portable
portavoz, *m*, mouthpiece

porte, *m*, bearing; gait
posaderas, *f, pl*, buttocks; backside *Anat*
posas, *f, pl*, buttocks; backside *Anat*
posibilidad, *f*, chance; ~ **de supervivencia** chance of survival
posible, *adj*, possible
posición, *f*, position; station; status; ~ **del cuerpo** body position; ~ **erecta** upright position; ~ **inclinada** tilted position
positivo, *adj*, positive (*contrario de negativo*)
poso, deposit (*sedimento*); ~**s de café**, coffee grounds
posoperatorio, *adj*, postoperative
posparto/postparto, *m*, postpartum; fourth stage of pregnancy
posponer, to put off
postcura, aftercare
postema, *Med*, abscess; tumor; *Mex*, pus; boil
postemilla, canker sore; dental abscess; *SpAm*, gumboil
posterior, *adj*, posterior
postilla, pock; scab
postizo, *adj*, artificial
post mortem, *f, adj*, postmortem
postración, *f*, languishment; prostration; ~ **por el calor** heat prostration
postrado, *adj*, prostrate; ~ **en cama**, *adj*, bedridden
postrar, to overwhelm (*con dolor, etc.*); *Med*, to weaken; to exhaust; to prostrate; ~**se** to prostrate oneself
postre, *m*, dessert
pot[1], marijuana
potasa, potash
potasio, potassium
potencia, potency; power; ~ **muscular** muscular strength
potencial, *m, adj*, potential; ~ **de reposo** resting potential; ~ **eléctrico** electric potential
potente, *adj*, powerful
potra, *Med*, hernia; rupture

potranca, **-co**, *PR*, large young girl/large young boy
potro, *SpAm, Med*, hernia; tumor
pozo de ventilación, ventilation shaft
práctica, practice; ~ **de un grupo** group practice/GP; ~ **impropia** malpractice; ~ **inhábil** malpractice
practicante general/P.G., *m/f*, general practitioner/GP
practicar, to practice
precalentar (**ie**), to preheat
precanceroso, *adj*, precancerous
precario, *adj*, precarious
precaución, *f*, precaution
precaucionar(se), to take precautions
precedencia, precedence
precedente, *m*, precedent
preceder a uno, to take precedence over s.o.
precepto, precept
precio, price; value; ~ **excesivo** overcharge (*caro*)
precipitado, precipitate; *adj*, rash (*acción*)
precipitar, to precipitate *Chem*; ~**se** to start
precisión, *f*, precision
preciso, *adj*, precise
precoz, *adj*, early; premature (*calvicie, etc.*)
precursor, **-ra**, *m/f*, precursor; *adj*, precursory
predecir, to predict
predisponer, to predispose
predisposición (**a**), *f*, predisposition (to); tendency *Med*
predispuesto, *adj*, prejudiced
prednisona, prednisone
predominante, *adj*, predominant
predominar, to predominate
preeclampsia, preeclampsia
preexistencia, preexistence
preexistente, *adj*, preexistent
preexistir, to preexist
preferencia, preference
preferencial, *adj*, preferential

preferente, *adj* preferential
preferible, *adj*, preferable
pregunta, question (*interrogativa*)
preguntar, to ask (questions); to question
prejuicio, prejudice (*falta de objetividad*)
preliminar, *m, adj*, preliminary
premadurez, *f*, prematurity
prematuro, *adj*, premature
premedicación, *f*, premedication
premioso, *adj*, tongue-tied; awkward (*habla*)
premolar, *m*, bicuspid tooth
prenatal, *adj*, prenatal
prender, ~ (*asir*) to seize; to grasp; ~ (**una vacuna/un transplante**) to take (*vacuna /transplante*); ~ [1] to hook on narcotics
prendido[1], *adj*, drugged; ~[1] *esp. Mex, adj*, hooked on drugs
prendimiento, *Chi*, constipation
preñada, *adj*, pregnant
preñar, *fam*, to get pregnant
preñez, *f*, gravidity; pregnancy
preocupación, *f*, disturbance; worry
preocupado, *adj*, concerned; worried; ~ **sin motivo** *adj*, overanxious (*perturbado*)
preocupante, *adj*, disturbing (*perturbador*); worrisome
preocupar, to absorb; to disturb (*molestar*); to worry (*inquietar*); ~**se** to be worried; to worry; ~**se por** to mind (*estar preocupado*)
preoperatorio, *adj*, preoperative
preparación, *f*, preparation
preparado, *Pharm*, preparation
preparar, to make up (*una receta*); to mix (bebidas); to prepare; ~ (*una receta*) to fill (*a prescription*); ~**se** to get ready
preparativo, arrangement
preparatorio, *adj*, preparatory
prepucio, *Anat*, foreskin; prepuce
prequirúrgico, *adj*, presurgical
presbicia, farsightedness; presbyopia
presbiopía/presbiopia, farsightedness; presbyopia

présbita/présbite, *adj*, farsighted; long-sighted
prescribir, to prescribe; ~ **un remedio** to prescribe
prescripción, *f*, prescription; ~ **facultativa** medical prescription
prescrito, prescribed
presencia, presence; ~ **de cetosa en la orina** ketosuria
presenciar, to witness
presentación, *f*, presentation; ~ **cefálica** cephalic presentation; head presentation; ~ **de cara** face presentation; ~ **de frente** brow presentation; ~ **de hombro** shoulder presentation; ~ **de la cabeza** head presentation; ~ **de nalgas** breech presentation; breechbirth; frank birth; ~ **de pies** footling presentation; ~ **de un caso** case report; ~ **franca de nalgas** frank breech presentation; ~ **pélvica** *form*, breech presentation; ~ **placentaria** placental presentation; ~ **transversa** transverse presentation; ~ **trasera** breechbirth
presentar, to introduce; to lay out; to put forward (*un prognóstico*); to present; to submit (*pruebas*); ~**se** to appear; to turn up (*aparecer*); to come up (*una dificultad*); to report (*para comenzar a trabajar*); ~**se (a)** to apply (for) (*para obtener un empleo*)
presente, *adj*, present
preservativo, rubber (*condón*); *slang*, condom
presión, *f*, press; pressure; ~ **alta** *fam*, hypertension (*hipertensión*); ~ **arterial** *form*, blood pressure; ~ **arterial alta** *fam*, high blood pressure; hypertension (*hipertensión*); ~ **arterial baja** *fam*, hypotension (*hipotensión*); low blood pressure; ~ **arterial elevada** *fam*, high blood pressure; ~ **atmosférica** air pressure;

~ **de sangre** blood pressure; ~ **del vapor** vapor pressure; ~ **diastólica** diastolic pressure; ~ **diferencial de la arteria pulmonar** pulmonary artery wedge pressure; ~ **intraocular** intraocular pressure/IOP; ~ **ocular** ocular pressure; ~ **parcial** partial pressure; ~ **sanguínea** blood pressure; B.P. (*presión arterial*); ~ **sistólica** systolic pressure; ~ **venosa** venous pressure/VP

presístole, *f*, presystole
préstamo, loan
prestar, to loan
presto, *adj, fam*, available
presunción, *f*, presumption; self-importance
pretender, to pretend (*reclamar*)
pretensión, *f*, pretense (*reclamación*)
pretexto, pretense (*excusa*); pretext
prevención, *f*, prevention
prevenible, *adj*, preventible
prevenir, to prevent
preventivo, *adj*, precautionary; preventive
prever, to foresee
previo, *adj*, previous
prima, premium (*en los negocios, seguro*); ~ **de seguro(s)** insurance premium; cousin
primario, *adj*, primary
primer[7]/**primero**, *adj*, first; **primer nombre** *m*, first name; **primer período del parto** *m*, first stage of labor; first stage of pregnancy; **primera ayuda** first aid; **primera circunvolución frontal** *f*, superfrontal convolution; **primera dentición** *f*, primary dentition; **primera fase del parto** *f*, first stage of pregnancy; **primera muela permanente** sixth-year molar; **primera regla** menarche; **primera señal de vida que da el feto** *f*, quickening; **primeros auxilios** acute care; first aid

primigrávida, primigravida
primípara, *f, adj*, primipara
primitivo, *adj*, primitive
primo, cousin; ~ **hermano** first cousin
primogénito, *adj*, first-born
principal, *adj*, main; *m, adj*, principal
principio, beginning; onset; principle
prioridad, *f*, precedence; priority
privado, toilet; *adj*, private
privar, to deprive
privilegiado, *adj*, privileged
probabilidad, *f*, chance (*esperanza*); ~ **de sobrevivir** chance of survival; ~**es de vida** life expectancy *sg*
probar (**ue**), to prove (*poner a prueba*); to taste; to test; to touch; to try (*experimentar; intentar*); ~ **su fuerza** to test one's strength
probeta, graduated cylinder
problema, *m*, issue (*cuestión que se trata de aclarar*); problem; ~**s cardíacos** cardiac problems; ~ **de las vías urinarias** urinary problem; ~ **familiar** family problem; ~**s físicos** physical problems; ~**s mentales** mental problems; ~ **personal** family problem
procaína, procaine
proceder, to proceed
procedimiento, procedure; ~ **clínico** clinical procedure; ~ **quirúrgico** surgical procedure; ~**s médicos** medical procedures
procesado de la dentadura, denture curing
proceso, event; process; ~ **alveolar** alveolar ridge
procreación planeada, *f*, planned parenthood
procrear, to procreate
proctitis, *f*, proctitis
proctología, proctology
proctólogo, proctologist

proctoscopio, proctoscope

producción energética, *f*, energy output

producir, to precipitate (*causar*); to produce; to raise (*Med*: *ampollas, etc.*); to yield; ~ **ampollas (en)** to blister; ~ **necrosis** to necrotize

producto, product; ~ **de desecho** end product; ~ **final** end product; ~ **lácteo** milk product

profesión, *f*, profession; ~ **de enfermería** nursing profession

profesional, *m/f, adj*, professional

profiláctica, prophylaxis

profiláctico, condom; *m, adj*, prophylactic; preventive; **medicamento** ~ preventive; prophylactic

profilaxis, *f*, prophylaxis

profundamente, *adv*, profoundly

profundidad, *f*, depth; ~ **focal** focal depth

profundo, *adj*, deep; lasting; sound (*dormir*)

profuso, *adj*, profuse

progenie, *f*, offspring; progeny

progenitor, *m*, forefather

progenitura, offspring

progesterona, progesterone

programa, *m*, program; schedule; ~ **de instrucción** educational program; ~ **de salud mental** mental health program; ~ **diario** daily schedule; ~ **educativo** educational program

programar, to schedule (*planificar*)

progresar, to progress *Med*

progresión, *f*, progression

progresivo, *adj*, advancing; progressive

progreso, progress

prohibida la entrada, no admittance

prohibido bañarse, no bathing

prohibir, to prohibit (*no permitir*)

prolapso, prolapse; ~ **de la matriz** prolapse of the uterus; ~ **de la válvula mitral** mitral valve prolapse/MVP; ~ **del cordón umbilical** prolapsed umbilical cord; ~ **del útero** prolapse of the uterus; ~ **valvular mitral** mitral valve prolapse/MVP

prole, *f*, progeny

prolífico, *adj*, prolific

prolongación, *f*, extension; prolongation

prolongado, *adj*, prolonged

prolongar, to prolong (*en el espacio*); ~**se** to lengthen

promedio, *m, adj*, average; ~ **de desviación** average deviation

promesa, promise

prominente, *adj*, prominent (*saliente*)

promiscuo, *adj*, promiscuous

pronosticar, to prognosticate

pronóstico, prognosis (*pl, prognoses*); **de ~ leve** not serious; **de ~ reservado** possibly serious; of uncertain gravity

pronto, *adv*, soon

pronunciación, *f*, enunciation

pronunciar mal, to slur (*palabras*)

propagación, *f*, propagation

propagar(se), to spread

propenso, *adj*, prone (*inclinado*); ~ **a constiparse** liable to catch cold

propiedad, *f*, property; ~ **indivisa** joint property

proporción, *f*, proportion; ~ **de excreción de urea** urea excretion ratio

proporcionar, to provide (*dar; proveer*)

proseguir (i), to proceed

prostaglandinas, prostaglandins

próstata, prostrate gland; prostate

prostático, *adj*, prostate; prostatic

prostatitis, *f*, prostatitis

prostético, *adj*, prosthetic

prostitución, *f*, prostitution

prostituta, prostitute

prostodoncia, prosthodontia; prosthodontics

protección, *f*, protection

proteccionista, *adj*, protective

protector, *m*, protector; defender; mouthpiece (*deportes*); ~ **cap** (*de una aguja*); ~ **del sol** sunscreen; **~ra** *adj*, protective

proteger, to protect; to shelter

protegido, *adj*, sheltered

proteína, protein; ~ **de la leche** milk protein

prótesis, *f*, prosthesis; ~ **acústica** hearing aid; ~ **auditiva** hearing aid; ~ **dental** dental prosthesis; bridgework; ~ **maxilofacial** maxillofacial prosthesis; ~ **posquirúrgica** postsurgical prosthesis

protética, prosthetics

protoplasma, *m*, protoplasm

protozoarios, protozoa (*sg, protozoo*)

protrombina, prothrombin

protrusión, *f*, protrusion

protuberancia, *form*, bump; lump (*hinchazón*); knob; ~ **lingual** lingual swelling; ~ **occipital** occipital protuberance

protuberante, *adj*, bulging

proveer, to provide (*suministrar*); ~ **con pañal** to diaper

provisión, *f*, provision; **~es** *pl*, provisions (*comida*)

provocar, to bring on; to provoke; to trigger; ~ **el parto** to induce labor; ~ **náuseas** to make gag; **~se el vómito** to cause vomiting

próximo, *adj*, next

proyección, *f*, projection; ~ **lateral** lateral view

proyectar, to project

proyecto, project (*plan*)

prudente, *adj*, safe (*cauto*); sane

prueba, proof; fitting (*de ropa*); tasting (*bebidas*); test (*parte de un examen*); test (*del laboratorio*); voucher; ~ **al azar** random test; **~s cruzadas** cross match; ~ **cualitativa** qualitative test; ~ **cuantitativa** quantitative test; ~ **cutánea** skin test; ~ **de compatibilidad** matching; ~ **de ejercicio** stress test; ~ **de embarazo** pregnancy test; ~ **de esfuerzo** stress test; ~

de esfuerzo graduado stress test; ~ **de función cardíaca** cardiac function test; ~ **de función pulmonar** pulmonary function test; ~ **de función respiratoria** respiratory function test; ~ **de la audición** hearing test; ~ **de la capacidad de aprendizaje** test of learning capacity; ~ **de la fuerza** treadmill test; ~ **de la orina** urinalysis test; ~ **de la tuberculosis** TB test; ~ **de las tiras mojadas** dip stick test; ~ **de posición** station test; ~ **de resistencia** endurance test; ~ **de sangre** blood test; ~ **de Schick** Schick test; ~ **de sobrecarga** load test; ~ **de tolerancia a la glucosa** glucose tolerance test; ~ **del diapasón** fork test; ~ **del glaucoma** glaucoma test; drinking test; ~ **del pañal** *fam*, phenylketonuria/PKU test; ~ **del parche** patch test; ~ **del saco amniótico** amniocentesis; ~ **del tiempo** test of time; ~ **ergométrica** stress test; ~ **evidente** positive proof; ~ **funcional del hígado** liver function test; ~ **funcional muscular** muscular function test; ~ **rutinaria** routine test; **~s sanguíneas cruzadas** cross matching; ~ **selecta de (la) sangre** blood screening; ~ **serológica** serology test; ~ **subsecuente** follow-up test; ~ **terapéutica** therapeutic test

prurito, itch (*sensación*); itching; pruritus (*picazón grave*); ~ **del baño** bath pruritus; ~ **vulvar** pruritus vulvae

(p)sicoanálisis[6], *f*, psychoanalysis

(p)sicoanalista[6], *m/f*, analyst; psychoanalyst

(p)sicoanalizar[6], to psychoanalyze

(p)sicodélico[6], *m*, *adj*, psychedelic

(p)sicodrama[6], *m*, psychodrama

(p)sicología[6], psychology

(p)sicológicamente[6], *adv*, psychologically

(p)sicológico[6], *adj*, psychological
(p)sicólogo[6], psychologist
(p)sicometría[6], *f*, psychometry
(p)sicomotor[6], *adj*, psychomotor
(p)siconeuroinmunología[6], psychoneuroimmunology
(p)siconeurosis[6], *f*, psychoneurosis
(p)sicópata[6], *m/f*, psycho; psychopath
(p)sicopatía[6], psychopathy
(p)sicopático[6], *adj*, psychopathic
(p)sicopatología[6], psychopathology
(p)sicosis[6] *f*, psychosis; ~ **de masas** mass psychosis; ~ **maníaco-depresiva** manic-depressive psychosis; ~ **situacional** situational psychosis
(p)sicosocial[6], *adj*, psychosocial
(p)sicosomático[6], *adj*, psychosomatic
(p)sicotecnia[6], psychotechnics
(p)sicoterapia[6], psychotherapeutics; psychotherapy
(p)sicoterapista[6], *m/f*, *fam*, therapist; psychotherapist
(p)sicótico[6], *adj*, psychotic
(p)sique[6], *f*, psyche
(p)siquiatra[6], *m/f*, psychiatrist
(p)siquiatría[6], *adj*, psychiatric
(p)siquiátrico[6], *adj*, psychiatric
(p)síquico[6], *adj*, psychic
(p)soríasis (**vulgar**)[6], *f*, psoriasis
pterigión, *m*, pterygium
ptomaína, ptomaine
ptosis, *f*, ptosis; ~ **mamaria** sagging breast
púber, *adj*, adolescent; *m/f*, child approaching puberty
pubertad, *f*, puberty
pubescencia, pubescence
púbico, *adj*, pubic
pubis, *m*, pubic region
público, *m*, *adj*, public
pudendo, *adj*, pudendal; pudendum
pudor, *m*, modesty
pudrido, *adj*, decayed
pudrir, to decay
puente, *m*, nosepiece (*de las gafas*);

Col, collarbone; *Mex*, *Carib*, *Riopl*, bridge *Dent*; ~ **coronario** (coronary) by-pass; ~ **de apoyo dental** abuttal; ~ **dental** dental bridge; ~ **externo** (coronary) by-pass; ~ **fijo** fixed bridge; ~ **movible** removable bridge
puerco, *adj*, *fam*, dirty
pueril, *adj*, babyish (*chiquillada*); puerile
puerperal, *adj*, puerperal
puerperio, confinement; lying-in; postpartum period; puerperium
puesto, place; position; ~ **de enfermeras** nursing station; ~ **de socorro** aid station; first aid post
pujar, to bear down; to push *Obst*, (*al expulsar el feto*); to strain (*al hacer de vientre*)
pujido, grunt
pujilateao, *adj*, *PR*, annoyed
pujo, tenesmus; ~**s** straining
pulga, flea; ~ **de mar** sand flea; ~ **penetrante** sand flea
pulgada, inch
pulgar, *m*, thumb; ~ **de tenista** tennis thumb
pulimento para muebles, furniture polish
pulir, to polish
pulmometría, spirometry
pulmón, *m*, lung; ~ **de acero** iron lung
pulmonar, *adj*, pulmonary
pulmonía, pneumonia; ~ **bronquial** broncho-pneumonia; ~ **estreptocócica** streptococcus pneumonia; ~ **neumocócica lobular** pneumococcal lobular pneumonia; ~ **por aspiración** aspiration pneumonia; ~ **por grasa** lipoid pneumonia; ~ **por lípidos** lipoid pneumonia; ~ **por virus** viral pneumonia; ~ **vírica** viral pneumonia
pulmotor, *m*, iron lung
pulpa, pulp; ~ **dental** dental pulp; ~ **dental desvitalizada** dead pulp; ~ **dentaria** dental pulp

pulpectomía, pulp extirpation
pulpejo, ball of finger/fingertip; ball of thumb; ear lobe
pulpotomía, pulpotomy
pulsación, *f*, throb(bing) (*del pulso*); pulsation; beating *Anat*; ~ **irregular** flutter (*del pulso*)
pulsar, to beat (*corazón*); to throb; ~ **a uno** to feel s.o.'s pulse; to take s.o.'s pulse
pulsátil, *adj*, throbbing
pulso, pulse; ~ **abdominal** abdominal pulse; ~ **arrítmico** irregular pulse; ~ **arterial** arterial pulse; ~ **capilar** capillary pulse; ~ **colapsante** collapsing pulse; ~ **espasmódico** jerky pulse; ~ **filiforme** threadlike pulse; ~ **fuerte** strong pulse; ~ **hipertenso** high-tension pulse; ~ **hipotenso** low-tension pulse; ~ **intermitente** intermittent pulse; ~ **lento** slow pulse; ~ **ondulante** threadlike pulse; ~ **rápido** quick pulse; ~ **saltón** jerky pulse; ~ **trémulo** running pulse; ~ **venoso** venous pulse; ~ **yugular** jugular pulse
pulverización, *f*, spray
pulverizador, *m*, spray
pulverizar, to spray (*un líquido*)
puna, *SpAm*, *Med*, mountain sickness
punción, *f*, puncture *Med*; ~ (**quirúrgica**) (surgical) tap; ~ **aspiradora** needle aspiration; ~ **biópsica** needle biopsy; ~ **de la médula ósea** marrow puncture; ~ **exploradora** exploratory puncture; ~ **lumbar** lumbar puncture; spinal tap
puncionar, *form*, to tap
pungitivo, **dolor**, punching pain
punta, point (*extremo agudo*); tip; top (*dirección*); ~[1] nail[2] (*aguja para inyectarse drogas*); needle; spike[2] (*aguja hipodérmica*); ~ **de la aguja** needle tip; ~ **de la lengua** tip of tongue; ~ **de la**

nariz tip of nose; ~ **del corazón** apex of the heart; ~ **del dedo** ball of finger/fingertip; tip of finger
puntada, stitch; suture; *SpAm*, *Med*, sharp pain; *fam*, flank pain
puntazo, stab wound; knife wound; *SpAm*, jab; poke
punto, period (*puntuación*); point; stitch; ~ **ciego de la retina** optic disc; ~ **de congelación** freezing point; ~ **de costado** *Med*, pain in the side; stitch; ~ **de ebullición** boiling point/b.p.; ~ **de fusión** melting point; ~ **de partida** base-line; ~ **de referencia** base-line; frame of reference; ~**s de referencia** landmarks; ~ **de salida** exit wound; ~ **de saturación** saturation point; ~**s de sutura hemostáticos** hemostatic sutures; ~ **de vista** viewpoint; ~ **doloroso** trigger point; ~ **luminoso** point of light; ~ **máximo** peak; ~**s negros** black spots
puntudo, *adj*, *SpAm*, sharp
puntura, puncture; prick
punzada, sharp pain; shooting pain; stab (*de dolor*); touch; twinge (*de dolor*); throb; prick; stabbing; spasm; sting (*de un insecto*); ~ **de dolor** grip (*dolor*)
punzante, *adj*, throbbing (*dolor*); nagging; stabbing
punzar, to sear (*de dolor, etc.*)
puñado, handful
puñalada, stab (*con un puñal*); stab wound
puñetazo, punch (*con los puños*); sock (*golpe*)
puño, fist; handgrip (*de una bicicleta, etc.*); ~ **apretado** tight fist
pupa, oral lesion; lip sore; blister; ulcer; pimple
pupila, pupil *Anat*
pupilente, *m*, contact lens
pupo, *Arg*, *Chi*, *Ec*, *Perú*, navel
pupú, *m*, *fam*, stool

purga, *Med*, purge; cathartic; purgative

purgación, *f*, purgation; *slang*, gonorrhea; **~es** *pl*, *slang*, gonorrhea

purgante, *m*, cathartic; laxative; purgative; purge

purgar, to defecate; *Med*, to purge; to administer a purgative to; **~se** *Med*, to take a purge

purificación, purification; **~ emocional** catharsis

purificar, to purify; to cleanse

puro, cigar

purple haze[1], LSD

púrpura visual, visual purple

purrete, *m*, *Ríopl*, child

purrón, *m*, *PR*, can (*generalmente para llevar la leche*)

purulento, *adj*, purulent

pus, *m*, matter (*supuración*); pus; **~ detrás de la córnea** hypopyon

pushar[1], to push[2] (*drogas*)

pusheador[1], *Chicano*, dope pusher[2]; peddler[2] (*distribuidor de drogas*)

pústula, pimple; pustule

puta, *vulg*, prostitute

putrefacción, *f*, putrefaction

putrescina, putrescine

puya, *PR*, black coffee without sugar

puyar, *PR*, to goad; *SpAm*, to jab; to prick; to wound; *CA*, to needle; to upset

puyón, *m*, *Col*, *Guat*, *PR*, jab; prick; *Mex*, sharp point; thorn

---

[1] Este vocabulario es nuevo y todavía no se encuentra en el *Diccionario de la lengua española*, publicado por la Real Academia Española. Forma parte del argot o la lengua de la calle. Se supone que el género es obvio a menos que sea indicado.

[2] Forma parte del vocabulario inglés actual de los drogadictos.

[4] El nombre viene del hecho de que originalmente el paquete de drogas tenía un valor de diez dólares.

[5] *Pasmo* es un tipo de enfermedad causada por un cambio de temperatura ambiente y caracterizada por hinchazón y una erupción cutánea.

[6] Hoy es aceptable deletrear las palabras que antes se escribían con *psi-* en español (o *psy-* en inglés) sin la *p* que es consonante silenciosa en este caso.

[7] Se usa *primer* antes de un sustantivo masculino y *primero* después de un sustantivo masculino.

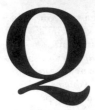

que, *pron. rel.*, who; whom; that; which; *conj*, (*se omite con frecuencia*) that; which; ~ **desaparece** evanescent; ~ **expulsa los gusanos intestinales** vermifuge; ~ **gime** moaning (*lamentar*); ~ **gotea** *adj*, dripping; ~ **indica la proximidad de la muerte** *adj*, thanatognomonic; ~ **mantiene el nivel del azúcar sanguíneo** glucokinetic; ~ **no puede sobrevivir** nonviable; ~ **no requiere receta médica** *adj*, over-the-counter; ~ **no tiene conducto excretor** ductless *Anat*,; ~ **pica(n)** *adj*, scratchy (*picante o irritado*); itchy; ~ **provoca flujo de lágrimas** dacryagogue; ~ **se cae** floppy; ~ **se explica por sí mismo** self-explanatory; ~ **tiene moretón** bruised (*equimosis*); ~ **va y viene** *adj phr*, intermittent; ~ **viene** next

qué, *adj interr y exclamat, pron interr,* what

quebradizo, *adj*, breakable; brittle; frail; sickly

quebrado, *adj*, broken; ruptured; *Med, m*, hernia

quebradura, break *Ortho* (*fractura*); ~ **de huesos** fracture; hernia; rupture (*hernia*); ~ **en la ingle** inguinal hernia

quebrantado, *adj*, broken (*salud*)

quebrantamiento, broken health; deterioration (*de la salud*); exhaustion (*agotamiento*)

quebrantarse, to break

quebranto, broken health; discouragement (*del ánimo*); distress (*dolor profundo*); exhaustion (*agotamiento*)

quebrar(se), to break *Ortho;* ~(se) *fam*, to fracture; ~se *Med*, to be ruptured; to have a rupture

quebraza, *Med*, crack (*en la piel*)

quedar, to remain; to stay (*permanecer*); ~ **en** to end up as; ~ **en** (+ *infinitive*) to agree to (+ *infinitivo*); ~se to stay; ~se **callado** to lapse into silence; ~se **dormido** to drop off into sleep; ~se **en cama** to keep in bed; to stay in bed; to lie in bed; ~se **en casa** to stay at home; ~se **levantado hasta muy tarde** to stay up late; ~se **sin aliento** to get out of breath; **quedársele pequeño** to grow out of

queilitis, *f*, cheilitis

queilosis, *f, form*, cheilosis (*llaga en la comisura de la boca*)

queja, complaint; moan (*de dolor*); ~ **principal** CC/chief complaint; **tener ~ de** to have a complaint about

quejarse, to complain; ~ (**de**) to grumble (at/about) (*lamentarse*); to moan

quejica, *adj*, nagging (*importunando*); grumpy; *m/f*, moaner

quejido, groan (*gemido*); moan

quejoso, *adj*, moaning (*de descontento*); querulous

queloide, *m*, keloid

quemado, *adj*, burned; burnt; ~ **del sol** *adj*, sunburned; ~[1] burned out[2]

quemadura, burn; ~ **de sol** sunburn; ~ **eléctrica** electrical burn; ~ **por ácido** acid burn; ~ **por álcali** alkali burn; ~ **por calor seco** dry heat burn; ~ **por explosión** flash burn; ~ **por fricción** friction burn; ~ **por frotamiento** friction burn; ~ **por llama** flame burn; ~ **química** chemical burn; ~ **térmica** thermal burn

quemante, *adj*, burning

quemao, *fam*, hangover

quemar, to bite (*hielo, escarcha*); ~(**se**) to burn (oneself); ~[1] to poke[2]; to smoke marijuana; to take a hit[2] (*dar chupadas de una abuja*); to toke up[2]

quemazón, *m*, burn; sunburn; ~ **al orinar** burning sensation when urinating

quemón[1], *m*, doper[2]; marijuana user

quemosis, *f*, chemosis

queratalgia, *form*, keratalgia

queratina, keratin

queratitis, *f*, keratitis

queratoconjuntivitis, *f*, keratoconjunctivitis

queratohipopión, *m*, keratohypopyon

queratoma, *m*, *form*, keratoma

queratoscopia, keratoscopy

queratotomía, keratotomy; ~ **radiada** radial keratotomy

querer (**ie**), to want/to love

querosén, *m*, kerosene

queso, cheese; *slang*, smegma

queta[1], marijuana

quetosis, *f*, ketosis

quetosuria, ketosuria

quevedos, spectacles (*con una montura de alambre*); eyeglasses

quieto, *adj*, still (*inmóvil*)

quijada, jaw *slang*; jawbone; ~ **rota** broken jaw

quilla, keel

quilosis, *f*, kyllosis

química, chemistry; ~ **aplicada** applied chemistry; ~ **física** physical chemistry; ~ **forense** forensic chemistry; ~ **mineral** inorganic chemistry; ~ **orgánica** organic chemistry

químico, *adj*, chemical; *m*, chemist

quimiocirugía, chemosurgery

quimioterapia, chemotherapy

quinesioterapeuta, *m/f*, kinesitherapist

quinesiterapia, kinesitherapy

quínico, *adj*, quinic

quinidamina, quinidamine

quinidina, quinidine

quinina, quinine

quinta de tos, fit of coughing

quintillizo, quint; quintuplet

quintípara, *f*, *adj*, quintipara

quíntuple, *m/f*, quintuplet

quiroespasmo, chirospasm

quirófano, operating room

quiropedia, chiropody

quiropodista, *m/f*, chiropodist; podiatrist

quiropráctico, chiropractor

quiropractor, chiropractor

quiropraxia, manipulation therapy

quirúrgico, *adj*, surgical

quirurgo, surgeon

quiste, *m*, cyst; ~ **de Baker** Baker's cyst; ~ **cutáneo** cutaneous cyst; ~ **láctico** milk cyst; ~ **mucoso** mucous cyst; ~ **ovárico** ovarian cyst; ~ **por distensión** distention cyst; ~ **pulmonar expansivo** expanding pulmonary cyst; ~ **radicular** periodontal cyst; ~ **sebáceo** sebaceous cyst; ~**s en los ovarios** cysts on the ovaries

quístico, *adj*, cystic

quitar, to remove; to take away/out; to relieve (*dolor*); ~ **el sarro a** to scale *Dent*; ~**le a alguien un peso de encima** to take a great weight off one's mind; ~**le el pecho al bebé** to wean; ~**se** to take off; to peel off (*ropa*); to take off (*desvestirse*); ~**se** (*a uno*) to grow out of (*una costumbre*)

quitear[1], to clear up[2]; to kick the habit[2]

quizá(s), *adv*, perhaps

---

[1] Este vocabulario es nuevo y todavía no se encuentra en el *Diccionario de la lengua española*, publicado por la Real Academia Española. Forma parte del argot o la lengua de la calle. Se supone que el género es obvio a menos que sea indicado.

[2] Forma parte del vocabulario inglés actual de los drogadictos.

R

R[1], *f*, artillery[2] (*término de las drogas*); gun[2]

rabadilla, *Anat*, coccyx; tail bone *fam*

rábano, radish

rabia, fury; rabies *Med*; *fam*, anger; hydrophobia

rabiar, to have rabies

rabioso, *adj*, rabid

rabo, tail

ración, *f*, intake (*de comida*); portion (*de comestibles*); ration

racional, *adj*, rational

racionalización, *f*, rationalization

radiación, *f*, radiation; ~ **inicial** initial radiation; **~es** radiation treatment

radiactividad, *f*, radioactivity

radiactivo, *adj*, radioactive

radiante, *adj*, radiant; radiating

radiar, to radiate; to treat with x-rays

radical, *adj*, radical

radicotomía, *f*, radicotomy

radio, radium *Chem*; radius *Anat*

radioactividad, *f*, radioactivity

radioactivo, *adj*, radioactive

radiobiólogo, radiation biologist

radiodiagnóstico, radiodiagnosis

radiografía, film (*imagen*); radiography; roentgenography; x-ray; ~ **de las venas** venogram; ~ **de (los) vasos sanguíneos** angiography test; vasography; ~ **de los ventrículos cerebrales** ventriculogram; ~ **de toda la boca** full mouth x-ray; ~ **del pecho** chest x-ray; ~ **del riñón** nephrogram; ~ **del tórax** chest x-ray; ~ **seccional** scan

radiografiar, to x-ray; to take an x-ray photo

radioisótopo, radioisotope

radiología, radiology

radiólogo, radiologist

radiolúcido, *adj*, radiolucent

radioondas, radiowaves

radiosensibilidad, *f*, radiosensibility

radioterapia, radiation therapy; radiotherapy; radium therapy; x-ray therapy; ~ **profunda** deep x-ray therapy

radiotermia, radiothermy

radiotransparente, *adj*, radiolucent

radiotrasparencia, radiolucency

radióxido de zinc, zinc oxide

radiumterapia, radiumtherapy

radón, *m*, radon

raedura, *Med*, abrasion

raer, *Med*, to abrade; to chafe

ráfaga, gust

raigón, *m*, stump (*de un diente; raíz grande*)

raíz, *f*, root; ~ **nerviosa** nerve root

raja, crack (*hendidura*); slice (*de queso, pescado, melón, etc.*);

rajada, *vulg*, vulva

rajao, *adj*, intoxicated

rajar, to crack (*vidrio, etc.*); **~se** *Arg, Col*, to be mistaken; *PR*, to get drunk

rajo, *SpAm*, tear; rip

rajuñar, *Arg*, (*Vea rasguñar.*)

ralo, *adj*, thin (*pelo*)

rama, branch; division; stick (*de apio*); ~ **de medicina** branch of medicine; ~ **fascicular** bundle branch

ramalazo, mark left by a lash; weal; bruise

ramificación, *f*, branch

ramificado, *adj*, branched

ramificar(se), to ramify

ramillete, *m*, bouquet

ramo, branch; *Med*, touch; slight attack (*de una enfermedad*); ~ **de locos** touch of madness; ~ **de locura** touch/streak of madness

rampa, charley horse cramp

rana, frog

ranchero, *adj, slang, Mex*, shy

rancio, *adj*, rancid; stale

rango, range; **~ de movimiento** range of motion

ranura, slot (*en que se introduce una moneda*)

rapiar, *Chicano*, to chat

rápidamente, *adv*, quickly

rápido, *adj*, fast (*veloz*); quick; rapid; *adv*, quick

rapo, *Chicano*, rape

rapto, kidnapping

raquialgia, rachialgia

raquiectomía, rachiectomy

raquiotomía, rachiotomy

raquis, *m*, backbone; vertebral column

raquisquisis, *f*, rachischisis *form*; spinal bifida

raquítico, *adj*, rachitic

raquitis, *f*, rachitis; rickets

raquitismo, rachitis; rickets

raro, *adj*, unusual

rascado, scratch (*en la piel*); *adj, Ven*, drunk

rascadura, scratch (*en la piel que pica*)

rascar(se), to scratch (*aliviar una picazón*); to tear; *slang, SpAm*, to be/get drunk; **~se** to pick (*una costra*)

rasgar, to tear; to rip; to tear to pieces (*papel*)

rasgo, line (*línea*); quirk (*de escritura*); trait; **~s** features

rasgón, *m*, rip; tear (*desgarrón*)

rasguñar, to scratch (*arañar*)

rasguño, nick; scratch (*en la piel*)

rasmillar, *Chi*, to scratch

rasmillón, *m, Chi*, scratch

raspa, *fam*, D & C

raspado, abrasion (*raspadura*); *fam*, curettage; **~ diagnóstico** D & C

raspado, *adj*, skinned (*desollado*)

raspadura, abrasion (*raspado*); scrape wound

raspar, to graze (*desollar*)

raspón, *m*, abrasion (*desolladura*); *SpAm*, bruise; scratch (*en la piel*)

rasquera, itching sensation

rasqueta, hair pick

rastro, vestige

rasurar(se), to shave

rata, rat

ratón, *m*, mouse; *Ven*, hangover

raya, line (*hecha por pluma o lápiz*); scratch (*en una superficie*); streak/part (*del pelo*); **hacerse la ~** to part one's hair

rayar, to scratch (*una superficie dura*); **~ en** to verge on; **~se** to bang; **~se**[1] to fix[2] (*inyectar drogas*); to inject oneself with drugs; to hit up[2]

rayo, beam (*de un rayo x, etc.*); ray; **~s catódicos** cathode rays; **~s cósmicos** cosmic rays; **~ equis / rayo x** x-ray (*un rayo de Roentgen—una película*); **~s equis** x-rays; **~ equis del pecho** chest x-ray; **~s infrarrojos** infrared rays; **~ láser** laser; **~s solares** solar rays; **~s ultravioletas** ultraviolet rays; **~s x** x-rays

raza, race; crack; fissure; slit

razón, *f*, reason

razpón, *m*, abrasion

reacción, *f*, reaction; response; **~ a la insulina** insulin reaction; **~ acelerada** accelerated reaction; **~ ácida** acid reaction; **~ adversa** adverse reaction; **~ alcalina** alkaline reaction; **~ alérgica** allergic reaction; **~ anafiláctica** anaphylactic reaction; **~ de alarma** emergency reaction; **~ de coloración** dye test; **~ de evitación** escape reaction; **~ de la piel** skin reaction; **~ de tipo diferido** delayed type reaction; **~ de Wassermann** (*prueba de la sífilis*) Wassermann's reaction; **~ en cadena** chain reaction; **~ falsa positiva** false positive reaction; **~-formación** reaction-formation; **~ generalizada** systemic reaction; **~ leucemoide**

leukemoid reaction; ~ **medicamentosa** drug reaction; ~ **tardía** delayed reaction; **tiempo de** ~ reaction time

reaccionar, to wince

reacio, *adj*, loath

reactivación, *f*, booster shot; flare up (*de una epidemia*)

reactivar, to reactivate

reactividad cardiovascular, *f*, cardiovascular reactivity

reactivo, reagent; *adj*, reactant

reactor nuclear, *m*, nuclear reactor

reagudizarse, *Med*, to become acute again; to get worse again

real, *adj*, actual (*auténtico*)

realidad, *f*, reality

realmente, *adv*, really

reanimación, *f*, resuscitation; ~ **cardiopulmonar** cardiopulmonary resuscitation/CPR

reaparecer, to reappear

reaparición, *f*, recurrence; ~ **local** local recurrence

rebajar, to downgrade

rebanada, slice (*de pan*)

rebase, *f*, rebase *Dent*

rebencudo, *adj*, *Cu*, stubborn

reborde, *m*, cushion; edge; ridge *Dent*; ~ **alveolar** alveolar ridge; ~ **bucocervical** buccocervical ridge; ~ **coronario** coronary cushion; ~**s dentales** dental ridges; ~ **linguocervical** linguocervical ridge; ~**s marginales** marginal ridges

rebosamiento, overflow

rebosar de, to shine (*de salud, etc.*); ~ **de alegría** to be overwhelmed with joy

rebote, *m*, rebound

recado, message

recaer, *Med*, to suffer a relapse

recaída, relapse (*de un enfermo*); setback *Med*

recalcarse un hueso, *SpAm*, to dislocate a bone

recámara, bedroom

recambio gaseoso, gas exchange

recao, *PR*, herb

recargo, *Med*, rise in temperature

recedente, *adj*, preceding

recelo, mistrust (*desconfianza*)

recepción, *f*, front desk; reception desk

recepcionista, *m/f*, receptionist

receptividad, *f*, receptivity

receptor, *m*, receiver; receptor; ~ **-ra universal** *m/f*, universal recipient (*que puede recibir sangre por transfusión de cualquiera de los 4 grupos*)

recesivo, *adj*, recessive

receta, prescription; ~ **médica** doctor's prescription; prescription

recetado, *adj*, prescribed

recetar, to order (*prescribir un medicamento*); to prescribe

rechazo, denial; rejection

rechinamiento de dientes, clenching; gnashing of the teeth

rechinar los dientes, to gnash; to grate one's teeth; to grit one's teeth

rechoncho, *adj*, chubby; heavyset; plump; squat

recibir, to receive

recibo, receipt

recidiva, recidivation; recurrence; relapse (*de un enfermo*)

recidivante, *adj*, relapsing

recien, *adv*, recently (+ *p.p.*); ~ **casado** newlywed; ~ **nacido** *m*, *adj*, baby (*infante*); newborn; ~ **viuda** recently widowed

reciente, *adj*, late; recent

recipiente, *m*, container (*vasija, etc.*); ~ **para guardar la dentadura** denture cup

recobrar, to recover (*voz, sentidos, etc.*); to recuperate (*la salud*); to regain; ~ **el aliento** to regain one's breath; ~ **el conocimiento** to regain consciousness; ~ **el juicio** to regain one's sanity; ~ **la respiración** to get one's breath back; ~ **la salud** to get back on one's legs; to pull through; ~se *Med*, to convalesce; to get over an illness; to regain consciousness

recoger, to pick up

recolección de la muestra, *f*, collection of the specimen urine

recomendar (ie), to recommend

recompensa, fee

reconfortar, *Med*, to strengthen; ~se con to fortify oneself with

reconocer, *Med*, to examine

reconocimiento, acknowledgment; examination; ~ médico check-up; medical examination; physical examination

recordar (ue), to remember; to reminisce

recorrer, to walk the length of

recreo, recreation

recrudecimiento, flare up (*nueva epidemia*); resurgence

rectal, *adj*, rectal

rectificar, to rectify

recto, *Anat*, rectum; *adj*, straight

rectocele, *m*, rectocele

rectoscopia, rectoscopy

rectoscopio, rectoscope

recuento, count; ~ de gérmenes bacteria count; ~ de glóbulos blancos white blood cell count; ~ de glóbulos rojos red blood count/RBC; ~ de leucocitos white cell count; ~ hemático blood count; ~ hemático completo complete blood count/CBC; ~ sanguíneo *fam*, blood count

recuperación, *f*, recovery

recuperar, to make up (*ganar*); to recover (*voz, sentidos, etc.*); to recuperate (*la salud*); ~se to bounce back; to get over an illness; to recover (*de una enfermedad*); to recuperate (*de una enfermedad*)

recurrente, *adj*, recurrent; recurring

recurrir (a), to resort (to)

recurso, resource; ~s finances; ~s de laboratorio laboratory facilities

red, *f*, net; network; ~ celular cell network; ~ neurofibrilar neurofibrillar network

reducción, *f*, abatement; reduction

reducir, to lessen; to reduce; ~ al mínimo to minimize; ~ la ansiedad to reduce anxiety; *Med*, to set (*un hueso*); ~ una fractura to set a fracture; ~(se) to shrink (*calidad*)

reductor, *adj*, reducing

reduplicar, to replicate

reeducación, *f*, reeducation

reemplazar, to replace (*sustituir a*)

reemplazo, replacement (*sustitución*); ~ parcial de la rodilla partial knee replacement; ~ total de la cadera total hip replacement; ~ total de la rodilla total knee replacement

referir (ie), to refer

refinado, *adj*, refined

reflejar, to reflect

reflejo, reflex; response; ~ aquíleo heel tap; Achilles tendon reflex; ~ condicionado conditioned reflex; trained reflex; ~ corneal eyelid closure reflex; ~ cremastérico cremasteric reflex; ~ de flexión de la pierna flexion reflex of the leg; ~ de prehensión grasping reflex; ~ del hociqueo rooting reflex; ~ del tendón de Aquiles Achilles tendon reflex; ~ exagerado increased reflex; ~ faríngeo gag reflex; ~ innato inborn reflex; ~ instintivo instinctive reflex; ~ lumbosacro back reflex; ~ nauseoso gag reflex; ~ no condicionado inborn reflex; ~ patelar knee jerk reflex; ~ retardado delayed reflex; ~ rotuliano knee jerk/kj; knee jerk reflex; patellar reflex; ~ tendinoso tendon jerk; tendon reflex

reflujo, reflux

reformatorio, house of correction

refracción, *f*, refraction

refractar, to refract

refractivo, *adj*, refractive
refregar, to scrub (*quirúrgicamente*)
refrescar, to refresh; *Mex, Med*, to get better; **~le la memoria a** to give s.o.'s memory a jog
refrigeración, *f*, refrigeration
refrigerador, *m*, refrigerator
refringente, *adj*, refractive
refuerzo, backing *Dent*; booster vaccination; **~ del ego** ego enhancement
refugio, shelter (*abrigo*)
refunfuñar, to grouch (*quejarse*); to grumble (*gemir*); to mutter (*con enojo*)
refunfuño, mumbling
refunfuñón, grouch/grumbling individual; *adj*, grouchy; grumbling
refutar, to disprove
regadera, *Mex*, shower
regaliz, *m*, licorice
regalo, present; gift
regazo, lap *Anat*
regeneración, *f*, regeneration
regenerar, to regenerate
régimen, (*pl*, **regímenes**) *m*, regime; system; diet *Med*; regimen *Med*; **~ alimenticio** diet; **~ de prueba** trial diet; **estar a ~** to be on a diet; **~ horario** time schedule; **~ pobre en grasas** low fat diet; **poner a uno a ~** to put s.o. on a diet
región, *f*, region; **~ glútea** gluteal region; **~ lumbar** small of the back
regional, *adj*, regional
registrar, to enter (*inscribir*); to record (*escribir en un registro*); to register (*matricular*); **~ el pulso** to take the pulse; **~ la señal** to pick up the signal
registro, entry; record (*de medicamentos, etc.*); tracing; **~ de defunciones** obituary; **~s médicos** medical records
regla, menstrual period; period; rule (*reglamento*); ruler (*utensilio para medir*); **~s** menses;

Mex, PR, menstruation; **~s muy abundantes** menorrhagia
reglamentos, regulations
reglar, to menstruate
regoldar, to belch
regordete, *adj*, chubby
regresar, to come back; to go back
regüeldo, burp
regulación, *f*, control; **~es** regulations; **~ de la natalidad** birth control; **~ de nacimientos** birth control; **~ refleja** reflex control
regular, *adj*, fair (*mediano*); regular
regular, to control; to regulate
regurgitación, *f*, regurgitation; **~ mitral** mitral regurgitation
regurgitar, to belch
regusto, aftertaste
rehabilitación, *f*, rehabilitation; **~ bucal** mouth rehabilitation; **~ de incapacitados** rehabilitation of the handicapped
rehabilitar, to rehabilitate
rehacer, to redo; to repair; **~ (la receta)**, to refill (*una prescripción*); **~se** *Med*, to recover; to regain one's strength
rehidratar, to rehydrate
reimplantación, *f*, reimplantation
reinervación, *f*, reinnervation
reinfección, *f*, reinfection
reinjertación, *f*, reimplantation
reinoculación, *f*, reinoculation
reintegrar, to reintegrate; to restore
reír (i), to laugh; **~ a carcajadas** to howl with laughter; to scream with laughter; **~ a mandíbula batiente** to laugh until one's sides ache; **~ con risa de conejo** to give a forced laugh; **~se** to laugh; **~se por nada** to giggle
rejilla de ventilación, vent (*de ventilador, etc.*)
rejuvenecimiento, rejuvenation
relación, *f*, relation; relationship; ratio; **~ bucolingual** buccolingual relation *Dent*; buccolingual relationship *Dent*; **~ cardiotorá-**

cica cardiothoracic ratio; ~ de reposo del maxilar inferior rest jaw relation *Dent* ; ~es dinámicas dynamic relations *Dent*; ~ estrecha close relationship; ~ mandibular jaw relation *Dent*; ~ maxilar jaw relation *Dent*; ~ oclusal de los maxilares occlusal jaw relation *Dent*; ~ peso-talla body-weight ratio; ~ sexual sexual intercourse; ~es sexuales sexual relations

relacionarse, to relate

relajación, *f, Med*, relaxation; hernia; rupture (*hernia*)

relajado, *m, Med*, hernia; *adj, Med*, ruptured

relajadores musculares, *m*, muscle relaxants

relajadura, *Mex*, hernia; rupture

relajamiento muscular, muscular relaxation

relajante, *m, adj, Med*, relaxant; laxative; ~ **muscular** muscle relaxant

relajar, to ease; ~ **el cuerpo** to relax; ~**se** to relax; ~**se un tobillo** *Med*, to lose the feeling in an ankle; ~**se un órgano** *Med*, to rupture an organ; ~**(se)** *fam*, to have a good time

relajo, disorderly conduct

relamerse, to smack one's lips

relámpago, lightning

relativamente, *adv*, relatively

relativo (a), *adj*, relative (to); ~ **la sangre** hematic; ~ **al embarazo o a la mujer preñada** gravidic

relieve, *m*, cushion; ~ **endocárdico** endocardial cushion

religar, to reattach

reliquias, *f, pl, Med*, after-effects; resultant weakness

rellenar, to fill *Dent*; to obturate; to pack *Med*; ~ **la herida con gasa** to pack the wound with gauze

relleno, dressing (*comestible*); filling (*cocina; empaste dental*); *adj*, stuffed

reloj, *m*, clock; watch; ~ **biológico** biological clock; ~ **de muñeca** wristwatch ; ~ **de pulsera** wristwatch

remedio, cure; drug; medicine; remedy; ~ **casero** home remedy

remisión, *f*, abatement; remission

remitencia, remittence

remitente, *adj*, remittent

remitir, to remit

remojar, to soak

remorder (ue), to nag (*la conciencia*); ~**se** to worry; to feel remorse

remover (ue), *Med*, to excise; to cut out

renal, *adj*, renal

rencor, *m*, anger

rendido de fatiga, *adj*, exhausted; worn out (*extenuado*)

rendija, crack (*hendidura*)

rendimiento, output (*de una máquina u obrero*)

rendir(se), to yield (*darse por vencido*)

renegar (ie), *Mex, Perú, Ríopl*, to get angry; to be upset

rengo, *adj*, lame

renguear, *SpAm*, to hobble; to limp (*renquear*)

renguera, *SpAm*, limp; limping

renina, renin

renovar (ue) el pañal (de), to diaper

renuncia, quitclaim; ~ **voluntaria** waiver

renunciar, to give up (*abandonar*)

reñir (i), to quarrel (*disputar*)

reóstato, rheostat

reparable, *adj*, mendable

reparar, to mend; to repair

reparo, *Med*, remedy

repaso de sistemas, review of systems

repelente, *m, adj*, repellent; ~ **contra insectos** insect repellent; ~ **de insectos** insect repellent

repelo, *Anat*, hangnail

repente, *m*, sudden movement

repentino, *adj*, sharp; sudden; unexpected (*inesperado*)

repetir (i), to belch; to repeat; *fam*, to burp; ~se to recur

repliegue, *m*, doubling; fold; replication; ~ **ungueal** nail wall

reponer, to replace (*poner de nuevo*); ~se **de una enfermedad** *Med*, to get over an illness

reposición, *f*, *Med*, recovery

reposo, rest; ~ **absoluto** *Med*, complete rest

representación esquemática, *f*, diagram

representar, to represent; ~ **la edad que se tiene** to look one's age

represión, *f*, repression

reprimir, to bottle up (*sentimientos*); to quench (*emociones*); to repress; to restrain (*refrenar*)

reproducción, *f*, reproduction

reproducirse, to recur *Med*

reproductivo, *adj*, reproductive

reproductor, *adj*, reproductive

repuesto, refill (*de una receta*); replacement (*recambio*)

repugnancia, aversion

reputación, *f*, reputation

requerimientos diarios mínimos, minimum daily requirements/ MDR

requerir (ie), to involve (*necesitar*); to request; to require

resbalar, to slide (*deslizar*); to slip (*dar traspiés*)

resbalón, *m*, slip (*involuntario*)

rescatar, to rescue; to save

rescate, *m*, rescue

resecar, *Med*, to amputate; to cut out; to exsiccate; to remove; to resect; ~sele **la boca a alguien** to have s.o.'s mouth parched

resección, *f*, resection; ~ **de una parte de intestino** enterectomy; ~ **de una raíz dental** root amputation; ~ **de una vena varicosa** varicotomy; ~ **gástrica** gastric resection; ~ **transuretral** transurethral resection

reseco, *adj*, dry; parched

resentimiento, hard feeling

resentirse (ie), to become resentful; to begin to weaken; to be affected; ~ **de** to suffer from; to feel the effects of

resequedad, *f*, extreme dryness; ~ **de la piel** dryness of the skin; ~ **de la piel causada por el viento** windburn; ~ **de los ojos** xerosis

reserpina, reserpine

reserva cardíaca, cardiac reserve

resfriado, cold (*enfermedad*); head cold; chill; **coger un** ~ to catch a cold; ~ **común** common cold; ~ **fuerte** bad cold

resfriar, *Med*, ~ **a uno** *Med*, to give s.o. a cold; ~se to catch a cold

resfrío, cold (*enfermedad*); head cold; *fam*, congestion

residencia, residence; ~ **para ancianos** old people's home; ~ **para jubilados** old people's home

residente, *m/f*, resident; ~ **en cirujía** surgical resident

residuo, debris; remnant; residue; ~s **atmosféricos** fallout; ~ **bajo** low residue

resina, resin; ~s **de intercambio** exchange resins

resistencia, endurance; resistance; ~ **bacteriana** bacterial resistance; ~ **globular** globular resistance

resistente, *adj*, lasting (*que resiste*); resistant; ~ **al calor** heat resistant; **hacerse** ~ (**a**) *Med*, to build up a resistance (to)

resistir, to resist

resollar (ue), to breathe heavily; to pant; to wheeze

resolución, *f*, resolution

resolver(se) (ue), to resolve; ~se to clear up (*una enfermedad, sarpullido, etc.*)

resonador, *m*, resonator

resonancia, resonance; ~ **magnética nuclear** magnetic resonance imaging/MRI

resonante, *adj*, resonant

resoplar, to breathe hard; (*Vea resollar.*)

resoplido, wheeze; noisy breathing; **dar ~s** to breathe heavily

resorción, *f*, resorption

respaldo, backing *Dent*; backup

respiración, *f*, breathing; respiration; **~ abdominal** abdominal respiration; **~ artificial** artificial respiration; **~ boca a boca** mouth-to-mouth breathing; **~ bucal** mouth-breathing; **~ dificultosa** difficulty in breathing; **~ entrecortada** jerky respiration; **~ estertorosa** stertorous respiration; **~ fetal** fetal respiration; **~ interrumpida** jerky respiration; **~ jadeante** labored breathing; **~ laboriosa** labored respiration; **~ sibilante** wheeze

respiradero, air vent; vent (*orificio de aeración*)

respirador, *m*, respirator

respirar, to inhale; *fam*, to breathe in; **~ asmáticamente** to wheeze; **~ con dificultad** to wheeze; **~ demasiado rápido** to hyperventilate; **~ hondo** to gulp for breath; **~ profundo** to take a deep breath; **~ (por la boca)** *fam*, to breathe; **~ cola**[1] to inhale glue[2]; to sniff glue[2]

respiratorio, *adj*, respiratory

respirómetro, respirometer

responder, to respond

responsabilidad, *f*, responsibility; legal responsibility; liability; **~ de la comunidad** community responsibility; **~ solidaria** joint responsibility

responsable, *adj*, accountable; responsible

respuesta, response

restablecer, to reestablish; **~se** *Med*, to recover (*de una enfermedad*)

restablecimiento, recovery

restar, to substract

restauración, *f*, restoration; **~ bucal** buccal restoration

restaurar, to repair; **~ las fuerzas a alguien** to restore s.o.'s strength

restaurativo, *adj*, restorative

restituir, to restore

resto, remnant; rest *Dent* (*lo que queda*)

restregar, to rub; to scrub (*ropa*)

restricción, *f*, limitation; restraint

restrictivo, *adj*, limiting

restricto, *adj*, limited

restringido, *adj*, restrictive

restringir, to restrict

resucitación, *f*, resuscitation; **~ boca a boca** mouth-to-mouth resuscitation; **~ cardiopulmonar/ RCP** cardiopulmonary resuscitation/ CPR

resucitador, *m*, resuscitator; **~ cardiopulmonar** cardiopulmonary resuscitator

resucitar, to bring (back) to life; to resuscitate

resudar, to sweat a little

resuello, breathing; **~ asmático** asthmatic wheeze; **corto de ~** short of breath; **~ ruidoso** wheeze

resultado, finding; outcome; result; score; **~ del análisis** laboratory finding; **~s a largo plazo** long term results; **~s de pruebas** test results

resultar, to turn out

resumen, *m*, summary

resurgir, *Med*, to recover

retardación, *f*, mental retardation; retardation; delay; **~ de crecimiento** growth retardation

retardado, *m*, *adj*, retarded; *adj*, mentally retarded; **~ mental** mentally retarded

retardar, to delay (*el desarrollo*)

retardo, delay (*del desarrollo*); mental retardation; retardation; **~ mental** mental retardation; **~ (p)sicomotor**[4] retención *f*, psychomotor retardation retention; **~ de (la) orina** retention of urine; **~ de la dentadura** denture retention; **~ de líquidos** liquid retention; **~ fecal** fecal retention; ~ **total** total retention; ~ **urinaria** retention of urine

retenedor, *m*, retainer *Dent*; safety catch (*en joyas*); ~ **por barra continua** continuous bar retainer

retener, to retain; ~ **el aliento** to hold one's breath

retícula, mesh; reticle; reticulum (*pl, reticula*) (*óptica*)

retículo, network; reticle; reticulum (*pl, reticula*)

reticulocito, reticulocyte

retina, retina; ~ **desprendida** detached retina

retinitis, *f*, retinitis; ~ **solar** eclipse blindness

retinocoroiditis, *f*, retinochoroiditis

retinopatía, retinopathy

retinoscopia, retinoscopy

retinoscopio, retinoscope

retintín, *m*, tinkle; tinkling; ringing (*en los oídos*)

retinto, *adj*, very dark-skinned lacking negroid features

retirada, withdrawal

retirarse, *m*, coitus interruptus

retirarse, to withdraw

retoque, *m*, *Med*, symptom

retorcer (**ue**), to kink (*dar vueltas a*); ~**se de dolor** to writhe in pain; ~**se de risa** to double up in laughter; ~**se las manos** to wring one's hands

retorcijón, *m*, *fam*, abdominal cramp; menstrual cramp

retorno, return

retortijón, *m*, abdominal cramp; ~ *m*, *fam*, menstrual cramp ~ **de tripas** stomach cramp

retracción, *f*, retraction; ~ **gingival** gingival retraction *Dent*; ~ **mandibular** mandibular retraction

retractor, *m*, retractor

retrasado, *adj*, late (*tarde*)

retrasar, to delay (*poco desarrollo*)

retraso, delay (*del desarrollo*); lag; ~ **mental** mental deficiency; mental retardation

retratao, *PR*, assault; beating

retrato del x-ray, *Chicano*, x-ray

retrete, *m*, latrine; lavatory (*cuarto de baño*); *Spain*, toilet

retroacción, *f*, feedback

retroceder, to drop back into; to regress

retroceso, *Med*, new outbreak; renewed attack; aggravation (*de una enfermedad*)

retroflexión, *f*, retroflexion

retrógrado, *adj*, retrograde

reuma/reúma, *m*, rheum; ~**s** rheumatism; *fam*, arthritis

reumático, *adj*, rheumatic

reumatismo, rheumatism; ~ **articular agudo** acute articular rheumatism; ~ **articular crónico** chronic rheumatism; ~ **subagudo** subacute rheumatism

reumatoide, *adj*, rheumatoid

reumatoideo, *adj*, rheumatoid

reumatología, rheumatology

reumatólogo, *adj*, rheumatologist

reunión, *f*, meeting

reunir, to gather together; ~**se** (**con**) to meet (*encontrarse*)

revacunación, *f*, booster shot; revaccination

revejido, *adj*, *Col*, weak; feeble

revelado de una radiografía, development of an x-ray film

revelador, *adj*, revealing; *m*, *Photo*, developer

revelar una radiografía, to develop an x-ray

reventar(se), to burst

reventazón, *f*, *Mex*, flatulence

reventón, *m*, rupture (*hernia*); *Chi*, *Med*, relapse

reversible, *adj*, reversible; reversal

reversión, *f*, reversion

revés, *m*, setback (*fracaso*)

revestir (**i**), to line; to sheathe

revisar, to examine; to review

revisión, *f*, examination; ~ **de sus partes** pelvic examination; ~ **médica** check-up; ~ **sistémica** review of systems

revista, magazine

revolver (ue), to stir; to turn; ~se to writhe; to squirm (*con dolor*)

revulsar, *Mex*, to vomit

rezumamiento, eczema; leak

rezumante, *adj*, weeping

rezumar, to exude; to ooze

Rh-negativo, *adj*, Rh negative

Rh-positivo, *adj*, Rh positive

riboflavina, riboflavin; vitamin B_2

rico, *adj*, rich (*adinerado; gustoso*)

ridículo, *adj*, sorry (*de poca estimación*)

riesgo, hazard; risk; ~ **de infección** risk of infection

rigidez, *f*, rigidity; ~ **cadavérica** rigor mortis; ~ **de nuca** neck stiffness

rígido, *adj*, rigid; stiff (*inflexible*)

rigor mortis, *m*, rigor mortis

rinconera, midwife

rinitis, *f*, rhinitis; ~ **catarral aguda** acute catarrhal rhinitis

rinofaringoscopia, rhinopharingoscopy

rinoplastia, rhinoplasty

rinopsia, internal strabismus

rinorragia, rhinorrhagia

rinoscopia, rhinoscopy

riña, quarrel

riñón, *m*, kidney; ~ **alargado** tandem kidney; ~ **anular** doughnut kidney; ~ **arteriosclerótico** arteriosclerotic kidney; ~ **artificial** artificial kidney; ~ **atrófico** atrophic kidney; chronic interstitial nephritis; ~ **cirrótico** cirrhotic kidney; ~ **contraído** chronic interstitial nephritis; ~ **ectópico** floating kidney; ~ **en herradura** horseshoe kidney; ~ **flotante** floating kidney; ~ **pélvico** pelvic kidney; ~ **poliquístico** polycystic kidney; ~ **quístico** cystic kidney; ~ **supernumerario** supernumerary kidney; ~ **único por fusión** fused kidney; ~, **uréter**, **vejiga** KUB/kidney, ureter, bladder

riñonera, emesis basin

risa, laugh; laughter

risueño, *adj*, laughing

ritmo, rhythm (*anticontraceptivo*); rhythm method; rate; ~ **alfa** alpha rhythm; ~ **beta** beta rhythm; ~ **biológico** biorhythm; ~ **circadiano** circadian rhythm; ~ **de galope** gallop rhythm; ~ **fetal** tick-tack sounds; ~ **respiratorio** respiratory rate; ~ **sinusal** sinus rhythm; ~ **sinusal normal** NSR / normal sinus rhythm

rizar, to curl; ~se to kink (*el pelo*)

rizo, curl of hair; kink (*de cabellos*)

robusto, *adj*, able-bodied

roce, *m*, rub; rubbing; ~ **pericárdico** pericardial rub; to and fro murmur; ~ **por fricción** friction rub

rociador, *m*, spray

rociar, to spray (*salpicar*)

rodeado, *adj*, surrounded

rodear, to surround

rodilla, knee; ~ **bloqueada** locked knee; ~ **de monja** housemaid knee

rodillera, knee bandage

rodio, rhodium

roentgen, *m*, roentgen

rogam, *m*, rhogam

rogar (ue), to beg

roja[1], seconal; ~s[1] devils[2] (*seconal, barbitúricos*)

rojizo, *adj*, reddish

rojo, *adj*, red; ~ **obscuro** maroon

rollo, roll; ~ **de gasa** gauze roll ; ~[1] marijuana

romadizo, head cold

romero, rosemary

romo, *adj*, blunt

romper, to break; to rupture; to tear; ~(se) *Carib*, to break *Ortho*; ~se to fracture; to go (*quebrantar*); to wear out

rompible, *adj*, breakable

rompimiento, break

ron, *m*, rum

roncar, to snore

roncha, efflorescence; hives; wheal swelling (*de una picadura*);

~ **hulera** leishmaniasis; ~ **mala** leishmaniasis

ronco, *adj*, hoarse; husky (*voz*)

ronquear, to be hoarse; to talk hoarsely

ronquera, aphonia (*de voz*); croup; hoarseness; huskiness

ronquido, snore; harsh, raucous sound; sound (*ronco, estridente*)

roña, mange; scab *Vet*; ~**s** *f, pl, fam*, hives

ropa, clothing; ~ **de cama** bedclothes; ~ **de dormir** nightclothes; ~ **de maternidad** maternity clothes; ~ **interior** underwear; ~ **limpia** clean laundry; ~ **sucia** dirty laundry

rosado, *adj*, pink

rosario raquítico, beading of the ribs

rosbif, *m*, roast beef

rosca, *Anat*, roll of fat

roséola, roseola; ~ **epidémica**[5] rubella

rostro, face

rotación, *f*, rotation; ~ **de la cabeza** head-rolling

rotadura, *Chicano*, rupture (*hernia*)

roto, *adj*, broken; ruptured; *vulg, PR*, ass

rótula, kneecap; patella

rotulador, *m*, felt-tipped pen

rotuliano, *adj*, patellar

rotundo, *adj*, outright (*categórico*)

rotura, break *Ortho*; rip; rupture (*de un hueso*); tear (*de un tejido*); *fam*, hernia

rozado, *adj*, chapped

rozadura, abrasion (*desolladura*); chafe; chafe wound; chafing; graze (*roce*)

rozar, to graze (*raer suavemente*); ~**(se)** to chafe; ~**se** to chap skin

rozón, *m*, graze (*roce*)

rubéola[5]/**rubeola**[5], *form*, German measles; roseola; rubella; threeday measles

rubio, *adj*, blond; fair (*pelo*); fairhaired

rubor, *m*, flush (*pudor; en las mejillas*); redness; ~ **atropínico** atropine flush; ~ **mamario** breast flush

ruborizarse, to blush; to flush

ruboroso, *adj*, bashful

ruda, rue

rugido, howl (*del viento*)

rugir, to howl (*el viento*)

ruibarbo, rhubarb

ruido, bruit; murmur; noise; row (*alboroto*); sound (*sonido*); ~**s aórticos** aortic sounds; ~ **áspero** rasping sound; ~**s cardíacos** heart sounds; ~ **chirrido** rasping sound; ~ **de bandera** flapping sound; ~ **de frotación** friction sound; ~ **de galope** gallop *Med*; ~ **de maullido** mewing murmur; ~ **de roce** friction murmur

ruidoso, *adj*, loud; noisy

ruptura, rupture (*hernia*)

rutina, routine

rutinario, *adj*, routine

---

[1] Este vocabulario es nuevo y todavía no se encuentra en el *Diccionario de la lengua española*, publicado por la Real Academia Española. Forma parte del argot o la lengua de la calle. Se supone que el género es obvio a menos que sea indicado.

[2] Forma parte del vocabulario inglés actual de los drogadictos.

[4] Hoy es aceptable deletrear las palabras que antes se escribían con *psi-* en español (o *psy-* en inglés) sin la *p* que es consonante silenciosa en este caso.

[5] *Rubéola/rubeola* es un término utilizado en los países de habla inglés como sinónimo de *measles* (sarampión) y de *rubella* (rubéola/rubeola o sarampión alemán). En español se usa de preferencia el término *rubéola/rubeola* para referirse a la *rubella* de los autores anglosajones.

S

sábana, sheet

sabañón, *m*, chilblain

saber, to find out; to know (*hechos, ser docto en algo*); ~ **a** to taste like; ~ **mal** to taste nasty

sabor, *m*, flavor; taste; ~ **a cereza** cherry flavor(ed); ~ **a menta** mint flavor(ed); ~ **a naranja** orange flavor(ed); ~ **de menta** mint flavor(ed)

saborear, to taste

sabrío, *adj, PR*, tasteless

sabroso, *adj*, rich (*comida*); *Mex, Perú, PR, RD*, talkative

saburra, fur (*en la lengua*); dental tartar

saburral, *adj*, furred; furry (*la lengua*); coated

sacada, *Arg, Col, Perú* (*Vea sacadura.*)

sacadura, *Col, Chi, Perú*, extraction

sacaleche, *m, inv*, breast pump

sacar, to dislodge (*quitar*); to extract; to pull (*extraer*); to remove; to take out; to stick out (*la lengua, el pecho*); to show (*los dientes*); to find; to get (*una respuesta*); to take (*un rayo x; una foto*); to have made (*una fotocopia*); ~ (**el**) **aire** *Chicano*, to burp (*un bebé*); ~ **aire** *Mex, CA, fam*, to breathe out; ~ **brillo** to shine (*pulir*); ~ **cuatro copias de** to quadruplicate; ~ **de paseo** to exercise (*un perro*); ~**le el nervio a alguien** to remove the nerve *Dent*; ~ **fotos** to take pictures; ~ **la lengua** to stick out one's tongue; ~ **leche del pecho** to express milk from the breast; ~ (**leche**) **por medio de una bomba** to pump (*leche*); ~ **los dientes** to show one's teeth; ~ **sangre** to draw blood; ~

un diente de un tirón to yank a tooth; ~ **una conclusión** to draw a conclusion

sacarina, saccharine

sacaromiceto, yeast fungus

sacerdote, *m*, priest

saco, bag; sac; jacket; jacket of a man's suit; ~ **amniótico** amniotic sac; ~ **vitelino** yolk sac

sacro, sacrum; *adj*, sacral

sacroilíaco, *adj*, sacroiliac

sacudida, jerk (*movimiento brusco, repentino*); jolt (*de un vehículo*); shake (*agitación*); tic; ~ **cruzada** crossed jerk; ~ **de Aquiles** Achilles jerk; ~ **de la rodilla** knee jerk; ~ **del tobillo** ankle jerk; ~ **maxilar** jaw jerk; ~ **muscular** muscular twitching; ~ **nerviosa** nervous jerk; ~ **tendinosa** tendon jerk

sacudir, to jerk (*dar una sacudida*); to shake (*agitar*)

sáculo, saccule

sádico, *adj*, sadistic; *m*, sadist

sadismo, sadism

sadista, *m/f*, sadist

safena, *adj, f, Anat*, saphenous; *f, Anat*, saphena

safenectomía, stripping; saphenectomy *form*

sajar, *Med*, to cut open; to lance

sajín, *m, CA*, underarm odor

sajino, *m, CA*, underarm odor

sal, *f*, salt; ~**es aromáticas** smelling salts; ~ **biliar** bile salt; ~ **corriente** noniodized salt; ~ **de Epsom** Epsom salt; ~ **de higuera** Epsom salt; ~**es perfumadas** smelling salts; ~ **yodada** iodized salt

sala, *form*, room; (hospital) ward; ~ **de cirugía** operating room; ~ **de disección** dissecting room; ~ **de emergencia** emergency room; ~

de espera reception room; waiting room; **~ de estar** waiting room; **~ de los médicos** doctors' lounge; **~ de los recién nacidos** newborn nursery; **~ de maternidad** maternity ward; **~ de operaciones** operating room; **~ de partos** delivery room; labor room; **~ de recepción** waiting room; **~ de recuperación** recovery room; **~ de restablecimiento** recovery room; **~ de terapéutica intensiva** intensive therapy room; **~ de urgencia** emergency room; **~ para puérperas** postdelivery room; **~ prenatal** labor room

salado, *adj*, saline (*con sabor de sal*); salty

salar, to salt (*para conservar o sazonar*)

salarete, *m*, bicarbonate of soda

salario, salary; **~ mínimo** minimum wage

salchicha, sausage

salicilato, salicylate

salida, efflux; electrical outlet; escape (*de un líquido*); exit; outlet; way out (*solución*); **~ de los dientes** teething

saliente, *adj*, outgoing (*que abandona o deja sus funciones*); prominent (*pómulo, diente, etc.*); *m*, protrusion

salino, *adj*, saline (*que contiene sal*)

salir, to drain (*pus, etc.*); to get out; to leave (*irse*); **~ bien** to turn out okay; **~ de lo normal** to deviate from the norm; **~ de su cuidado** *Chicano*, to give birth; **~ de una larga enfermedad** to recover from a long illness; **~ dientes** to cut teeth; **~ sangre** to hemorrhage; **~le barros** to break out; **~le granos** to break out; **~le leche** *fam*, to lactate; **~le sangre de la nariz** to have a nosebleed; **~se** to withdraw (sexually); **~se** *m*, *slang*, coitus interruptus

saliva, saliva; spit (*en la boca*); sputum

salivación, *f*, salivation

salivazo, spit (*expulsado por o de la boca*)

salmón, *m*, salmon

salmonela, salmonella

salmonelosis, *f*, salmonellosis

salón, *m*, hall (*sala grande*); **~ de entrada** lounge; **~ principal** lobby

salpingectomía, salpingectomy

salpingitis, *f*, salpingitis

salpullido, diaper rash; rash; swelling (*de una picadura*); fleabite; **~s** *m*, *pl*, *fam*, hives

salsa, sauce; **~ para ensalada** salad dressing; **~^{1}** gravy^2 (*una mezcla de sangre y heroína*)

saltar, to hop; to jump

salto, leap; **~ atrás** throw-back

saltón, *adj*, protruding (*dientes*); bulging (*ojos*); popping (*ojos*)

salubridad, *f*, healthiness; health statistics; **~ pública** public health

salud, *f*, health; state of health; *fig*, welfare; wellbeing; **¿Cómo vamos de ~?** How are we today?; **devolverle (ue) la ~ a uno** to give s.o. back his/her health; to restore s.o. to health; **estar bien de ~** to be in good health; **estar mal de ~** to be in bad/poor health; **~ física** physical health; **mejorar de ~** to improve one's health; **~ mental** mental health; **~ pública** public health

saludable, *adj*, healthy

saludar, to greet

saludo, greeting

salvado, bran

salvamento, rescue

salvar, to rescue; to save

salvavidas, *m/f*, lifeguard; *m*, *inv*, life preserver; *adj*, lifesaving

salvo, *adj*, safe (*seguro*)
salvohonor, *m*, *fam*, buttock
sampullido, eruption of the skin
samurar, *Ven*, to walk with bowed head
sanar, to heal (*una herida*); to recover (*de una enfermedad*); *Chicano*, *euph*, to give birth; ~**se** to get well; to heal
sanatorio, sanitarium (*lugar para tratamientos*); clinic; nursing home
sangradera, *Med*, lancet
sangrado, bleeding; *fam*, hemorrhage; ~ **por la nariz** bloody nose; ~ **vaginal** bloody show
sangrador, *m*, bleeder
sangradura, *Anat*, bend of the elbow; *Med*, cut made into a vein
sangramiento, hemorrhage
sangrante, *adj*, bleeding
sangrar, to bleed; to hemorrhage; to let bleed
sangre, *f*, blood; ~ **clara** *fam*, anemia; ~ **completa** whole blood; ~ **débil** *fam*, anemia; weak blood; ~ **desecada** dry blood; ~ **en el orín** blood in the urine; hematuria; ~ **en la orina** blood in the urine; hematuria; ~ **entera** whole blood; ~ **mala** *slang*, syphilis; ~ **oculta** occult blood; ~ **oxalatada** oxalated blood; ~ **pobre** *fam*, anemia; weak blood; ~ **pura** whole blood; ~ **umbilical** cord blood
sangrear, to bleed
sangría, bleeding; ~ **suelta** *Med*, excessive flow of blood
sangriento, *adj*, bleeding; bloody
sanguijuela, leech (*parásito*)
sanguíneo, *adj*, bleeding; blood; **vaso** ~ blood vessel
sanguinolento, *adj*, blood-stained; bloody; tinged with blood; bloodshot (*ojos*)
sanidad pública, *f*, public health (department)
sanitario, *adj*, sanitary
sano, *adj*, able-bodied; healthy; sane (*persona*: *mente*); sound (*saludable*); whole (*entero*); wholesome (*sin vicios*)
santo, saint's day
santos óleos, extreme unction; last rites
sapeta, *Chicano*, diaper
sapo, *PR*, *SD*, thrush
sarampión, *m*, measles; morbilli; ~ **alemán** German measles; rubella; ~ **bastardo** German measles; rubella; ~ **de tres días** *fam*, German measles; three-day measles; ~ **malo** hard measles (*rubeola*); measles
saraviado, *adj*, *Col*, freckled (*persona*)
sarcoma, *m*, sarcoma; ~ **de células gigantes** giant cell sarcoma; ~ **de Kaposi** Kaposi's sarcoma
sardina, sardine
sarna, itch; scabies; mange *Vet*
sarpullido, eruption of the skin; rash; ~ **causado por exceso de calor** prickly heat
sarro, dental calculus; dental tartar; film (*en los dientes*); plaque; scale (*en los dientes*); tartar; fur (*de la lengua*)
sarroso, *adj*, covered with tartar (*dientes*); furry (*lengua*)
sartorio, sartorius muscle
satisfacer, to satisfy
saturación, *f*, saturation
saturnismo, lead poisoning
saúco, elder (*árbol*)
sauna, sauna
sazonar con pimienta, to pepper
scanner, *m*, scanner
se prohibe, it is prohibited; ~ **fumar** smoking is prohibited; ~ **la entrada** no admittance
sebáceo, *adj*, fatty; sebaceous
seborrea, seborrhea
seca, *fam*, bubo
secado al frío, freeze drying
secador, *m*, dryer; ~ **de cabello/de pelo** hair dryer; ~ **para el pelo** hair dryer

secadora, clothes dryer
secante, *adj*, drying
secar, to bake; to dry
sección, *f*, division; section; ~ cesárea caesarean section; ~ transversal cross section
seccionar, to divide
seco, *adj*, dry (*no mojado*); extracto ~ de hígado (dry) liver extract
seconal, *m*, seconal
secreción, *f*, discharge (*fluido*); secretion; ~ excesiva de moco o jugo gástrico gastrorrhea; ~ mucosa mezclada con sangre bloody show; ~ vaginal vaginal discharge (*sin sangre*)
secreta, *slang*, venereal disease
secretar, to secrete; ~ leche to lactate
secretaria de sala, ward clerk
secretina, secretin
secuela, complication; sequela; ~s after-effects
secuestro, kidnapping; sequestrum; ~ óseo bone sequestrum
secundario, *adj*, minor; secondary
secundinas, placenta; *pl*, *Mex*, afterbirth
sed, *f*, thirst
seda encerada, dental floss
sedante, *m*, *adj*, calmative; depressant; pain killer; sedative; ~ ligero mild sedative
sedativo, downer[2] (barbitúrico); sedative; sleeping pill
sedentario, *adj*, sedentary
sedimentación, *f*, sedimentation; ~ de eritrocitos erythrocyte sedimentation
sedimento, deposit; dregs; sediment; ~ urinario urinary sediment
seducción, *f*, abuse
segmento, segment
segregación, *f*, *Anat*, secretion
segregado, *Anat*, secretion
segregar, *Anat*, to secrete
seguido, *adj*, continuous

seguir (i), to continue; to follow; to go after; ~ trabajando to continue working; ~ un tratamiento médico to be under doctor's care; ~ una dieta to follow a diet
segundo, *m*, *adj*, second; segunda dentición *f*, secondary dentition; segunda fase del parto *f*, second stage of pregnancy; segunda muela permanente twelfth-year molar; segunda opinión *f*, second opinion; ~ nombre *m*, middle name; ~ parto *Chicano*, afterbirth; placenta; ~ período del parto second stage of labor; second stage of pregnancy
seguridad, *f*, safety; security; ~ pública public safety
seguro, insurance; safety catch (*de armas*); security; *Mex*, safety pin; *adj*, positive (*cierto*); reliable (*de fiar*); safe (*firme*); secure (*inestable*); sure; póliza de ~ insurance policy; prima de ~ insurance premium; ~ a todo riesgo fully comprehensive insurance; ~ colectivo group insurance; ~ contra accidentes accident insurance; ~ de hospitalización hospitalization insurance; ~ de sí mismo *adj*, self-confident; ~ de vida life insurance; ~ médico health insurance; ~ sobre la vida life insurance; ~ social Social Security
selección, *f*, screening; selection; ~ multifásica multiphasic screening
seleccionar, to choose; to select; ~ para detectar (+ *enfermedad*) to screen for (+ *illness*)
selenio, selenium
sellar, to seal (*cerrar*); to stamp (*estampar un sello*)
sello, seal; stamp; *Med*, capsule; pill
semana, week
semanalmente, weekly
semejante, *adj*, similar

semejanza, similarity
semen, *m*, semen; seminal fluid; sperm
semicomatoso, *adj*, semicomatose
semicupio, sitz bath
semidesintegración, *f*, half-life
semilla, seed; *Chi*, baby; child; *slang*, *Mex*, sperm; **~s de dondiego de día**[1] blue star[2]; flying saucers[2]; morning glory seeds[2]
semilunar, *adj*, semilunar
seminífero, *adj*, seminiferous; **túbulos ~s** seminiferous tubules
seminoma, *m*, seminoma
sencillo, *adj*, plain (*sin adorno*); simple
senda, path
senectud, *f*, old age; senility
senil, *adj*, senile
senilidad, *f*, senility
seno, breast; sinus; **~s** *pl*, bosom; **~ auricular** pacemaker; **~ doloroso** painful breast; **~ occipital** occipital sinus; **~s pesados** heaviness in breasts
sensación, *f*, feeling; sensation; sense; **~ de ahogo** shortness of breath; **~ de desmayo** light-headedness; **~ de dolor** sense of pain; **~ de mareo** sensation of dizziness; **~ de pesantez en el perineo** bearing-down pain; **~ de placer** sense of pleasure; **~es de ser apretado** *adj*, pressure sensations
sensato, *adj*, sane (*persona: de buen juicio*)
sensibilidad, *f*, feeling; sensitivity; tenderness; **~ gustativa** taste sensitivity; **~ táctil** tactile sensibility
sensibilización, *f*, sensitization; **~ a proteínas** protein sensitization; **~ al factor Rh** Rh sensitization
sensibilizado, *adj*, sensitized
sensibilizar, to sensitize
sensible, *adj*, responsible; sensitive; tender; **~ (sitio)** *Med*, sore; tender
sensitivo, *adj*, sore; touchy

sensorial, *adj*, sensorial
sensorio, sensorium
sentadera, buttock; **~s** *fam*, bottom (*trasero*)
sentarse (**ie**), to sit down
sentido, hearing; feeling (*sentimiento*); sensation; sense; meaning; sense (*significado*); **~ de la vista** sense of sight (*visual*); **~ de orientación** sense of direction; **~ del gusto** sense of taste (*sabor*); **~ del humor** sense of humor; **~ del oído** sense of hearing (*auditivo*); **~ del olfato** sense of smell (*olor*); **~ del tacto** sense of feeling (*táctil*); **~ muscular** kinesthesia
sentimiento, feeling; sentiment; **~ de culpabilidad** guilt feelings
sentir (**ie**), to feel (*afligirse; tocar*); **~ bascas** to feel nauseated; to gag (*dar náuseas a*); **~ nostalgia** to be homesick; **~ calor** to feel warm; **~(se) caluroso** to feel hot; **~(se) sofocado** to feel hot; **~lo** to be sorry (*afligirse*); **~se en forma** to feel up to scratch; **~se mal** to feel ill; **~se molesto** to be embarrassed; **~se solo** to feel lonely; **~se** to feel (*emoción/dolor; salud*); to suffer (*de una enfermedad*)
seña, sign
señal, *f*, sign; signal; **~ (luminosa) de peligro** danger light
señalar, to mark; to point to
señor, *m*, man; gentleman; Sir
señora, lady; woman; Madam
señorita, young lady; Miss
separación, *f*, separation
separado, *adj*, separated
separar, to divide; to hold away from; to single out; to spread apart
sepsis, *f*, blood poisoning; sepsis
septicemia, blood poisoning; sepsis; septicemia
séptico, *adj*, septic
sequedad, *f*, dryness; **~ de boca** dry mouth

sequiar, (*Arg*: *fumadores*) to inhale (*tabaco, etc.*)

ser, to be; ~ arrestado *adj*, to be busted *slang*; ~ compatible con to match (*sangre, tejidos, etc.*); ~ demasiado joven to be underage; ~ duro de oído to have a dull sense of hearing; ~ garantizado *adj*, to be guaranteed; ~ herido *adj*, to get hurt (*herirse*); ~ humano *m*, human being; ~ indiferente a to be apathetic towards; ~ internado, *adj*, to be admitted; ~ mayor de edad to be of age; ~ menor de edad to be underage; ~ torcido *adj*, to be busted; ~ un manojo de nervios to be a mass of nerves; ~ uña y carne to be close to each other

serenarse, to regain one's composure

sereno, *adj*, serene

serie, *f*, series

serio, *adj*, serious

seroaglutinación, *f*, seroagglutination

seroalbúmina, seroalbumin

serodiagnóstico, serodiagnosis

serología, serology

serorresistente, *adj*, serum-fast

serosa, serosa

seroso, *adj*, serous

serpiente, *f*, snake; ~ de cascabel rattlesnake; ~ del pasto grass snake

serpigo, ringworm; tinea

servicio, lavatory (*cuarto de baño*); service; ~s *pl*, restroom; toilet; ~ de ambulancias ambulance service; ~ de consulta externa outpatient department; ~ de cuidados intensivos intensive care; ~s de salud pública public health services; ~s domiciliarios de salud home health services; ~s médicos healthcare; ~ médico de guardia medical duty; ~ médico de urgencia EMS/emergency medical service; ~s profesionales professional services; ~ social social service

servilleta, napkin; ~ sanitaria sanitary napkin; sanitary pad; ~s faciales facial tissues

servir (i), to serve; ~le de desahogo a alguien to be an outlet

sésamo, sesame

sesentón, -tona, *m/f*, person about sixty; *adj*, sixtyish

sesión, *f*, session

sesonar[1], to sniff glue[2]

sesos, *fam*, brain

seta, *fam*, mushroom

setentón, -tona, *m/f*, person about seventy; *adj*, seventyish

seudociesis, *f*, pseudocyesis

severamente enflaquecido, *adj*, emaciated

severidad, *f*, severity

severo, *adj*, severe

sevillana, switchblade knife

sexo, sex; ~ oral oral sex

sexual, *adj*, sexual

Sherm[1], PCP

shock, *m*, shock

shockterapia, shock therapy

shootear[1], to bang[2]; to fix[2] (*inyectar drogas narcóticas*); to hit up[2]; to inject o.s. with drugs; ~ salsa[1] to shoot gravy[2] (*sangre aspirada por la aguja, mezclada con drogas narcóticas, calentada e inyectada*)

shunt, *m*, shunt

sí, yes

si, if; ~ es necesario *s.o.s./si opus sit*/if necessary

sicoanálisis, *f*, psychoanalysis

sicoanalista, *m/f*, psychoanalyst

sicoanalizar, to psychoanalyze

sicodélico, *m*, *adj*, psychedelic

sicodrama, *m*, psychodrama

sicología, psychology

sicológico, *adj*, psychological

sicólogo, psychologist

sicometría, *f*, psychometry

sicomotor, *adj*, psychomotor

siconeuroinmunología, psycho-neuroimmunology
siconeurosis, *f*, psychoneurosis
sicópata, *m/f*, psycho; psychopath
sicopatía, psychopathy
sicopatología, psychopathology
sicosis, *f*, psychosis; ~ **maníaco-depresiva** manic-depressive psychosis; ~ **maniacodepresiva** manic-depressive insanity
sicosocial, *adj*, psychosocial
sicosomático, *adj*, psychosomatic
sicoterapia, psychotherapeutics; psychotherapy
sicótico, *m*, *adj*, psychotic
SIDA/síndrome de inmuno(logía) deficiencia adquirida *m*, AIDS/acquired immune deficiency syndrome
sidoso, *fam*, sufferer of AIDS
siempre joven, *adj*, ageless
sien, *f*, temple
sierra, saw
siesta, nap
siete días/7 días, *m*, infantum tetanus
sietecueros, *m*, *inv*, *fam*, blister on sole of foot; *SpAm*, gumboil
sietemesino, *m*, *adj*, (*lit. seven months*) premature fetus
sífilis, *f*, syphilis; ~ **congénita** congenital syphilis; ~ **conyugal** marital syphilis; ~ **primaria** early syphilis; ~ **terciaria** tertiary syphilis
sifilítico, *m*, *adj*, syphilitic
sigla, abbreviation
sigma cólico, sigmoid colon
sigmoide, *adj*, sigmoid
sigmoideo, *adj*, sigmoid
sigmoidoscopia, sigmoidoscopy
sigmoidoscopio, sigmoidoscope
significado, meaning; sense
significar, to imply
signo, sign; ~ **característico** hallmark; ~ **de advertencia** warning sign; ~ **físico** physical signs; ~**s vitales** vital signs
siguetear, *Perú*, (*Vea seguir.*)

siguiente, *adj*, next
silbar, to hiss; to wheeze; to whistle
silbido, hiss (*de abucheo; vapor, gas*); souffle; wheeze; whistle
silencioso, *adj*, mute; quiet; silent; still
silice, *f*, silica
silicio, silicon
silicona, silicone
silla, chair; ~ **de dentista** dentist's chair; ~ **de operaciones** operating chair; ~ **de ruedas** wheelchair
silleta, *Med*, bedpan
sillón de ruedas, *m*, wheelchair
silueta, profile (*del cuerpo*)
simbiosis, *f*, symbiosis
símbolo, symbol
simetría, symmetry
simétrico, *adj*, symmetrical
similñoco, *PR*, gadget; *PR*, *fam*, amputee
simpatía, sympathy
simpático, *adj*, nice; sympathetic (*nervio, dolor*)
simple, *adj*, *euph*, mentally retarded
sin, s/*sans*/without; ~ **azúcar** sugarless; ~ **cobro** no charge; ~ **complicaciones** uneventful; ~ **cordón umbilical** efuniculate; ~ **cura** past recovery; ~ **dificultad** painless (*nada difícil*); ~ **dolor** painless (*físicamente*); ~ **esperanza** hopeless; ~ **éxito** unsuccessful; ~ **hijos** childless; ~ **hogar** homeless; ~ **importancia** irrelevant; ~ **olor** odorless; ~ **pagar** outstanding (*pendiente*); ~ **querer** involuntarily; ~ **relieve** dull (*sin brillo*); ~ **sabor fuerte** bland; ~ **sentido** senseless; ~ **utilidad** obsolete; ~ **vida** lifeless; dull (*sin animación*); ~ **zapatos** barefoot
sinapismo, mustard plaster; poultice
sinapsis, *f*, synapsis
síncope, *m*, exanimation; faint; fainting spell; syncope

síndrome, *m*, syndrome; ~ **agudo por radiación** acute radiation syndrome; ~ **alcohólico fetal** fetal alcohol syndrome; ~ **asmático** asthmatic syndrome; ~ **carotídeo** carotid sinus syndrome; ~ **de ansiedad** anxiety syndrome; ~ **de asfixia traumática** ecchymotic mask syndrome; ~ **de choque tóxico** toxic shock syndrome; ~ **de deficiencia de** ___ ___ deficiency syndrome; ~ **de dificultad respiratoria del adulto** adult respiratory distress syndrome/ARDS; ~ **de dificultad respiratoria del recién nacido** hyaline membrane syndrome; ~ **de Down** Down's syndrome; ~ **de Dressler** Dressler's syndrome; ~ **de estómago de vaciamiento rápido** dumping stomach syndrome; ~ **de insuficiencia respiratoria del adulto** adult respiratory distress syndrome/ ARDS; ~ **de insuficiencia respiratoria del recién nacido** hyaline membrane syndrome; ~ **de Klinefelter** Klinefelter's syndrome; ~ **de la membrana hialina** hyaline membrane syndrome; ~ **de la muerte súbita del lactante** SIDS/sudden infant death syndrome; crib death; ~ **de la piel escaldada** scalded skin syndrome; ~ **de las piernas inquietas** restless legs syndrome; ~ **de muerte infantil repentina** sudden infant death syndrome/SIDS; crib death; ~ **de muerte súbita en la cuna** crib death; SIDS; ~ **de muerte súbita del lactante** crib death; SIDS; ~ **de muerte súbita infantil** crib death; SIDS; ~ **de shock tóxico/SST** *Spain*, toxic shock syndrome/TSS; ~ **del canal del carpo** carpal tunnel syndrome; ~ **del climaterio femenino** menopausal syndrome; ~ **del colon irritable** irritable bowel syndrome; ~ **del lóbulo medio del pulmón** middle lobe syndrome; ~ **del niño golpeado** battered child syndrome; ~ **del seno carotídeo** carotid sinus syndrome; ~ **del túnel carpiano** carpal tunnel syndrome; ~ **del túnel del carpo** carpal tunnel syndrome; ~ **fetal alcohólico** fetal alcohol syndrome; ~ **funcional doloroso miofacial** myofacial pain disfunction; ~ **menopáusico** menopausal syndrome; ~ **por aplastamiento** compression syndrome; ~ **por compresión** compression syndrome; ~ **posinfarto de miocardio** Dressler's syndrome; ~ **premenstrual** premenstrual syndrome/PMS

sinequia, synechia

sinergía, synergy

sinergismo, synergism

sínfisis, *f*, symphysis

siniestrado, victim (*de un accidente, etc.*)

sinoatrial, *adj*, sinoatrial

sinoauricular, *adj*, sinoauricular

sinoventricular, *adj*, sinoventricular

sinovia, synovial liquid

sinovial, *adj*, synovial

sinsemilla[1], Acapulco gold[2] (*mariguana*)

sintético, *adj*, synthetic

sintetizar, to synthesize

síntoma, *m*, complaint; diagnostic (symptom); sign; symptom; ~ **característico** characteristic symptom; ~ **de advertencia premonitorios** warning symptom; ~**s de supresión** withdrawal symptoms; ~ **demorado** delayed symptom; ~ **equívoco** equivocal symptom; ~ **general** general symptom; ~**s objetivos** objective symptoms; ~ **por simpatía** sympathetic symptom; ~ **presente**

presenting symptom; ~ **principal** chief complaint

sintomático, *adj*, symptomatic

sinusitis, *f*, sinus congestion; sinusitis

sipo, *adj*, *Ec*, pockmarked

siquiatra, *m/f*, psychiatrist

siquiatría, psychiatry

síquico, *adj*, psychic

SIRA/síndrome de insuficiencia respiratoria del adulto, *m*, ARDS/adult respiratory distress syndrome

siriasis, *f*, sunstroke

sirimba, *Cu*, faint; fainting fit

sisear, to hiss

siseo, hiss (*para llamar la atención*)

sisote, *m*, boil; *Chicano*, ringworm; tinea

sistema, *m*, system; ~ **alimentario** digestive system; ~ **alimenticio** alimentary system; ~ **biológico** biological system; ~ **bulboespiral** bulbospiral system; ~ **C.G.S.** centimeter-gram-second system; ~ **cardiovascular** cardiovascular system; circulatory system; ~ **cegesimal** centimeter-gram-second system; ~ **cerebro(e)spinal** central nervous system; ~ **cerrado** closed system; ~ **cinesódico** kinesodic system; ~ **circulatorio** circulatory system; hematologic system; ~ **de inmunidad** immune system; ~ **de oxidación-reducción** oxidation-reduction system; ~ **digestivo** digestive system; ~ **ecológico** ecological system/ecosystem; ~ **endocrino/endócrino** endocrine system; ~ **esquelético** skeletal system; ~ **estático** static system; ~ **gastrointestinal** gastrointestinal system; ~ **genitourinario** genitourinary system; ~ **hematicovascular** blood-vascular system; ~ **hematológico** circulatory system; hematologic system; ~ **hematopoyético** hematopoietic

system; ~ **inmune** immune system; ~ **integumentario** integumentary system; ~ **laceríntico** vestibular system; ~ **linfático** lymphatic system; ~ **masticatorio** masticatory system; ~ **métrico** metric system; ~ **muscular** muscular system; ~ **musculoesquelético** musculoskeletal system; ~ **nervioso** nervous system; ~ **nervioso autónomo** autonomic nervous system; ~ **nervioso central** central nervous system; ~ **nervioso craneosacral** parasympathetic nervous system; ~ **nervioso de la vida orgánica** autonomic nervous system; ~ **nervioso de los ganglios** autonomic nervous system; ~ **nervioso idiotropo** autonomic nervous system; ~ **nervioso involuntario** autonomic nervous system; ~ **nervioso parasimpático** parasympathetic nervous system; ~ **nervioso periférico** peripheral nervous system; ~ **nervioso simpático** sympathetic nervous system; ~ **nervioso vegetativo** autonomic nervous system; vegetative nervous system; ~ **neurovegetativo** autonomic nervous system; ~ **postural** static system; ~ **quinesódico** kinesodic system; ~ **reproductivo** reproductive system; ~ **respiratorio** respiratory system; ~ **reticuloendotelial** reticuloendothelial system; ~ **urogenital** urogenital system; ~ **vascular** vascular system; ~ **vascular sanguíneo** blood-vascular system; ~ **vasomotor** vasomotor system; ~ **vestibular** vestibular system

sistemático, *adj*, systemic

sístole, *f*, systole; ~ **abortada** aborted systole; ~ **anticipada** anticipated systole; ~ **arterial** arterial systole; ~ **auricular** auricular systole; ~ **prematura** anticipated systole; ~ **ventricular** ventricular systole

sistólico, *adj*, systolic

sitio para las piernas, leg room

situación, *f*, lie *Obst*; situation; ~ **longitudinal** longitudinal lie; ~ **oblicua** oblique lie; ~ **transversa** transverse lie

situado, *adj*, located

sobaco, *fam*, armpit

sobador, -ra, *m/f*, *Col*, *Mex*, bonesetter; quack

sobandero, *Col*, *Ven*, bonesetter; quack

sobaquera, *fam*, crutch; *CA*, *Mex*, *PR*, underarm odor

sobaquina, underarm odor

sobar, to massage; *SpAm*, to set (*huesos*)

sobasquera, *CA*, *Mex*, *PR*, underarm odor

sobras, leftovers

sobre, *m*, envelope (*para cartas*); *prep*, on; over

sobreañadido, *adj*, superimposed

sobrecargar, to overload

sobrecorreción, *f*, overcorrection

sobrecubierta, jacket (*de un libro*)

sobredentellada, overbite

sobredosis[1], *f*, *inv*, hot shot[2] (*sobredosis muchas veces fatal*); overdose; ~ **de drogas** drug overdose; ~ **tóxica**[1] hot shot[2] (*sobredosis muchas veces fatal*); overdose

sobreexcitado, *adj*, overwrought

sobreextensión, *f*, overextension

sobremordida, overbite

sobrenatural, *adj*, supernatural

sobreparto, afterbirth; confinement; lying-in; **morir (ue) de** ~ to die in childbirth

sobrepeso, excess weight; overweight

sobreprecio, overcharge (*precio excesivo*)

sobresaliente, *adj*, outstanding

sobresaltar, to shock (*asustar*)

sobresalto, scare; shock; start (*movimiento nervioso*)

sobresanar, *Med*, to heal superficially

sobreviviente, *m/f*, survivor

sobrevivir, to outlive (*una persona; vergüenza*); to survive

sobrina, niece

sobrino, nephew

sobrio, *adj*, sober

socarse, *CA*, to get drunk

socarrar, to singe

social, *adj*, social

sociedad, *f*, society

socioeconómico, *adj*, socioeconomic

socioterapia, sociotherapy

socorrer, to relieve

socorrista, *m/f*, paramedic

socorro, assistance; help; ~ **inmediato** immediate help

sodio, sodium

sodoku, *m*, rat bite fever

sofocación, *f*, suffocation

sofocante, *adj*, oppressive (*atmósfera*); sweltering (*día, oficina, etc.*)

sofocar, to asphyxiate; to choke (*debido a una falta de aire, vapores, etc.*); ~**(se)** to suffocate; ~**se de calor** to swelter

sofoco, choking sensation (*ahogo*); flash; flush (*enfermedad, fiebre*); ~ **de calor** hot flush; ~**s de calor** hot flashes

sofocón, *m*, *fam*, shock (*gran disgusto*); ~**es** *pl*, *fam*, hot flashes

solanera, sunburn (*insolación*); sunstroke

solar, *adj*, solar

soldarse, *Med*, to fuse (*huesos quebrantados*); to knit (*huesos*)

soleada, *SpAm*, sunstroke

soledad, *f*, privacy

sóleo, soleus (muscle)

soler (ue), to be accustomed to; to be in the habit of

solicitar, to ask (for); ~ **admisión a** to apply for admission

solicitud, *f*, application; request

solidez, *f*, massiveness; solidity

sólido, *m*, *adj*, solid

solitaria, solium; tapeworm
sollozar, to whimper
sollozo, whimper
solo, *adj*, alone
soltar (**ue**), to let go of; to release; ~**se del estómago** to have diarrhea
soltera, spinster
soltero, bachelor; *adj*, single (*no casado*)
soltura, loose bowels; *Chicano, cult,* diarrhea; ~ **de vientre** *Med,* diarrhea
soluble en agua caliente, *adj,* HWS/hot water soluble
solución, *f,* solution; ~ **de Ringer** Ringer's solution; ~ **endovenosa** IV/intravenous solution; ~ **fijadora** fixing solution; ~ **fisiológica** physiological solution; ~ **normal** normal solution; ~ **normal salina** normal saline solution; ~ **salina** saline solution; ~ **salina normal** NSS/normal saline solution; Ringer's solution
solvente, *m,* solvent
sombra, shade
sombrero, hat; ~ **de Panamá**[1] *slang,* rubber (*condón*)
sombrío, *adj,* gloomy; glum
someter, to submit
somnífero, sleeping pill
somnolencia, drowsiness; sleepiness
somnoliento, *adj,* drowsy (*soñoliento*)
sonado[1], *adj,* high on[2] (*drogas narcóticas*)
sonambulismo, nightwalking; somnambulism
sonámbulo, nightwalker; ~[1] *adj,* high on[2] (*drogas narcóticas*)
sonar (**ue**), to blow; to ring; to sound; ~ (**las narices**) **a un niño** to blow a child's nose; ~**se la nariz** to blow one's nose; ~**se las narices** to wipe one's nose; ~**se**[1] to have a buzz[2] (*efecto de una droga*); to get high[2]; to get loaded[2]; to trip out[2]

sonda, catheter; probe; sound *Med*; tube (*para alimentación*); ~ **a permanencia** indwelling catheter; ~ **acodada** elbowed catheter; ~ **biacodada** elbowed catheter; ~ **de doble corriente** two-way catheter; ~ **de Foley** Foley catheter; ~ **flexible** flexible catheter; ~ **gástrica** stomach tube; ~ **nasogástrica** nasogastric tube; ~ **para alimentación** feeding tube; ~ **tejana** Texas catheter; ~ **uretral** urethral sound
sondaje, *m,* catheterization; ~ **anal** rectal catheterization; ~ **duodenal** duodenal catheterization; ~ **esofágico** esophageal catheterization; ~ **gástrico** gastric catheterization; stomach tube; ~ **rectal** rectal catheterization; ~ **ureteral** vesical catheterization; ~ **vesical** vesical catheterization
sondar, to sound (*con una sonda*)
sondear, to catheterize; to probe *Med*
sondeo, catheterization; probing
sonido, sound (*ruido*); ~ **auscultatorio** auscultatory sound; ~ **hueco** hollow sound; ~ **metálico** metallic tinkling; ~ **sordo** muffled sound; ~ **valvular** flapping sound
sonograma, *m,* sonogram
sonreír (**i**), to smile
sonriente, *adj,* smiling
sonrisa, smile
soñador, **-ra**, *m/f,* daydreamer; dreamer
soñar (**ue**) (**con**), to dream (of); ~ **despierto** *adj,* to daydream
soñoliento, *adj,* drowsy (*somnoliento*); sleepy
soplar, to blow (*exhalar aire con fuerza*); ~**se la nariz** *Carib,* to blow one's nose
soplo, blow (*de aire*); bruit; murmur *Med*; souffle; *fam,* heart murmur; ~ **aneurismático**

aneurysmal bruit; aneurysmal murmur; ~ **aórtico** aortic murmur; ~ **arterial** arterial murmur; ~ **cardíaco** cardiac murmur; heart murmur; ~ **cardiopulmonar** cardiopulmonary murmur; ~ **cardiorrespiratorio** cardiorespiratory murmur; ~ **de fuelle** bellows murmur; ~ **diastólico** diastolic murmur; ~ **endocardíaco** endocardial murmur; ~ **estenósico** stenosal murmur; ~ **funcional** functional murmur; innocent murmur; ~ **mitral** mitral murmur; ~ **orgánico** organic murmur; ~ **pansistólico** pansystolic murmur; ~ **placentario** bruit placentaire; ~ **prediastólico** prediastolic murmur; ~ **presistólico** presystolic murmur; ~ **regurgitante** regurgitant murmur; ~ **sistólico** systolic bruit; systolic murmur; ~ **tricuspídeo** tricuspid murmur

sopor, *m*, *Med*, drowsiness
soporífera, sleeping pill
soporífero, *m*, *adj*, sedative; soporific; sleeping pill
soporífico, *m*, *adj*, soporific
soportar, to bear; to endure; to hold up; to support; ~ **bien la enfermedad** to fight the disease
soporte, *m*, support; ~ **de la base de la dentadura** denture base foundation; ~ **de piernas** leg rest; ~ **para el arco del pie** arch support
sorber, to lap (*beber rápidamente con mucho ruido*); to sip; ~ **por las narices** to sniff (in, up); ~ **por las narices** *Med*, to inhale
sorbete, *m*, sherbet
sorbeto, *slang*, drinking straw
sorbo, gulp (*trago*); sip
sordera, deafness; ~ **para los sonidos altos** high tone deafness
sordo, *adj*, deaf; dull (*dolor, sonido*); muffled; still (*ruido*); held back; pent-up; *m*, deaf person

sordomudo, *adj*, deaf and dumb; deaf mute
sordomudez, *f*, deaf-mutism
soríasis, *f*, psoriasis
sorocharse, *Bol, Chi, Ec, Perú*, to get mountain sickness
soroche, *m*, *SpAm*, mountain sickness
sortija, ring (*anillo*)
sosiego, calmness
sospechar, to suspect
sostén, *m*, backing *Dent;* brassiere; maintenance; support; ~ **de maternidad** nursing bra; ~ **oclusal** occlusal rest
sostener, to bear (*aguantar*); to hold (*sujetar*); to support (*defender*); to sustain (*peso; esfuerzo*); ~ **la respiración** to hold one's breath
sotabarba, double chin; jowl
sótano, basement
staturnos[1], LSD
struma, goiter
stufa[1], heroin
suave, *adj*, easy; gentle (*de carácter; voz, sonido, movimiento*); mild (*medicina, tabaco, sabor, etc.*); soft (*color, luz*)
suavemente, *adv*, mildly; softly
subagudo, *adj*, subacute
subclase, *f*, subclass
subconsciencia, subconsciousness
subconsciente, *m*, *adj*, subconscious
subcutáneo, *adj*, subcutaneous
subespecialidad, *f*, subspecialty
subida, rise (*temperatura, etc.*); ~ **de la leche** postpartum flow of milk
subir, to go up; to rise; ~ **a la mesa** to get up on the table; ~ **la escalera** to go up the stairs; ~**se** to climb up; ~**se la manga** to roll up one's sleeve
súbito, *adj*, sudden
subrogado, *adj*, surrogate
subrogar, to surrogate
su(b)scribir, to subscribe
subsidio, subsidy (*a una persona*);

Col, Ec, anxiety; worry; ~ **de enfermedad** sick benefit; ~ **de paro** unemployment benefit

substancia[4], substance; ~ **adamantina** enamel; ~ **gris** gray matter/grey matter; ~ **radi(o)activa** radioactive substance

su(b)stitutivo[4], *m, adj,* substitute (*cosa*); ~ **de plasma** plasma substitute

su(b)stituto[4], substitute; ~ **de sal** salt substitute

subvención, *f,* grant (*donación de dinero*); subsidy (*a una empresa*)

subvencionado, *adj,* subsidized (*una empresa*)

subvencionar, to subsidize (*una empresa*)

succinilcolina, succinylcholine

succión, *f,* suction; ~ **del pulgar** thumb-sucking

suceder, to happen

sucesivo, *adj,* successive

suceso, event

suche, *m, Arg,* pimple

sucho, *adj, Arg, Ec,* maimed; paralytic

suciedad, *f,* dirt

sucio, *adj,* dirty; soiled

sudación, *f,* sweating; transpiration

sudar, to perspire; to sweat

sudón, sudona, *adj, SpAm,* sweaty

sudor, *m,* perspiration; sweat; ~ **nocturno** night sweats; ~**es a chorros** *pl,* diaphoresis; ~**es fríos** cold sweats; **chorrear de ~** to be dripping with sweat

sudorífico, sweater (*persona que suda*) *Med*

suegro, father-in-law

suela, sole of the shoe

sueldo, salary

suelo, floor (*interior*); ground

suelto, *adj,* fluent (*conversación*); free; lax (*el vientre*); loose (*pelo; ropa*); undone (*sin atar*); agile; daring (*atrevido*)

sueñera, *SpAm,* drowsiness; sleepiness

sueño, dream; sleep; ~ **crepuscular** twilight sleep anesthesia; ~ **malo** nightmare; ~ **paroxístico** sleep apnea

suero, *Med,* serum; ~ **antialacrán** black widow spider antivenin serum; ~ **antiviperino** antivenin serum; ~ **de leche** whey; ~ **de sangre** blood serum; ~ **fisiológico** physiological saline solution; ~ **glucosado** IV/intravenous solution; ~ **por la vena** IV/intravenous solution; ~ **sanguíneo** blood serum

suerofisiológico, IV/intravenous solution

suerte, *f,* fate; luck

suficiencia, competence

suficiente, *adj,* adequate; enough; *adv,* sufficient

sufrimiento, affliction (*dolor*); distress (*dolor*); hardship; misery (*miseria*); suffering

sufrir, to endure; to go through; to suffer (*experimentar*); to sustain (*una herida, un ataque, etc.*); to undergo/to take (*un examen*); ~ **de** to be afflicted with; to suffer from; ~ **un accidente** to meet with an accident; ~ **un colapso** to collapse; ~ **un tirón** to pull a muscle; strain (*un músculo*)

sufusión hemorrágica, *f,* hemorrhagic suffusion

sugar[1], LSD

sugerencia, suggestion

sugerir (ie), to suggest

sugestión, *f,* suggestion (*psiquiátrica*); ~ **hipnótica** hypnotic suggestion; ~ **poshipnótica** posthypnotic suggestion

suicidarse, to commit suicide

suicidio, suicide

sujetar, to embed; to hold down (*a la fuerza*); to hold (*fijar*); to restrain; to seize (*agarrar*); to tie tightly (*atar*); ~ **con correa** to strap down

sulfamida, sulfa drug; sulphamide
sulfatiazol, *m*, sulfathiazole
sulfato, sulfate; ~ **de bario** barium sulfate; ~ **de cadmio** cadmium sulfate; ~ **de cobre** copper sulfate; ~ **de magnesia** Epsom salt; ~ **de magnesio** magnesium sulfate; ~ **de quinina** quinine sulfate; ~ **de sodio** (*in toilet cleaners*) sodium sulfate (*en limpiadores de inodoros*); ~ **ferroso** ferrous sulfate; iron vitamin
sulfoniluria, sulfonyluria
sulfuro, sulfide; ~ **de carbono** carbon sulfide; ~ **de hidrógeno** hydrogen sulfide
suma, sum
sumersión, *f*, drowning
suministro, provisions (*víveres*); supply
sunco, *adj*, *Col*, (*Vea manco.*)
sunshine[1], LSD
superar, to ooze
superficial, *adj*, superficial
superficie, *f*, surface; ~ **bucal** buccal surface *Dent*; ~ **corporal** body surface; corporal surface; ~ **de ajuste** fitting surface *Dent*; ~ **de impresión** (*denture, tooth*) impression surface (*de la dentadura*); ~ **inferior** underside; ~ **oclusal** occlusal surface; ~**s oclusales de balance** balancing occlusal surfaces; ~ **oclusal funcional** working occlusal surface; ~ **pulida** (*tooth, denture*) polished surface (*de la dentadura*)
superior, *adj*, superior; upper
supermercado, supermarket
superpoblado, *adj*, overpopulated
supervisar, to oversee; to supervise
supervisión, *f*, oversight; supervision
supervivencia, survival
supino, *adj*, supine
suplementario, *adj*, supplementary
suplemento, supplement; ~**s de antibióticos** antibiotic supplements; ~**s minerales** mineral supplements
suplicante, *adj*, imploring
suplicar, to implore
suponer, to assume; to involve (*implicar*); to make believe; to presume
supositorio, suppository
suprarrenal, *adj*, adrenal; suprarenal
supresión, *f*, withdrawal; ~ **de un narcótico** drug withdrawal
suprimir, to cut out; to stop; to suppress; ~ (**un tratamiento**) to discontinue (a treatment)
supuración, *f*, discharge (*flúido*); drainage; suppuration
supurar, to suppurate; to weep (*herida*); ~ (**un absceso**) to come to a head
surco, furrow; groove; ~ **alveololingual** alveololingual groove; ~ **bicipital** bicipital groove; ~ **dental primitivo** primitive dental groove; ~ **genital** genital groove; ~ **interventricular anterior** anterior interventricular groove; ~ **interventricular posterior** posterior interventricular groove; ~ **medular** medullary groove; ~ **paramedio anterior de la médula espinal** anterior paramedian groove; ~ **paramedio posterior de la médula espinal** posterior paramedian groove; ~ **ungueal** nail groove
surtidor, *m*, pump (*gasolina*); ~ **de gasolina** gas pump
surtir efecto, to take effect
surumpe, *m*, *Bol*, *Perú*, inflammation of the eyes (*causada por lo fuerte de la nieve*)
susceptible, *adj*, susceptible
suspender, to delay; to hold up (*pagos*); ~ (**un tratamiento**) to discontinue (a treatment)
suspensión, *f*, suspension
suspensorio, athletic supporter; jockstrap

suspicaz, *adj*, jealous
suspirar, to sigh
suspiro, sigh
sustancia[4], substance; ~ **áspera** roughage; ~ **de desecho** residue substance; ~ **nutritiva** nutriente; ~ **química** chemical
sustentar, to support (*sostener*); to sustain (*vida*)
sustituir[4], to replace (*reemplazar*); to substitute
sustituto[4], replacement (*suplente*)
susto[5], fright; jolt; scare; shock; start; trauma; *fam*, emotional shock; ~ **con resuello duro** *fam*, shock and hyperventilation
sustraer, to subtract
sutura, seam *Anat*; stitch; suture; dental suture; ~ **abotonada** knotted suture; ~ **absorbible** absorbable suture; dissolving suture; ~ **circular** circular suture; ~ **continua** continuous suture; running suture; uninterrupted suture; ~ **de punto sobre punto** over-and-over suture; ~ **de puntos separados** interrupted sutures; ~ **emplumada** quilled suture; ~ **en ángulo recto de colchonero** right angle mattress suture; ~ **en bolsa de tabaco** purse-string suture; ~ **en cadena** chain suture; ~ **en punto de ojal** lockstitch suture; ~ **horizontal de colchonero** horizontal mattress suture; ~ **incluida** buried suture
suturar, to suture

---

[1] Este vocabulario es nuevo y todavía no se encuentra en el *Diccionario de la lengua española*, publicado por la Real Academia Española. Forma parte del argot o la lengua de la calle. Se supone que el género es obvio a menos que sea indicado.

[2] Forma parte del vocabulario inglés actual de los drogadictos.

[4] Las palabras que se deletreaban con<<subst...>>también hoy en día se deletrean <<sust...>>.

[5] En las regiones rurales la gente nombra *susto* a un tipo de miedo causado por el diablo sí mismo, o por lo menos una bruja. También ellos dicen que *susto* puede ser causado por algo que asusta de repente. Los síntomas que la víctima sufre incluyen: la pérdida del peso, la pérdida del sueño, el, temblor, y hasta la muerte.

Tratan de curarlo usando remedios caseros, como remedios mágicos, cenizas, oraciones, cruces, etc. Muchas personas adultas que sufren del *susto* tienen susceptibilidad a la mala sugestión. A veces los adultos padecen de hiperventilación (resuello duro) además del susto. En los niños que sufren del *susto*, la causa no se debe a la mala sugestión, sino a otras cosas, como pesadillas, fiebres, o la desnutrición. Cuando los niños se mueven de una manera extraña, puede ser causado por *delirio*.

Lo importante es tratar de calmar a la persona y buscar tratamiento médico si es necesario, o si se debe a la sugestión, ayudar a la persona a vencer su miedo y a calmarse.

T

taba, *Anat*, ankle bone
tabaco, tobacco; ~ **de mascar** chewing tobacco; *esp. Carib*, cigar; (*common*) marijuana
tabacón, *m*, *Mex*, marijuana
tabacosis, *f*, tabagism
tábano, cattle fly
tabaquismo, tabagism
tabardillo, epidemic typhus
tabes, *f*, tabes
tabique, *m*, septum; ~ **auriculoventricular** atrioventricular septum of heart; ~ **bronquial** bronchial septum; ~ **cervical intermedio** intermediate cervical septum; ~ **de la nariz** bridge of the nose; ~ **desviado** deviated septum; ~ **gingival** gingival septum; ~ **interauricular del corazón** interatrial septum of heart; ~ **interventricular** interventricular septum; ~ **nasal** nasal septum; bridge of the nose; ~ **orbitario** orbital septum
tabla expediente, chart
tableta, (solid) pill; tablet
tablilla, splint
taboparálisis, *f*, taboparalysis
tabú, *m*, taboo
TAC/tomografía axial computarizada, *f*, CAT scan/computerized axial tomography
tacañoso, *adj*, stingy
tacatosa[1], LSD
tachar, to efface; to scratch out
tacho, *Ríopl*, washbasin
tachón, *m*, *Med*, effacement
tachuela, *Arg, Chi, Guat, Mex*, short, stocky person
taciturno, *adj*, morose (*triste*)
tacón, *m*, heel (*de calzado*); ~ **alto** high heel
tacote, *m*, *Mex*, marijuana
tacotillo, *Chicano*, boil; tumor

táctil, *adj*, tactile
tacto, touch (*sentido*); ~ **abdominal** abdominal touch; ~ **rectal** rectal examination; rectal touch; ~ **vaginal** vaginal touch; ~ **vaginal y rectal simultáneos** double touch
tacuache, *adj*, drunk
tafetán inglés, *m*, adhesive plaster
tagarnina, *Col, Guat, Mex*, drunkenness
tajada, slice (*porción de carne*); *Med*, hoarseness
tajarrazo, *CA, Mex*, slash; wound
tajeadura, *Chi, Ríopl*, long scar
tajear, to cut up s.o. with a knife/ switchblade
tajo, cut (*corte*); slash; *slang*, episiotomy
tal vez, *adv*, perhaps
taladrar, to bore; to drill
taladro, dental drill; drill
tálamo, thalamus; ~ **óptico** thalamus
talao, *adj*, *PR*, easy
talasanemia, thalassanemia
talasemia, thalassemia; thalassanemia; ~ **mayor** thalassemia major; ~ **menor** thalassemia minima
talasoterapia, *form*, thalassotherapy
talco, talc; talcum powder; ~[1] *Texas, Cu*, big C[2] (*cocaína*); candy[2] (*cocaína*); cocaine
talega, diaper
talidomida, thalidomide
talio, thallium; **electrocardiograma de esfuerzo con ~** *m*, thallium stress test
talipédico, *adj*, clubfooted
talipes, *m*, *form*, talipes; clubfoot
talismo, talipes
talla, *Med*, gallstone operation; ~ (*de ropa*) size
talle, *m*, *Anat*, waist; figure (*de una mujer*); physique (*de un hombre*)

tallo, stem; stalk; ~ **cerebral** brainstem; ~ **del pelo** hair shaft

talón, *m*, heel (*de pie, calzado, media, etc.*)

tamaño, size; ~ **grande** large size; ~ **pequeño** small size; ~ **surtido** assorted size

tambalearse, to stagger

tambor, *m*, *Anat*, eardrum; ~ **roto** perforated eardrum

tampax, *m*, Tampax

tampón, *m*, buffer; plug; **ta(m)pón** tampon

tamponamiento, tamponade; ~ **cardíaco** cardiac tamponade

tanatognomónico, *adj*, thanatognomonic

tanque, *m*, tank; ~ **de oxígeno** oxygen tank; ~ **séptico** septic tank

tapa, cap (*de una botella*); lid (*de baúl*); lift (*capa del tacón*); top (*lid*); ~ **de los sesos** *fam*, top of skull; ~ **de seguridad** safety cap

tapado, *adj*, constipated; ~ **de orín** *m*, prostatitis

tapadura, filling *Dent*

tapaojo, *m*, *SpAm*, eye patch; (eye) bandage

tapar, to cover; to fill *Dent*; to obturate; *fam*, to block *Anat*; ~**se la nariz** to hold one's nose

tapetillo de los niños, *fam*, measles

tapón, *m*, stopper; ~ **de cera** impacted earwax; ~ **de moco** *Mex*, bloody show

taponado, *adj*, stuffy (*congestionado*)

taponamiento nasal, nasal packing

taponar los oídos, to stop up one's ears

taquicardia, *form*, rapid heartbeat; tachycardia; ~ **auricular** auricular tachycardia; ~ **auricular paroxística** auricular paroxysmal tachycardia; ~ **paroxística** paroxysmal tachycardia; ~ **sinusal** sinus tachycardia; ~ **ventricular paroxística** ventricular paroxysmal tachycardia

taquicardíaco, *adj*, tachycardiac

taranta, *Mex*, drunkenness; *CR, Ec*, mental disturbance; ~**s** *Chicano, Mex, Hond*, dizziness; *Hond*, bewilderment

taranto, *adj*, *Col*, dazed; bewildered

tarántula, tarantula; ~ *adj*, *Chicano*, hairy

tararear, to hum (*un aire*)

tarareo, hum (*de una canción*); humming (*un aire*)

tardar en (+ *infinitive*), to be late in (+ *gerundio*)

tarde, *adv*, late

tardío, *adj*, late (*desarrollo, etc.*); overdue (*embarazo*)

tardo, *adj*, backward; sluggish; ~ **de oído** hard of hearing

tarea, task

tarjeta, card

tarrajazo, *Guat*, blow; wound

tarsal, *adj*, tarsal

tarso, *m*, *adj*, tarsus

tartajoso, *adj*, stammering; tongue-tied

tartamudear, to falter; to stammer; to stutter

tartamudeo, lisp (*ceceo*); stammer

tartamudez, *f*, stuttering

tartamudo, stutterer

tártaro, dental tartar

tasa, rate; ~ **de accidentes** accident rate; ~ **de colesterol** cholesterol level; ~ **de mortalidad** mortality rate; ~ **de natimortalidad** stillbirth rate

tatarabuelo, great-great-grandfather

tataranieto, great-great-grandson

tatas, andar a, to crawl; to toddle

tatuaje, *m*, tattoo(ing)

taza, cup; cupful; *Chi*, washbasin; ~ **de medir** measuring cup; ~ **de té** teacupful; ~ **del excusado** toilet bowl; ~ **del inodoro** toilet bowl; ~ **para té** teacup

tazón, *m*, basin

TBC/tuberculosis, *f*, TBC/tuberculosis

TC/tomografía computada, *f*, CT scan/computed tomography té, *m*, tea; ~[1] marijuana; ~ **borde** wormseed tea; (*Vea té de epazote*); ~ **cargado** strong tea; ~ **de arnica** arnica flower tea (*se usa en casos de golpes internos, bronquitis, neumonía, tónico muscular*); ~ **de azahar** orange blossom tea (*se usa para problemas de los nervios y del corazón*); ~ **de barba de elote** corn tassel tea (*se usa para problemas de los riñones, para cálculos biliares, la hinchazón de piernas durante el embarazo y para la gota*); ~ **de baqueña** *PR*, medicinal tea (*se usa para los cálculos renales*); ~ **de borraja** borage tea (*se usa para tos, para ayudar a orinar y sudar, para eliminar la infección en fiebres eruptivas como varicela, sarampión, etc.*); ~ **de canela** cinnamon tea (*se usa para tos y como tónico con anemia; ayuda a la digestión y para combatir los gases*); ~ **de canutillo** (**del campo**) *Mormon* tea (*ayuda contra la anemia*); ~ **de careaquillo** *PR*, medicinal tea (*se usa para resfriados*); ~ **de cocolmeca** sarsaparilla tea (*se usa para problemas de los riñones*); ~ **de damiana** damiana tea (*se usa o como té o como lavado vaginal para tratar frío en la matriz; también ayuda contra la diabetes, la inflamación de los riñones y los problemas en la vejiga*); ~ **de epazote** wormseed tea (*se usa para eliminar parásitos y para ayudar a la menstruación*); ~ **de estafiate** wormwood tea; Rocky Mountain sage tea; black sage tea (*ayuda contra los parásitos, la mala digestión y para cólico*); ~ **de flor de sauz y hojas de alhucema** elderberry and lavender tea (*se usa para sarampión y fiebre*); ~ **de flores de tilo** linden tea (*para calmar los nervios, toses espasmódicas y*

fiebres por infección); ~ **de hierba del indio** desert milkweed tea (*se usa para trastornos de los riñones*); ~ **de hierba del manzo** swamp root tea (*se usa para dolores de estómago*); ~ **de hierba del pasmo** spasm herb tea (*se usa en el tratamiento de pasmo*); ~ **de hinojo** fennel tea (*se usa para gases, cólico de bebés, flemas y vómitos*); ~ **de inmortal** spider milkweed tea; ~ **de malva** mallow tea (*como té se usa en casos de disentería y dolor de estómago en los niños*); ~ **de manzanilla** camomile tea (*sirve para la diarrea verde de los niños y para regularizar la menstruación*); ~ **de maví** *PR*, medicinal tea made from bark of soldierwood tree; ~ **de México** wormseed tea; (*Vea té de epazote.*); ~ **de naranja** orange leaves tea (*se usa para cólico*); ~ **de negrita** elderberry tea (*se usa para cólico*); ~ **de orégano** wild marjoram tea (*se usa para combatir infecciones intestinales, disentería, y gases así como para regularizar la menstruación*); ~ **de oshá** parsley tea (*se usa para ayudar a curar la inflamación de los riñones*); ~ **de pamita** tansy mustard herb tea; ~ **de pionillo** croton tea; ~ **de quinino de pobre** *PR*, medicinal tea (*se usa para la diabetes*); ~ **de romero** rosemary tea (*se usa para regularizar la menstruación y estimular la digestión*); ~ **de rosa de Castilla** herb rose tea (*se usa para cólicos infantiles, empacho así como una purga, y en caso de conjuntivitis como un lavaojos*); ~ **de ruda** rue tea (*para aliviar la presión alta, jaquecas, y para la menstruación y partos difíciles o abortos*); ~ **de sacabuche** *PR*, medicinal tea (*se usa para tratar la indigestión y* *trastornos estomacales*); ~ **de sangrededrago** limberbush tea (*se usa para la anemia*); ~ **de yerbabuena** (spear)mint tea (*se usa para el cólico*); ~ **fuerte** strong tea

tecata[1], cocaine; heroin

tecato[1], (drug) addict; junkie[2] (*un adicto a las drogas narcóticas*); heroin user (*adicto*); hype[2] (*un adicto que se da inyecciones subcutáneas*); sleep walker[2] (*un adicto a la heroína*); user[2]

techo, roof

tecla, key (*de una máquina de escribir*); ~[1] cigarette butt[2]; roach[2] (*colilla de un cigarrillo de mariguana*)

técnica, technique; ~ **de enrojecimiento** flush technique; ~ **de tiempo de difusión** time diffusion technique

técnico, technician; ~ **de laboratorio** laboratory technician; *adj*, technical

tecnología, technology

teco[1], heroin user (*adicto*)

tecolota[1], cigarette butt[2]; roach[2] (*colilla de un cigarrillo de mariguana*)

tecunda, *Mex*, chicken pox

tejido, tissue; ~ **adiposo** adipose tissue; ~ **blando** soft tissue; ~ **canceroso** cancerous tissue; ~ **celular** cell tissue; ~ **cerebral** brain tissue; ~ **cicatrizal** scar tissue; ~ **conectivo** connective tissue; ~ **conjuntivo** connective tissue; ~ **eréctil** erectile tissue; ~ **nervioso** nerve tissue; ~ **óseo** bony tissue; ~ **vascular** vascular tissue

tela, film (*en el ojo; en la superficie de un líquido*); membrane; tape (*para vendajes, etc.*); ~ **adhesiva** adhesive tape

tele, *f, Chicano*, baby bottle; breast

telefonear, to telephone

teléfono, telephone; ~ **móvil** car telephone; cellular phone

telenque, *adj, Chi*, weak; feeble

telepatía, telepathy

telescopio, telescope

televisión, *f*, television

temascal, *m, CA, Mex*, bathroom

temblar, to quake (*moverse violentamente*); to quaver (*la voz*); to shiver; to tremble; ~ **de frío** to shake with cold; ~ **de miedo** to quake with fear; ~**le a uno las rodillas** to quake at the knees

temblón, *adj*, shaky (*la escritura*)

temblor, *m*, quake; quiver; tremor; ~ **de párpado** *Sp, SpAm*, kyllosis

tembloroso, *adj*, shaky (*la voz, la mano*); tremulous

temer, to be afraid; to fear

temor, *m*, fear; ~ **morboso** morbid fear

temperamento, makeup (*manera de ser*); temperament

temperatura, fever; temperature; ~ **ambiente** room temperature; ~ **corporal basal** BBT/basal body temperature; ~ **de la habitación** room temperature; ~ **del cuerpo** body temperature; ~ **interna del cuerpo humano** internal temperature of the human body

tempestuoso, *adj*, rough (*tiempo*)

templado, *adj*, temperate; warm; lukewarm

templarse, to act with restraint; *Col, Perú, PR*, to get drunk; *Ec, Guat, Hond*, to die; ~ **en la comida** to eat frugally

temporada, season (*espacio de tiempo impreciso*); spell (*un período de tiempo*); ~ **de la gripe** flu season; ~ **de los catarros** cold season

temporal, *adj*, temporary

temporero, *adj*, temporary

temporomandibular, *adj*, temporomandibular

temporomaxilar, *adj*, temporomaxillary

temporooccipital, *adj*, temporooccipital

tempozonte, *adj*, *Mex*, hunchbacked
temprano, *adj*, early
tenacillas, nippers; *Med*, tweezers; forceps
tenaz, *adj*, tenacious; tough
tenazas, forceps; tongs; ~ **de extracción** dental forceps
tendencia, liability (*propensión*); tendency; trend; ~s **a sangrar** bleeding tendencies
tender (**ie**), to stretch (*extender*); ~ (**con**) to spread (out)
tendón, *m*, tendon; ~ (**del hueso**) **poplíteo** hamstring; ~ **de Aquiles** Achilles tendon; ~ **de la corva** hamstring; ~ **externo de la corva** outer hamstring; ~ **interno de la corva** inner hamstring
tenedor, *m*, fork
tener, to have; to hold; to own; ~ ____ **años** to be ___ years old; ~ **a alguien al corriente** to keep s.o. informed; ~ **adormecido** to be numb; ~ **angustia** *fam*, to be anxious; ~ **ansias** *fam*, to be anxious; ~ **ayuntamiento carnal fuera del matrimonio** to fornicate; ~ **basca** *fam*, to throw up; to vomit; ~ **buen** (**mal**) **sabor** to taste good (bad); ~ **buen aspecto** (*cosas*) to look/appear well; ~ **buena cara** (*persona*) to look/appear well; ~ **calor** *m*, (*personas*) to be hot; to be warm; ~ **carraspera** to have a frog in one's throat; ~ **catarro** to have a cold; ~ **comezón** to itch; ~ **confianza en** to trust; ~ (**mucho**) **cuidado** to be (very) careful; to exercise (a lot of) care; ~ **cuidado con** to look out for (*ejercer cuidado*); ~ **deseos** (**de**) to desire (to); ~ **dolor** to be in pain ~ **dolor de** (+ *parte del cuerpo*) to ache; to be sore; ~ **el mes** to menstruate; ~ **el moño parao** *fam*, to get angry; ~ **el niño** to deliver; ~ **en cuenta** to allow for; ~ **enfriamiento de los pies** (**o las**

manos) to have cold extremities; ~ **eructos** to belch; ~ **éxito** to be successful; ~ **frío** (*persona*) to be cold; ~ **ganas** (**de**) to feel like; ~ **gas** to have gas; ~ (**mucha**) **hambre** *f*, to be (very) hungry; ~ **hip** to have the hiccoughs, hiccups; ~ **inconveniente** to object; ~ **la buena vista** to have good vision; ~ **la cara picada de viruelas** to mark (by smallpox); ~ **la congestión** to be congested; ~ **la culpa** to be guilty; to be at fault; ~ **la garra** to menstruate; ~ **la regla** to have the (monthly) curse; ~ **la vista normal** to have normal vision; ~ **las piernas entumecidas** to be stiff in the legs; ~ **las piernas poco firmes** to be shaky on one's legs; ~ **lástima a uno** to be sorry for s.o.; ~ **los grifos parao** *fam*, to get angry; *PR*, *vulg*, to get mad; ~ **los ojos a millón** *fam*, to have bloodshot eyes; *PR*, to have bloodshot eyes from smoking or drinking; ~ **los ojos de pescao de nevera** *fam*, to have bloodshot eyes from smoking or drinking; *fam*, to have bloodshot eyes; ~ **los ojos de un gato que lambe aceite** *PR*, to have bloodshot eyes from smoking or drinking; ~ **los ojos de un gato que lambe aceite** *fam*, *PR*, to have bloodshot eyes; ~ **los pies fríos** (**o las manos frías**) to have cold extremities; ~ **lugar** to take place; ~ **mal aspecto** (*cosas*) to look (appear) bad; ~ **mal sabor** to taste nasty; ~ **mala cara** (*personas*) to look (appear) bad; ~ **miedo** to be afraid; to be scared; to fear; ~ **mucha voluntad** to have a strong will; ~ **murria** to be blue; ~ **náusea(s)** to be nauseated; ~ **náuseas** to gag (*basca*); to have a queasy stomach; to wamble; ~ **permiso** to have permission; ~ **picazón** to itch; ~ **prisa** to be in a hurry; ~ **que** (+ *infinitive*) to have to (*deber*); ~ **razón** *f*, to be right; ~ **relaciones sexuales** to have sexual relations; ~ **retraso** to be late; ~ **sangramiento** *fam*, to hemorrhage; ~ **sed** *f*, to be thirsty; ~ **sello** *PR*, to have the looks of homosexual; ~ **sentido** to make sense; ~ **sofocos** to flush; ~ **sueño** to be sleepy; ~ **tapado algo** *adj*, (*los oídos, la nariz*) to be congested; ~ **un corazón de piedra** to be as hard as nails; ~ **un hambre**[3] **canina** to be ravenous; ~ **un resfriado** to have a cold; ~ **un sapo en la mano** *PR*, to have butterfingers; to be a clutz; ~ **un tirón en un músculo** to have a pulled muscle; ~ **una cruda** *Mex*, to be hungover; ~ **una nota** to be higher than a kite; ~ **una opinión errónea** to misjudge; ~ **una resaca** to be hungover; ~ **una tranca**, *SpAm*, to be drunk; ~ **vasca** to barf *vulg* (*vomitar*); ~ **vergüenza** *f*, to be ashamed; ~ **vértigo** to feel dizzy

tenesmo, *form*, tenesmus; ~ **anal** anal tenesmus; ~ **rectal** rectal tenesmus; ~ **vesical** vesical tenesmus

teni, *m*, *Chicano*, tennis shoe

tenia, *form*, tapeworm

teniasis, *f*, teniasis

tenotomía, tenotomy

tensiómetro, blood pressure cuff

tensión, *f*, tension; pressure *Med*; strain (*nerviosa, mental*); ~ **alta** *fam*, hypertension/high blood pressure; ~ **arterial** blood pressure; ~ **arterial elevada** hypertension/high blood pressure; ~ **de la sangre** blood tension; ~ **de la sangre arterial** arterial blood tension; ~ **de la sangre capilar** capillary blood tension; ~ **de la sangre venosa** venous blood tension; ~ **del cuello** neck strain; ~ **del líquido** (*cefalorraquídeo*) liquor tension; ~ **emocional** emotional stress; ~ **nerviosa** nervous tension

tenso, *adj*, tense; strained (*nervios*)

tentador, *adj*, tempting

tentar (**ie**), to feel (*examinar por tacto*); to probe; to tempt

teñir (**i**), to dye

teofilina, theophylline

teoría, theory; ~ **atómica** atomic theory; ~ **germinal** germ theory

TEP/tomografía por emisión de positrones, *f*, PET/positron emission tomography

terapeuta, *m/f*, *form*, therapist; ~ **ocupacional** occupational therapist

terapéutica, *form*, therapeutics; therapy; ~ **alimenticia** alimentary therapeutics; ~ **física** physical therapy; ~ **por electrochoque** electroshock therapy/EST

terapéutico, *adj*, therapeutic

terapia, therapy; ~ **de grupo** group therapy; ~ **de inhalación** inhalation therapy; ~ **de oxígeno** oxygen therapy; ~ **del habla**[3] speech therapy; ~ **electrochoque/TEC** ECT/electroconvulsive therapy; ~ **electroconvulsiva/TEC** ECT/electroconvulsive therapy; ~ **en grupo** group therapy; ~ **física** physical therapy; ~ **inmunizante** immunization therapy; ~ **intensiva** intensive therapy; ~ **laboral** occupational therapy; ~ **masiva por gota a gota intravenosa** massive drip intravenous therapy; ~ **ocupacional** occupational therapy; ~ **profesional** occupational therapy; ~ **respiratoria** respiratory therapy; ~ **sustitutoria con estrógeno** estrogen replacement therapy; ~ **tiroidea** thyroid therapy

terapista, *m/f*, therapist; ~ **físico**, physical therapist

tercer(o), **-ra**, *adj*, third; **tercer molar** *m*, third molar; **tercer período del parto** third stage of labor; third stage of pregnancy; **tercera circunvolución temporal** *f*, subtemporal convolution; **tercera fase del parto** *f*, third stage of pregnancy

terciario, *adj*, tertiary

tere, *adj*, *Col*, weak; sickly; weepy

terebrante, *adj*, boring; piercing; sharp (*dolor*)

termal, *adj*, thermal

termalgesia, thermalgesia

term(o)analgesia, therm(o)analgesia

térmico, *adj*, thermal

terminación, *f*, ending; **~ del nervio** nerve ending; **~ nerviosa** nerve ending

terminal, *adj*, terminal

terminar, to end; to finish

término, term

terminología, terminology

termoanalgesia, thermoanalgesia

termoanestesia, thermoanesthesia

termocauterización, *f*, thermocauterization

termodinámica, thermodynamics

termómetro, thermometer; **~ bucal** oral thermometer; **~ centígrado** centigrade thermometer; **~ clínico** clinical thermometer; **~ de Fahrenheit** Fahrenheit thermometer; **~ de superficie** surface thermometer; **~ oral** oral thermometer; **~ rectal** rectal thermometer

termorregulación, *f*, thermoregulation

termorregulador, *m*, thermostat

termorresistente, *adj*, thermoresistant

termostato, thermostat

termoterapia, heat therapy; thermotherapy

ternera, calf (*pl, calves*) (*animal*)

terneza, tenderness

ternilla, *Cu*, *Mex*, *Nic*, cartilage of the nose

ternilloso, *adj*, cartilaginous

terramicina, Terramycin

terrones[1], LSD

terror nocturno, *m*, night screaming; **~es nocturnos** night terrors

test de apercepción temática/ TAT, *m*, thematic apperception test/TAT

testamento, will (*un documento*)

testarada, *fam*, bump on the head; **darse una ~** to bump one's head

testarazo, *fam*, bump on the head

testarudo, *adj*, hard-headed (*obstinado*)

testicular, *adj*, testicular

testículo, orchis *form*; testicle; testis; **~ no descendido** undescended testicle; **~s** balls *slang*

testigo, witness; **~ ocular** eyewitness

testosterona, testosterone

teta, *slang*, breast; **quitar la ~ a** to wean

tetar, to suckle

tétano(s), lock jaw/lockjaw; tetanus; **~ del recién nacido** infantum tetanus; **~ medicamentoso** drug tetanus

tetera, nursing bottle; *Mex, Cu, PR*, nipple (*de un biberón*)

tetero, *Col, PR, Ven*, nursing bottle

tetilla, *Anat*, nipple (*de un hombre o de un biberón*)

tetina, nipple (*de un biberón*)

teto, nipple (*de un biberón*)

tetraciclina, tetracycline

tetracloruro, tetrachloride; **~ de carbón** carbon tetrachloride; **~ de carbono**, carbon tetrachloride

tetralogía, tetralogy; **~ de Fallot** tetralogy of Fallot

tetraplejía, quadriplegia; tetraplegia

tetrapléjico, *m, adj*, quadriplegic

tetravalente, *adj*, tetravalent

tetuda, *adj, fam*, big breasted

textura, texture

tez, *f*, complexion; ~ **blonda** light complexion

tiabendazol, *m*, thiabendazole

tiamina, thiamine; vitamin B_2

tiberio, *adj*, *Guat*, *Mex*, drunk

tibia, shinbone; tibia; ~ **dirigida hacia dentro** tibia varus; ~ **en sable** saber tibia; ~ **valga** tibia valga; ~ **vara** tibia vara

tibio, *adj*, lukewarm; tepid; warm

tic, *m*, tic; ~ **degenerativo** degenerative tic; ~ **doloroso de la cara** tic douloureux; ~ **(p)sicomotor**[6] psychomotor tic; ~**s** *pl*, twitching

tiempla, *Chi*, drunkenness

tiempo, time; ~ **de circulación** circulation time; ~ **de coagulación (de sangre)** blood coagulation time; clotting time; coagulation time; ~ **de exposición** exposure time; ~ **de hemorragia** bleeding time; ~ **de hemorragia secundaria** secondary bleeding time; ~ **de internamiento** length of hospital stay; ~ **de irradiación** exposure time; ~ **de latencia** time lag; ~ **de muerte térmica** thermal death time; ~ **de protrombina** prothrombin time; ~ **de reacción** reaction time; ~ **de retracción del coágulo** (blood) clot reaction time; ~ **de sangrar** bleeding time; ~ **de sedimentación** sedimentation time; ~ **de semidesintegración** half-life time; ~ **del mes** *fam*, menstruation; ~ **parcial** *adv*, part-time; ~ **parcial de tromboplastina** partial thromboplastin time/PTT

tienda, store; tent; ~ **de oxígeno** oxygen tent; ~ **de refrescos** snack shop; ~ **de vapor** steam tent

tienta, *Med*, probe

tiento, *Arg*, *PR*, snack

tierno, *CA*, baby (*infante*)

tierra, earth

tieso, *adj*, stiff (*Med: pierna*); stiff (*tenso*); rigid; erect; taut

tiesto, *Chi*, chamberpot

tiesura, stiffness (*rigidez*)

tifo, typhus fever; *fam*, typhus; ~ **de América** yellow fever; ~ **asiático** cholera; ~ **de Oriente** bubonic plague

tifus, *m*, typhus (fever); ~ **abdominal** typhoid fever; abdominal typhus; ~ **clásico** epidemic typhus; ~ **de los nudos linfáticos** scrofula; ~ **epidémico** spotted fever; ~ **exantemático** camp fever; exanthematous fever; spotted fever; typhus fever; epidemic typhus; ~ **icteroides** yellow fever

tijeras, *f*, *pl*, scissors; ~ **de cura** dressing scissors; ~ **de vendaje** bandage scissors; dressing scissors; ~ **grandes** shears; ~ **para las uñas** nail scissors

tijeretas, earwigs

tijerillas, earwigs

timba[1], heroin capsule

timbebe, *adj*, *Chi*, weak; trembling

timbre, *m*, bell

tímido, *adj*, bashful; shy

timo, thymus; ~ **accesorio** accessory thymus; ~ **persistente** persist thymus

timpánico, *adj*, tympanic

tímpano, tympanum *form*; drum *Anat*; eardrum (*tympanic membrane*); ~ **perforado** perforated eardrum; ~ **roto** perforated eardrum

tina, bathtub; ~ **de baño** tub

tinción, *f*, stain/staining

tinea, tinea (*tiña*); ~ **de la cabeza** tinea capitis; ~ **de la pierna** tinea cruris; ~ **del cuerpo** tinea corporis; ~ **del pie** tinea pedis; ~ **inguinal** tinea cruris

tiniado[1], *adj*, high from sniffing paint thinner[2]

tinitus, *m*, tinnitus

tinta, ink

tinte, *m*, dye; hue (*color*)

tintura, dye; tincture; ~ **de genciana compuesta** gentian tincture compound; ~ **de yodo** tincture of iodine

tiña, *form*, ringworm; tinea; ~ **crural** jock(ey) itch *fam*; ringworm of the groin; ~ **de la barba** barbers' itch; ringworm of the beard; ~ **de la cabeza** tinea capitis; ~ **del cuerpo** ringworm of the body; tinea corporis; ~ **del pie** tinea pedis; ~ **inguinal** tinea cruris; jock(ey) itch *fam*

tiñoso, *adj*, *Med*, scabby

típico, *adj*, typical

tipificación, *f*, typing (*clasificación*); ~ **de la sangre** typing of blood

tipo, kind; type; *fam*, well-dressed, well educated guy; ~ **atlético** athletic type; ~ **corporal** body type; ~ **de sangre** blood type; ~ **inestable** unstable type; ~ **sanguíneo** blood type

tira, strap; ~ **de cuero** (leather) strap; ~ **reactiva** dip stick; test strip

tirabuzón, *m*, curl of hair

tiraleche, *m*, breast pump

tirante, *m*, shoulder strap

tirar, to hurl; ~ (**de**) to pull (*estirar*); ~ (**el**) **agua**[3] *slang*, to urinate; ~ **gases** to pass gas; ~ **la cadena** to flush the toilet; ~ **las tripas** to throw up; to vomit; ~ **moco** *slang*, *Chicano*, to cry (*con lágrimas*); ~ **viento(s)** *slang*, to pass gas; ~**se flato** to expel anal gas; ~**se un pedo** to expel anal gas

tiritar, to shiver

tiritón, *m*, *fam*, tremor; ~**es** *pl*, chills; ~**es** *pl*, *fam*, convulsions

tiro, gunshot; *fam*, well-dressed, well educated guy

tiroidectomía, thyroidectomy

tiroideo, *adj*, thyroid

tiroides, *m/f*, thyroid; ~ **aberrante** aberrant thyroid

tiroidina, thyroid extract

tirón, *m*, jerk (*sacudida*); tic; yank

tirotropina, thyrotropin

tis, *f*, *Chicano*, *fam*, tuberculosis

tisana, (medicinal) tea; tisane; infusion

tísico, tuberculous patient; *fam*, tuberculosis; *adj*, tubercular

tisis, *f*, consumption; phthisis; *fam*, tuberculosis; ~ **galopante** *f*, galloping consumption

tisiqu(i)ento, *adj*, *Ríopl*, pale and thin

tisuria, weakness caused by excessive urination

titanio, titanium

titrato, titrate

titubear, to vacillate (*vacilar*)

titulable, *adj*, *Chem*, titratable

titulación, *f*, *Chem*, titration

titulado, *adj*, qualified (*profesionalmente*)

título, heading; qualification (*diploma*); titer/titre

tiznarse, *Chi*, *Guat*, *Mex*, to get drunk

tlacote, *m*, *Mex*, tumor; growth

tlacuache, *adj*, drunk

toalla, towel; ~ **de baño** bath towel; ~ **de felpa** Turkish towel; ~ **femenina** *Mex*, sanitary napkin; ~**s en los ojos** eyepads

toallero, towel rack

toallita, washcloth

tobillera, ankle support

tobillo, ankle

tobogán, *m*, slide (*para niños*)

tocar, to feel; to touch (manually) (*rozar*); to ring

tocino, bacon

tocola[1], roach[2] (*colilla de un cigarrillo de mariguana*)

tocología, midwifery; tocology

tocólogo, obstetrician; tocologist

tocón, *m*, stump (*de un árbol*)

todavía, *adv*, still

todos los días, every day

tolerancia, tolerance; ~ **adquirida** acquired tolerance

tolerar, to bear (*soportar*); to tolerate

tolondro, *Med*, bump; lump; swelling

toma, intake (*de agua, etc.*); ~ **de aire** air intake; outlet *Elect*; *Med*, dose; ~ **de la muestra** collection of the urine specimen

tomacorriente, *f*, *SpAm*, electric socket; outlet *Elect*

tomado, estar, *SpAm*, to be drunk

tomaína, ptomaine

tomar, to drink; to take; to take (*drogas*); ~ **aire** to catch one's breath; ~ **aire** *fam*, to breathe in; ~ **drogas**[1] to get down[2] (*obtener drogas*); ~ **el sol** to sunbathe; ~ **la presión** to take the blood pressure; ~ **las huellas digitales a** to fingerprint; ~ **medicinas** to doctor (*a un paciente*); ~ **menos** to cut down (on); ~ **píldoras** to be on pills; ~ **una dosis excesiva** to take an overdose; ~ **una radiografía (de)** to x-ray (*sacar un rayo x*); ~ **una siesta** to take a nap; ~**selo con calma** to take it easy

tomate, *m*, tomato; *slang, Chicano*, eyeball

tomillo, thyme

tomodesintometría, CAT scan/computerized axial tomography

tomografía, body section roentgenography; tomography; ~ **axial computarizada / TAC**, *f*, computerized axial tomography/CAT; ~ **computada/TC**, *f*, computerized tomography/CT; ~ **por emisión de positrones/TEP** positron emission tomography/PET; ~ **transaxial de emisión de positrones/TEP** positron emission tomography/PET

tomógrafo, tomograph

tomograma, *m*, tomogram

tongonear, *PR*, to cuddle; to indulge someone

tónico, tonic

tono, pitch; tone; ~ **cardíaco fetal** fetal heart tone; ~ **de la voz** tone of voice; ~ **doble** double murmur; ~ **grave** low-pitched (*voz*); ~ **muscular** muscle tone; ~**s cardíacos** heart tones

tonsil(s), *m*, *Chicano*, tonsil(s)

tonsila, tonsil

tonsilitis, *f*, *Chicano*, tonsillitis

tonsilotomía, tonsillectomy

tontería, foolishness; ~**s** drivel (*bobería*)

tonto, *adj*, dull (*intelectualmente*)

topar, to butt *Dent*

tópico, *adj*, topical; local; for external application

toque, *m*, dab; trait; ~[1] drag[2] (*bocanada de un cigarrillo de mariguana*); hit of marijuana[2]; marijuana; ~[1] *Chicano*, toke of marijuana or hashish[2]

toracentesis, *f*, pleural tap; thoracentesis

torácico, *adj*, thoracic

toracotomía, thoracotomy

tórax, *m*, *form*, chest; thorax; ~ **en quilla** chickenbreast thorax; ~ **en tonel** barrel chest; barrel-shaped thorax; ~ **globoso** barrel chest

torcedura, sprain; strain *Med;* wrench

torcer (ue), to sprain; to twist (*dar la vuelta*); to wrench; ~**se (ue)** to strain (*la espalda, músculos, etc.*); ~**se (ue) el tobillo** to sprain one's ankle; ~**se (ue) la muñeca** to strain one's wrist

torcido, *adj*, crooked; strained (*tobillo, muñeca, espalda*); twisted

torcijón cólico, *m*, *Mex*, stomach cramp

torcimiento, sprain

tórico, *adj*, toric

torniquete, *m*, tourniquet; ~ **de campo** field tourniquet

torno, dental drill; drill

torombolo, *adj*, *Cu*, pot-bellied

torpe, *adj*, dull (*necio*); slow (*en comprender o en movimientos*)
torpeza intelectual, intellectual slowness; obtusion
torpor mental, *m*, clouding of consciousness
torrente, *m*, flow (*de lágrimas*); stream (*de lágrimas*); ~ **circulatorio** bloodstream; ~ **de sangre** bloodstream; ~ **sanguíneo** bloodstream
torsión, *f*, torsion
torso, torso
torsón, *m*, *fam*, abdominal cramp
tortícolis, *m/f*, [*Ú.m.c.f.*], *form*, stiff neck; torticollis *form*; wryneck; ~ **congénita** congenital torticollis; ~ **espasmódica** intermittent torticollis
torunda de algodón, *Mex*, *CA*, cotton ball
torzón, *m*, *fam*, abdominal cramp; sharp internal pain
tos, *f*, cough; ~ **ahogana** *Mex*, whooping cough; pertussis; ~ **auricular** ear cough; ~ **blanda** wet cough; ~ **bronca** brassy cough; ~ **con flema** cough with phlegm; ~ **convulsiva** pertussis; whooping cough; ~ **desgarrando** cough with phlegm; ~ **emetizante** emetic cough; ~ **ferina**[4] whooping cough; pertussis; ~ **fuerte** hacking cough; ~ **húmeda** loose cough; productive cough; wet cough; ~ **metálica** brassy cough; ~ **perruna** barking cough; ~ **por fumar** smoker's cough; ~ **productiva** productive cough; wet cough; ~ **seca** dry cough; hack; hacking cough
tosecilla, hacking cough
toser, to cough
tosferina[5], whooping cough; pertussis
tosido, *Chi*, *Guat*, *Mex*, cough
tostado, *adj*, suntanned
tostao, *adj*, crazy

tostar[1], to smoke marijuana; ~**(se)** to crack up[2]
total, *adj*, complete; total; ~ **expedito** *m*, output; ~ **producido** *m*, output
totalidad, *f*, whole
totuma, *Chi*, bump; bruise; abscess; bump on the back
totumo, *Chi*, bump on the head; bump on the back
toxemia, blood poisoning; septicemia; toxemia; ~ **del embarazo** toxemia of pregnancy; ~ **eclámptica** eclamptic toxemia; ~ **gravídica** pregnancy toxemia; toxemia of pregnancy
toxémico, *adj*, toxemic
toxicidad, *f*, toxicity
tóxico, *adj*, poison (*gas*, *droga*, *etc.*); toxic
toxicología, toxicology
toxicólogo, toxicologist
toxicomanía, (drug) addiction[2]; (drug) dependence; drug habit; habit[2]
toxicómano[1], (drug) addict[2]; dope fiend *fam*; junkie[2] (*un adicto a las drogas narcóticas*); user[2]
toxina, toxin; ~ **bacteriana** bacterial toxin; ~ **estafilocócica** staphylococcal toxin; ~ **estreptocócica** streptococcal toxin
toxoide, *m*, toxoid; ~ **diftérico** diphtheria toxoid; ~ **tetánico** tetanus toxoid
toxoplasmosis, *f*, toxoplasmosis
traba, *fam*, obstacle
trabajador, -ra, *m/f*, worker; ~ **de salud** health care worker; ~ **social** social worker
trabajar, to work; ~ **demasiado** to overwork; ~ **por turnos** to work in shifts
trabajo, employment; job; occupation; work; ~ **de equipo** team effort; ~ **de parto** labor; ~ **en equipo** teamwork; ~ **fijo** steady job

trabajoso, *adj*, laborious; painful; *adj*, *Med*, pale; sickly

tracción, *f*, traction

tracoma, *m*, conjunctivitis; pinkeye; trachoma

tracto, tract *Anat*; ~ **alimentario** alimentary tract; ~ **alimenticio** alimentary tract; ~ **gastrointestinal** gastrointestinal tract; ~ **genitourinario** genitourinary tract; ~ **respiratorio** respiratory tract; ~ **urinario** urinary tract

traducción libre, *f*, loose translation

traducir (al), to translate (into)

traer, to bring; ~ **carga**[1] to be carrying narcotic drugs

traficante, *m/f*, dealer; ~[1] peddler[2] (*vendedor de drogas*); trafficker[2] (*de drogas, etc.*)

traficar, to traffic in drugs

tráfico, traffic

tragadero, *fam*, esophagus; throat

tragante, *m*, *fam*, *Chicano*, esophagus

tragar, to gulp; to swallow; to inhale (*humo de tabaco*); *vulg*, to practice cunnilingus; to go down on someone; ~**se las lágrimas** to hold back one's tears

trago, gulp (*bebida*); shot (*porción de una bebida*); swallow; tragus; ~ **de ron** shot of rum; *Anat*, tragus (*de la oreja*)

traguear, *CR*, to drink; *Ven*, to get drunk; ~**se** *CA, Col, Mex*, to get drunk

traje, *m*, outfit (*ropa*); suit

trakes[1], *m*, *Chicano*, tracks[2] (*marcas y cicatrices causadas por el uso de agujas hipodérmicas*)

trama vascular, *m*, vascular markings

tramo de escalera, flight of stairs

trancarse, *Cu, Ven*, to get drunk; *Chi, Mex, Ríopl*, to be constipated

trancazo, *fam*, bends; *fam*, *Med*, flu *fam*

trance, *m*, trance; ~ **alcohólico** alcoholic trance; ~ **hipnótico** hypnotic trance; ~ **histérico** ecstatic trance

tranquilidad, *f*, calmness; ~ **de espíritu** peace of mind

tranquilizante, *m*, downer (*barbitúrico*); tranquilizer

tranquilizar, to reassure; to tranquilize; ~**se** to calm down

tranquilo, *adj*, calm (*persona*); easy (*conciencia*); quiet (*quieto; libre de preocupación*); still

transcultural, *adj*, cross-cultural

transcurrir, to elapse

transección, *f*, transection

transexual, *adj*, *m/f*, transsexual

transferencia, transfer

transferir (ie), to carry over; to transfer

transformación, *f*, transformation; ~ **de impulsos en acción directa** acting-out

transformar, to transform; ~**se** to become transformed; to change (*convertirse*); to evolve

transfusión, *f*, transfusion; ~ **de sangre incompatible** mismatched blood transfusion; ~ **directa** direct transfusion; ~ **intravenosa** IVT/intravenous transfusion; ~ **placentaria** placental transfusion; ~ **sanguínea** blood transfusion; ~ **sanguínea incompatible** mismatched blood transfusion

transido, *adj*; ~ **de angustia** beset with anxiety; ~ **de dolor** racked with pain; ~ **de frío** frozen to the bone; ~ **de hambre** overcome with hunger

transitorio, *adj*, fleeting; temporary; transient

tra(n)smisible, *adj*, communicable; transmittable

transmisión, *f*, transmission; ~ **mediante contacto** transmission by contact; ~ **mediante vector** vector transmission; ~ **por gotillas** droplet transmission

transmisor, *m*, transmitter; ~ **ultrasonido**, ultrasound transmitter
transmitido, *adj*, transmitted; ~ **a través de la sangre** *adj*, blood borne; ~ **por el agua**[3] *adj*, waterborne; ~ **por vía sanguínea** *adj*, transmitted through the blood
tra(n)smitir, to transmit; *Med*, to carry (*microbios*); to infect with
transparencia, slide *Photo*
transparente, *adj*, clear; transparent
tra(n)spiración, *f*, transpiration
tra(n)splantación, *f*, transplantation
tra(n)splante, *m*, transplantation
transportar, to carry over; to transport
transporte, *m*, transportation; ~ **subvencionado** subsidized transport
transverso, *adj*, transverse
transvestido, transvestite
transvestista, *m/f*, transvestite
trapecio, *m*, *adj*, trapezius; trapezium
tráquea, trachea; windpipe
traqueítis, *f*, tracheitis
traqueobronquial, *adj*, tracheobronchial
traqueobronquitis, *f*, tracheobronchitis
traqueoesofágico, *adj*, tracheoesophageal
traqueofaríngeo, *adj*, tracheopharyngeal
traqueolaríngeo, *adj*, tracheolaryngeal
traqueoscopia, tracheoscopy
traqueostomía, tracheostomy
traqueotomía, tracheotomy
traques[1], *m*, *Chicano*, tracks[2] (*marcas y cicatrices causadas por el uso de agujas hipodérmicas*)
traquetero[1], heroin pusher
trasbocar, *Arg, Col, Chi*, to vomit
trasero, anus; hams *fam*; *m*, *adj*, rear
trasladar, to transfer (*a un paciente*)
traslúcido, *adj*, translucent
traspatio, backyard

traspié, *m*, slip (*tropezón*)
trasplantar, to transplant
trasplante, *m*, transplant; ~ **de corazón** heart transplant; ~ **de la médula** marrow transplant; ~ **de riñón** kidney transplant
trastornado, *adj*, deranged
trastornante, *adj*, disturbing (*mentalmente*)
trastornar, to disturb (*la paz, el orden*); to upset
trastorno, disorder (*malestar*); problem; upset; ~ (**mental**) disturbance (*mental*); ~ **alérgico** allergic reaction; ~ **bilioso** bilious attack; ~ **de la personalidad** personality disorder; ~ **del estrés postraumático** post-traumatic stress disorder; ~ **del sueño** sleep disorder; sleep disturbance; ~ **estomacal** stomach upset; ~ **gástrico** stomach upset; ~ **menstrual** menstrual disorder; ~ **mental** derangement *Med*; mental disorder; mental disturbance; ~ **nervioso** nervous disorder; ~**s de coordinación** coordination problems; ~**s del ritmo cardíaco** irregular heart rhythms; ~**s ováricos** ovarian disorders
tratamiento, management; therapy; treatment; ~ **complementario** follow-up care; ~ **con rayos x** x-ray treatment; ~ **de choque eléctrico** shock treatment; ~ **de urgencia** first aid treatment; ~ **hormonal** hormone treatment; ~ **medicamentoso** drug therapy; ~ **médico** medical treatment; ~ **naturista** nature treatment; ~ **por baños de mar** thalassotherapy; ~ **postoperatorio** aftercare; ~ **precoz** early treatment; ~ **térmico** heat therapy
tratar, to treat; ~ (**de/por** *a specific ailment*) (**con**) to treat (for *una enfermedad*) (with); ~ **con rayos x** to x-ray (*en una pantalla*

fluorescente); **~le a uno con un nuevo fármaco** to treat s.o. with a new drug; **~ de** (*book, meeting, report, etc.*) to be about; to discuss; to talk about; **~ de** (*+ infinitive*) to try to (*+ infinitivo*); **~se de** to have to do with

trato, manner; **~ carnal** sexual intercourse; **~ preferente** preferential treatment; **~ sexual** sexual intercourse

trauma, *m, form*, trauma; **~ del nacimiento** birth trauma; **~ (p)síquico**[6] psychic trauma

traumático, *adj*, traumatic

traumatismo, trauma; traumatism; **~ de la pierna** leg injury

traumatizar, to traumatize

traumatología, traumatology

traumatólogo, traumatologist

travesura, mischief

travieso, *adj*, mischievous

trayecto del proyectil, track of bullet wound

trazado, tracing; **~ electrocardiográfico** electrocardiographic pattern

trazador, *m/f*, tracer

trazo, tracing; line; **~ de lápiz** pencil mark

trementina, turpentine

tremor, *m*, tremor

trémulo, *adj*, shaky (*voz*)

trenzar, to braid

trepado, *m, adj*, tear-off; perforation

trépano, dental drill; drill; trepan

tres veces, three times; **~ a la semana** *t.i.w*/three times a week; **~ al por día** *t.i.d./ter in die*/three times a day

trespata, *vulg*, penis (*lit. 3ª pierna*)

tríceps, *m*, triceps

tricloroetileno, trichloroethylene

tricobezoar, *m*, hairball

tricocéfalo, trichocephalus

tricomonas, trichomonas; **~ vaginales** Trichomonas vaginalis

tricúspide, *adj*, tricuspid

trigémino, *m, adj*, trigeminal; trigeminus

triglicéridos, triglicerides; **~ elevados** high triglycerides

trigo entero, whole wheat

trigueño, *adj*, bronze-skinned; olive-skinned (*persona, rostro*); *PR*, swarthy; *m, adj*, brunette; *SpAm, euph*, African-American

trillizo, triplet

trimestral, *adj*, quarterly

trimestre, *m*, trimester; quarter (*trimestre*)

trimo, tetanus

trinca, *Cu, Mex, PR*, drunkenness

trinco, *Mex, PR*, drunkard

trip[1], LSD

tripa, *Anat, fam, often pl*, bowels; insides; **~ ida** *slang*, blocked intestine; **~s** *pl*, guts *fam*; **dolerle (ue) las ~s** to have a stomachache; **echar las ~s** to retch violently; to vomit violently

tripeando[1], in transit[2]

tripear[1], to trip[2]

tripeo, *Chicano*, trip on drugs[2]

tripita, *fam*, appendix

triple, *f*, vaccination, DPT

tripleto, triplet

tripón, -na, *m/f, Mex*, little child

triptófano, tryptophan

triquinosis, *f*, trichinosis

trismo, lockjaw; trismus

triste, *adj*, blue (*melancólico*); glum; sad; sorry (*situación*)

triturar, to crush (*pulverizar*); to grind (*moler*)

trivalente, *adj*, trivalent

trocánter, *m*, trochanter; **~ mayor** greater trochanter; **~ menor** lesser trochanter

trocisco, lozenge; tablet; troche; **~ para la tos** cough lozenge

tromadora[1], marijuana

trombo, thrombus

trombocito, plaque; thrombocyte

tromboflebitis, *f, form*, thrombophlebitis; phlebitis

trombógeno, *m, adj*, prothrombin; thrombogen; thrombogenic

trombosis, *f*, thrombosis; ~ **coronaria** coronary thrombosis

trompa, tube *Anat*; duct *Anat*; *fam*, mouth; ~ **de Eustaquio** Eustachian tube; otosalpinx; ~ **de Falopio** Fallopian tube

tronado, *adj*, drunk

tronar[1], to blow weed[2] (*fumar mariguana*); ~**(se)**[1] to smoke marijuana; to take a hit[2] (*dar chupadas de una abuja*); ~**sela**[1] to take a hit[2] (*dar chupadas de una abuja*)

tronco, trunk; ~ **cerebral** brainstem; ~ **del haz auriculoventricular** trunk of atrioventricular bundle

troquel, *m*, die *Dent*

trotador, **-ra**, *m/f*, jogger

trotar, to jog

trote corto, *m*, jog (*paso*)

trozo, slip (*de papel, etc.*); chunk; piece

truncar, to truncate

trusas, *PR*, shorts (*traje de baño de hombres*)

tuberculina, tuberculin test

tuberculinorreacción, *f*, tuberculin reaction

tuberculosis, *f*, consumption; TB/tuberculosis; phthisis; ~ **de huesos y articulaciones** tuberculosis of bones and joints; ~ **de la piel** skin TB; ~ **de los pulmones** tuberculosis of the lungs; ~ **intestinal** tuberculosis of the intestines; ~ **osteoarticular** tuberculosis of bones and joints; ~ **pulmonar** pulmonary tuberculosis

tuberculoso, *m*, *adj*, tubercular; tuberculous patient

tubería, *f*, tubing

tuberosidad, *f*, tuberosity

tubo, catheter; duct; passage *Anat*; pipe (*tubería*); tube *Anat*; ~ **capilar** capillary tube; ~ **de drenaje** drain; drain tube; drainage tube; ~ **de ensayo** test tube; ~ **de Falopio** Fallopian tube; ~ **de intubación** intubation tube; ~ **de jeringuilla** ampoule/ampule; ~ **de plástico** coil (*anticontracepción*); ~ **de respiración** breathing tube; ~ **de traqueotomía** tracheotomy tube; ~ **de ventilación** air duct; ventilating tube; vent (*conducto de ventilación*); ~ **digestivo** alimentary canal/tract; digestive tube; gastrointestinal tract; ~ **embriológico** embryologic lumen; ~ **endotraqueal** endotracheal tube; ~ **esofágico** esophageal tube; ~ **gástrico** stomach tube; ~ **intestinal** intestinal tract; ~ **nasogástrico** nasogastric tube; NG tube; ~ **nutricio** feeding tube; ~ **otofaríngeo** otopharyngeal tube; ~**s** Fallopian tubes; ~**s falopios** Fallopian tubes

tubular, *adj*, tubular

túbulos seminíferos, seminiferous tubules

tuco, *fam*, amputee; *SpAm*, stump *Anat*; *SpAm*, *adj*, maimed; lacking a finger/hand

tuerca, nut (*para tornillo*)

tuerto, *adj*, blind in one eye; one-eyed; *m*, one-eyed person; person blind in one eye

tuétano, *Anat*, bone marrow

tufo, *PR*, bad breath from alcohol

tularemia, rabbit fever

tullido, *m*, *adj*, cripple; crippled; disabled; maimed

tullir, to cripple; to maim

tumbar, to have sexual relations

tumefacción, *f*, swelling; tumefaction

tumor, *m*, growth (*tumor*); tumor; *fam*, swelling; ~ **benigno** benign tumor; ~ **canceroso** cancerous tumor; ~ **cerebral** brain tumor; ~ **de células de la granulosa** granulosa cell tumor; ~ **de teji-**

do **conectivo** connective tissue tumor; ~ **del riñón** nephroma; ~ **fibroideo** fibroid tumor; ~ **fibroso** fibrous tumor; ~ **maligno** malignant tumor; malignancy; ~ **sebáceo** sebaceous tumor

tumorcito, lump

túnel, *m*, tunnel; ~ **del carpo** carpal tunnel

tupición, *f*, *SpAm*, blockage; obstruction; *SpAm*, *Med*, catarrh; *Ven*, blocking (of nose with mucus)

turbar, to embarrass (*dejar perplejo*)

turbieza de la orina, cloudiness of urine

turbio, *adj*, turbid

turista, *slang*, diarrhea

turma, *Anat*, testicle

turnio, *adj*, cross-eyed

turno, appointment; shift (*al trabajo*); spell (*turno de vigilancia*); ~ **de día** day shift; ~ **de noche** night shift

tuso, *adj*, *Col*, *Ven*, pockmarked

---

[1] Este vocabulario es nuevo y todavía no se encuentra en el *Diccionario de la lengua española*, publicado por la Real Academia Española. Forma parte del argot o la lengua de la calle. Se supone que el género es obvio a menos que sea indicado.

[2] Forma parte del vocabulario inglés actual de los drogadictos.

[3] Se emplean el artículo definido e indefinido masculinos en español delante de esta palabra con la *ha* o con la *a* inicial acentuada aunque se usan adjetivos calificativos femeninos para modificarla.

[4] Esta palabra, que también se escribe *tosferina*, muchas veces se refiere a cualquier tos que los niños tienen.

[5] *Tosferina* también puede ser una tos persistente.

[6] Hoy es aceptable deletrear las palabras que antes se escribían con *psi-* en español (o *psy-* en inglés) sin la *p* que es consonante silenciosa en este caso.

U

ubrera, *Med*, thrush

úlcera, sore (*lesión*); ulcer; ~ catarral cold sore; ~ de estrés stress ulcer; ~ del estómago stomach ulcer; ~ del Yemen Yemen ulcer; ~ duodenal duodenal ulcer; ~ dura hard ulcer; (*Vea chancro.*); ~ en los labios cold sore; ~ gangrenosa canker sore; ~ gástrica gastric ulcer; ~ indolente indolent ulcer; ~ inflamada inflamed ulcer; ~ maligna canker; ~ oculta concealed ulcer; ~ péptica peptic ulcer; ~ perforante perforating ulcer; ~ por decúbito bedsore; decubital/decubitus ulcer; decubital necrosis; ~ por presión pressure sore; ~ rebelde intractable ulcer; ~ redonda peptic ulcer; round ulcer; ~ sangrante bleeding ulcer; ~ superficial fester; ~ trófica trophic ulcer; ~ venérea venereal lesion

ulceración, *f*, canker sore; ulceration; ~ bucal canker

ulcerarse, to fester; to ulcerate

ulceroso, *adj*, festering; ulcerous

último sueño, last sleep

ultrasonda, ultrasound

ultrasonografía, ultrasonography

ultrasonoterapia, ultrasonotherapy

ultravioleta, ultraviolet

umbilicado, *adj*, umbilicated; vesículas ~ umbilicated vesicles

umbral, *m*, threshold; ~ de conciencia threshold of consciousness

un, a; an; one; ~ cuarto de hora quarter of an hour; ~ día sí, otro no every other day; ~ hombre vigoroso (a) vigorous man; ~ masaje enérgico vigorous massage; ~ par de a couple of; ~ par de medias a pair of stockings; ~ sabor agradable pleasant flavor(ed)

una vez por semana, once a week

unas tijeras, a pair of scissors

uncinaria, hookworm; uncinaria *form*

ungir, *Med*, to put ointment on; to rub ointment on; to anoint

ungüento, balm; balsam; ointment; salve; unguent; ~ para los labios lip balm; ~ para los ojos eye salve

único, *adj*, only

unidad, *f*, unit; ~ de aislamiento isolation unit; ~ de cuidados intensivos/UCI intensive care unit; ~ de peso igual a 480 gramos troy ounce; ~ de sangre unit of blood; ~ de vigilancia intensiva/UVI intensive care unit/ICU; ~ reductora de enturbiamiento TRU/turbidity reducing unit

unido, *adj*, bound; close-knit (*familia, etc.*); linked

uniforme, *m*, *adj*, uniform; even (*superficie*)

unión, *f*, bond; junction; ~ de alta energía high energy phosphate bond; ~ de hidrógeno hydrogen bond; ~ emocional emotional bond; ~ peptídica peptid bond

unir, to attach; to bind (*atar*); to join; to link; to merge

universal, *adj*, universal; antídoto ~ universal antidote

untadura, *Med*, ointment

untar, to paint *Med*; ~ (de) to smear

unto, ointment; smear; ~s de Papanicolaou *m*, Pap smear

uña, fingernail; nail (*de un dedo*); ~ (de los dedos del pie) toenail; ~ en cáscara de huevo eggshell nail; ~ **encarnada** ingrown toenail; ~ **enterrada** ingrown toenail; ingrown nail

uñero, ingrown toenail

urea, urea (*componente de la orina*)

uremia, blood urea; uremia

urente, *adj*, *Med*, burning; stinging

uréter, *m*, nephric duct; ureter

ureteritis, *f*, ureteritis

ureterolitotomía, ureterolithotomy

ureteropielitis, *f*, ureteropyelitis

ureterostomía, ureterostomy

uretra, urethra

uretritis, *f*, urethritis; ~ **inespecífica** nonspecific urethritis; ~ **no específica** *f*, nonspecific urethritis (*enfermedad venérea*); ~ **no gonococal** *f*, nongonococcal urethritis (*enfermedad venérea*)

uretrocele, *m*, urethrocele

urgencia, emergency; urgency

urgente, *adj*, urgent

úrico, *adj*, uric

urinálisis, *m*, *inv*, urinalysis test; urinalysis

urinario, urinal; *adj*, urinary

urobilina, urobilin (*componente de la orina*)

urobilinógeno, urobilinogen

urobilirrubina, urobilirubin (*componente de la orina*)

urocele, *m*, urocele

urocultivo, urine culture

urogenital, *adj*; **aparato** ~ urogenital apparatus

urología, urology

urólogo, urologist

urticaria, hives; nettle-fever; urticaria

urticariano, *adj*, urticarial

urticariformes, *adj*, urticarial

urutar, *Chicano*, to burp

úrzula, *Chicano*, typhus fever

usar, to use; ~ **drogas** to get down[2] (*adquirir drogas*)

uso, use; ~ **irregular de drogas** ice cream habit[2]

usted/Vd./Ud., you *form*, *sg*

ustedes/Vds./Uds., you *form*, *pl*

usual, *adj*, usual

útero, matrix; uterus; womb

uterosalpingografía, uterosalpingography

útil, *adj*, effective; useful

utilizable, *adj*, usable; fit for use (*que puede servir*); ready for use (listo para ser utilizado); *fam*, available

utizable, *adj*, *fam* available

úvula, uvula

uvular, *adj*, uvular

uvulitis, *f*, uvulitis

---

[2] Forma parte del vocabulario inglés actual de los drogadictos.

vacante, *adj*, vacant; void (*posición*)
vaccineo, *adj*, vaccinal
vaciado, casting; ~ **uterino** uterine curettage
vaciar, to drain (*no dejar lleno*); to empty (out)
vacilación, *f*, vacillation
vacilar, to hesitate; to vacillate (*hesitar*); to wobble
vacío, *m*, vacancy; void; *adj*, empty; vacuum; hollow (*hueco*)
vacuna, immunization (*inmunización*); vaccination; vaccine; ~ **anticarbuncosa** anthrax vaccine; ~ **anticolérica** cholera vaccine; ~ **antisarampión de virus vivo** live measles virus vaccine; ~ **bacteriana** bacterial vaccine; ~ **contra la rabia** rabies vaccine; ~ **contra la viruela** smallpox vaccine; ~ **contra las paperas** mumps vaccine; ~ **contra parotiditis** mumps vaccine; ~ **de Sabin por vía bucal** Sabin's oral polio vaccine; ~ **de virus sarampionoso inactivado** inactivated measles virus vaccine; ~ **de virus sarampionoso vivo atenuada** live attenuated measles virus vaccine; ~ **oral contra polio** Sabin's oral polio vaccine; ~ **triple** DPT/diphtheria/pertussis/tetanus
vacunación, *f*, vaccination
vacunal, *adj*, vaccinal; **profilaxis ~** *f*, vaccinal prophylaxis
vacunar, to immunize; to vaccinate
vacunoprofilaxis, *f*, vaccinal prophylaxis
vacunoterapia, vaccinotherapy
vacuola, vacuole; ~ **alimenticia** food vacuole; ~ **de aire** air vacuole
vagabundo, *adj*, vagrant
vagal, *adj*, vagal

vagina, *form*, vagina; **prolapso de la ~** vagina prolapse
vaginal, *adj*, vaginal
vaginalitis, *f*, vaginalitis
vaginismo, vaginismus
vaginitis, *f*, *inv*, vaginitis
vaginodinia, vaginodynia
vaginoperineotomía, vaginoperineotomy
vaginopexia, vagina prolapse; vaginopexy *form*,
vaginoplastia, vaginoplasty
vago, *adj*, vague; **nervio ~** vagus nerve
vagotomía, vagotomy; ~ **completa** complete vagotomy; ~ **médica** medical vagotomy; ~ **quirúrgica** surgical vagotomy
vaguedad, *f*, vagueness
vaguido, dizzy spell
vahído, dizziness; dizzy spell; giddiness; faint
vahos, *m*, *pl*, *Med*, inhalation
vaina, sheath; ~ **neural** neural sheath; ~ **sinovial** synovial sheath
vale, *m*, voucher
valgo/valgus, *adj*, valgus (*dirigido hacia afuera*)
válido, *adj*, *Med*, strong; robust
valioso, *adj*, valuable
valor, *m*, value; **~es de la sociedad** societal values; ~ **globular** globular value; ~ **hematócrito** hematocrit value
valoración de Apgar, *f*, Apgar score
valuación del metabolismo basal/V.M.B., *f*, basal metabolic rate/B.M.R.
valva, valva; ~ **aórtica** aortae valva
valvotomía, valvotomy
válvula, valve; valvula; (*pl*, *valvulae*); electric valve; **~s anales** anal valves; ~ **auriculoventricular**

derecha right atrioventricular valve; ~ **auriculoventricular izquierda** left atrioventricular valve; ~ **bicúspide** bicuspid valve; ~**s cardíacas** cardiac valves; ~ **coronaria** coronary valve; ~ **de la vena cava inferior** valve of the inferior vena cava; ~ **del corazón** heart valve; ~ **del seno coronario** valve of coronary sinus; ~ **mitral** mitral valve; ~ **pequeña** valvula; ~ **pilórica** pyloric valve; ~ **pulmonar** pulmonary valve; ~ **reductora** reducing valve; ~ **sigmoidea aórtica** aortae valva; ~ **tricúspide** tricuspid valve

valvular, *adj*, valvular

valvulitis, *f*, valvulitis

vapor, *m*, fumes; steam; vapor; ~ **de agua** water vapor; *Med*, dizzy spell; faintness

vaporizador, *m*, vaporizer

vaporizar, to vaporize

vaporizo, *Mex*, *PR*, steamy heat; *Med*, inhalation

vapoterapia, vapotherapy

vareta, **estar de**, *Med*, *fam*, to have diarrhea

variabilidad, *f*, variability

variable, *f*, *adj*, variable; variant (*cambiable*)

variación, *f*, range; variance; variation

variado, *adj*, varied

variante, *f*, *adj*, variant (*que es diferente*)

variar, to vary

várice/varice, *f*, varicose veins; varix (*pl*, *varices*) (*en inglés casi siempre se usa la forma plural*); ~**s** varicose veins; ~**s** *fam*, enlargement of the veins; ~ **esofágicas** esophageal varices

varicela, chicken pox; varicella

varicocele, *m*, varicocele

varicosidad, *f*, varicosity

varicoso, *adj*, varicose

varicotomía, varicotomy

variedad, *f*, variety

varilla, rod (*vara pequeña*); jawbone *Anat*; ~ **de metal** metal rod

varioloso, *adj*, *form*, variolous (*picado de viruelas*)

varios, *adj*, several

variz, *m*, varicose veins; (*Vea várice/varice.*)

varo, *adj*, bent inward; varus

varón, *m*, *adj*, male; *Col*, husband

varonil, *adj*, viril

varus, *adj*, varus

vasca(s), *fam*, vomit

vascular, *adj*, vascular

vascularización, *f*, vasculature

vasculatura, vasculature

vasectomía, vasectomy

vaselina, vaseline

vaselinoma, *m*, paraffinoma

vasija, basin; receptacle; ~ **para vomitar** emesis basin

vasín de cama, *m*, bedpan

vaso, drinking glass; glass (*recipiente para beber*); vessel; *Anat*, duct; tube; vessel; ~ **arterial** artery; ~ **capilar** capillary; ~ **linfático** lymph duct; ~ **quilífero** lymph duct; ~ **sanguíneo** blood vessel; ~ **venoso** vein

vasoconstricción, *f*, vasoconstriction

vasoconstrictor, *m*, *adj*, vasoconstrictor

vasodepresión, *f*, vasodepression

vasodepresor, *m*, *adj*, vasodepressor

vasodilatación, *f*, vasodilation

vasodilatador, *m*, *adj*, vasodilator

vasoestimulante, *m*, *adj*, vasostimulant

vasografía, vasography

vasomoción, *f*, vasomotion

vasomotilidad, *f*, vasomotion

vasomotor, *m*, *adj*, vasomotor

vasomovimiento, vasomotion

vasorreflejo, vasoreflex

vástago, offspring

vatio, watt

vecindad, *f*, neighborhood; vicinity

vecino, neighbor; *adj*, neighboring

vegetación adenoide, *f*, adenoid

vegetal, *m*, vegetable
vegetariano, *m*, *adj*, vegetarian
vegetativo, *adj*, vegetative
vehículo, transmission vehicle; vehicle; ~ (**de**) *Med*, carrier (of); transmitter (of)
vejez, *f*, old age
vejiga, bleb; blister; bladder; ~ (**de la orina**) bladder; urinary bladder; ~ **de la bilis** gall bladder/gallbladder; ~ **urinaria** urinary bladder
vela, candle; *CA*, *RD*, funeral wake
velar, *f*, *adj*, *Anat*, velar
velar, to veil; to stay awake (*no dormir*); to keep watch; ~ **por la salud de un enfermo** to watch over a sick person; ~ **a un enfermo** to sit up with a sick person
vello, hair (*del cuerpo, especialmente el de la región púbica*); vellus hair; villus (*pl*, *villi*); ~ **púbico** pubic hair
vellosidad, *f*, villus; downiness; ~ **coriónica** chorionic villus; ~ **pericárdica** pericardial villus; **~es del intestino delgado** villi of small intestine
velloso, *adj*, fuzzy; hairy
velo, veil; ~ **del paladar** *Anat*, soft palate; velum; ~ **humeral** humeral veil; ~ **palatino** soft palate
velocidad, *f*, rate; ~ **de eritrosedimentación** erythrocyte sedimentation rate; ~ **de sedimentación** sedimentation rate; ~ **de sedimentación globular/VSG** global sedimentation rate
vena, blood vessel; vein; vena (*pl*, *venae*); ~ **cava** (**inferior**) (**superior**) (inferior) (superior) vena cava; ~ **coronaria** (**mayor**) (**menor**) (great) (small) cardiac vein; ~ **mamaria** (**interna**) (**externa**) (internal) (lateral) mammary/thoracic vein; ~ **portal** portal vein; ~ **subclavia** subclavian vein; **~s varicosas** varicose veins; ~ **yugular** jugular; jugular vein

vencer, to overcome (*algo dificultoso*)
vencido, *adj*, outdated (*medicinas*)
venda, band; bandage (*material*); Bandaid; dressing (*vendaje*); fascia; ~ **Ace** Ace bandage; ~ **adhesiva** adhesive bandage; ~ **de gasa** gauze bandage; ~ **elástica** elastic bandage; ~ **floja** loose bandage; ~ **umbilical** naval truss
vendaje, *m*, bandage; dressing (*venda*); fascia; ligamentum; ~ **a presión** pressure bandage; ~ **abdominal** abdominal bandage; abdominal binder; binder; ~ **circular** circular bandage; ~ **compresivo** compression bandage; ~ **de yeso** gypsum cast; ~ **elástico** elastic bandage; ~ **en T** T bandage; ~ **enyesado** plaster bandage; cast (*un vendaje hecho con vendas de yeso, destinado a inmovilizar una parte del cuerpo*); plaster cast; ~ **inmóvil** immobilizing bandage; ~ **protectivo** protective bandage; ~ **provisional** first-aid bandage; ~ **quirúrgico** surgical dressing; **quitar el ~ de** to undress (*una herida*)
vendar, to band; to bandage; to bind (up) (*envolver en vendajes*); to dress (*una herida*)
vendedor, -ra de drogas, *m/f*, peddler[2] (*narcotraficante*)
vender, to sell
veneno, poison; venom; ~ **aspirado** inhaled poison; ~ **común** common poison; ~ **inyectado** injected poison; ~ **tomado por la boca** oral poison
venenoso, *adj*, poison (*culebras, etc.*); poisonous; venomous
venéreo, *adj*, venereal
venereología, venereology
venereólogo, venereologist
venir, to come; **~se** slang, to climax (*sexual*); to ejaculate; to come (*sexualmente*); *vulg*, to reach sexual climax
venograma, *m*, venogram

venoso, *adj*, venous
venta y tráfico de drogas, drug traffic
ventaja, advantage
ventana, window; **~ de la nariz** nostril; **~s nasales** nostrils
ventanilla de la nariz, nostril
ventilación, *f*, ventilation; **~ ascendente** upward ventilation; **~ descendente** downward ventilation; **~ natural** natural ventilation; **~ por escape** exhausting ventilation; **~ pulmonar** pulmonary ventilation
ventilador, *m*, ventilator
ventilar, to air (*exponer al aire*); to ventilate
ventosa[4], cup (*del curanderismo y remedios caseros*); cupping glass; glass cup; leech; vacuum chamber; **~ húmeda** wet cup; **~ seca** dry cup
ventosearse, *Chicano*, to expel anal gas
ventosidad, *f*, flatus
ventostomía, cutdown
ventricular, *adj*, ventricular; **extrasístole ~** *f*, ventricular escape
ventrículo, ventricle; **~ (primero) (lateral) (segundo) (tercero) del cerebro** (first) (lateral) (second) (third) ventricle of the cerebrum; **~ de la médula espinal** ventricle of the cord; **~ del cerebro** ventricle of the brain; **~ del corazón** ventricle of the heart
ventriculografía, ventriculography
ventriculograma, *f*, ventriculogram
ventriculostomía, ventriculostomy
ver, to meet (*dar a conocer*); to see
verbal, *adj*, verbal
verde, *m*, *adj*, green
verdón, *m*, *Arg*, bruise; welt
verdosa[1], marijuana; *adj*, greenish
verdugo, weal; welt
verdugón, *m*, weal; large welt
verdura, vegetable
vereda, *Ec*, *Peru*, *Bol*, *Chi*, sidewalk

vergüenza, embarrassment; shame (*humillación*); **~s** *pl*, genitals
verijas, *f*, *pl*, genitals; pubic region
veringo, *adj*, *Col*, naked; nude
veringuearse, to undress
verme, *m*, intestinal worm (*parásito*); vermin; **~ cilíndrico** roundworm; **~ solitario** solitary vermin
vermicida, *m*, vermicide
vermifugo, *m*, *adj*, vermifuge
vernix caseosa, *f*, vernix caseosa
verruga, (*Vea wart.*) verruga; wart; **~ de brea** tar wart; **~ genital** genital wart (*enfermedad venérea*); **~ plantar** *form*, plantar wart; **~ venérea** genital wart (*enfermedad venérea*)
verrugoso, *adj*, verrucous; covered in warts; warty
versión, *f*, version (*del feto*)
vértebra, vertebra (*pl*, *vertebrae*); **~ cervical** cervical vertebra; **~s coccígeas** coccygeal vertebrae; **~s dorsales** dorsal vertebrae; **~s lumbares** lumbar vertebrae; **~s sacras** sacral vertebrae
vertebral, *adj*, vertebral; **columna ~** vertebral column; **discos ~es** vertebral discs
vértice, *m*, top (*dirección*); vertex; **~ de la cabeza** top of head
vertiginoso, *adj*, dizzy; giddy
vértigo, dizziness; fainting spell; giddiness; Ménière's disease; vertigo; **~ auricular** aural vertigo; **~ de la altura** height vertigo
vesicación, *f*, blistering
vesicante, *m*, *adj*, vesicant
vesícula, bladder; blister; vesicle; **~ biliar** gall bladder/gallbladder; **~ en escama de pescado** fish-scale gallbladder; **~ en fresa** strawberry gallbladder; **~ en papel de lija** sandpaper gallbladder; **~s de la fiebre** fever blisters; **~ febril** fever blister; **~ seminal** seminal vesicle
vestíbulo, hall (*de una casa*); lobby (*de un edificio*); vestibule/

vestibulum *Anat*; ~ **bucal** buccal vestibule; ~ **de la aorta** vestibule of aorta; ~ **de la faringe** vestibule of pharynx; ~ **de la laringe** vestibule of larynx; ~ **de la vagina** vestibule of vagina; ~ **labial** labial vestibule

vestigio, track; vestige

vestirse (i), to dress oneself; to get dressed; ~ **de bata de hospital** to be gowned

vestuario, changing room

veterano, *m*, *adj*, veteran

veterinaria, veterinary medicine

veterinario, *m/f*, *adj*, veterinarian; veterinary surgeon

vía, path; track; tract *Anat*; passage; ~**s aéreas** air passages; ~**s biliares** biliary tract; ~ **central del trigémino** central tract of trigeminal nerve; ~ **corticoespinal** corticospinal tract; ~ **de entrada** route of entry (*de un parásito*); ~**s digestivas** digestive tract; ~ **oclusal** occlusal path; ~ **parenteral** parenteral route; **por** ~ **bucal** through the mouth; orally; **por** ~ **interna** internally; ~ **respiratoria** airway; ~**s respiratorias** respiratory tract; ~**s urinarias** urinary tract

viable, *adj*, viable

viaje, *m* trip; ~¹ *slang*, trip on drugs; ~ **(en las nubes)**¹ LSD

vial, *m*, vial

viaraza, *Col*, *Guat*, *Ríopl*, fit of anger; **estar con la** ~ to be in a bad mood

víbora, viper

vibración, *f*, vibration

vibrador, *m*, vibrator

vibrante, *adj*, vibrating

vibrar, to throb; to vibrate

vibratorio, *adj*, vibrating

vibromasaje, *m*, vibromassage

vicio, bad habit (*mala costumbre*); vice

vicioso, *adj*, vicious

víctima, *f*, victim

victimar, *SpAm*, to wound

vida, life; living; ~ **conyugal** married life; ~ **matrimonial** married life; ~ **media** half-life; ~ **sexual** sex life

vidrio, glass (*cristal*); ~ **inastillable** safety glass

vieja, old woman

viejo, *m*, old man; *adj*, old

viento, wind; *slang*, fart *slang*; flatus; gas (*flato*)

vientre, *m*, abdomen; stomach; womb (*cavidad pelviana*)

vigilancia, surveillance

vigilar (de cerca), to watch (closely); to guard (closely)

vigilia, vigil

vigoroso, *adj*, vigorous

VIH/Virus de (la) Inmunodeficiencia Humana, *m*, HIV/Human Immunodeficiency Virus

vinagre, *m*, vinegar

vinculado, *adj*, related

vincular, to bind (*atar*)

vínculo, bond

vinilo, vinyl

vino, wine

violación, *f*, abuse; rape; violation (*de una mujer*)

violador, *m*, rapist

violar, to outrage (*cometer una violación*); to rape; to violate (*a una mujer*)

violencia, violence

violento, *adj*, violent

violeta, *adj*, violet; ~ **de genciana** gentian violet

vípora, snake

viral, *adj*, viral

virar, to turn over

virgen, *f*, *adj*, virgin

virginal, *adj*, virginal; maidenly

virginidad, *f*, virginity; maidenhood

viril, *adj*, viril

virilidad, *f*, virility; manhood

viringo, *adj*, *Col*, *Ec*, bare; naked

virología, virology

virtud curativa, *f*, healing power

virucida, *m, adj*, virucide
viruela, pock; ~ **caprina** goatpox; ~ **de gallina** *slang*, chicken pox; ~ **loca** varicella; **~s** smallpox; **~s locas** *Mex, CA, fam*, chicken pox
virulencia, virulence
virulento, *adj*, virulent
virulo, *adj, Chicano*, one-eyed
virus, *m, inv*, virus; ~ **de Epstein-Barr/VEB** EB virus; EBV/Epstein-Barr virus; ~ **de (la) inmunodeficiencia humana/VIH** human immunodeficiency virus /HIV; ~ **de la fiebre de garrapata del Colorado** Colorado tick fever virus; ~ **de la hepatitis** hepatitis virus; ~ **de la rabia** rabies virus; ~ **de papiloma humano** human papilloma virus; ~ **enmascarado** masked virus; ~ **herpético** herpes virus; ~ **transmitido por garrapatas** tick-borne virus
víscera, viscus (*pl, viscera*); *f, pl*, entrails; organ meats; viscera
visceral, *adj*, visceral
viscómetro, viscometer
viscosidad, *f*, thickness (*consistencia*); viscosity
visera, vizor
visibilidad, *f*, visibility
visible, *adj*, visible
visiblemente, *adv*, visibly
visión, *f*, hallucination; sight (*vista*); vision; ~ **(a)cromática** (a)chromatic vision; ~ **binocular** binocular vision; ~ **borrada** blurred vision; ~ **borrosa** blurred vision; ~ **central** central vision; ~ **con un solo ojo** monocular vision; ~ **crepuscular** twilight vision; ~ **diurna** day vision; ~ **doble** double vision; ~ **emborronada** blurred vision; ~ **en túnel** tunnel vision; ~ **estereoscópica** depth perception (*stereopsis*); ~ **monocular** monocular vision; ~ **nocturna** night vision; ~ **ocular** ocular vision; ~ **periférica** peripheral vision; ~ **profunda** depth perception; **~es** *pl*, visions

visita, call; visit; visitor; ~ **al consultorio** office call; ~ **al hogar** house call; *Perú, PR*, enema
visitador, **-a**, *m/f*, (frecuent) visitor; inspector; **~ra** *f, SpAm*, enema; syringe
visitante, *m/f*, visitor; *adj*, visiting
visitar, to visit
visitas, rounds (*del doctor*)
vista, eyesight; sight (*sentido*); view; vision; *fam*, eye; ~ **borrosa** blurred vision; ~ **cansada** eyestrain; presbyopia; farsightedness; ~ **corta** nearsightedness; ~ **doble** double vision; ~ **empañada** blurred vision; foggy vision; ~ **larga** *fam*, farsightedness; ~ **nocturna** night vision; ~ **nublada** *fam*, blurred vision
vistazo, glance
visto, check mark
visual, *adj*, visual
vital, *adj*, vital
vitamina, vitamin; ~ **hidrosoluble** water-soluble vitamin; ~ **liposoluble** fat-soluble vitamin
vitaminado, *adj*, enriched with vitamins
vitamínico, *adj*, enriched with vitamins
vitaminología, vitaminology
vitelo, yolk; vitellus
vitíligo, vitiligo
vitola, cigar band
vítreo, *m, adj*, vitreous; **cuerpo ~** vitreous body; **cámara ~** vitreous chamber; **cápsula ~** vitreous chamber
vitropresión, *f*, vitropression
viuda, widow; ~ **negra** black widow spider
viudez, *f*, widowhood
viudo, widower
vivacidad, *f*, vivaciousness; liveliness
vivaracho, *adj*, alert
vivaz, *adj*, alert; vivacious
viveza, alertness
viviente, *adj*, living
vivíparo, *adj*, viviparous

vivir, to live
vivisección, *f,* vivisection
vivo, *adj,* alive; vivid; live; nasty (*que se enoja fácilmente*); raw (*la piel, etc.*); rich (*color*)
vocabulario, vocabulary
vocación, *f,* vocation
vocal, *adj,* vocal
vodka, *m/f,* vodka
volar (ue), to fly
volátil, *adj,* volatile
volcao, *adj,* extremely high on[2] (*drogas narcóticas*); *adj, PR,* (severely) intoxicated
voltaje, *m,* voltage
voltearse, to roll over; to turn around (over)
voltio, volt
volubilidad, *f,* volubility
volumen, *m,* volume; ~ atómico atomic volume; ~ corriente en reposo tidal volume; ~ de reserva espiratoria expiratory reserve volume; ~ de reserva inspiratoria inspiratory reserve volume; ~ de ventilación pulmonar VT/tidal volume; ~ pulmonar lung capacity; ~ respiratorio tidal volume; ~ sanguíneo blood volume; ~ sistólico systolic discharge; ~ y tensión V and T/volume and tension (*refiriéndose al pulso*)
voluntad, *f,* will
voluntario, volunteer; *adj,* voluntary
voluptuoso, *m, adj,* voluptuous; sensualist
volver (ue), to come back; to return (*regresar*); ~ a emplear to reuse; ~ a ocurrir to recur; ~ andando to walk back; ~ el estómago to have nausea; ~ en sí to regain consciousness; ~se to

turn (over); ~ gris to turn grey; ~ loco to crack up; to go crazy; to flip; to go mad
vólvulo, volvulus
vomitar, to barf *slang* (*tener vómitos*); to disgorge; to throw up; to vomit
vomitera, *Cu, PR,* retching
vomitivo, *m, adj,* emetic; vomitive
vómito, vomit; vomiting; ~ bilioso bilious vomit; ~ de sangre bloody vomit; ~s de sangre vomiting blood; ~s del embarazo morning sickness; vomiting of pregnancy; ~ en poso de café coffee-ground vomit; ~ histérico hysterical vomiting; ~ matutino morning-after vomiting; morning vomiting; ~ negro yellow fever; black vomit; ~ nervioso nervous vomiting; ~ pernicioso pernicious vomiting; ~ seco retching; ~s secos dry vomiting
voraz, *adj,* voracious
voyurismo, voyeurism
voz, *f,* voice; ~ aguda high-pitched voice; ~ apagada dull voice; muffled voice; ~ bronca cracked voice; ~ cuchicheada whispered voice; ~ embargada por el dolor inarticulate with grief; ~ gangosa nasal voice; ~ temblorosa quavering voice; ~ vibrante de emoción voice vibrating with emotion; forzar (ue) la ~ to strain one's voice
vudú, *m,* voodoo
vuelta, lap (*en una carrera*); turn
vulnerable, *adj,* vulnerable
vulva, vulva
vulvitis, *f,* vulvitis
vulvovaginitis, *f,* vulvovaginitis

---

[1] Este vocabulario es nuevo y todavía no se encuentra en el *Diccionario de la lengua española,* publicado por la Real Academia Española. Forma parte del argot o la lengua de la calle. Se supone que el género es obvio a menos que sea indicado.
[2] Forma parte del vocabulario inglés actual de los drogadictos.
[4] Es una de las técnicas que se usan para curar el empacho. Vea la nota 4 en la página 357.

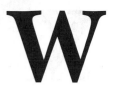

W

wáter, *m,* lavatory; water closet
WC, *m,* restroom; water closet

whiskey, *m,* whisk(e)y
white[1], LSD

---

[1] Este vocabulario es nuevo y todavía no se encuentra en el *Diccionario de la lengua española,* publicado por Real Academia Española. Forma parte del argot o la lengua de la calle. Se supone que el género es obvio a menos que sea indicado.

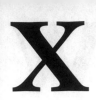

xantoma, *m, form,* xanthoma
xantosis, *f, form,* xanthosis

xerografía, xerox copy
xerosis, *f, inv, form,* xerosis

y otros, et al.

ya, *adv*, already ~ **oído** déjà entendu; ~ **probado** déjà éprouve; ~ **visto** déjà vu

yarda, yard (*medida*)

yaya, *m*, *CA*, *Col*, wound; *Chi*, *Col*, *Cu*, *Perú*, scar; slight wound; small pain

yedo[1], marijuana

yedra, ivy; ~ **venenosa** poison ivy

yel, *f*, *Chicano*, gall

yema, bud; fleshy tip of the finger; yolk; ~ **de(l) huevo** egg yolk; ~ **del dedo** ball of finger/fingertip; tip of finger; ~ **terminal** end bud

yerba, herb; Acapulco gold[2] (*mariguana*); marijuana (*muy común*); ~ **de oro**[1] marijuana; ~ **del diablo**[1] marijuana; ~ **santa**[1] marijuana; ~ **verde**[1] marijuana

yerbabuena, mint; ~[1] marijuana

yerno, son-in-law

yerto de frío, *adj*, stiff with cold

yesca[1], Acapulco gold[2] (*mariguana*); marijuana

yesco[1], doper[2]; marijuana smoker; marijuana user

yeso, cast (*un vendaje hecho con vendas de yeso, destinado a inmovilizar una parte del cuerpo*); plaster (*sulfato de calcio dihidratado*); ~ **de descarga** nonweight bearing plaster; ~ **mate/~ de Paris** plaster of Paris; ~[1] (drug) addict; junkie[2] (*adicto a las drogas narcóticas*); user[2]

yeyunal, *adj*, jejunal

yeyunitis, *f*, jejunitis

yeyuno, jejunum

yodo, iodine; ~ **radiactivo** RAI/radioactive iodine

yodurar, to iodize

yoduro, iodide; ~ **de cadmio** cadmium iodide; ~ **de etilo** ethyl iodide; ~ **de potasio** potassium iodide

yoga, *m*, yoga

yogur, *m*, yogurt

yonquearse, *Chicano*, to be exhausted

yugular, *adj*, jugular

yunque, *m*, anvil of middle ear; incus *form*

yustaarticular, *adj*, juxta-articular

yuxtaposición, *f*, juxtaposition

[1] Este vocabulario es nuevo y todavía no se encuentra en el *Diccionario de la lengua española*, publicado por la Real Academia Española. Forma parte del argot o la lengua de la calle. Se supone que el género es obvio a menos que sea indicado.
[2] Forma parte del vocabulario inglés actual de los drogadictos.

Z

zacate[1], *m*, Acapulco gold[2] (*mariguana*); marijuana (*variedad de baja calidad*)

zafacón, *m*, *PR*, garbage can

zafado, *adj*, *SpAm*, dislocated

zafadura, *Chicano*, *fam*, dislocation

zafar, to release; ~**se** to get loose; *Bol*, *Col*, *Ec*, *Peru*, *Ven*, to dislocate

zaguán, *m*, lobby

zambo, *adj*, *fam*, bow-legged; twisted

zancajo, heel *Anat*

zancudo, *Chicano*, *SpAm*, mosquito

zangarri(an)a, headache *Med*; migraine *Med*

zapatilla, slipper

zapato, shoe

zapeta, *Chicano*, diaper

zarasa, semi-erection

zigoto, zygote

zinc, *m*, zinc0

ziper, *m*, *Chicano*, zipper

zocato, *Mex*, sickly child

zodíaco, zodiac

zona, shingles; zoster; zone; ~ **ciliar** ciliary zone; ~ **neutra** neutral zone; ~ **postal** postal zone/zip code; ~ **reflexógena** trigger area; ~**s moteadas** mottled areas

zoología, zoology

zoster[4], *f*, herpes zoster; shingles; *m*, *fam*, herpes

zumaque venenoso, *m*, poison ivy

zumbar, to buzz; to hum (*una canción*); to ring (*los oídos*)

zumbido, buzz; hum (*de una máquina, insectos, etc.*); humming (*de un motor, insectos, etc.*); ringing (*en los oídos*); ~ **de (los) oídos** buzzing in the ears; ~ **del oído** tinnitus

zumo, juice

zurdería, left-handedness

zurdo, *adj*, left-handed

zurra, spanking

---

[1] Este vocabulario es nuevo y todavía no se encuentra en el *Diccionario de la lengua española*, publicado por la Real Academia Española. Forma parte del argot o la lengua de la calle. Se supone que el género es obvio a menos que sea indicado.

[2] Forma parte del vocabulario inglés actual de los drogadictos.

[4] Según el *Diccionario de la lengua española*, la palabra aparece sin acento. Sin embargo, hoy en día se usa acento también, *zóster*. En cuanto a su género, puede ser o masculino o femenino.